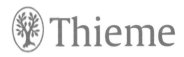

Clinical Anatomy Q&A

Mark H. Hankin, PhD
Professor and Senior Anatomist
Director of the Anatomical Services Center
Oregon Health & Science University
Portland, Oregon

Dennis E. Morse, PhD
Visiting Professor of Anatomy
Department of Physiology and Cell Biology
University of Nevada-Reno School of Medicine
Reno, Nevada

Judith M. Venuti, PhD, FAAA
Professor and former Chair
Department of Foundational Medical Studies
Oakland University William Beaumont School of Medicine
Rochester, Michigan

Malli Barremkala, MBBS
Assistant Professor
Department of Foundational Medical Studies
Oakland University William Beaumont School of Medicine
Rochester, Michigan

563 illustrations

Thieme
New York • Stuttgart • Delhi • Rio de Janeiro

Library of Congress Cataloging-in-Publication Data is available from the publisher.

© 2020. Thieme. All rights reserved.

Thieme Publishers New York
333 Seventh Avenue, New York, NY 10001 USA
+1 800 782 3488, customerservice@thieme.com

Thieme Publishers Stuttgart
Rüdigerstrasse 14, 70469 Stuttgart, Germany
+49 [0]711 8931 421, customerservice@thieme.de

Thieme Publishers Delhi
A-12, Second Floor, Sector-2, Noida-201301
Uttar Pradesh, India
+91 120 45 566 00, customerservice@thieme.in

Thieme Publishers Rio de Janeiro, Thieme Publicações Ltda.
Edifício Rodolpho de Paoli, 25º andar
Av. Nilo Peçanha, 50 – Sala 2508
Rio de Janeiro 20020-906, Brasil
+55 21 3172 2297

Cover design: Thieme Publishing Group
Cover illustration
Front: Steve Debenport
Back: Karl Wesker, Berlin

Typesetting by Thomson Digital

Printed in USA by King Printing Company, Inc.   5 4 3 2 1

ISBN 978-1-62623-421-5

Also available as an e-book:
eISBN 978-1-62623-422-2

Important note: Medicine is an ever-changing science undergoing continual development. Research and clinical experience are continually expanding our knowledge, in particular our knowledge of proper treatment and drug therapy. Insofar as this book mentions any dosage or application, readers may rest assured that the authors, editors, and publishers have made every effort to ensure that such references are in accordance with **the state of knowledge at the time of production of the book.**

Nevertheless, this does not involve, imply, or express any guarantee or responsibility on the part of the publishers in respect to any dosage instructions and forms of applications stated in the book. **Every user is requested to examine carefully** the manufacturers' leaflets accompanying each drug and to check, if necessary in consultation with a physician or specialist, whether the dosage schedules mentioned therein or the contraindications stated by the manufacturers differ from the statements made in the present book. Such examination is particularly important with drugs that are either rarely used or have been newly released on the market. Every dosage schedule or every form of application used is entirely at the user's own risk and responsibility. The authors and publishers request every user to report to the publishers any discrepancies or inaccuracies noticed. If errors in this work are found after publication, errata will be posted at www.thieme.com on the product description page.

Some of the product names, patents, and registered designs referred to in this book are in fact registered trademarks or proprietary names even though specific reference to this fact is not always made in the text. Therefore, the appearance of a name without designation as proprietary is not to be construed as a representation by the publisher that it is in the public domain.

Illustrations

Schuenke M, Schulte E, Schumacher U. THIEME Atlas of Anatomy. Illustrations by M. Voll and K. Wesker
Gilroy A, Atlas of Anatomy, based on the work of Schuenke M, Schulte E, Schumacher U. Illustrations by M. Voll and K. Wesker

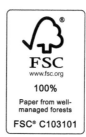

The authors have served (and continue to serve) as anatomy instructors for thousands of medical, dental, and allied health students over a combined 100 years. Our greatest rewards have been the privilege to interact with these students, follow their career development, and be reminded that not only do students remember their course in medical gross anatomy, but they also actually use what they learn. This book is, in large part, due to student expectation that questions on examinations be relevant to their professions, clearly formulated, and representative of the information they were given in the classroom and dissection laboratory. Thus, it is appropriate that we, collectively, dedicate this book to our students.

We are particularly indebted to the many individuals who have donated their body for the purpose of educating health care professional students. Without these altruistic gifts, our students—and, indeed, anatomists—would be without the most critical learning resource: a real human body.

I have been fortunate to have learned from many talented teachers, all of whom shared a depth of knowledge and passion for anatomy, and a commitment to educating students for clinical practice: the late Ronald Singer at the University of Chicago who introduced me to human anatomy; my long-time mentor, colleague, and friend Raymond Lund, at the University of Pittsburgh who encouraged my passion for anatomy education; and wonderful colleagues at the University of Toledo including Dennis Morse, Carol Bennett-Clarke, Carlos Baptista, and Richard Yeasting, all of whom were part of an "anatomy dream team" with whom I spent 22 happy years.

My contributions to this book are dedicated to my wife, Sharyl, whose support, patience, and constant love have helped me through many long projects. This book is one more milestone in our shared journey.

—*Mark H. Hankin*

While I did not always appreciate it at the time, I had the great fortune to be taught gross anatomy by two very demanding, "go look it up," pedantic, classical anatomists. They were not well-known outside of the university but their commitment and passion for knowledge of the anatomy of the human body was exemplary and respected by all who interacted with them. Thank you Christopher J. Hamre (deceased) and Jean Colville Oberpriller (deceased). I dedicate my contribution to this book in your memories.

And, most of all, thank you, Jayne.

—*Dennis E. Morse*

It has been my privilege to learn anatomy from so many wonderful teachers, colleagues, and students over the years. They have taught me how little I know and how much more I wish to learn. It is my hope that I have, in some way, helped them understand and appreciate the beauty and intricacies of the human body so that they too may share their knowledge and appreciation with others.

Special thanks goes to all of my family for their continued love and support.

—*Judith M. Venuti*

It is an honor to learn anatomy from all the donors that have dedicated their bodies for the advancement of the anatomical education and research. To my parents, Chandrasekhar and Nirmala, and my brother, Siva, for their lifelong support and love; my wonderful daughters, Eesha and Laasya; and my loving wife, Raga, for her support and patience.

—*Malli Barremkala*

Contents

Preface ix

Acknowledgments x

About the Authors xi

How to Use This Series xii

1 Nervous System 1

2 Musculoskeletal System 39

3 Cardiovascular System 143

4 Respiratory System 189

5 Urinary System 215

6 Digestive System 237

7 Female Reproductive System 275

8 Male Reproductive System 303

9 Endocrine System 333

10 Lymphatic System 357

Index 389

Preface

In contemporary medical curricula, students studying gross anatomy must learn not only the "what" and "why" of anatomy, but also "how" anatomical information is used in the development of a differential diagnosis. With this fundamental precept in mind, the questions in this book are designed to provide students with practice in answering multiple choice questions with a USMLE format. The anatomical information covered is intended to be similar to that encountered in assessments in any curriculum or in the USMLE Step 1 examination. More importantly, this work offers our colleagues teaching medical anatomy a database of case-based questions that can be used and adapted for their curriculum.

Book organization: This book is organized by organ system so that students in systems-based undergraduate medical curricula will find it correlates better with their learning and review. As such, the book is intended primarily for students who are in the preclinical portion of their training, either for review and preparation for course assessments or for the basic science portion of licensure examinations (e.g., USMLE Step 1, COMLEX-USA Level 1, NCCPA).

Chapter organization: Each chapter begins with a list of broad *learning objectives*. These are designed to encourage the learner to consider not only the anatomy of the structures within a system but also to include anatomical relationships, surface projections, landmarks for identification, as well as common clinical problems associated with the organs and tissues forming that system. For each question, the *level of difficulty* (easy, medium, or hard) is indicated. In many cases, questions are presented with *clinical images* from which information must be extracted to answer the question.

Question format: The questions in this book reflect actual clinical cases (many adapted from the clinical literature) to illustrate how anatomical knowledge is used in medical practice. All questions in this book are presented in a multiple-choice format similar to that found in USMLE Step 1, COMLEX-USA Level 1, NBME, and NBOME examinations: a clinical scenario, which often includes photographic or imaging evidence, is followed by a question (occasionally more than one) that requires understanding of fundamental or applied anatomy. Each question is provided with four or more (usually five) alphabetized choices from which the learner chooses the best response. Explanations are provided for the correct answer and all incorrect answers, and illustrations or clinical images are provided for many questions to explain visually the anatomy that provides the foundation for the clinical scenario.

In most chapters, the questions are randomized in terms of anatomical region and level of difficulty. In the Musculoskeletal chapter, however, the questions are broadly grouped by anatomical region (back and upper limb, head and neck, trunk, and lower limb) because the anatomy of these regions is still presented regionally in most systems-based curricula.

Online version: We are pleased that Thieme will provide an online resource for this book that will allow students to create customized learning tools that will help students find what they need and use their time to the best advantage.

Mark H. Hankin, PhD
Dennis E. Morse, PhD
Judith M. Venuti, PhD, FAAA
Malli Barremkala, MBBS

Acknowledgments

The authors are grateful to numerous individuals who reviewed many questions, provided feedback in terms of the scope and accuracy of the clinical scenarios, and offered their assessment of the level of difficulty for each question.

Basic Science Faculty
- William Cameron, PhD, Associate Professor Emeritus, Oregon Health and Science University, Portland, Oregon
- William Forbes, DDS, Associate Professor, Department of Foundational Medical Studies, Oakland University William Beaumont School of Medicine, Rochester, Michigan
- Douglas Gould, PhD, Chair and Professor, Department of Foundational Medical Studies, Oakland University William Beaumont School of Medicine, Rochester, Michigan
- Keith Metzger, PhD, Assistant Dean of Undergraduate Medical Education and Learning Strategies, Seton Hall University, South Orange, New Jersey
- Peter Ward, PhD, Associate Professor, Department of Biomedical Sciences, West Virginia School of Osteopathic Medicine, Lewisburg, West Virginia
- Tim Wilson, PhD, Associate Professor, Department of Anatomy and Cell Biology, University of Western Ontario, London, Ontario

Attending Physicians
- David Bloom, MD, Department of Radiology, Beaumont Health Systems and Oakland University William Beaumont School of Medicine, Royal Oak, Michigan
- Dawn Jung, MD, Department of Emergency Medicine, Beaumont Health Systems and Oakland University William Beaumont School of Medicine, Royal Oak, Michigan

Residents at Oregon Health and Science University
- Megan Cohen, MD (Obstetrics and Gynecology)
- Cate Edgell, MD (Internal Medicine)
- Sarah Hecht, MD (Urology)
- Justine Hum, MD (Internal Medicine)
- Curtis Lachowiez, MD (Internal Medicine)
- Taylor C. Myers (Locke), MD (Internal Medicine)
- Drew Oehler, MD (Internal Medicine)
- Mario Padilla, MD (Internal Medicine)
- Meryl Paul, MD (Internal Medicine)
- Travis Philipp, MD (Orthopaedics)
- Zhuyi Elizabeth Sun, MD (Neurology)
- Celine Zhou, MD (Internal Medicine)

Second-Year Medical Students at Oregon Health and Science University
- Kimberly Bullard
- Trevor Feldman
- Carter Haag
- Phoebe Hammer

Fourth-Year Medical Students at Oakland University William Beaumont School of Medicine
- Renee M. Choloway (Residency: General Surgery)
- Rachel Hunt (Residency: Neurosurgery)
- Tania Kohal (Residency: Internal Medicine)
- Karis E. Stevenson (Residency: Urology)
- Lauren M. Quinn (Residency: Emergency Medicine)
- Alexa M. Shepherd (Residency: Obstetrics and Gynecology)
- Nico B. Volz (Residency: Emergency Medicine)

The authors are indebted to the remarkable original three volume *Thieme Atlas of Anatomy* by Michael Schuenke, Erik Schulte, and Udo Schumacher, all supported by the brilliant illustrations of Markus Voll and Karl Wesker. The adaptation of their work by Anne Gilroy and Brian MacPherson into the single volume *Thieme Atlas of Anatomy* also provided further insight. Illustrations from all of these works provided invaluable enhancement for explanations of the anatomy associated with the clinical scenarios in the book. We also thank Richard Gunderman for numerous clinical images in *Thieme Essential Radiology*, as well as other authors of Thieme publications for clinical insights and additional images. We also wish to thank our colleagues at Thieme Publishers for their steadfast encouragement, support, and patience, without whose efforts this resource would not have been realized. We are particularly grateful to:

- Delia K. DeTurris (Acquisitions Editor)

- Gaurav Prabhu (Project Manager)

About the Authors

Mark H. Hankin earned a BA in biological sciences from The University of Chicago and a PhD in developmental neurobiology and human anatomy from Case Western Reserve University. After postdoctoral training at The University of Pittsburgh, Dr. Hankin was on the faculty for 22 years at the Medical College of Ohio (now the University of Toledo College of Medicine). He was Professor and Director of Anatomy Education at the new Oakland University William Beaumont School of Medicine in Rochester, Michigan. He is currently Professor and Senior Anatomist, and Director of the Anatomical Services Center at the Oregon Health & Science University in Portland, Oregon.

Dennis E. Morse earned a BA in biology from Hastings College (Nebraska) and MS and PhD in human anatomy from the University of North Dakota. He is Visiting Professor of Anatomy in the Department to Physiology and Cell Biology at the University of Nevada-Reno School of Medicine, Reno, Nevada.

Judith M. Venuti received a BS in biology and an MS in developmental biology from Northeastern University in Boston. Her PhD in anatomical sciences was from the State University of New York at Buffalo School of Medicine. She has taught anatomy and embryology to dental students, medical students, physical therapy students, and nursing and undergraduate students over the course of her career, and also at the College of Physicians and Surgeons, Columbia University and the Louisiana State University Health Sciences Center. She is currently Professor and former Chair in the Department of Foundational Medical Studies at Oakland University William Beaumont School of Medicine in Rochester, Michigan.

Malli Barremkala earned an MBBS (MD) from NTR University of Health Sciences, India, holds an active medical licensure in India, and is registered with the Medical Council of India. He taught anatomy and medical simulation to medical students at Ross University School of Medicine, Dominica. He is currently Assistant Professor of Biomedical Sciences at Oakland University William Beaumont School of Medicine in Rochester, Michigan.

How to Use This Series

Question Difficulty Key

Green box = Easy question
Yellow box = Medium question
Red box = Hard question

Chapter Head

Section Header

Question Stem

Answer Options

1 Nervous System

1.1 Questions

| Easy | Medium | Hard |

1. A 28-year-old woman is admitted to the obstetric service for caesarean section delivery of a fetus that is in the breech position. The patient elects to have a transverse, suprapubic (Pfannenstiel or "bikini") incision (refer to the dashed line in the accompanying image). Which of the following nerves is most likely to be injured during this procedure?

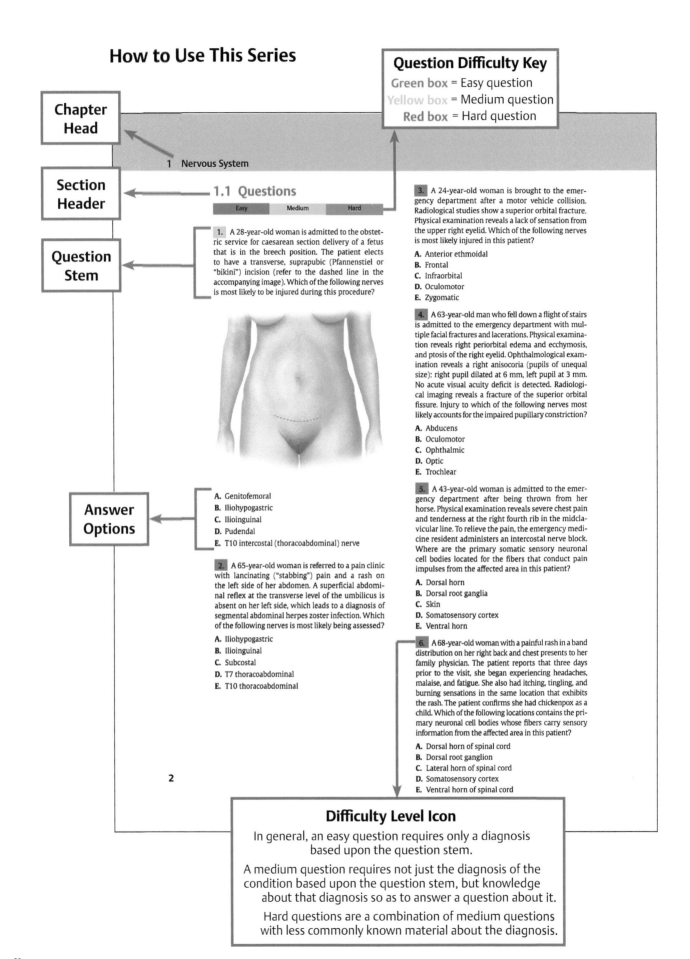

A. Genitofemoral
B. Iliohypogastric
C. Ilioinguinal
D. Pudendal
E. T10 intercostal (thoracoabdominal) nerve

2. A 65-year-old woman is referred to a pain clinic with lancinating ("stabbing") pain and a rash on the left side of her abdomen. A superficial abdominal reflex at the transverse level of the umbilicus is absent on her left side, which leads to a diagnosis of segmental abdominal herpes zoster infection. Which of the following nerves is most likely being assessed?

A. Iliohypogastric
B. Ilioinguinal
C. Subcostal
D. T7 thoracoabdominal
E. T10 thoracoabdominal

3. A 24-year-old woman is brought to the emergency department after a motor vehicle collision. Radiological studies show a superior orbital fracture. Physical examination reveals a lack of sensation from the upper right eyelid. Which of the following nerves is most likely injured in this patient?

A. Anterior ethmoidal
B. Frontal
C. Infraorbital
D. Oculomotor
E. Zygomatic

4. A 63-year-old man who fell down a flight of stairs is admitted to the emergency department with multiple facial fractures and lacerations. Physical examination reveals right periorbital edema and ecchymosis, and ptosis of the right eyelid. Ophthalmological examination reveals a right anisocoria (pupils of unequal size): right pupil dilated at 6 mm, left pupil at 3 mm. No acute visual acuity deficit is detected. Radiological imaging reveals a fracture of the superior orbital fissure. Injury to which of the following nerves most likely accounts for the impaired pupillary constriction?

A. Abducens
B. Oculomotor
C. Ophthalmic
D. Optic
E. Trochlear

5. A 43-year-old woman is admitted to the emergency department after being thrown from her horse. Physical examination reveals severe chest pain and tenderness at the right fourth rib in the midclavicular line. To relieve the pain, the emergency medicine resident administers an intercostal nerve block. Where are the primary somatic sensory neuronal cell bodies located for the fibers that conduct pain impulses from the affected area in this patient?

A. Dorsal horn
B. Dorsal root ganglia
C. Skin
D. Somatosensory cortex
E. Ventral horn

6. A 68-year-old woman with a painful rash in a band distribution on her right back and chest presents to her family physician. The patient reports that three days prior to the visit, she began experiencing headaches, malaise, and fatigue. She also had itching, tingling, and burning sensations in the same location that exhibits the rash. The patient confirms she had chickenpox as a child. Which of the following locations contains the primary neuronal cell bodies whose fibers carry sensory information from the affected area in this patient?

A. Dorsal horn of spinal cord
B. Dorsal root ganglion
C. Lateral horn of spinal cord
D. Somatosensory cortex
E. Ventral horn of spinal cord

2

Difficulty Level Icon

In general, an easy question requires only a diagnosis based upon the question stem.

A medium question requires not just the diagnosis of the condition based upon the question stem, but knowledge about that diagnosis so as to answer a question about it.

Hard questions are a combination of medium questions with less commonly known material about the diagnosis.

1.2 Answers and Explanations

Easy	Medium	Hard

1.   Correct: Iliohypogastric (B)

Refer to the following image for answer 1:

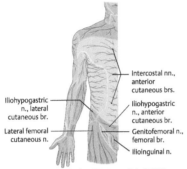

Source: Gilroy AM et al. Atlas of Anatomy. 3rd ed. 2016. Based on: Schuenke M, Schulte E, Schumacher U. THIEME Atlas of Anatomy. Volumes 1-3. Illustrations by Voll M and Wesker K. 2nd ed. New York: Thieme Medical Publishers; 2016

(**B**) The iliohypogastric nerve (L1) provides sensory innervation from suprapubic skin. (**A**) The genitofemoral nerve (L1–L2) provides sensory innervation in females from skin over the mons pubis and labium majus, as well as from the anteromedial thigh. (**C**) The ilioinguinal nerve (L1) provides sensory innervation from skin over the mons pubis and labium majus, as well as the proximal medial thigh. (**D**) The pudendal nerve (S2–S4) provides sensory innervation from skin of the perineum. (**E**) The T10 intercostal (thoracoabdominal) nerve provides sensory innervation from skin around the umbilicus.

2.   Correct: T10 thoracoabdominal (E)

(**E**) The dermatome that includes the umbilicus is supplied by the T10 thoracoabdominal nerve (refer to the accompanying image). By definition, the superficial abdominal reflex assesses the T8–T12 spinal cord levels. It is one of four superficial cutaneous reflexes: abdominal, cremaster, plantar, and the anocutaneous ("anal wink"). (**A**) The iliohypogastric nerve contributes to the L1 dermatome, which includes the suprapubic skin. (**B**) The ilioinguinal nerve contributes to the L1 dermatome, which includes the skin over the mons pubis and labium majus, as well as the proximal medial thigh. (**C**) The subcostal nerve is the ventral ramus of the T12 spinal nerve. (**D**) On

the anterior (and lateral) body wall, the T7, as well as the T8–T9, thoracoabdominal nerves carry sensory information from skin located between the xiphoid process (which is generally included in the T6 dermatome) and the umbilicus.

Refer to the following image for answer 2:

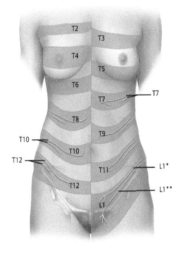

T7 Thoracoabdomial nerve

T10 Thoracoabdomial nerve

T12 Subcostal nerve

L1* Iliohypogastric nerve

L1** Ilioinguinal nerve

3.   Correct: Frontal (B)

(**B**) Branches of the ophthalmic nerve (CN V1) provide sensory innervation from the upper eyelid. Within the orbit, the frontal nerve (a branch of CN V1) courses immediately inferior to the periorbita. Branches of this nerve (supraorbital and supratrochlear) along with infraorbital (from nasociliary) and lacrimal supply the upper eyelid. (**A**) The anterior ethmoidal nerve is a branch of CN V1, but it does not provide sensory innervation from the upper eyelid. (**C**) The infraorbital nerve is a branch of the maxillary division of the trigeminal nerve (CN V2). It provides sensory innervation from the lower eyelid (refer to the following image). (**D**) The oculomotor nerve (CN III) provides motor innervation to most of the extraocular muscles. (**E**) The zygomatic nerve is a branch

16

Chapter 1

Nervous System

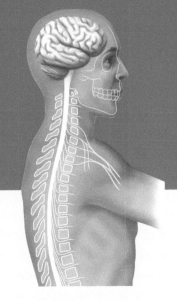

ANATOMICAL LEARNING OBJECTIVES

▶ Describe the anatomy of the:
- Spinal cord and the spinal meninges
- Typical spinal nerve, including its roots and rami
- Somatic cervical, brachial, and lumbosacral nerve plexuses, including their contributing nerve roots and the distribution of their branches
- Fascial compartments of the upper and lower limbs, including the muscle groups contained within each and their innervation and action(s)
- Organs of the special senses of smell, vision, hearing, balance, and taste
- Carotid sinus and carotid body, including their function and associated neural components
- Orbit and associated neurovasculature and musculature (including their attachments, action(s), and innervation)
- Enteric nervous system and its developmental origins
- Organs and structures of the head and neck, including their neurovasculature and anatomical relationships
- Thoracic, abdominal, and pelvic walls, including their skeleton, muscles, fascial layers, and neurovasculature
- Thoracic organs, including their neurovasculature and anatomical relationships
- Abdominal, pelvic, and perineal organs and structures, including their neurovasculature and anatomical relationships

▶ Describe the distribution of somatic sensory nerve distribution in dermatomes on the head, trunk, and limbs, and the trigeminal nerve in the face.

▶ Describe the anatomical bases of the corneal, gag, cremasteric, anal, and tendon reflexes.

▶ Describe the anatomy of each cranial nerve, including their functional composition, origin, course, and distribution.

▶ Describe the common defects arising from abnormal nervous system development and explain their embryonic origins.

1.1 Questions

Easy	Medium	Hard

1. A 28-year-old woman is admitted to the obstetric service for caesarean section delivery of a fetus that is in the breech position. The patient elects to have a transverse, suprapubic (Pfannenstiel or "bikini") incision (refer to the *dashed line* in the accompanying image). Which of the following nerves is most likely to be injured during this procedure?

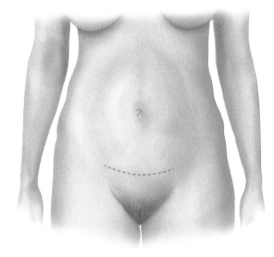

A. Genitofemoral
B. Iliohypogastric
C. Ilioinguinal
D. Pudendal
E. T10 intercostal (thoracoabdominal) nerve

2. A 65-year-old woman is referred to a pain clinic with lancinating ("stabbing") pain and a rash on the left side of her abdomen. A superficial abdominal reflex at the transverse level of the umbilicus is absent on her left side, which leads to a diagnosis of segmental abdominal herpes zoster infection. Which of the following nerves is most likely being assessed?

A. Iliohypogastric
B. Ilioinguinal
C. Subcostal
D. T7 thoracoabdominal
E. T10 thoracoabdominal

3. A 24-year-old woman is brought to the emergency department after a motor vehicle collision. Radiological studies show a superior orbital fracture. Physical examination reveals a lack of sensation from the upper right eyelid. Which of the following nerves is most likely injured in this patient?

A. Anterior ethmoidal
B. Frontal
C. Infraorbital
D. Oculomotor
E. Zygomatic

4. A 63-year-old man who fell down a flight of stairs is admitted to the emergency department with multiple facial fractures and lacerations. Physical examination reveals right periorbital edema and ecchymosis, and ptosis of the right eyelid. Ophthalmological examination reveals a right anisocoria (pupils of unequal size): right pupil dilated at 6 mm, left pupil at 3 mm. No acute visual acuity deficit is detected. Radiological imaging reveals a fracture of the superior orbital fissure. Injury to which of the following nerves most likely accounts for the impaired pupillary constriction?

A. Abducens
B. Oculomotor
C. Ophthalmic
D. Optic
E. Trochlear

5. A 43-year-old woman is admitted to the emergency department after being thrown from her horse. Physical examination reveals severe chest pain and tenderness at the right fourth rib in the midclavicular line. To relieve the pain, the emergency medicine resident administers an intercostal nerve block. Where are the primary somatic sensory neuronal cell bodies located for the fibers that conduct pain impulses from the affected area in this patient?

A. Dorsal horn
B. Dorsal root ganglia
C. Skin
D. Somatosensory cortex
E. Ventral horn

6. A 68-year-old woman with a painful rash in a band distribution on her right back and chest presents to her family physician. The patient reports that three days prior to the visit, she began experiencing headaches, malaise, and fatigue. She also had itching, tingling, and burning sensations in the same location that exhibits the rash. The patient confirms she had chickenpox as a child. Which of the following locations contains the primary neuronal cell bodies whose fibers carry sensory information from the affected area in this patient?

A. Dorsal horn of spinal cord
B. Dorsal root ganglion
C. Lateral horn of spinal cord
D. Somatosensory cortex
E. Ventral horn of spinal cord

7. A 45-year-old man presents to the emergency department after a high-speed automobile accident. Coronal CT imaging shows a fracture of the ethmoid bone. At a follow-up visit, the patient complains of a loss of taste. At the location indicated by the *circle* in the accompanying image, which of the following nerves is most likely injured?

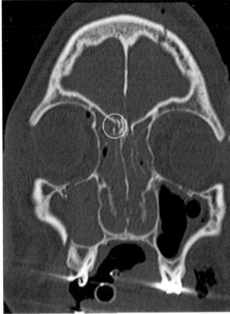

Source: Anzai Y, Tozer-Fink K, Imaging of Traumatic Brain Injury. 1st Edition. Thieme; 2015.

A. Anterior ethmoidal
B. Lacrimal
C. Nasociliary
D. Olfactory
E. Posterior ethmoidal

Consider the following case for questions 8 and 9:

A 54-year-old woman with sudden loss of vision in her left eye presents to the emergency department. The patient has a history of coronary artery disease and recently had coronary artery bypass graft surgery, balloon angioplasty, and a left carotid endarterectomy. A cherry-red spot is seen in the macula of the affected (right) eye by ophthalmoscopic examination (refer to the accompanying image).

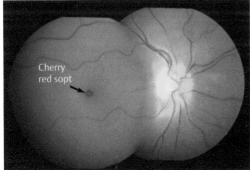

Cherry
red sopt

Source: Image provided courtesy of Dr. Aristomenis Thanos, Associated Retinal Consultants, Oakland University William Beaumont School of Medicine, Royal Oak, MI.

8. Flow in which of the following blood vessels is most likely disrupted in this patient?

A. Central retinal artery
B. Internal carotid artery
C. Internal jugular vein
D. Middle meningeal artery
E. Ophthalmic artery

9. Which of the following cells are most directly affected by the vascular occlusion in this patient?

A. Cone photoreceptor cells
B. Retinal ganglion cells
C. Retinal pigment epithelium cells
D. Rod photoreceptor cells
E. Scleral cells

10. A 20-year-old man replaces his contact lenses but accidentally uses ear drops to lubricate his eyes. This results in acute eye pain and blurred vision. He is brought to the emergency department where he is diagnosed with corneal abrasion caused by the introduction of toxic compounds in the ear drops. Which of the following nerves transmits the pain from this part of the eye?

A. Frontal
B. Infraorbital
C. Lacrimal
D. Nasociliary
E. Optic

11. A 37-year-old woman with difficulty closing her right eye, drooping of the right side of her mouth, and a change in taste sensation presents to the emergency department. On physical examination, the patient has difficulty raising her right eyebrow and right side of her forehead. When the physician gently strokes the cornea, a corneal reflex is not elicited. Injury to which of the following nerves most likely accounts for the absence of this reflex?

A. Facial
B. Infraorbital
C. Lacrimal
D. Nasociliary
E. Supraorbital

12. A 37-year-old telemarketing worker with sudden, left-sided, facial paralysis that involves her forehead and lower face visits the emergency department fearing she is having a stroke. She reports that her taste is altered such that hot and spicy foods taste metallic and she is experiencing excessive drooling. With a diagnosis of Bell's palsy, at which location is the lesion in this patient?

A. Cavernous sinus
B. Facial canal, proximal to chorda tympani
C. Internal acoustic meatus
D. Jugular foramen
E. Stylomastoid foramen

13. A 21-year-old woman presents with headache, esotropia (medial deviation of one eye relative to the other), and diplopia. A patient history reveals that the headache began 5 days, and the diplopia 3 days, previously. Neurological examination shows an ophthalmoplegia of the left eye (refer to the accompanying image) and papilledema. Lumbar puncture reveals an opening pressure of 40 cm H_2O (normal: 10–20 cm H_2O). In the absence of a detectable cause, the patient is diagnosed with idiopathic intracranial hypertension (pseudotumor cerebri). Injury to which of the following nerves is responsible for the visual deficit in this patient?

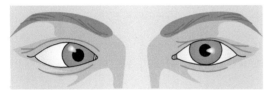

Source: Gilroy AM et al. Atlas of Anatomy. 3rd ed. 2016. Based on: Schuenke M, Schulte E, Schumacher U. THIEME Atlas of Anatomy. Volumes 1-3. Illustrations by Voll M and Wesker K. 2nd ed. New York: Thieme Medical Publishers; 2016

A. Abducens

B. Long ciliary

C. Nasociliary

D. Oculomotor

E. Trochlear

14. An 18-year-old female soccer player presents to the emergency department after she is hit in the right side of her head by an opponent while heading the ball. Physical examination reveals that the patient tilts her head to the left side. A patient history reveals that she had initially lost consciousness, and then experienced headache, dizziness, and diplopia. During neurological examination, the diplopia is exacerbated with gaze downward and to the patient's right. The position of the eye in primary gaze is shown in the accompanying image. Which of the following extraocular muscles is paralyzed in this patient?

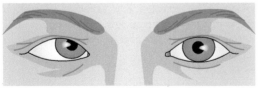

Source: Gilroy AM et al. Atlas of Anatomy. 3rd ed. 2016. Based on: Schuenke M, Schulte E, Schumacher U. THIEME Atlas of Anatomy. Volumes 1-3. Illustrations by Voll M and Wesker K. 2nd ed. New York: Thieme Medical Publishers; 2016

A. Inferior oblique

B. Inferior rectus

C. Medial rectus

D. Superior oblique

E. Superior rectus

15. A 45-year-old woman with headache, diplopia, and ptosis presents to the emergency department. A patient history reveals that the headache came on suddenly about 2 weeks previously, and the double vision and "droopy eyelid" about 1 week afterward. Neurological examination shows a ptosis of the right eyelid, and the right eye is hypotropic and exotropic (i.e., deviated downward and outward, respectively as seen in the accompanying image). A right-sided mydriasis (a dilated pupil) is detected. Paralysis of which of the following muscles most likely accounts for the ptosis in this patient?

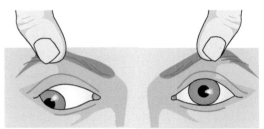

Source: Gilroy AM et al. Atlas of Anatomy. 3rd ed. 2016. Based on: Schuenke M, Schulte E, Schumacher U. THIEME Atlas of Anatomy. Volumes 1-3. Illustrations by Voll M and Wesker K. 2nd ed. New York: Thieme Medical Publishers; 2016

A. Levator labii superioris

B. Levator palpebrae superioris

C. Superior oblique

D. Superior rectus

E. Superior tarsal

16. A 40-year-old man with sudden onset of a severe, sustained headache is admitted to the emergency department. A patient history reveals that the pain is of several-days duration and is localized immediately posterior to the right orbit. He also reports that 3 days after the headache started, he experienced "double vision." Neurological examination reveals impaired adduction and upward gaze of the right eye and mydriasis (a dilated pupil). Ptosis is not observed. A palsy of which of the following nerves accounted for the signs and symptoms in this patient?

A. Abducens

B. Deep petrosal

C. Long ciliary

D. Nasociliary

E. Oculomotor

17. An adult patient visits her primary care physician for an annual physical examination. During neurological examination, the primary care physician visualizes the retina through his ophthalmoscope. Which of the following structures is found at the position indicated by *white circle* in the accompanying image?

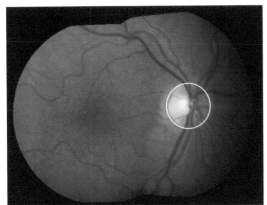

Source: Image provided courtesy of Dr. Aristomenis Thanos, Associated Retinal Consultants, Oakland University William Beaumont School of Medicine, Royal Oak, MI.

A. Ciliary body

B. Cone photoreceptors

C. Lens

D. Retinal ganglion cell axons

E. Rod photoreceptors

Consider the following case for questions 18 and 19:

A 21-year-old man presents to the emergency department after being punched in the left eye. Physical examination reveals ecchymosis (bruising) and enophthalmos (sinking in) of the left eye. Radiological imaging shows an orbital floor fracture (*arrows* in the accompanying image).

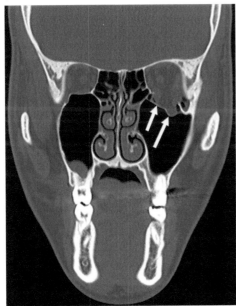

Source: Yu E, Jaffer N, Chung T et al. RadCases. Emergency Radiology. 1st Edition. Thieme; 2015.

18. Which of the following clinical signs would be most likely in this patient?

A. Diplopia with lateral gaze

B. Diplopia with medial gaze

C. Diplopia with upward gaze

D. Mydriasis

E. Ptosis

19. Which additional symptom would be possible in this patient?

A. Dry eye

B. Dry mouth

C. Hypesthesia (diminished sensation) from the cheek

D. Lack of corneal reflex

E. Miosis

20. A 24-year-old man developed right shoulder pain after a day of lifting heavy objects at work. Three weeks later, he presents to his family physician with shoulder weakness on the right side. Physical examination reveals atrophy of the trapezius muscle, weakness of abduction of the right arm (which is limited to 90 degrees), lateral scapular winging, and depression of the right shoulder. Which nerve is most likely affected in this patient?

A. Accessory

B. Dorsal scapular

C. Long thoracic

D. Lower subscapular

E. Suprascapular

Consider the following case for questions 21 and 22:

A 45-year-old woman with spasmodic rotational movements of her head and neck toward the right side presents to the neurology clinic. A patient history indicates that the condition has progressed over time, although she reports that the symptoms are less severe in the morning and that she has had spontaneous remissions that have lasted a few weeks to a few months. The neurologist diagnoses idiopathic cervical dystonia (commonly referred to as torticollis or spasmodic torticollis).

21. Which of the following nerves innervates the affected muscle?

A. Left accessory

B. Left dorsal scapular

C. Right accessory

D. Right dorsal scapular

E. Right suprascapular

22. Where are the cell bodies located for the nerve affected in this patient?

A. Facial motor nucleus

B. Nucleus ambiguus

C. Solitary tract nucleus

D. Trigeminal motor nucleus

E. Ventral horn of the spinal cord

23. A 67-year-old man with severe headache that had started 10 days previously and had worsened progressively is admitted to the emergency department. He reports that he has difficulty swallowing (dysphagia) and slurred speech (dysarthria). A neurological examination showed unilateral tongue atrophy, with deviation toward the right side when protruded. No other neurological deficits were observed. Which of the following nerves is most likely injured in this patient?

A. Left hypoglossal

B. Left lingual

C. Right hypoglossal

D. Right inferior alveolar

E. Right lingual

24. During a routine physical examination of a 58-year-old man, the physician taps the tendon of the triceps brachii muscle with a reflex hammer. Which of the following spinal cord levels provides the predominant innervation for this reflex?

A. C5

B. C6

C. C7

D. C8

E. T1

25. A 68-year-old woman with symptoms of low back pain with weakness and numbness in her right leg presents to the orthopaedic clinic. Physical examination reveals weakness in knee extension and sensory loss over the medial leg. Radiological imaging shows a herniated intervertebral disc (*black arrow* in the accompanying image). Which of the following deep tendon reflexes would most likely be diminished in this patient?

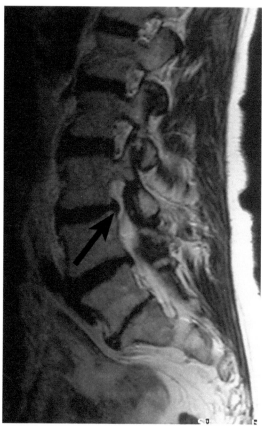

Source: Uhlenbrock D. MR Imaging of the Spine and Spinal Cord. 1st Edition. Thieme; 2003.

A. Calcaneal (Achilles') tendon reflex

B. Patellar reflex

C. Superficial anal reflex

D. Tibialis posterior reflex

26. A 72-year-old woman is struck by an automobile while crossing a street and thrown to the roadway onto the left side of her body and head. Which of the following would most likely result from fracture of the opening indicated by the *yellow arrow* in the accompanying coronal CT image of this patient?

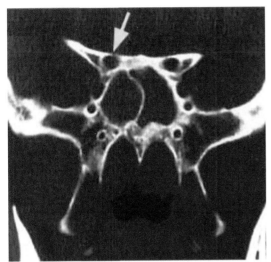

Source: Valvassori G, Mafee M, Becker M. Imaging of the Head and Neck. 2nd Edition. Stuttgart: Thieme; 2004.

A. Bell's palsy

B. Bilateral blindness

C. Ipsilateral blindness

D. Oculomotor nerve palsy

E. Trochlear nerve palsy

27. A 40-year-old woman with unilateral, stabbing pain on the right side of her face presents to the emergency department. A patient history reveals that the pain was initially vague and episodic, but has become worse over the past several days. She reports that the pain can be triggered by chewing, speaking, or by touching the affected areas, and that she lives in fear that pain can strike at any time. Physical examination shows that the pain is localized to the mandibular and maxillary regions. Sensory nerve cell bodies for fibers conducting the pain will be located in which ganglion?

A. Geniculate

B. Otic

C. Pterygopalatine

D. Superior cervical

E. Trigeminal

Consider the following case for questions 28 and 29:

A 32-year-old man is admitted to the emergency department after being punched in the left eye. Physical examination reveals ecchymosis of the upper eyelid and loss of sensation from the dorsum of the nose, and limited abduction of the left eye.

28. Injury to which of the following nerves most likely accounted for the sensory loss?

A. Anterior ethmoidal

B. Infraorbital

C. Posterior ethmoidal

D. Supraorbital

E. Supratrochlear

29. Which of the following bones was most likely fractured?

A. Ethmoid bone (lamina papyracea)

B. Lacrimal

C. Orbital surface of maxilla

D. Sphenoid

E. Zygomatic

Consider the following case for questions 30 and 31:

A 54-year-old woman with left facial pain for the past month visits the neurology clinic. The patient describes having sharp, lancinating ("shooting") pain across her left upper jaw, and that the pain is aggravated by chewing, brushing her teeth, and talking. The patient has not undergone any dental work or has a history of dental caries. She reports having lost 15 lbs in the past month from not wanting to eat for fear of exacerbating the pain.

30. Which of the following nerves is most likely involved?

A. Chorda tympani

B. Facial

C. Mandibular

D. Maxillary

E. Ophthalmic

31. Which of the following is the location of the sensory ganglion for the affected nerve?

A. Cochlea

B. Facial canal

C. Jugular foramen

D. Middle cranial fossa

E. Pterygopalatine fossa

32. A 30-year-old man visits his dentist for extraction of his right maxillary second molar. Prior to the procedure, the dentist injects lidocaine into the buccal gingiva to achieve local anesthesia. Which of the following nerves is targeted?

A. Anterior superior alveolar

B. Buccal

C. Greater palatine

D. Nasopalatine

E. Posterior superior alveolar

7

33. A 28-year-old woman visits the dentist for extraction of her left third mandibular molar. Prior to the procedure, the dentist performs an inferior alveolar nerve block to achieve local anesthesia. Which anatomical feature would be specifically targeted for the injection to anesthetize this nerve?

A. Foramen ovale

B. Foramen rotundum

C. Infratemporal fossa

D. Lingula of mandible

E. Pterygopalatine fossa

34. A 72-year-old woman with right facial numbness presents to the otolaryngology clinic. Physical examination demonstrates that the patient has hypesthesia on the superior aspect of her ear where her glasses rest (*arrow* in the accompanying image). MRI imaging reveals a perineural tumor adjacent to foramen ovale. Based on this patient's symptoms, which of the following nerves is most likely involved?

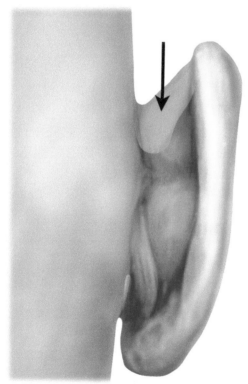

Source: Gilroy AM et al. Atlas of Anatomy. 3rd ed. 2016. Based on: Schuenke M, Schulte E, Schumacher U. THIEME Atlas of Anatomy. Volumes 1-3. Illustrations by Voll M and Wesker K. 2nd ed. New York: Thieme Medical Publishers; 2016

A. Auriculotemporal

B. Facial

C. Great auricular

D. Lesser occipital

E. Vagus

35. A 32-year-old man visits his dentist for removal of his mandibular third molar. An inferior alveolar nerve block near the mandibular foramen is performed to achieve local anesthesia. In addition to anesthesia related to the mandibular teeth, which of the following symptoms could occur in this patient?

A. Decreased salivation only

B. Loss of general sensation and taste from the anterior two-thirds of the tongue

C. Loss of general sensation only from the posterior one-third of the tongue

D. Loss of general sensation and taste from the anterior two-thirds of the tongue and decreased salivation

E. Loss of taste only from the anterior two-thirds of the tongue

Consider the following case for questions 36 and 37:

A 49-year-old man with a 3-month history of hyperacusis in his left ear presents to the otolaryngology clinic. An MRI (refer to *arrows* in the accompanying images) reveals a tumor in the posterior cranial fossa.

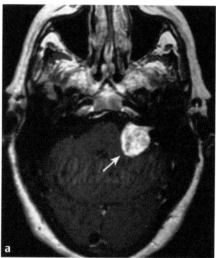

Source: Burgener F, Meyers S, Tan R et al. Differential Diagnosis in Magnetic Resonance Imaging. 1st Edition. Thieme; 2002.

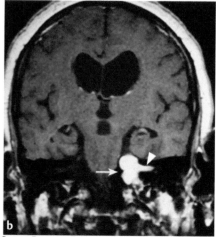

Source: Burgener F, Meyers S, Tan R et al. Differential Diagnosis in Magnetic Resonance Imaging. 1st Edition. Thieme; 2002.

36. Injury to which of the following nerves is most likely responsible for this clinical symptom?

A. Chorda tympani
B. Lesser petrosal
C. Greater petrosal
D. Nervus intermedius
E. Nerve to stapedius

37. Which opening is occupied by the contrast material in this MRI from the same individual (*arrowhead*)?

A. Cavernous sinus
B. External acoustic meatus
C. Internal acoustic meatus
D. Jugular foramen
E. Mastoid air cells

38. A 42-year-old man is referred to the audiology clinic with "ringing" (tinnitus) in both ears after spending the weekend with college friends at a rock concert. The group had seats close to the stage, right in front of a set of speakers. Physical examination shows the external ear canal and tympanic membrane, vestibular function, and peripheral neuromuscular function are normal. Tympanometry reveals dysfunction of the stapedius muscle. Which of the following nerves is most likely injured in this patient?

A. Cochlear
B. Facial
C. Ophthalmic
D. Nervus intermedius
E. Vestibular

39. A 58-year-old woman visits her prosthodontist complaining of difficulty inserting her upper dentures because it makes her gag. Examination of the patient confirms a hyperactive gag reflex. Which of the following nerves carries general somatic afferents in this reflex?

A. Facial
B. Glossopharyngeal
C. Mandibular
D. Maxillary
E. Vagus

40. A 45-year-old man is admitted to the hospital after suffering a severe head injury. A neurological examination shows an absent gag reflex on the left side and the uvula is deviated to right side. Laryngoscopy reveals paralysis of the left vocal fold, and his ability to elevate his left shoulder is weak. The rest of the examination is normal. Which of the following is most likely fractured in this patient?

A. Left hypoglossal canal
B. Left internal acoustic meatus
C. Left jugular foramen
D. Right hypoglossal canal
E. Right jugular foramen

41. A 42-year-old woman visits the orthopaedics clinic with neck and arm pain. She describes a dull, aching pain that radiates to the shoulder. Physical examination reveals weakness in elbow extension, and hypesthesia and paresthesia from the middle finger. Which of the following nerve roots is most likely involved in this patient?

A. C4
B. C5
C. C6
D. C7
E. T1

42. A 33-year-old woman visits the orthopaedics clinic with left-sided neck pain radiating along her left upper extremity from her deltoid to her middle finger. The patient is referred for radiological examination of a suspected herniated intervertebral disc and the MRI reveals a posterior herniation of the C5–C6 intervertebral disc (*yellow arrow* in the accompanying image). Based on the MRI, which of the following symptoms would be most likely in this patient?

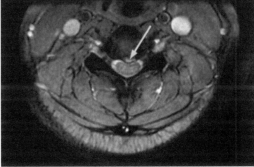

Source: Image provided courtesy of William Beaumont Hospital.

A. Bilateral hypesthesia from skin over the deltoid muscles
B. Bilateral paresis of the biceps brachii muscles
C. Unilateral hypesthesia from the great toe
D. Unilateral hypesthesia from the middle finger
E. Unilateral paresis of thumb abduction

43. A 60-year-old woman visits her primary care physician with radicular symptoms from her left upper limb, including hypesthesia from the proximal medial forearm and weakened abduction and adduction of the fingers. Biceps, triceps, and brachioradialis deep tendon reflexes are within normal limits. Radiological examination reveals the presence of an osteophyte (bone spur) that is narrowing the intervertebral foramen on the left side. Which of the following spinal nerves is most likely compressed in this patient?

A. C5

B. C6

C. C7

D. C8

E. T1

Consider the following case for questions 44 and 45:

A 45-year-old man visits his primary care physician with severe chronic low back pain of 6-month duration. Physical examination shows weakness and sensory deficits in his lower extremity. An MRI demonstrates a posterolateral lumbar herniated disc with nerve compression (*white circle* in the accompanying image).

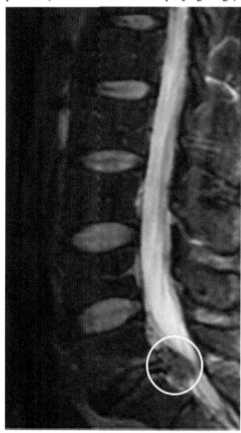

Source: Gunderman R. Essential Radiology. Clinical Presentation, Pathophysiology, Imaging. 3rd Edition. Thieme; 2014.

44. Which of the following signs or symptoms would be most likely in this patient?

A. Hypesthesia from the lateral foot

B. Hypesthesia from the medial foot

C. Weakened dorsiflexion and inversion

D. Weakened knee extension

E. Weakened knee flexion

45. Which of the following deep tendon reflexes would most likely be diminished in this patient?

A. Biceps femoris

B. Calcaneal (Achilles')

C. Patellar

D. Tibialis anterior

E. Tibialis posterior

46. A 12-year-old boy is brought to the emergency department with acute, severe right testicular pain. Physical examination reveals scrotal swelling and elevation of his right testicle. In addition, the cremasteric reflex is absent on the affected side. Which of the following nerves provides the efferent (motor) limb for this reflex?

A. Genital branch of genitofemoral

B. Iliohypogastric

C. Ilioinguinal

D. Obturator

E. Sympathetic

47. A 49-year-old woman presents to the emergency department with an attack of crushing retrosternal pain that radiates to her left shoulder and upper arm, and her back and neck. A patient history reveals that she has had attacks daily for the past 10 days, and that physical exertion precipitates the attacks and ceasing physical activity relieves the symptoms within a couple of minutes. Elevated cardiac enzymes and ECG changes are consistent with myocardial infarction and coronary angiography demonstrates a 90% stenosis of the left coronary artery. Which of the following nerves is responsible for the pain that is referred to the upper arm in this patient?

A. Lateral cutaneous nerve of the forearm

B. Lateral pectoral

C. Long thoracic

D. Medial cutaneous nerve of the forearm

E. Phrenic

48. A 40-year-old woman is admitted to the urology service for augmentation cystoplasty (bladder enlargement). Following the procedure, she experiences severe pain, itching, and numbness from her medial thigh and a "waddle" gait. Which of the following nerves was most likely injured iatrogenically during the procedure?

A. Femoral

B. Genitofemoral

C. Ilioinguinal

D. Lumbosacral trunk

E. Obturator

49. A 56-year-old woman with advanced pancreatic adenocarcinoma is admitted for palliation of pain in the epigastrium and back. A celiac plexus neurolysis (block) is performed, which involves injection of alcohol into the celiac ganglia and a neurectomy of associated nerves that carry visceral afferent fibers. Which of the following nerves most likely carries the majority of visceral afferent fibers associated with this ganglion?

A. Greater splanchnic

B. Hypogastric

C. Least splanchnic

D. Lumbar splanchnic

E. Vagus

50. A 44-year-old woman is admitted to the emergency department with a 2-week history of intermittent epigastric pain that also extends to the middle of her back. The patient describes a burning pain that is present at night, and is relieved by eating but recurs after several hours. She claims not to have lost weight during the period since the pain began. An abdominal CT reveals a pneumoperitoneum with extravasation of contrast into the omental bursa (lesser sac), which is consistent with duodenal perforation. Which of the following additional symptoms is most likely in this patient?

A. Pain in left upper limb

B. Shoulder pain

C. Suprapubic pain

D. Weakness in hip flexion

E. Weakness in shoulder abduction

51. A 54-year-old man presents with difficulty defecating to his family physician. A patient history reveals that passing stool is difficult and painful for him, and that he has found blood on the toilet paper. During a rectal examination, the physician evaluates the anocutaneous reflex in which the perianal skin is touched with the gloved finger to elicit a brief contraction of the external anal sphincter (often referred to as an anal "wink"). Which of the following nerves provides the efferent (motor) limb for this reflex?

A. Cavernous nerves

B. Inferior rectal

C. Pelvic splanchnic

D. Perineal

E. Rectal plexus

52. A 59-year-old man is referred to the urology clinic with a prostate specific antigen level that had risen from 2.1 to 8.6 ng/mL over five years (normal: < 4 ng/mL). Firm nodules suggestive of cancer are palpable by digital rectal examination from the peripheral zone (posterior lobe) of the prostate. Following robotic radical prostatectomy, the patient experiences erectile dysfunction in which he is unable to attain or maintain a penile erection sufficient for satisfactory sexual performance. Which of the following nerves was most likely damaged in this patient?

A. Cavernous nerves

B. Dorsal nerve of the penis

C. Hypogastric

D. Perineal

E. Sacral splanchnic

53. A 46-year-old man is admitted to the urology clinic with fever, chills, and body ache. He indicates he is experiencing painful urination, the need to urinate frequently, and that he has to get up one or more times at night to urinate (nocturia). Upon admission, his pulse is 104, temperature is 37.9 °C (100.2 °F), and blood pressure is 132/88 mm Hg. Physical examination reveals a distended bladder and a tender, enlarged prostate. Urinalysis and urine culture show an elevated white blood cell count and positive *Escherichia coli*, respectively. To which of the following regions will pain be referred in this patient?

A. Epigastric

B. Left lumbar

C. Penis and scrotum

D. Right lumbar

E. Umbilical

54. A 43-year-old woman presents to the physician with a chronic cough and chest pain. Physical examination reveals that she has severe, sharp chest pain on the right side when breathing deeply or coughing, but the pain subsides when she holds her breath. Auscultation of her lungs reveals a friction rub (rough scratching sound) with inspiration and expiration. In order to reduce the pain, her physician could anesthetize which of the following nerves?

A. Greater splanchnic

B. Intercostal

C. Phrenic

D. Pulmonary plexus

E. Vagus

55. A 35-year-old man is admitted to the emergency department after a fishbone becomes lodged in this throat. The patient is experiencing considerable pain with each attempt to swallow and laryngoscopy reveals that the bone is lodged in the piriform fossa. Which of the following nerves is responsible for the pain in this patient?

A. External laryngeal

B. Internal laryngeal

C. Pharyngeal plexus

D. Recurrent laryngeal

E. Sympathetic

56. During unilateral thyroidectomy in a 34-year-old man, the blood vessels to the inferior pole of the thyroid gland are identified and ligated. Which of the following nerves is most vulnerable during the surgery?

A. External laryngeal

B. Internal laryngeal

C. Recurrent laryngeal

D. Superior laryngeal

E. Vagus

57. A 4-month-old boy is admitted to the pediatric urological surgery clinic with hypospadias in which the external urethral orifice is ectopically located proximal to the tip of the glans penis on the ventral aspect of the penis. General anesthesia combined with caudal epidural anesthesia is used for the hypospadias repair surgery. Which of the following spinal nerves will be targeted for this procedure by the anesthetic injected through the sacral hiatus?

A. T9–T12

B. T11–T12

C. T12

D. L2–L4

E. S2–S4

Consider the following case for questions 58 and 59:

A 68-year-old woman presents to the emergency department with pain, deformity, and swelling of her right arm after she slipped and fell on ice. Radiological examination reveals a fracture of the middle third of the humerus.

58. Which of the following nerves is most vulnerable to injury in this patient?

A. Axillary

B. Musculoskeletal

C. Radial

D. Median

E. Ulnar

59. Which of the following clinical signs would most likely be seen in this patient?

A. Hypesthesia from the palm

B. Hypesthesia from the tip of the thumb

C. Inability to extend the elbow

D. Inability to extend the wrist

E. Inability to supinate the forearm

60. A 20-year-old man presents with a 2-month history of decreasing function of his right hand. A patient history reveals no previous hand trauma. Physical examination of the right hand shows atrophy of the first dorsal interosseous muscle. MRI shows a ganglion cyst arising from the third carpometacarpal joint that is compressing the deep branch of the ulnar nerve. Which of the following additional signs or symptoms actions would be likely in this patient?

A. Abduction and adduction of the medial four digits

B. Abduction of the thumb

C. Flexion of the distal interphalangeal joint of the little finger

D. Hypesthesia from the skin over the medial hand

E. Hypesthesia from the thenar eminence

61. A 42-year-old woman presents in the orthopaedic clinic with a painful, palmar wrist mass and numbness over the left thenar eminence (*large shaded area* in the accompanying image). Physical examination shows a 1 cm mass proximal to the wrist, adjacent to the ulnar side of the flexor carpi radialis tendon (*small shaded area* in the accompanying image). Which of the following nerves is most likely affected in this patient?

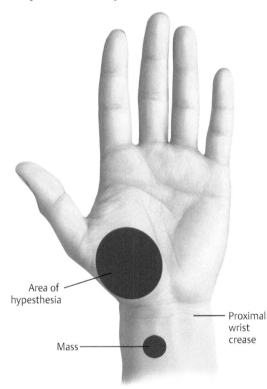

Area of hypesthesia

Proximal wrist crease

Mass

Source: Gilroy AM et al. Atlas of Anatomy. 3rd ed. 2016. Based on: Schuenke M, Schulte E, Schumacher U. THIEME Atlas of Anatomy. Volumes 1-3. Illustrations by Voll M and Wesker K. 2nd ed. New York: Thieme Medical Publishers; 2016

A. Median
B. Palmar cutaneous branch of median
C. Palmar cutaneous branch of ulnar
D. Recurrent branch of median
E. Superficial branch of ulnar

62. A 63-year-old woman presents for her 1-month follow-up after coronary bypass surgery. She relates that she is experiencing burning and tingling sensations along her right medial leg. The vein for the coronary bypass was harvested from the medial side of her right knee and ankle. Which nerve has been traumatized to account for the symptoms?

A. Obturator
B. Posterior femoral cutaneous
C. Saphenous
D. Superficial fibular
E. Tibial

63. A 52-year-old man presents with burning, tingling, and numbness on the sole of his right foot. Physical examination reveals indistinct longitudinal and transverse plantar arches. He relates that he has always had flat feet. Which nerve is being compressed to produce the symptoms?

A. Deep fibular
B. Saphenous
C. Superficial fibular
D. Sural
E. Tibial

64. A 71-year-old man presents for his 1-month follow-up appointment following placement using the anterior approach of a right hip prosthesis. Physical examination reveals weak knee extension on the right side and his patellar reflex is absent. Which nerve was traumatized during the surgery?

A. Anterior branch of obturator
B. Femoral
C. Posterior branch of obturator
D. Sciatic
E. Superficial fibular

65. A 16-year-old girl presents to her orthopedist for removal of a plaster cast from her leg 7 weeks after she fractured her tibia. Physical examination of the limb after cast removal reveals weak dorsiflexion and eversion, along with sensory loss along the anterior and lateral leg and on the dorsum of her foot. Which nerve has been compressed by the cast to account for the symptoms?

A. Deep fibular
B. Common fibular
C. Saphenous
D. Superficial fibular
E. Tibial

Consider the following case for questions 66 to 68:

A 22-year-old man presents to the emergency department with anorexia (lack of appetite), vomiting, and diffuse abdominal pain. The patient tells the examining physician that the pain began in the periumbilical region but is now localized to the right lower part of his abdomen. Physical examination reveals right lower quadrant tenderness and a temperature of 39.5°C (103°F). The physician suspects acute appendicitis and, after the patient is admitted to the hospital for further evaluation, the patient undergoes an appendectomy.

13

66. The initial pain around the umbilicus is most likely transmitted via which of the following nerves?

A. Greater splanchnic
B. Inferior hypogastric
C. Least splanchnic
D. Lesser splanchnic
E. Superior hypogastric

67. The pain from the right lower quadrant is most likely transmitted via which of the following structures?

A. Greater splanchnic nerve
B. Least splanchnic nerve
C. Lumbar sympathetic ganglia
D. Superior cervical ganglion
E. Superior mesenteric plexus

68. At surgery, it is noted that the appendix had perforated and there is pus within the abdominal cavity. The abdomen is irrigated with warm saline solution. The patient initially makes an uneventful recovery, but by postoperative day 7 he is experiencing pain over his right shoulder and is spiking temperatures. Involvement of which nerve is mediating the referred shoulder pain?

A. Iliohypogastric
B. Pelvic splanchnic
C. Phrenic
D. Subcostal
E. T10 thoracoabdominal

69. A 37-year-old woman is seen in the gastroenterology clinic because of painful bowel movements associated with pain, itching, and burning of the rectum. The patient typically has one bowel movement each day and she has occasionally noted bright red blood on the toilet paper. She has experienced frequent constipation and hard stools have been streaked with blood. Physical examination reveals a tender, bluish-black nodule at the anal margin characteristic of an external hemorrhoid. Which of the following nerves most likely transmits the pain described by this patient?

A. Hypogastric
B. Ilioinguinal
C. Pelvic splanchnic
D. Pudendal
E. Sacral splanchnic

Consider the following case for questions 70 and 71:

A 2-day-old male infant presents with bilious vomiting and has not yet passed meconium. Physical examination reveals a distended abdomen. Intestinal imaging with contrast (refer to the accompanying image) reveals dilated loops of colon and segmental narrowing of the sigmoid colon (*black arrows*) with an abrupt transition to a markedly dilated, prestenotic colon (*white arrow*). A rectal mucosal suction biopsy reveals an absence of ganglion cells below the transition zone.

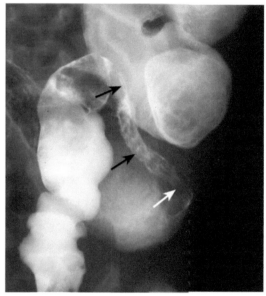

Source: Burgener F, Kormano M, Pudas T. Differential Diagnosis in Conventional Radiology. 3rd Edition. Stuttgart: Thieme; 2007.

70. Which of the following diagnoses is consistent with the signs and symptoms in this infant?

A. Cloacal extrophy
B. Duodenal atresia
C. Hirschsprung's disease
D. Imperforate anus
E. Meckel's diverticulum

71. A failure of migration of which cell type results in this developmental anomaly?

A. Endoderm
B. Intermediate mesoderm
C. Neural crest
D. Paraxial mesoderm
E. Visceral (splanchnic) mesoderm

72. An ultrasound reveals that a fetus has a defect in his lower vertebral column. At birth, the defect appears as a fluid-filled out-pocketing and ultrasound reveals that neural tissue is involved in the defect. Which of the following conditions exists in this neonate?

A. Meningoencephalocele

B. Spina bifida occulta

C. Spina bifida with meningocele

D. Spina bifida with meningomyelocele

Consider the following case for questions 73 and 74:

A 12-year-old girl presents to the emergency department with fever, headache, myalgia, and multiple episodes of vomiting over the course of the day. To rule out meningitis, a lumbar puncture (LP) is performed to obtain a sample of cerebrospinal fluid for analysis.

73. Between which of the following vertebrae, or into which space, would the physician insert the needle during this procedure?

A. L1–L2

B. L2–L3

C. L3–L4

D. Sacral foramina

E. Sacral hiatus

74. Which of the following developmental events explains why the above procedure is unlikely to injure the spinal cord?

A. Neural tissue is not present in the lumbar cistern.

B. Spinal nerves do not exit the vertebral column inferior to L2.

C. The developing vertebral column elongates faster than the spinal cord, creating the lumbar cistern with nerve roots that form the cauda equina.

D. The length of the vertebral column shortens relative to the developing neural tube.

E. The spinal cord is not present in the lumbar region of the vertebral column.

75 A 2-day-old male infant is in the neonatal unit with shoulder dystocia resulting from birth trauma. In the immediate postnatal period, he presents with the right arm adducted and medially rotated at the shoulder, the elbow extended and forearm pronated, and the fingers flexed. Which of the following roots of the brachial plexus are most likely injured in this patient?

A. C2–C4

B. C5–C6

C. C5–T1

D. C7 only

E. C8–T1

76. A 27-year-old woman, para 3, presents to the women's health clinic with pain, amenorrhea, and vaginal bleeding. She reports a positive result from a home urine pregnancy test. Physical examination reveals mild lower abdominal tenderness and pelvic exam reveals fullness and tenderness of the left adnexa on bimanual palpation. A vaginal speculum examination reveals bleeding from the cervical os. Diagnostic laparoscopy identifies a hemoperitoneum from a rupture of a left, ampullary tubal pregnancy requiring peritoneal lavage and a left salpingectomy. Which of the following nerves would transmit the pain from the affected organ in this patient?

A. Greater splanchnic

B. Hypogastric

C. Pelvic splanchnic

D. Sacral splanchnic

E. Sacral sympathetic trunk

77. A 60-year-old man presents to the emergency department with sudden, recurrent episodes of syncope (loss of consciousness). During an episode in the emergency department, his pulse is noted to decrease to 35 beats per minute (normal: 60–100) and his blood pressure decreases to 75/40 mm Hg (normal: 120/80). His pO_2, pCO_2, and pH are normal. MRI reveals a mass that is compressing the proximal portion of the left internal carotid artery. Which of the following structures is most likely affected in this patient?

A. Carotid body

B. Carotid sinus

C. Otic ganglion

D. Stellate ganglion

E. Superior cervical ganglion

78. A 6-year-old otherwise healthy girl with a 10-day history of nasal discharge, nasal congestion and cough is brought to a primary care physician. Her parents report she has had daily fever spikes to 38.7 °C (101.7 °F) and the cough is worse at night. Physical examination shows that her lungs and tympanic membranes are clear. Her nasal conchae (turbinates) are erythematous (reddened) and swollen, and she has thick, yellow purulent mucus in her nasal cavity and nasopharynx. She has mild tenderness to palpation of her cheeks and halitosis (bad breath). The patient is diagnosed with acute bacterial sinusitis and prescribed amoxicillin for 10 days. Which of the following nerves is most likely responsible for the tenderness in the involved paranasal sinus in this patient?

A. Mandibular

B. Maxillary

C. Olfactory

D. Ophthalmic

E. Vagus

1.2 Answers and Explanations

Easy	Medium	Hard

1. Correct: Iliohypogastric (B)

Refer to the following image for answer 1:

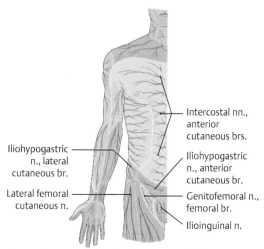

Intercostal nn., anterior cutaneous brs.

Iliohypogastric n., lateral cutaneous br.

Iliohypogastric n., anterior cutaneous br.

Lateral femoral cutaneous n.

Genitofemoral n., femoral br.

Ilioinguinal n.

Source: Gilroy AM et al. Atlas of Anatomy. 3rd ed. 2016. Based on: Schuenke M, Schulte E, Schumacher U. THIEME Atlas of Anatomy. Volumes 1-3. Illustrations by Voll M and Wesker K. 2nd ed. New York: Thieme Medical Publishers; 2016

(**B**) The iliohypogastric nerve (L1) provides sensory innervation from suprapubic skin. (**A**) The genitofemoral nerve (L1–L2) provides sensory innervation in females from skin over the mons pubis and labium majus, as well as from the anteromedial thigh. (**C**) The ilioinguinal nerve (L1) provides sensory innervation from skin over the mons pubis and labium majus, as well as the proximal medial thigh. (**D**) The pudendal nerve (S2–S4) provides sensory innervation from skin of the perineum. (**E**) The T10 intercostal (thoracoabdominal) nerve provides sensory innervation from skin around the umbilicus.

2. Correct: T10 thoracoabdominal (E)

(**E**) The dermatome that includes the umbilicus is supplied by the T10 thoracoabdominal nerve (refer to the accompanying image). By definition, the superficial abdominal reflex assesses the T8–T12 spinal cord levels. It is one of four superficial cutaneous reflexes: abdominal, cremaster, plantar, and the anocutaneous ("anal wink"). (**A**) The iliohypogastric nerve contributes to the L1 dermatome, which includes the suprapubic skin. (**B**) The ilioinguinal nerve contributes to the L1 dermatome, which includes the skin over the mons pubis and labium majus, as well as the proximal medial thigh. (**C**) The subcostal nerve is the ventral ramus of the T12 spinal nerve. (**D**) On

the anterior (and lateral) body wall, the T7, as well as the T8–T9, thoracoabdominal nerves carry sensory information from skin located between the xiphoid process (which is generally included in the T6 dermatome) and the umbilicus.

Refer to the following image for answer 2:

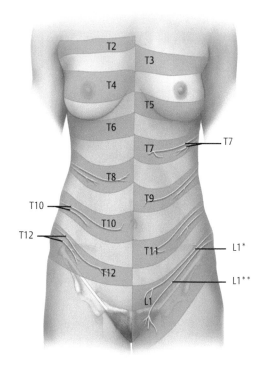

T7 Thoracoabdomial nerve
T10 Thoracoabdomial nerve
T12 Subcostal nerve
L1* Iliohypogastric nerve
L1** Ilioinguinal nerve

3. Correct: Frontal (B)

(**B**) Branches of the ophthalmic nerve (CN V1) provide sensory innervation from the upper eyelid. Within the orbit, the frontal nerve (a branch of CN V1) courses immediately inferior to the periorbita. Branches of this nerve (supraorbital and supratrochlear) along with infraorbital (from nasociliary) and lacrimal supply the upper eyelid. (**A**) The anterior ethmoidal nerve is a branch of CN V1, but it does not provide sensory innervation from the upper eyelid. (**C**) The infraorbital nerve is a branch of the maxillary division of the trigeminal nerve (CN V2). It provides sensory innervation from the lower eyelid (refer to the following image). (**D**) The oculomotor nerve (CN III) provides motor innervation to most of the extraocular muscles. (**E**) The zygomatic nerve is a branch of CN V2, which provides sensory innervation from the lower eyelid.

Refer to the following image for answer 3:

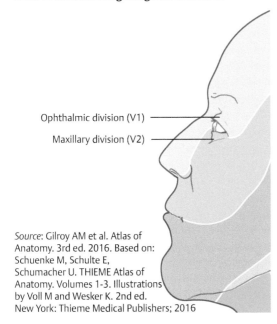

Ophthalmic division (V1)

Maxillary division (V2)

Source: Gilroy AM et al. Atlas of Anatomy. 3rd ed. 2016. Based on: Schuenke M, Schulte E, Schumacher U. THIEME Atlas of Anatomy. Volumes 1-3. Illustrations by Voll M and Wesker K. 2nd ed. New York: Thieme Medical Publishers; 2016

4. Correct: Oculomotor (B)

Refer to the following image for answer 4:

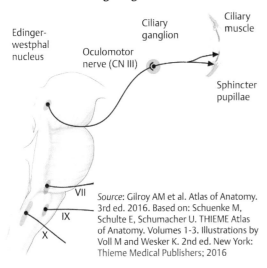

Edinger-westphal nucleus

Oculomotor nerve (CN III)

Ciliary ganglion

Ciliary muscle

Sphincter pupillae

VII

IX

X

Source: Gilroy AM et al. Atlas of Anatomy. 3rd ed. 2016. Based on: Schuenke M, Schulte E, Schumacher U. THIEME Atlas of Anatomy. Volumes 1-3. Illustrations by Voll M and Wesker K. 2nd ed. New York: Thieme Medical Publishers; 2016

(**B**) The ophthalmic veins and CNs III (oculomotor), IV (trochlear), V1 (ophthalmic), and VI (abducens) pass through the superior orbital fissure. Of these, only the oculomotor nerve (CN III) contains preganglionic parasympathetic fibers that synapse in the ciliary ganglion on cells whose postganglionic axons innervate the sphincter pupillae muscle (refer to the accompanying image). Injury to the oculomotor nerve in the superior orbital fissure may result in mydriasis (pupillary dilation) in the affected eye, which would lead to anisocoria (pupils of unequal size). (**A**) While the abducens nerve (CN VI) does pass through the superior orbital fissure, it does not contain fibers that regulate pupil size. (**C**) While the

ophthalmic nerve (CN V1) does pass through the superior orbital fissure, it does not contain fibers that regulate pupil size. (**D**) The optic nerve (CN II) passes through the optic canal and does not contain fibers that regulate pupil size. (**E**) While the trochlear nerve (CN IV) does pass through the superior orbital fissure, it does not contain parasympathetic fibers that regulate pupil size.

5. Correct: Dorsal root ganglia (B)

(**B**) Neuronal cell bodies for primary sensory neurons related to somatosensation from the body wall are located in dorsal (posterior) root ganglia. (**A**) The dorsal horn of the spinal cord contains the terminal dendrites of primary sensory neurons, as well as the cell bodies of interneurons. (**C**) The skin contains the peripheral axon terminals of primary sensory neurons. (**D**) The somatosensory cortex contains tertiary neurons that receive information relayed from primary sensory neurons. (**E**) The ventral horn contains the neuronal cell bodies of somatic motor neurons.

6. Correct: Dorsal root ganglion (B)

(**B**) Primary sensory neuronal cell bodies related to dermatomes of the body are located in the dorsal root ganglia. Infection with varicella zoster virus may presents as two distinct entities: (1) chickenpox as the primary infection, which usually manifests in children, and (2) herpes zoster or shingles, which is a secondary condition that develops when the virus is reactivated in primary sensory neurons located in all sensory ganglia (except special sensory ganglia) and then migrates along cutaneous (sensory) nerves in associated dermatomes, causing sensory disturbances and, eventually, a rash. (**A**) The dorsal horn of the spinal cord contains second order sensory neuronal cell bodies. (**C**) The lateral horn of the spinal cord contains preganglionic sympathetic neuronal cell bodies. (**D**) The somatosensory cortex contains higher order sensory neurons. (**E**) The ventral horn of the spinal cord contains motor neuron cell bodies.

7. Correct: Olfactory (D)

(**D**) The unmyelinated axons of the bipolar olfactory neurons traverse the cribriform plate and synapse on mitral and tufted cells in the olfactory bulb. Fractures of the cribriform plate (which forms the roof of the nasal cavity) can, therefore, disturb olfaction. Patients may be unaware of a unilateral deficit because the contralateral receptors can compensate, whereas those with bilateral involvement may complain of decreased ability to taste (olfaction plays a role in taste). (**A–C, E**) The anterior and posterior ethmoidal, lacrimal, and nasociliary nerves do not pass through the cribriform plate, nor are they related to olfaction or taste.

8. Correct: Central retinal artery (A)

Refer to the following image for answer 8:

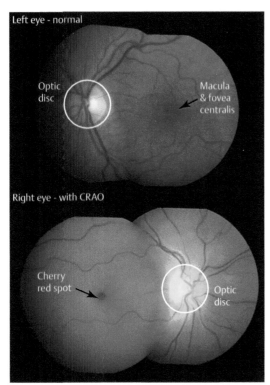

Source: Image provided courtesy of Dr. Aristomenis Thanos, Associated Retinal Consultants, Oakland University William Beaumont School of Medicine, Royal Oak, MI.

(**A**) The central retinal artery, a branch of the ophthalmic, enters the optic nerve and passes through the optic disc where it divides to supply the inner layers of the retina. Normally, the macular region appears slightly yellowish, while the fovea appears red due to the underlying choroidal vessels. With occlusion of the central retinal artery, the surrounding retina undergoes infarction and appears milky, enhancing the appearance of the choroid vessels and leading to a prominent "cherry-red spot." (**B, E**) The internal carotid artery and its ophthalmic branch indirectly supply the retina via central retinal and ciliary branches. While their occlusion will likely lead to visual deficits, only occlusion of the central retinal artery will lead to the formation of a cherry-red spot. (**C, D**) Neither the internal jugular vein nor the middle meningeal artery supply the retina.

9. Correct: Retinal ganglion cells (B)

(**B**) The retina has a dual blood supply: the central retinal artery supplies its inner layers (layers 6–9: inner nuclear layer through the nerve fiber layer), while the outer layers (layers 1–5: pigment epithelium through outer plexiform layers) are avascular and are supplied indirectly by blood in the choroid (choriocapillary layer). The retinal ganglion cells, as well as cells in the inner nuclear layer, are part of the inner retina. (**A, C–E**) Cone photoreceptor cells, retinal pigment epithelium cells, rod photoreceptor cells, and scleral cells are all located in the outer retina and are supplied by the choriocapillaris in the choroid.

Refer to the following image for answer 9:

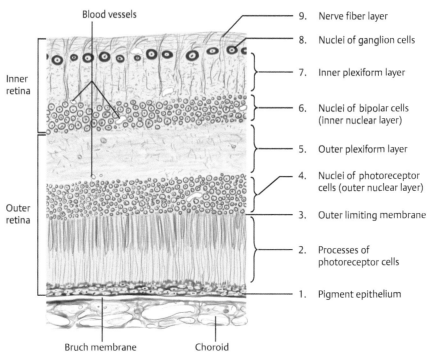

Source: Schuenke M, Schulte E, Schumacher U. THIEME Atlas of Anatomy. Head, Neck, and Neuroanatomy. Illustrations by Voll M and Wesker K. 2nd ed. New York: Thieme Medical Publishers; 2016

10. Correct: Nasociliary (D)

(**D**) In addition to somatic afferents from the face, the nasociliary nerve also contains sensory fibers that either pass directly to the eye via long ciliary nerves, or through the ciliary ganglion and then to the eye via short ciliary nerves. These fibers supply sensory innervation from the cornea, as well as the iris and ciliary body. (**A–C**) These frontal, infraorbital, and lacrimal nerves carry afferent fibers from the face, including the eyelids (upper lid via the frontal and lacrimal nerves; lower lid via the infraorbital nerve) but not from the eye. (**E**) The optic nerve, formed by the axons of the retinal ganglion cells, carries visual information from the eye to subcortical nuclei.

11. Correct: Facial (A)

(**A**) The corneal reflex (blink reflex) involves gently stroking the cornea with fibers of a sterile cotton swab which is followed under normal conditions by eyelid closure (action of orbicularis oculi). The afferent arm of this reflex is mediated by the nasociliary nerve (which provides sensory innervation from the cornea) while the efferent arm is mediated by the facial nerve (which innervates the orbicularis oculi muscle). Patients with hemifacial paralysis (Bell's palsy) have impairment of the facial nerve, which interrupts the efferent arm of the corneal reflex, and results in the inability to close the eyelids. (**B–E**) The infraorbital, lacrimal, nasociliary, and supraorbital nerves are all branches of the trigeminal nerve and are generally not affected in Bell's palsy patients.

12. Correct: Facial canal, proximal to chorda tympani (B)

(**B**) Bell's palsy is a unilateral facial paralysis that involves the facial nerve (CN VII), with symptoms depending on the location of the facial nerve lesion. In this patient, the unilateral facial paralysis and alteration in taste indicates that the facial nerve lesion must be in the facial canal, proximal to the origin of the chorda tympani, but distal to the origin of the greater petrosal nerve and nerve to stapedius since there is no dry eye (greater petrosal nerve) or hyperacusis (nerve to stapedius). (**A**) The facial nerve does not pass through the cavernous sinus; therefore, the sinus is not involved in Bell's palsy. (**C**) A lesion of the facial nerve at the internal acoustic meatus would likely include dysfunction of hearing and balance (CN VIII), as well as hemifacial paralysis and disturbances in taste, salivation, and lacrimation. (**D**) The facial nerve does not pass through the jugular foramen; therefore, the foramen is not involved in Bell's palsy. (**E**) A lesion of the facial nerve at the stylomastoid foramen would present as hemifacial paralysis only.

Refer to the following image for answer 12:

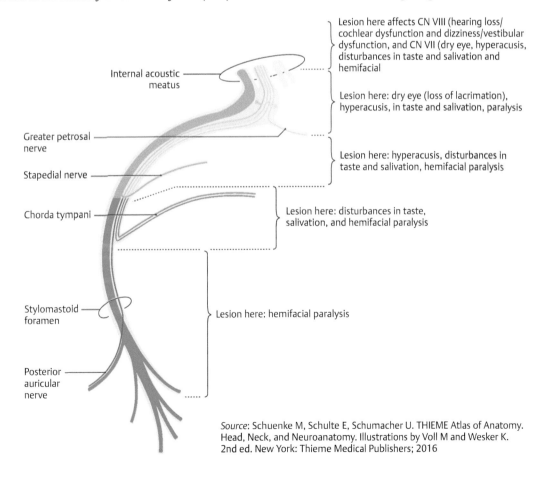

Lesion here affects CN VIII (hearing loss/cochlear dysfunction and dizziness/vestibular dysfunction, and CN VII (dry eye, hyperacusis, disturbances in taste and salivation and hemifacial

Lesion here: dry eye (loss of lacrimation), hyperacusis, in taste and salivation, paralysis

Lesion here: hyperacusis, disturbances in taste and salivation, hemifacial paralysis

Lesion here: disturbances in taste, salivation, and hemifacial paralysis

Lesion here: hemifacial paralysis

Internal acoustic meatus

Greater petrosal nerve

Stapedial nerve

Chorda tympani

Stylomastoid foramen

Posterior auricular nerve

Source: Schuenke M, Schulte E, Schumacher U. THIEME Atlas of Anatomy. Head, Neck, and Neuroanatomy. Illustrations by Voll M and Wesker K. 2nd ed. New York: Thieme Medical Publishers; 2016

13. Correct: Abducens (A)

(**A**) The abducens nerve (CN VI) innervates the lateral rectus, which is the primary abductor of the eye. Increased intracranial pressure can result in inferior displacement of the brainstem, which may stretch the abducens nerve as it passes from the brainstem to its exit through the dura mater (via Dorello's canal). This results in an abduction deficit, with patients experiencing diplopia ("double vision") with attempted lateral gaze ipsilateral to the affected eye. (**B–E**) The long ciliary, nasociliary, oculomotor, and trochlear nerves do not innervate extraocular muscles that are primary abductors of the eye.

14. Correct: Superior oblique (D)

(**D**) The superior oblique, which is innervated by the trochlear nerve (CN IV), intorts, depresses, and abducts the eye. With paralysis of the superior oblique, the affected eye is hypertropic (elevated) and adducted due to the unopposed actions of the eye adductors—the medial rectus and the vertical recti (i.e., the superior and inferior rectus muscles) and the inferior oblique and superior rectus, which elevate the eye. The patient may tilt their head to the side contralateral to the affected side in order to eliminate the diplopia. (**A**) The inferior oblique, which is innervated by the oculomotor nerve (CN III), extorts, elevates, and abducts the eye. Its ability to elevate the eye, which is unopposed by the superior oblique, accounts for the hypertropic (elevated) eye position in this patient. (**B**) The inferior rectus, which is innervated by the oculomotor nerve (CN III), depresses, adducts, and extorts the eye. Its ability to adduct the eye, which is unopposed by the superior oblique, accounts for the esotropic (adducted) eye position in this patient. (**C**) The medial rectus, which is innervated by the oculomotor nerve (CN III), adducts the eye. Its ability to adduct the eye, which is unopposed by the superior oblique, accounts for the esotropic (adducted) eye position in this patient. (**E**) The superior rectus, which is innervated by the oculomotor nerve (CN III), elevates, adducts, and intorts the eye. Its ability to elevate the eye, which is unopposed by the superior oblique, accounts for the hypertropic (elevated) eye position in this patient.

15. Correct: Levator palpebrae superioris (B)

(**B**) The levator palpebrae superioris, which is innervated by the oculomotor nerve (CN III), elevates the upper eyelid. Ptosis in the presence of ophthalmoplegia (i.e., paralysis of extraocular muscles responsible for eye movements) suggests involvement of the levator palpebrae superioris. (**A, C, D**) The levator labii superioris, superior oblique, and superior rectus muscles do not elevate the eyelid. (**E**) The superior tarsal muscle, which receives sympathetic innervation via the nasociliary nerve and ciliary nerves (long and short), elevates the upper eyelid to widen the palpebral fissure during a sympathetic response. While interruption of sympathetic innervation to the eye would likely result in ptosis, miosis (i.e., a constricted pupil due to paralysis of the dilator pupillae), rather than mydriasis, would also likely be observed.

16. Correct: Oculomotor (E)

(**E**) The oculomotor nerve (CN III) carries preganglionic parasympathetic fibers to the ciliary ganglion. Postganglionic fibers travel to the eye via short ciliary nerves to innervate the sphincter pupillae muscle. Mydriasis indicates parasympathetic involvement, which could be affected in any of the structures involved in this pathway, that is, the accessory oculomotor nucleus (Edinger–Westphal), the oculomotor nerve, the ciliary ganglion, and short ciliary nerves. The impaired adduction and upward gaze implicate the medial and vertical (superior and inferior) rectus muscles, as well as the inferior oblique, indicating that the lesion is in the oculomotor nerve. (**A**) The abducens nerve (CN VI) innervates the lateral rectus, which is the primary abductor of the eye. It does not carry parasympathetic fibers, so a lesion would not affect pupillary function. (**B**) The deep petrosal nerve contains postganglionic sympathetic fibers from the internal carotid plexus. The nerve joins the greater petrosal nerve, which carries preganglionic parasympathetic fibers, to form the nerve of the pterygoid canal (Vidian nerve). After synapsing in the pterygopalatine ganglion, the postganglionic parasympathetic fibers innervate the lacrimal gland and glands of the nasal cavity, palate, and superior portion of the pharynx. (**C**) Long ciliary nerves, which branch from the nasociliary nerve, carry postganglionic sympathetic fibers to the iris and cornea. (**D**) The nasociliary nerve, a branch of the ophthalmic (CN V1), carries sensory fibers and postganglionic sympathetic fibers to the eye via long ciliary nerves.

17. Correct: Retinal ganglion cell axons (D)

(**D**) The structure indicated by the white circle is the optic disc, the position at which the axons of retinal ganglion cells leave the eye to form the optic nerve (CN II); no photoreceptors are found in this region. (**A**) The ciliary body is located in the anterior part of the eye. (**B**) Cone photoreceptors are concentrated in the fovea centralis, a structure of the retina located temporal to the optic disc. There are almost no rods in the fovea. (**C**) The lens is located in the anterior part of the eye. (**E**) Rod photoreceptors are located primarily in the periphery of the retina.

18. Correct: Diplopia with upward gaze (C)

(**C**) Blowout fractures result from a forceful blow to the orbital rim (i.e., frontal, zygomatic, and maxillary bones). The sudden force transmitted to bones within the orbit commonly causes a fracture of the floor of the orbit, and less commonly a fracture of the medial wall. Although orbital edema may affect the function of extraocular muscles, entrapment of muscles in close apposition to the fracture may limit eye movement away from the muscle. With an orbital floor fracture, the inferior rectus may be trapped, directing the gaze downward. Consequently, the elevation action of superior rectus may be limited (relative to the unaffected eye), leading to diplopia with attempted upward gaze. (**A, B**) The primary muscles responsible for lateral gaze (lateral rectus) and medial gaze (medial rectus) are not related to the orbital floor. (**D**) Mydriasis indicates involvement of parasympathetic fibers, either in the accessory oculomotor (Edinger–Westphal) nucleus or along their pathway to the eye (i.e., in the oculomotor nerve, the ciliary ganglion, or short ciliary nerves). (**E**) The levator palpebrae superioris is not related to the orbital floor. It elevates the upper eyelid and is responsible for ptosis when paralyzed.

19. Correct: Hypesthesia (diminished sensation) from the cheek (C)

(**C**) The infraorbital nerve passes through the infraorbital groove (in the floor of the orbit) and exits the infraorbital foramen to reach the skin over the maxilla. The nerve is commonly injured in a blowout fracture and can result in sensory deficits (e.g., hypesthesia/hypoesthesia, anesthesia) from the cheek. (**A**) The nerve fibers that innervate the lacrimal gland do not pass through the floor of the orbit and are not likely to be injured in a blowout fracture. (**B**) The nerve fibers that innervate the salivary glands do not pass through the orbit and are not likely to be injured in a blowout fracture. (**D**) The corneal reflex is mediated by the nasociliary nerve (the afferent arm, which provides sensory innervation to the cornea) and by the facial nerve (the efferent arm, which innervates the orbicularis oculi muscle). These nerves are not likely to be injured in a blowout fracture. (**E**) Miosis (a constricted pupil) occurs when sympathetic innervation to the dilator pupillae is interrupted. The postganglionic sympathetic fibers arise from cells in the superior cervical ganglion and enter the internal carotid plexus to reach the eye via the nasociliary nerve, and then long ciliary nerves or via the ciliary ganglion and short ciliary nerves. These fibers are unlikely to be injured in a blowout fracture.

20. Correct: Accessory (A)

(**A**) The accessory nerve (CN XI) innervates the trapezius and sternocleidomastoid. The trapezius elevates, adducts and retracts the scapula, and rotates the glenohumeral fossa upward. The trapezius, serratus anterior, and rhomboids hold the scapula against the posterior thoracic wall and, therefore, paralysis of one of these muscles with the unopposed contraction of the other functioning scapular muscles may result in medial (serratus anterior paralysis) or lateral (trapezius or rhomboid paralysis) scapular winging. In this case, the clinical signs indicate paralysis of the trapezius. (**B**) The long thoracic nerve innervates the serratus anterior, which protracts the scapula, contributes to its upward rotation, and holds it against the thoracic wall. Paralysis of this muscle results in limited abduction of the arm and medial scapular winging, but not lateral scapular winging or depression of the shoulder. (**C**) The dorsal scapular nerve innervates the rhomboids, which retract and rotate the scapula to direct the glenoid cavity inferiorly (also known as lateral rotation due to the lateral movement of the inferior scapular angle). (**D**) The lower subscapular nerve innervates subscapularis and teres major. Both of these muscles medially rotate and adduct the arm. Paralysis of these muscles would not result in the clinical presentation of this patient. (**E**) The suprascapular nerve innervates supraspinatus and infraspinatus. Supraspinatus abducts the arm, whereas infraspinatus laterally rotates the arm. Paralysis of these muscles would not result in the clinical presentation of this patient.

21. Correct: Left accessory (A)

(**A**) The accessory nerve (CN XI) innervates the sternocleidomastoid and trapezius. Acting unilaterally, the sternocleidomastoid rotates the head to the opposite side and laterally flexes ("tilts") the head to the same side. Thus, the left sternocleidomastoid—innervated by the left accessory nerve—rotates the head to the right side. (**B–E**) The dorsal scapular and suprascapular nerve nerves do not innervate muscles that rotates the head to the opposite side (dorsal scapular nerve innervates the rhomboid muscles; the suprascapular nerve innervates the supra- and infraspinatus muscles).

22. Correct: Ventral horn of the spinal cord (E)

(**E**) Axons of the accessory nerve (CN XI) arise from neuronal cell bodies in the ventral horn of the spinal cord and innervate the sternocleidomastoid and trapezius. (**A**) Motor axons arising from neuronal cell bodies in the facial motor nucleus contribute to the facial nerve and innervate the muscles of facial expression. (**B**) Branchial motor axons arising from neuronal cell bodies in the nucleus ambiguus innervate muscles of the soft palate (CN IX and X), pharynx (CN IX and X), and larynx (CN X). (**C**) The solitary tract nucleus (nucleus solitarius) is a sensory nucleus for the synapse of visceral afferent axons from the facial, glossopharyngeal, and vagus nerves. These nerves supply sensation from a variety of structures, including the tongue (CN VII and IX), the ear (CN X), the carotid sinus and body (CN IX), and thoracic and abdominal viscera supplied by afferent fibers in the vagus nerve. The afferent arms of important reflexes are mediated through this nucleus, including the gag reflex, baroreceptor and chemoreceptor reflexes, and respiratory and GI reflexes. (**D**) Axons arising from neuronal cell bodies in the trigeminal motor (masticator) nucleus innervate the muscles of mastication, as well as tensor tympani and veli palatini, mylohyoid, and the anterior digastric muscles.

23. Correct: Right hypoglossal (C)

(**C**) The genioglossus, the primary muscle that protrudes the tongue, is innervated by the hypoglossal nerve (CN XII). With a unilateral lesion of the hypoglossal nerve, the unaffected (opposite) genioglossus will force the protruded tongue toward the affected side. Thus, a right hypoglossal palsy will result in deviation of the protruded tongue toward the right side. (**A**) A left hypoglossal palsy will result in deviation of the protruded tongue toward the left side. (**B, E**) The lingual nerve, a branch of the mandibular nerve, carries general and special (taste) sensory information from anterior two-thirds of the tongue and does not innervate muscles. (**D**) The inferior alveolar nerve, a branch of the mandibular nerve, carries general sensory information from the mandible, mandibular teeth, and skin over the mandible.

24. Correct: C7 (C)

(**C**) The C7 spinal cord provides the predominant innervation for the triceps brachii tendon reflex. (**A–B**) The commonly agreed upon spinal cord levels for deep tendon reflexes that are routinely tested in a physical examination are: C5(C6)—biceps brachii reflex; C6—brachioradialis reflex; C7—triceps brachii reflex; L4—patellar tendon ("knee jerk") reflex (mediated through the quadriceps muscle); and S1—calcaneal (Achilles') tendon reflex (mediated through the triceps surae muscle). (**D–E**) The C8 and T1 spinal cord levels are not associated with elicited deep tendon reflexes.

25. Correct: Patellar reflex (B)

Refer to the following image for answer 25:

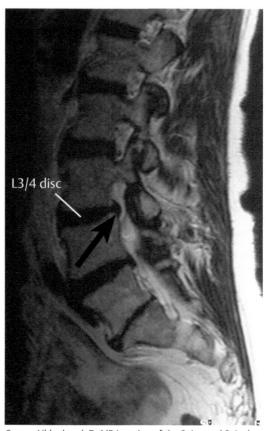

Source: Uhlenbrock D. MR Imaging of the Spine and Spinal Cord. 1st Edition. Thieme; 2003.

(**B**) The MRI shows a herniation of the L3 to L4 intervertebral disc, which will affect the L4 spinal nerve. The L4 spinal nerve is the predominant contribution to the patellar reflex. The L4 spinal nerve contributes to the femoral nerve (L2–L4) and, thereby, to innervation of the quadriceps muscle (L2–L4), whose primary function is knee extension. The L4 dermatome includes the medial leg, which is supplied by the saphenous nerve (the terminal branch of the femoral nerve). (**A**) The calcaneal (Achilles') tendon reflex is mediated by the S1 spinal nerve. (**C**) The superficial anal reflex is mediated by the pudendal nerve (S2–S4). (**D**) The tibialis posterior reflex, which is not easily elicited, is mediated by the L5 spinal nerve.

26. Correct: Ipsilateral blindness (C)

(**C**) The optic canal is indicated by the arrow in the CT image. Since this passageway transmits the optic nerve (CN II) from one eye, a fracture of this opening would likely damage the ganglion cell axons in the optic nerve, which transmit visual signals from the retina. (**A**) Bell's palsy involves a lesion of the facial nerve (CN VII), which is transmitted via the facial canal. (**B**) Bilateral blindness may result from a number of conditions, including damage of the retina and or optic nerves of both eyes. (**D**) The oculomotor nerve (CN III) passes through the superior orbital fissure and would, therefore, not be involved in a fracture of the optic canal. It is not involved in vision. (**E**) The trochlear nerve (CN IV) passes through the superior orbital fissure and would, therefore, not be involved in a fracture of the optic canal.

27. Correct: Trigeminal (E)

(**E**) The trigeminal ganglion contains sensory cell bodies of the ophthalmic (CN V1), maxillary (CN V2), and mandibular (CN V3) nerves. (**A**) The geniculate ganglion contains sensory cell bodies for fibers associated with the facial nerve, and is carried via nervus intermedius, chorda tympani, and the lingual nerve. (**B, C**) The otic and pterygopalatine ganglia contain postganglionic parasympathetic neuronal cell bodies. (**D**) The superior cervical ganglion contains postganglionic sympathetic neuronal cell bodies.

28. Correct: Anterior ethmoidal (A)

(**A**) Sensation from the dorsum of the nose is supplied by the external nasal nerve, the terminal branch of the anterior ethmoidal nerve (a branch of the nasociliary nerve from CN V1). The anterior ethmoidal nerve also supplies sensory innervation to the anterior and middle ethmoidal air cells and most of the anterior nasal cavity. This patient sustained an orbital blowout fracture that involved the medial wall of the orbit, which is traversed by the anterior ethmoidal nerve. While this type of fracture usually does not directly affect nerves that supply extraocular muscles (i.e., CNs III, IV, VI), the fracture may entrap the medial rectus muscle in its fragments, which can limit adduction or abduction. (**B**) The infraorbital nerve does not pass through the medial wall of the orbit and would not be affected in this patient. It is the terminal branch of the maxillary nerve (CN V2). It supplies sensory innervation from the ala of the nose, the upper lip, and lower eyelid. (**D**) The posterior ethmoidal nerve, like the anterior ethmoidal, passes through the medial wall of the orbit and would likely be affected in this patient. However, it provides sensory innervation from the posterior ethmoidal air cells and sphenoidal sinus. (**E**) The supraorbital nerve does not pass through the medial wall of the orbit and would not be affected in this patient. It branches from the frontal nerve, which is a branch of the ophthalmic nerve in the orbit. It supplies sensory innervation from the upper eyelid and from the forehead. (**C**) The supratrochlear nerve does not pass through the medial wall of the orbit and would not be affected in this patient. It is the smaller medial branch of the frontal nerve and supplies sensory innervation from the medial aspect of the upper eyelid and from the forehead (medial to the supraorbital nerve).

29. Correct: Ethmoid bone (lamina papyracea) (A)

(**A**) This patient has a blowout fracture of the medial orbital wall that is formed by the orbital plate of the ethmoid bone, also known as lamina papyracea (Latin, *paper-thin*). The loss of sensation from the dorsum of the nose was due to injury of the anterior ethmoidal nerve, which passes through the medial wall of the orbit. This type of fracture typically does not directly affect the nerves that supply extraocular muscles (i.e., CNs III, IV, VI), but it may entrap the medial rectus muscle in its fragments, which can limit adduction or abduction. Such entrapment of the medial rectus likely presents with the eye in an esotropic (adducted) position because the eye becomes "caught" by the fragments and is retained in a medially deviated position by the fracture fragments. From this position, therefore, limited abduction is apparent. (**B**) The lacrimal bone is not typically involved in an orbital blowout fracture. (**C**) The orbital surface of the maxilla is commonly fractured in an orbital blowout fracture. While it often results in entrapment of the inferior rectus (resulting in a superior gaze palsy), it would not affect sensation from the distribution of the anterior ethmoidal nerve. Rather, sensory changes would involve the distribution of the infraorbital nerve, which passes through the infraorbital canal in this bone. (**D**) The sphenoid bone is not typically involved in an orbital blowout fracture. (**E**) The zygomatic bone is not typically involved in an orbital blowout fracture.

30. Correct: Maxillary (D)

(**D**) This patient has trigeminal neuralgia (also known as tic douloureux), a facial pain syndrome that involves dysfunction of the trigeminal nerve or one of its divisions (ophthalmic, maxillary, mandibular). Most often, trigeminal neuralgia involves the maxillary (CN V2) and/or mandibular (CN V3) nerves, with symptoms related to the distribution of the affected nerve. In this patient, the symptom of lancinating pain from her upper jaw (maxilla) is related to that transmitted by the maxillary nerve. (**A**) Chorda tympani carries two types of nerve fibers: (1) sensory fibers that convey taste from the anterior two-thirds of the tongue, and (2) preganglionic parasympathetic fibers that synapse with postganglionic neurons in the submandibular ganglion that innervate the submandibular and sublingual glands. (**B**) The symptoms in this patient are not related to the facial nerve (CN VII), which provides motor innervation to the muscles of facial expression, as well as preganglionic parasympathetic and special sensory (taste) fibers. (**C**) The symptom of lancinating pain from her upper jaw (maxilla) in this patient is not related to the distribution of the mandibular nerve. (**E**) The symptoms in this patient are not related to the distribution of the ophthalmic nerve (CN V1).

23

31. Correct: Middle cranial fossa (D)

(**D**) The neuronal cell bodies whose peripheral processes form the ophthalmic, maxillary, and mandibular divisions of the trigeminal nerve reside in the trigeminal ganglion, which is located in the trigeminal (Meckel's) cave in the middle cranial fossa. (**A**) The cochlea contains the organ of hearing, including the spiral ganglion whose fibers form the cochlear nerve. (**B**) The facial canal contains the geniculate ganglion that contains sensory neuronal cell bodies whose peripheral processes pass through chorda tympani to the anterior two-third of the tongue. (**C**) The jugular foramen contains the sensory neuronal cell bodies within ganglia of the glossopharyngeal nerve (CN IX) and the superior (sensory) ganglion of the vagus nerve (CN X). (**E**) The pterygopalatine fossa contains the pterygopalatine ganglion, which contains postganglionic neuronal cell bodies whose fibers innervate the lacrimal gland and glands of the nasal cavity, palate, and superior pharynx.

32. Correct: Posterior superior alveolar (E)

(**E**) The posterior superior alveolar nerve, a branch of the maxillary nerve (CN V2), innervates the posterior maxillary teeth (especially the molars). (**A**) The anterior (and middle) superior alveolar nerve, also a branch of the maxillary nerve, supplies more anterior maxillary teeth. (**B**) The buccal nerve, a branch of the mandibular nerve (CN V3), provides sensory innervation from the mucous membrane of the cheek and overlying skin. (**C**) The greater palatine nerve, which carries both sensory fibers from the maxillary nerve and postganglionic parasympathetic fibers from the pterygopalatine ganglion), provides sensory innervation from the palatal mucous membrane (including lingual gingivae). It anastomoses with the branches of the nasopalatine nerve. It does not supply the teeth. (**D**) The nasopalatine nerve, a branch of the maxillary nerve, distributes to portions of the nasal septum and anterior hard palate. It does not supply the teeth.

Refer to the following image for answer 32:

33. Correct: Lingula of mandible (D)

(**D**) The inferior alveolar nerve passes through the mandibular foramen and into the mandibular canal, where it distributes to the mandibular teeth. The lingula is a small process that lies on the medial side of the mandible, anterior to the mandibular foramen. Anesthetic injection near the lingula would best target the inferior alveolar nerve, although the lingual nerve would also likely be affected. (**A**) The mandibular nerve (CN V3) passes through the foramen ovale, and its branches (e.g., inferior alveolar, lingual, auriculotemporal, and numerous other muscular branches) arise distal to this opening. Anesthetic injection at this location would likely affect more than the inferior alveolar nerve. (**B**) The maxillary nerve (CN V2) passes through the foramen rotundum. Anesthetic injection at this location would not specifically target the inferior alveolar nerve. (**C**) Numerous nerves traverse the infratemporal fossa, including the inferior alveolar, lingual, auriculotemporal, and chorda tympani. Thus, anesthetic injection in this location would not specifically target the inferior alveolar nerve. (**E**) The parasympathetic pterygopalatine ganglion and the maxillary nerve are located in the pterygopalatine fossa. Thus, anesthetic injection in this location would not specifically target the inferior alveolar nerve.

34. Correct: Auriculotemporal (A)

(**A**) The auriculotemporal nerve, a branch of the mandibular nerve (CN V3), innervates anterior and superior portions of the auricle (this includes the area of skin involved in this patient). This nerve also supplies a band of skin anterior and superior to the auricle. (**B**) Most of the facial nerve supplies the muscles of facial expression. A small, cutaneous portion of the nerve supplies skin of the concha and posterior aspect of the auricle. It does not supply the area of skin involved in this patient. (**C, D**) The great auricular and lesser occipital nerves are branches of the cervical plexus. They supply skin inferior and posterior to the auricle, but not the area of skin involved

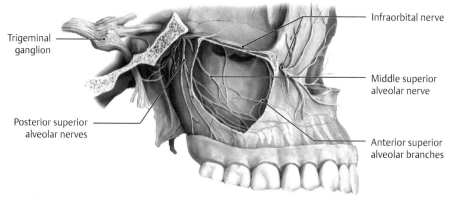

Labels: Trigeminal ganglion; Posterior superior alveolar nerves; Infraorbital nerve; Middle superior alveolar nerve; Anterior superior alveolar branches

Source: Schuenke M, Schulte E, Schumacher U. THIEME Atlas of Anatomy. Head, Neck, and Neuroanatomy. Illustrations by Voll M and Wesker K. 2nd ed. New York: Thieme Medical Publishers; 2016

in this patient. (**E**) The vagus nerve carries sensation from skin posterior to the auricle, from the external acoustic meatus, and part of the external surface of the tympanic membrane.

Refer to the following images for answer 34:

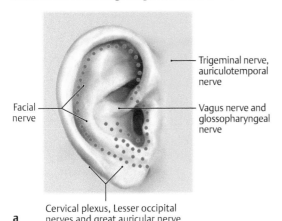

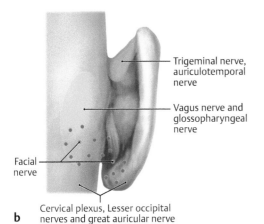

a Cervical plexus, Lesser occipital nerves and great auricular nerve

b Cervical plexus, Lesser occipital nerves and great auricular nerve

Source: Gilroy AM et al. Atlas of Anatomy. 3rd ed. 2016. Based on: Schuenke M, Schulte E, Schumacher U. THIEME Atlas of Anatomy. Volumes 1-3. Illustrations by Voll M and Wesker K. 2nd ed. New York: Thieme Medical Publishers; 2016

35. Correct: Loss of general sensation and taste from the anterior two-thirds of the tongue and decreased salivation (D)

(**D**) Injection of anesthetic to the inferior alveolar nerve near the mandibular foramen could also affect the lingual nerve. At this location, the lingual nerve contains sensory fibers related to general sensation (CN V3) and taste from the anterior two-thirds of the tongue (CN VII, chorda tympani). In addition, preganglionic parasympathetic fibers passing in the lingual nerve to the submandibular ganglion may also be affected, resulting in decreased salivation (dry mouth) from the submandibular and sublingual glands. (**A**) Decreased salivation would implicate the chorda tympani, lingual nerve, and/or the submandibular ganglion, but no other branches. As the injection is likely to bathe the area, an effect restricted to salivation is unlikely. (**B**) Loss of general sensation and taste from the anterior two-thirds of the tongue would involve taste fibers from chorda tympani and general sensory fibers from the trigeminal nerve. The proximity of the submandibular ganglion to the mandibular foramen makes it likely that salivation would also be affected. (**C**) Loss of only general sensation from the posterior one-third of the tongue would involve the glossopharyngeal nerve, but this nerve is not found near the mandibular foramen. (**E**) Loss of only taste from the anterior two-thirds of the tongue would involve taste fibers from the chorda tympani. This is unlikely since these fibers and general sensory fibers from the trigeminal nerve are bound together in the lingual nerve. In addition, the proximity of the submandibular ganglion to the mandibular foramen makes it likely that salivation would also be affected.

Refer to the following image for answer 35:

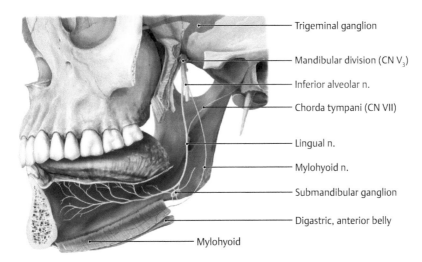

Source: Gilroy AM et al. Atlas of Anatomy. 3rd ed. 2016. Based on: Schuenke M, Schulte E, Schumacher U. THIEME Atlas of Anatomy. Volumes 1-3. Illustrations by Voll M and Wesker K. 2nd ed. New York: Thieme Medical Publishers; 2016

36. Correct: Nerve to stapedius (E)

(**E**) The nerve to stapedius, a branch of the facial nerve (CN VII) that arises in the facial canal, innervates the stapedius muscle. This muscle helps to prevent excessive movement of the stapes and thereby limits oscillation of the oval (vestibular) window. Injury to this nerve prevents the dampening effects of the muscle on the stapes and oval window and results in hyperacusis (increased sensitivity to sound). In this patient, compression of the facial nerve in the internal acoustic meatus impacted the nerve to stapedius. (**A**) The chorda tympani, a branch of the facial nerve, carries preganglionic parasympathetic fibers to the pterygopalatine and submandibular ganglia, as well as special sensory fibers that join the lingual nerve and innervate the anterior two-thirds of the tongue. It is distinct from, and does not give rise to, the nerve to stapedius. (**B**) The lesser petrosal nerve is a branch of the glossopharyngeal nerve (CN IX) that carries preganglionic parasympathetic fibers to the otic ganglion. (**C**) The greater petrosal nerve is a branch of the facial nerve that carries preganglionic parasympathetic fibers to the pterygopalatine ganglion. (**D**) The nervus intermedius joins the motor root of the facial nerve in the internal acoustic meatus. This nerve carries primarily special sensory and preganglionic parasympathetic fibers to the facial nerve within the facial canal. These special sensory fibers and some of the preganglionic parasympathetic fibers leave the facial nerve as the chorda tympani; other preganglionic parasympathetic fibers leave the facial nerve as the greater petrosal nerve.

37. Correct: Internal acoustic meatus (C)

(**C**) The contrast material outlines an acoustic neuroma that occupies the internal acoustic meatus. This opening in the temporal bone transmits the facial nerve (CN VII) and vestibulocochlear nerve (CN VIII). (**A, B, D, E**) The cavernous sinus, external acoustic meatus, jugular foramen, and mastoid air cells are not outlined by the contrast material.

38. Correct: Facial (B)

(**B**) The branchial motor component of the facial nerve (CN VII) supplies the muscles of facial expression, as well as the stylohyoid, the posterior digastric, and stapedius. Paralysis of the stapedius allows greater movement of the stapes, which is attached to the oval window and transmits vibrations of the tympanic membrane to the oval window. This overreaction of the auditory ossicles may lead to tinnitus (ringing in the ear) and/or hyperacusis (in which normal sounds are uncomfortably loud). Branchial motor fibers in the mandibular nerve (CN V3) also supply tensor tympani the muscle, which attaches to the malleus and serves a similar function to the stapedius in that it controls excessive responses to auditory vibrations. (**A**) The cochlear nerve, a part of

the vestibulocochlear nerve (CN VIII), conveys auditory information from the cochlea. Specific damage to this nerve would likely result in hearing loss. (**C**) The ophthalmic nerve (CN V1) is a sensory nerve that supplies the forehead, frontal sinuses, a portion of the nasal cavity and external nose, conjunctiva, eye and cornea, and orbit. (**D**) The nervus intermedius is a distinct portion of the facial nerve that carries visceral motor and sensory (general and special) information. (**E**) The vestibular nerve, a part of the vestibulocochlear nerve (CN VIII), conveys balance information from the semicircular canals and other vestibular structures. Physical examination shows vestibular functions are intact in this individual.

39. Correct: Glossopharyngeal (B)

(**B**) The glossopharyngeal nerve (CN IX) conveys general sensation from the mucosa of the oropharynx and oropharyngeal isthmus (isthmus of the fauces), including the palatine tonsils, soft palate, and posterior one-third of the tongue. Although the gag reflex is typically elicited by touching the posterior pharyngeal wall, the posterior third for the tongue and palatoglossal arches receive sensory innervation from the glossopharyngeal nerve and are, therefore, also sensitive in stimulating a gag reflex. (**A**) The facial nerve (CN VII) provides general sensation only from a small area of skin near the external acoustic meatus. It is not involved in the gag reflex. (**C**) The mandibular nerve (CN V3) provides general sensation from the face, anterior two-thirds of the tongue, portions of the oral cavity, parts of the nasal cavity and paranasal sinuses, and part of the cranial dura mater. It is not involved in the gag reflex. (**D**) The maxillary nerve (CN V2) provides general sensation from the face, portions of the oral cavity, and parts of the external ear. It is not involved in the gag reflex. (**E**) The vagus nerve (CN X) carries the motor limb of the gag reflex. It innervates most pharyngeal muscles (except stylopharyngeus, innervated by CN IX), muscles of the soft palate (except tensor veli palatini, innervated by CN V3), and all intrinsic muscles of the larynx.

40. Correct: Left jugular foramen (C)

(**C**) This patient presents with symptoms consistent with a skull base fracture that involved the jugular foramen. The glossopharyngeal (CN IX), vagus (CN X), and accessory (CN XI) nerves pass through this opening. The absence of a gag reflex on the left indicates interruption of either the afferent (sensory) limb of this reflex (carried by the glossopharyngeal nerve), or the efferent (motor) limb of this reflex (carried by the vagus nerve), or both. Involvement of the left vagus nerve is confirmed by the deviation of the uvula (soft palate) toward the unaffected side—the right side in this patient. Paralysis of the left vocal fold is also consistent with involvement of the vagus nerve as its laryngeal branches supply intrinsic laryngeal muscles that regulate the vocal folds. Weakened shoulder elevation on the left indicates involvement of the left accessory nerve (trapezius). (**A, D**) The hypoglossal nerve (CN XII) passes through the hypoglossal canal. This nerve controls movements of the tongue, which are not affected in this patient. (**B**) The facial (CN VII) and vestibulocochlear (CN VIII) nerves pass through the internal acoustic meatus. Lesion of the facial nerve at the internal acoustic meatus would likely result in facial paralysis, a loss of taste from the anterior two-thirds of the tongue and decreased salivation (chorda tympani), and dry eye (greater petrosal nerve). A lesion of the vestibulocochlear nerve at the internal acoustic meatus would likely result in disturbances of hearing and/or balance. (**E**) Fracture of the right jugular foramen is not indicated because all of the deficits are related to nerve lesions on the left.

41. Correct: C7 (D)

(**D**) The most common level of cervical disc herniation is C6–C7 (approximately two-thirds of cases), and the remaining cases involve the C5–C6 disc. The C7 dermatome includes the middle finger, and motor fibers in the radial nerve from the C6 to C8 spinal cord levels innervate the triceps brachii muscle that extends the elbow (C7 fibers also predominate in the triceps tendon reflex). The clinical symptoms are, therefore, consistent with herniation of the C6–C7 intervertebral disc.

42. Correct: Bilateral paresis of the biceps brachii muscles (B)

(**B**) Cervical myelopathy (compression of the cervical spinal cord) in this patient is caused by the posterior herniation of the C5–C6 intervertebral disc causing focal compression of the anterior corticospinal tract, as well as a mass effect on the anterior spinal cord. The neck and upper extremity pain is likely related to mass effects due to the disc degeneration and accompanying loss of disc height. Because this lesion likely affects the anterior spinal cord at adjacent C5 and C6 levels, it is likely that motor functions of muscles innervated by these levels (e.g., biceps brachii) would be affected. In addition, since the herniated disc projects paracentrally (posteriorly from the midline), the cord compression is likely bilateral, resulting in bilateral paralysis or paresis. In contrast, the effects of a posterolateral herniation are more likely to result in unilateral compression of a spinal nerve in the intervertebral foramen, leading to radicular pain and level-specific symptoms (radiculopathy). (**A**) Bilateral hypesthesia from skin over the deltoid (C5 dermatome) could result from a lesion that affects the C5 spinal cord. (**C**) Unilateral hypesthesia from the great toe (L4 and L5 dermatomes) would likely occur as a result of posterolateral L3–L4 and/or L4–L5 disc herniations that resulted in radiculopathy. (**D**) Unilateral hypesthesia from the middle finger (C7 dermatomes) would likely occur as a result of posterolateral C6 to C7 disc herniation that resulted in radiculopathy. (**E**) Unilateral paresis of thumb abduction (C7 abductor pollicis longus; C8–T1 abductor pollicis brevis) would likely occur as a result of posterolateral disc herniation that resulted in C7, C8, or T1 radiculopathies.

43. Correct: T1 (E)

(**E**) The T1 dermatome is located along the distal medial arm and medial forearm, and the muscles responsible for finger abduction and adduction, the interossei and abductor pollicis brevis, are innervated by nerves carrying fibers from the T1 spinal cord level. (**A**) The C5 dermatome is located on the skin over the deltoid muscle and motor axons from this spinal level innervate proximal muscles of the upper limb, including serratus anterior, deltoid, rotator cuff, and biceps brachii. The C5 spinal cord provides the predominant innervation for the biceps brachii tendon reflex. (**B**) The C6 dermatome is located along the lateral forearm and hand. The C6 spinal cord provides the predominant innervation for the brachioradialis tendon reflex. (**C**) The C7 dermatome is represented in the arm, forearm, and hand; it is, however, commonly tested on the middle finger. Motor axons from this spinal level contribute to innervation of shoulder and arm muscles. The C7 spinal cord provides the predominant innervation for the triceps brachii tendon reflex. (**D**) The C8 dermatome is located along the medial aspect of the hand. Motor axons from this spinal level contribute to innervation of forearm and intrinsic hand muscles.

44. Correct: Hypesthesia from the lateral foot (A)

(**A**) In this patient, the L5–S1 disc is herniated and is compressing the S1 spinal nerve. The S1 dermatome is located along the lateral aspect of the leg and foot and, thus, the clinical symptom in this patient would be hypesthesia from the lateral foot. (**B**) The L4 dermatome is located along the medial aspect of the foot. (**C**) Dorsiflexors and inverters of the foot (extensor digitorum longus, extensor hallucis longus, tibialis anterior and posterior) are supplied by nerves that have contributions from the L4 and L5 spinal levels. (**D**) Muscles that extend the knee (quadriceps femoris) are supplied by nerves that have contributions from the L2–L4 spinal levels. (**E**) Muscles that flex the knee (hamstrings, biceps femoris short head, and gastrocnemius) are supplied by nerves that have contributions from the L5 and S1 spinal levels. However, since the L5 spinal nerve would not be compressed by the posterolateral herniation of the L5–S1 disc, these muscles would not be involved.

45. Correct: Calcaneal (Achilles') (B)

(**B**) The S1 spinal cord provides the predominant innervation for the calcaneal (Achilles') tendon reflex. (**A**) The biceps femoris muscle is not associated with a deep tendon reflex. (**C**) The L4 spinal cord provides the predominant innervation for the patellar tendon reflex. (**D**) The tibialis anterior muscle is not associated with a deep tendon reflex. (**E**) The L5 spinal cord provides the predominant innervation for the tibialis posterior tendon reflex (this reflex is difficult to elicit).

46. Correct: Genital branch of genitofemoral (A)

(**A**) The genital branch of genitofemoral nerve (L1) provides the efferent limb of the cremasteric reflex; the ilioinguinal nerve (L1), and to a lesser extent the femoral branch of the genitofemoral, provides the afferent limb of the cremasteric reflex. This reflex is elicited by stroking or pinching the medial thigh, causing contraction of the cremaster muscle, which elevates the testis (the reflex is considered positive if the testicle moves at least 0.5 cm). An absent cremasteric reflex is one of the most sensitive physical findings in cases of testicular torsion. (**B**) The iliohypogastric nerve (L1) supplies suprapubic skin near the anterior midline. (**C**) The ilioinguinal nerve (L1), and to a lesser extent the femoral branch of the genitofemoral, provides the afferent limb of the cremasteric reflex. (**D**) The obturator nerve, derived from the L2–L4 spinal cord levels, supplies skin of the medial thigh. (**E**) Sympathetic fibers do not innervate the cremaster muscle.

47. Correct: Medial cutaneous nerve of the forearm (D)

(**D**) Visceral afferent fibers from the heart travel through the cardiac plexus, sympathetic chain, and ultimately through the T1–T4 dorsal root ganglia. The medial cutaneous nerve of the forearm (T1) carries somatic afferent fibers from the upper arm that would converge with the T1 visceral afferents from the heart. (**A**) Somatic afferent fibers in the lateral cutaneous nerve of the forearm pass through the C6 dorsal root ganglion and would not be involved in referred pain from the heart (T1–T4). (**B, C, E**) The lateral pectoral (C5–C6), long thoracic (C5–C7), and phrenic (C3–C5) nerves are motor nerves that arise from upper parts of the brachial plexus. Because they arise from the upper brachial plexus, and do not carry somatic afferent fibers, they would not be involved in referred pain from the heart (T1–T4).

48. Correct: Obturator (E)

(**E**) The location of the obturator nerve (L2–L4) along the lateral pelvic wall makes it susceptible to iatrogenic injury during genitourinary surgical procedures (e.g., direct compression or stretching during surgery, or postoperative compression from local edema). The obturator nerve innervates skin of the upper medial thigh and muscles of the adductor compartment. The most prominent symptoms of obturator neuropathy are sensory deficits in the medial upper thigh and difficulty adducting the thigh. A characteristic "waddle" gait may result from adductor weakness and/or as a reaction to pain caused by moving hip joint (the nerve passes through both the psoas major and obturator externus muscles and, consequently, hip motions can often be painful when there is nerve injury). The "waddle" gait is also present because the adductor muscles assist gluteus medius and minimus to stabilize the hip on the weight-bearing side during locomotion. When driving, patients may also report difficulty moving their right foot from the accelerator to brake pedal, an action that involves thigh adduction. (**A**) Other than pectineus (commonly supplied by the obturator and femoral nerves), the femoral nerve does not innervate any muscles with a primary action of adduction of the thigh. (**B, C**) The distribution of the genitofemoral and ilioinguinal nerves in the thigh is only sensory. (**D**) The lumbosacral trunk (L4–L5) itself does not innervate any muscles. It joins the sacral plexus and its fibers are distributed with branches of that plexus to the posterior thigh, leg, and foot.

49. Correct: Greater splanchnic (A)

(**A**) As seen in the accompanying image, the greater splanchnic nerve (T5–T9) carries preganglionic sympathetic fibers from the sympathetic chain to the celiac ganglion, where they synapse on postganglionic neuronal cell bodies that innervate foregut structures, including the pancreas. Visceral afferent fibers in the celiac plexus transmit sensory innervation from foregut structures, including the distal esophagus stomach, proximal duodenum, liver, gallbladder, spleen, and pancreas. Visceral pain from the pancreas is referred to the T5–T9 dermatomes of the anterior and posterior trunk, including the epigastric area. (**B**) The hypogastric nerves contain primarily postganglionic sympathetic fibers from T10–L2 spinal cord levels that pass through the inferior hypogastric (pelvic) plexus to pelvic organs. The hypogastric nerves also contain preganglionic sympathetic fibers that synapse on small ganglia in the inferior hypogastric plexus, as well as visceral afferents from the upper parts of the uterine body (including its fundus). (**C**) The least splanchnic nerve (T11–T12) passes to the renal plexus to synapse in the aorticorenal ganglion. It does not transmit afferent information from viscera innervated by the celiac plexus. (**D**) Lumbar splanchnic nerves arise from the L1–L4 sympathetic ganglia and pass medially to join the intermesenteric (aortic), inferior mesenteric, and superior hypogastric plexuses. Postganglionic, and accompanying visceral afferent, fibers supply the hindgut (upper lumbar splanchnics) and pelvic viscera (lower lumbar splanchnics). (**E**) Fibers from the vagus nerves, which pass through the celiac ganglion and plexus, do not transmit afferent information from viscera innervated by the celiac plexus.

Refer to the following image for answer 49:

50. Correct: Shoulder pain (B)

(**B**) The presence of contrast in the omental bursa (lesser sac) indicates that duodenal contents/fluid and extravasated blood would also likely be found in this potential space. Because the diaphragm and its peritoneal lining limit this space superiorly, duodenal contents/fluid and extravasated blood would likely stimulate sensory fibers in the phrenic nerve (C4–C5), resulting in referred pain from these dermatomes, which are located in the lower neck and shoulder regions. (**A**) Pain radiating to the upper limb would be more consistent with cardiac referred pain, which is mediated by visceral afferents in sympathetic nerves to the T1–T4 spinal cord. (**C**) Suprapubic pain would most likely be related to genitourinary tract causes (e.g., urinary tract infection, kidney stones, cystitis) and mediated by visceral afferents in sympathetic nerves to the T10–L1 spinal cord. (**D**) Weakness in hip flexion suggests injury to the iliopsoas muscle, which is innervated by axons from L1–L3 spinal cord. (**E**) Weakness in shoulder abduction suggests injury to nerves that supply one or more muscles, primarily supraspinatus (suprascapular nerve, C4–C6) and deltoid (axillary nerve, C5–C6). Signal in visceral afferent fibers would not affect motor innervation to these muscles.

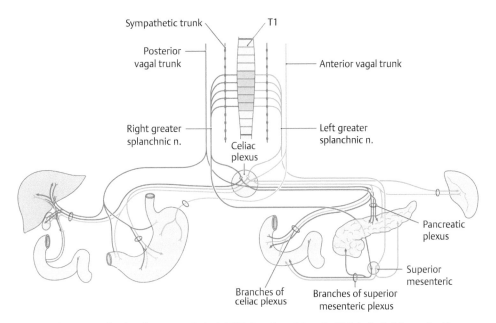

Source: Gilroy AM et al. Atlas of Anatomy. 3rd ed. 2016. Based on: Schuenke M, Schulte E, Schumacher U. THIEME Atlas of Anatomy. Volumes 1-3. Illustrations by Voll M and Wesker K. 2nd ed. New York: Thieme Medical Publishers; 2016

51. Correct: Inferior rectal (B)

(**B**) The anocutaneous reflex (anal reflex, anal "wink") occurs when a tactile or noxious stimulus of the perianal region causes a brief contraction of the external anal sphincter. The afferent and efferent limbs of this reflex are provided by the inferior rectal nerve (a branch of the pudendal nerve, S2–S4) that supplies the perianal skin, mucous lining of the lower anal canal, and the external anal sphincter. (**A, C–E**) The cavernous, pelvic splanchnic, and perineal nerves, and the rectal plexus do not innervate the external anal sphincter, although some cutaneous branches of the perineal nerves (**E**) may overlap the distribution of the inferior rectal nerves.

52. Correct: Cavernous nerves (A)

(**A**) Erection and detumescence is controlled via cavernous nerves that contain both parasympathetic (S2–S4) and sympathetic (T11–L2) fibers. Respectively, these nerves regulate relaxation and contraction of smooth muscle in cavernous and arteriolar and arterial walls of penile erectile tissue. In the flaccid penis, these smooth muscles are tonically contracted and allow only a small amount of arterial flow into cavernous blood sinuses. Stimulation of parasympathetic fibers in the cavernous nerves during sexual arousal results in smooth muscle relaxation, arterial/arteriolar dilation, and flow of blood into cavernous sinusoids. At the same time, compression of the venous channels deep to the deep penile fascia (Buck's)—especially the deep dorsal and its circumflex venous channels—impedes venous outflow to help attain and maintain erection. (**B, D**) Branches of the perineal nerve and dorsal nerve of the penis, both branches of the pudendal nerve, provide sensory innervation from the penis. They do not carry parasympathetic and sympathetic fibers that control erection. (**C**) The hypogastric nerves convey preganglionic sympathetic fibers from T11–L2 spinal cord to the pelvic plexus, where they synapse in small ganglia. Some parasympathetic fibers ascend from the pelvic plexus to supply portions of the hindgut. None of these fibers are involved with erection. (**E**) Sacral splanchnic nerves (usually S1–S2 sympathetic ganglia) pass into the pelvic plexus and then to pelvic viscera.

Refer to the following image for answer 52:

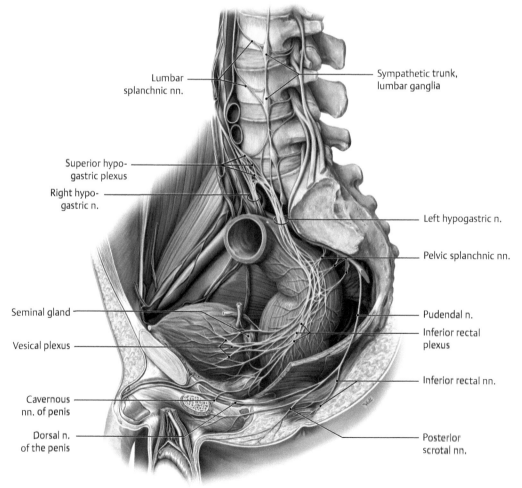

Lumbar splanchnic nn.

Sympathetic trunk, lumbar ganglia

Superior hypo-gastric plexus

Right hypo-gastric n.

Left hypogastric n.

Pelvic splanchnic nn.

Seminal gland

Vesical plexus

Pudendal n.

Inferior rectal plexus

Inferior rectal nn.

Cavernous nn. of penis

Dorsal n. of the penis

Posterior scrotal nn.

Source: Gilroy AM et al. Atlas of Anatomy. 3rd ed. 2016. Based on: Schuenke M, Schulte E, Schumacher U. THIEME Atlas of Anatomy. Volumes 1-3. Illustrations by Voll M and Wesker K. 2nd ed. New York: Thieme Medical Publishers; 2016

53. Correct: Penis and scrotum (C)

(C) Since the prostate is not in contact with the peritoneum, that is, below the pelvic pain line, pain associated with prostatitis is referred to the S2–S4 dermatomes. This includes the inguinal region, the perineum (e.g., scrotum, testes, penis and perianal region), and lower back, and/or in the suprapubic area above the bladder. (A, B, D, E) The dermatomes related to the epigastric, lumbar, and umbilical regions are above the pelvic pain line. Therefore, they would be involved with referred pain (visceral afferents involved with pain) from pelvic organs that are in contact with peritoneum (e.g., superior surface of the bladder, upper, and portions of the uterine body).

54. Correct: Intercostal (B)

(B) Pleuritic (sharp) chest pain experienced with breathing reflects inflammation of the parietal pleura and the friction rub is caused by the roughened pleural surfaces (parietal and visceral) as they rub against each other. The parietal pleura is innervated by somatic nerves: intercostal nerves supply costal parietal and peripheral diaphragmatic pleura and the phrenic nerves supply mediastinal and central diaphragmatic pleura. Because the patient experiences chest pain, and not shoulder or neck pain, this indicates that the intercostal nerves should be targeted. (A, D, E) The greater splanchnic, pulmonary plexus, and vagus nerves do not innervate pleura. (C) While the phrenic nerve does supply sensory innervation to mediastinal and central diaphragmatic pleura, it is not appropriate to perform a nerve block because it would impair the motor function of the diaphragm.

55. Correct: Internal laryngeal (B)

(B) The internal laryngeal nerve, a branch of the superior laryngeal from the vagus, provides sensory innervation from the mucous membrane of the piriform fossa, and from laryngeal membranes *superior* to the vocal fold. (A) The external laryngeal nerve, also a branch of the superior laryngeal, provides motor innervation to the cricothyroid and inferior pharyngeal constrictor muscles. (C) The pharyngeal plexus is formed by branches from the glossopharyngeal and vagus nerves, as well as postganglionic sympathetic fibers from superior sympathetic ganglion. It provides most of the sensory and motor supply to the pharynx. (D) The recurrent laryngeal nerve provides sensory innervation from the mucous membrane *inferior* to the vocal fold (including the vocal fold itself). (E) Sympathetic fibers do not provide sensory innervation from the pharynx or larynx.

56. Correct: Recurrent laryngeal (C)

Refer to the following images for answer 56:

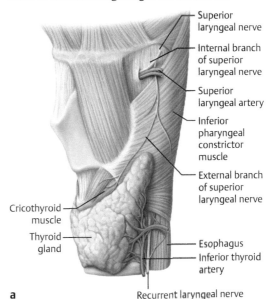

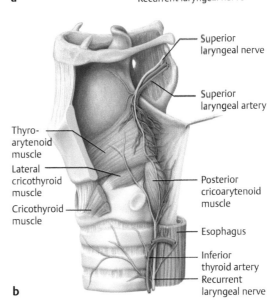

Source: Schuenke M, Schulte E, Schumacher U. THIEME Atlas of Anatomy. Head, Neck, and Neuroanatomy. Illustrations by Voll M and Wesker K. 2nd ed. New York: Thieme Medical Publishers; 2016

(C) The recurrent laryngeal nerve passes superiorly in the tracheoesophageal groove. Near the thyroid gland, it is closely associated with the inferior laryngeal artery and vein and must be isolated before ligating these vessels. Since this nerve supplies all intrinsic laryngeal muscles except the cricothyroid, its injury will result in paralysis or paresis of the vocal fold. (A) The external laryngeal nerve, a branch of the superior laryngeal from the vagus, provides motor innervation to the cricothyroid and inferior pharyngeal constrictor muscles. Only the terminal portion of this nerve may be associated with the thyroid gland and its injury will not lead to paralysis or paresis of the vocal fold (since the cricothyroid muscles increases tension of the vocal fold, an inability to reach high pitches may be apparent). (**B**) The internal laryngeal nerve, also a branch of the superior laryngeal from the vagus, provides sensory innervation from the mucous membrane of the piriform fossa and from the larynx as far inferior as the vestibular fold. It does not innervate any laryngeal muscles and, therefore, its injury would not result in paralysis or paresis of the vocal fold. (**D**) The superior laryngeal nerve branches from the inferior vagal (nodose) ganglion in the neck near the jugular foramen. It is not likely to be injured directly during thyroidectomy surgery. (**E**) At the level of the thyroid gland, the vagus nerve is within the carotid sheath and not susceptible to injury.

57. Correct: S2–S4 (E)

(**E**) The penis is innervated by the dorsal nerve of the penis, a branch of the pudendal (S2–S4). Although the extent of caudal epidural anesthesia depends on the amount of anesthetic injected and the position of the patient, the nerves that innervate the perineum in general, and the penis specifically—namely spinal nerves that contribute to the pudendal nerve (S2–S4)—are targeted. (**A–D**) None of these spinal nerves contribute to the pudendal nerve.

58. Correct: Radial (C)

(**C**) In the middle third of the humerus, the radial nerve courses in the radial (spiral) groove. Because of its close apposition to the humeral shaft, the nerve is at risk of injury in fractures of this portion of the bone. Injury of the radial nerve at this position most often results in "wrist drop" caused by weakness in wrist extensors. (**A, B, D, E**) Branches of the T9–T12, L2–L4, and S2–S4 spinal nerves do not innervate extensor muscles, nor are they adjacent to the shaft of the humerus (and, therefore, are unlikely to be injured by a fracture in its middle third).

59. Correct: Inability to extend the wrist (D)

(**D**) Distal to the middle third of the humerus, the radial nerve innervates muscles of the posterior forearm (extensor-supinator), including those that extend the wrist. Thus, injury of the radial nerve in the middle third of the humerus results in an inability to extend the wrist, leading to the characteristic clinical sign of "wrist drop." (**A**) Sensory innervation from the palm is provided by the median and ulnar nerves. (**B**) Sensory innervation from the tip of the thumb is provided by the median nerve. (**C**) Injury to the radial nerve in the middle third of the arm does not paralyze the triceps muscle completely because its lateral and long heads receive

their radial innervation in the proximal arm. Thus, elbow extension is only weakened. (**E**) While injury to the radial nerve will affect the supinator muscle, supination is only weakened because the musculocutaneous nerve is not affected and the biceps brachii remains functional.

60. Correct: Abduction and adduction of the medial four digits (A)

(**A**) The deep branch of the ulnar nerve supplies most intrinsic hand muscles, including all interosseous and hypothenar muscles. As a result, injury to this branch of the ulnar nerve would result in paresis or paralysis of abduction and adduction of the medial four digits. (**B**) Abduction of the thumb is produced by the abductor pollicis longus (radial nerve) and abductor pollicis brevis, which are innervated by the recurrent branch of median nerve. (**C**) Flexion of the distal interphalangeal joint of the little finger is produced by the medial part of flexor digitorum profundus, which is innervated in the forearm by the ulnar nerve. (**D**) The skin over the medial hand, the C8 dermatome, is supplied by the superficial branch of the ulnar nerve. (**E**) Hypesthesia from the thenar eminence, part of the C6 dermatome, is supplied primarily by the median nerve. The superficial branch of the radial nerve supplies the lateral-most portion of the skin over the eminence.

61. Correct: Palmar cutaneous branch of median (B)

Refer to the following image for answer 61:

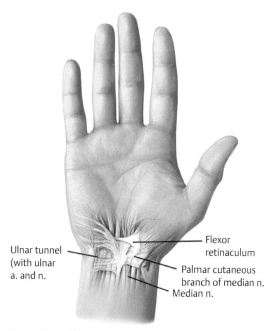

Source: Gilroy AM et al. Atlas of Anatomy. 3rd ed. 2016. Based on: Schuenke M, Schulte E, Schumacher U. THIEME Atlas of Anatomy. Volumes 1-3. Illustrations by Voll M and Wesker K. 2nd ed. New York: Thieme Medical Publishers; 2016

(**B**) In this patient, the palmar cutaneous branch of the median nerve is compressed between the flexor carpi radialis tendon and a ganglion cyst, which likely arose from within the tendon sheath. This nerve supplies the proximal palm over the thenar eminence. (**A**) Just proximal to the wrist, the median nerve becomes superficial and lies between the tendons of flexor digitorum superficialis and flexor carpi radialis. Signs and symptoms of a median nerve injury at this location, including sensory deficits from its distal distribution in the hand and weakness of the thenar muscles and lateral two lumbricals, were not seen in this patient. (**C**) The palmar cutaneous branch of the ulnar nerve supplies the proximal palm over the hypothenar eminence. (**D**) The recurrent branch of the median arises from the median nerve immediately distal to the carpal tunnel. It supplies the thenar muscles, but does not have a cutaneous distribution. (**E**) The superficial and deep branches of the ulnar nerve arise in the ulnar tunnel (of Guyon) on the medial side of the wrist. The superficial branch is primarily a sensory nerve for skin on the medial side of the hand and fingers.

62. Correct: Saphenous (C)

(**C**) The saphenous nerve, the largest cutaneous branch of the femoral, accompanies the great saphenous vein along much of its course in the distal thigh and leg. It is distributed to the anteromedial leg (including the knee) and foot. It may be injured when the great saphenous vein is harvested for coronary artery bypass grafting procedures. (**A, B, D, E**) The superficial fibular, obturator, posterior femoral cutaneous, and tibial nerves are not related anatomically to the great saphenous vein and are not distributed to the anteromedial leg and foot.

Refer to the following image for answer 62:

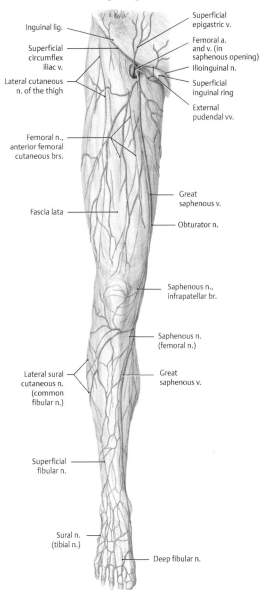

Source: Gilroy AM et al. Atlas of Anatomy. 3rd ed. 2016. Based on: Schuenke M, Schulte E, Schumacher U. THIEME Atlas of Anatomy. Volumes 1-3. Illustrations by Voll M and Wesker K. 2nd ed. New York: Thieme Medical Publishers; 2016

63. Correct: Tibial (E)

Refer to the following image for answer 63:

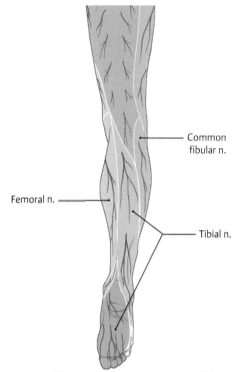

Source: Gilroy AM et al. Atlas of Anatomy. 3rd ed. 2016. Based on: Schuenke M, Schulte E, Schumacher U. THIEME Atlas of Anatomy. Volumes 1-3. Illustrations by Voll M and Wesker K. 2nd ed. New York: Thieme Medical Publishers; 2016

(**E**) The tibial nerve, through its medial and lateral plantar branches, carries sensation from the sole of the foot. This nerve can be compressed in the tarsal tunnel (the canal formed between the medial malleolus and the flexor retinaculum) and by flat feet or fallen arches. (**A–D**) The deep fibular, saphenous, superficial fibular, and sural nerves do not supply sensory innervation to the sole of the foot.

64. Correct: Femoral (B)

(**B**) The femoral nerve (L2–L4) passes deep to the inguinal ligament to enter the thigh anterior and slightly medial to the hip joint. Weakened knee extension (femoral nerve supplies the quadriceps, whose main action is knee extension) and an absent patellar reflex (the L4 spinal nerve is the predominant contribution to this reflex) indicate involvement of the femoral nerve. Although rare, femoral neuropathy may occur as a complication of anterior hip arthroplasty. (**A, C**) The obturator nerve passes through the obturator canal to enter the medial thigh. Muscles innervated by this nerve are not involved in knee extension. (**D**) The sciatic nerve enters the thigh posterior to the hip and muscles it innervates are not involved in knee extension. (**E**) The superficial fibular

nerve arises at the fibular neck as a branch of the common fibular. It innervates muscles in the lateral compartment of the leg and is distributed to skin on the dorsum of the foot.

65. Correct: Common fibular (B)

(**B**) When the leg is placed in a cast, it is common for the upper edge of the cast to lie at the level of the fibular neck. This corresponds to the subcutaneous position of the common fibular nerve and a cast that is initially too tight, or one that does not allow for posttraumatic swelling, may lead to the common fibular nerve being compressed between the cast and the fibula. Patients with this type of injury typically present with high-stepping gait to compensate for the non-weight-bearing foot assuming plantarflexion (foot drop) caused by weak muscles of dorsiflexion (deep fibular nerve to anterior leg compartment muscles). Eversion will also be compromised (superficial fibular nerve to lateral leg compartment muscles), as well as sensory loss along the anterior and lateral leg and on the dorsum of the foot. (**A, D**) The main branches of the common fibular nerve, the superficial and deep fibular, would not individually account for all of the symptoms. (**C**) The saphenous nerve is a cutaneous branch of the femoral that innervates skin along the medial leg and foot. It would not be involved in this type of casting injury. (**E**) The tibial nerve is part of the sciatic that innervates muscles in the posterior compartments and skin along the posterior aspect of the lower limb. It would not be involved in this type of casting injury.

66. Correct: Lesser splanchnic (D)

(**D**) Diffuse, periumbilical pain that gradually migrates to the right lower quadrant is a classic sign of appendicitis. In the early stages of acute appendicitis, only the visceral peritoneum around the appendix is inflamed and the pain is more generalized (visceral pain). In advanced stages, when the parietal peritoneum around the appendix is inflamed, the pain becomes localized (somatic pain) to the right lower quadrant. Visceral afferent fibers from the appendix travel via the superior mesenteric plexus and lesser splanchnic nerve (sympathetic nerves) to reach neuronal cell bodies in the T10–T11 dorsal root ganglia. Fibers from the T10 dorsal root ganglia converge centrally with somatic afferent fibers from the umbilicus (T10 dermatome) to refer pain from the appendix to the periumbilical region. (**A–C, E**) The greater splanchnic, inferior hypogastric, least splanchnic, and superior hypogastric nerves do not carry visceral afferents from the appendix.

67. Correct: Superior mesenteric plexus (E)

(**E**) Visceral afferent fibers from the appendix travel via the superior mesenteric plexus and lesser splanchnic nerve (sympathetic) to neuronal cell bodies in the

T10–T11 dorsal root ganglia. (**A, B–D**) Visceral afferent fibers from the appendix do not travel via the greater splanchnic nerve, least splanchnic nerve, lumbar sympathetic ganglia, or superior cervical ganglion.

68. Correct: Phrenic (C)

(**C**) Although the pus from the ruptured appendix was irrigated during the appendectomy, the development of postoperative referred shoulder pain and spiking temperatures indicates that infectious material remained in the peritoneal cavity. This likely led to collection of fluid in the hepatorenal (Morrison's) pouch that, in turn, stimulated somatic afferent fibers in the phrenic nerve along the adjacent parietal peritoneum on the abdominal aspect of the right diaphragm. Involvement of this nerve will have led to the referred right shoulder pain. (**A, B, D, E**) The iliohypogastric, pelvic splanchnic, subcostal, and T10 thoracoabdominal nerves are not involved with somatic sensation from the shoulder.

69. Correct: Pudendal (D)

(**D**) The signs and symptoms in this patient (notably, the perianal venous nodules and the type of pain described) support a diagnosis of external hemorrhoids. The pudenal nerve, via its inferior rectal (anal) branches, supplies somatic pain receptors in perianal skin and anal canal inferior to the pectinate line, activation of which results in sharp pain, itching and burning that is most often associated with external hemorrhoids. In contrast, patients with internal hemorrhoids often describe only vague anal discomfort consistent with visceral afferent innervation of the mucosa that overlies the internal rectal venous plexus. (**A**) The hypogastric nerves convey preganglionic sympathetic fibers from T11–L2 spinal cord to the pelvic plexus, where they synapse in small ganglia. (**B**) The ilioinguinal nerve carries sensation from the L1 dermatome, which does not contribute to the perianal skin. (**C**) Pelvic splanchnic nerves carry preganglionic parasympathetic fibers from the S2–S4 spinal cord. Visceral afferent fibers that convey pain from organs below the pelvic pain line, including most of the rectum and anal canal superior to the pectinate line, travel with these parasympathetic fibers. (**E**) Sacral splanchnic nerves (usually from the S1–S2 sympathetic ganglia) pass into the pelvic plexus and then to pelvic viscera. They do not supply sensory innervation to the perianal skin.

70. Correct: Hirschsprung's disease (C)

(**C**) This infant has Hirschsprung's disease. The absence of ganglion cells and the presence of a distended bowel immediately above the transition zone indicates that the enteric nervous system has not developed in the distal gastrointestinal tract. Transition zone refers to the region where a marked change in caliber occurs, with the dilated, normal colon above and the narrowed, aganglionic colon below. The absence of ganglion cells results in a constricted segment where the neurons are absent and a distended area of intestine immediately distal. (**A**) Cloacal extrophy is a rare congenital anomaly where much of pelvic viscera are exposed and external genitalia may be split in the midline. It is caused by a defect in mesodermal migration into the lower abdominal wall and cloacal region and defective body wall formation. (**B**) Duodenal atresia is a result of the failure of the endodermal epithelium to recanalize and form a lumen in the duodenum. It classically presents with the "double bubble sign" seen on radiographs or ultrasound where two air filled bubbles are seen, representing the two discontiguous loops of bowel. While the failure to pass meconium might be seen in duodenal atresia, the lack of ganglion cells is indicative of Hirschsprung's disease. (**D**) An imperforate anus is a congenital malformation where no opening exists where the anus should be. The portion of the cloaca where the hindgut endoderm meets the ectoderm of the cloacal membrane normally breaks down to allow the formation of the anal opening and anal canal. (**E**) A Meckel's diverticulum is a finger-like projection located in the distal ileum, usually within 5 cm of the ileocecal valve, is about 5 cm long and 2 cm wide. It is considered a true diverticulum as it contains all layers of the intestinal wall. It forms from the persistence of the proximal part of the vitelline duct.

71. Correct: Neural crest (C)

(**C**) Hirschsprung's disease, also called congenital megacolon, is due to the failure of neural crest cells to migrate into the distal bowel as it develops, resulting in the absence of ganglion cells in both Auerbach's and Meissner's plexuses of the bowel wall. (**A, B, D, E**) The endoderm, intermediate mesoderm, paraxial mesoderm, and visceral (splanchnic) mesoderm do not contribute to the ganglion cell population of the gut wall.

72. Correct: Spina bifida with meningomyelocele (D)

(**D**) Spina bifida with meningomyelocele (myelomeningocele) is a neural tube defect that occurs when a sac containing both meninges and neural tissue protrudes through a vertebral defect (-*cele* refers to a hernia or swelling; -*myelo* refers to the spinal cord; and -*meningo* refers to the meninges). The hernia sac in a myelomeningocele contains cerebrospinal fluid (CSF), as well as meninges and portions of the spinal cord and nerve roots. Myelomeningoceles can occur anywhere along the spinal cord, but are most common in the lumbar and sacral regions. Loss of function may occur below the level of the defect. (**A**) A meningoencephalocele involves protrusion of part of the brain (*encephelo*), as well as meninges and skin. It occurs in the cranial region. (**B**) Spina bifida occulta is the mildest form of neural tube defect. It does not usually present with a noticeable vertebral defect or outpocketing, hence the term "occulta." Signs of spina bifida occulta can sometimes be seen on the newborn's skin dorsal to the spinal defect: these include an abnormal tuft of hair, a fatty bulge, and a small dimple or birthmark. (**C**) Spina bifida with meningocele would involve meninges and no neural tissue.

73. Correct: L3–L4 (C)

(**C**) The lumbar puncture needle can be safely inserted in the midline *below* the level of the conus medullaris, which usually occurs at the level of the L2–L3 intervertebral disc. Thus, the lumbar puncture needle would typically be inserted between the L3–L4 or L4–L5 spinous processes. The supracristal plane (i.e., the superior-most aspect of the iliac crest) usually passes through the L4 spinous process and serves as a landmark for a lumbar puncture. Because the vertebral canal below L3 usually contains only the cauda equina bathed in CSF, damage to neural tissue is less likely because, in addition to being inferior to the spinal cord, it is relatively difficult to damage the nerve roots in the lumbar cistern—somewhat analogous to trying to hit a piece of cooked spaghetti in a pot of water. (**A, B**) The space between the L1–L2 or L3–L3 vertebral levels would be too close to the conus medullaris and injury to the spinal cord is possible. (**D, E**) Neither the sacral hiatus nor the sacral foramina are used for a lumbar puncture.

74. Correct: The developing vertebral column elongates faster than the spinal cord, creating the lumbar cistern with nerve roots that form the cauda equina (C)

(**C**) At birth, the caudal end of the spinal cord is located at the level of L2–L3 intervertebral disc. Due to the differential growth of the vertebral column, however, the conus medullaris (the caudal end of the spinal cord) often comes to lie at a more superior level in the adult—at the level of the L1–L2 intervertebral disc, although it may be found as high as the T12 vertebra or as far inferior as the L3 vertebra. Given the uncertainty of the exact location of the conus at a given age, a lumbar puncture needle inserted into the subarachnoid space below the L2–L3 IV disc will most likely encounter only the spinal nerve roots that form the cauda equina inferior to the conus medullaris. (**A**) Neural tissue is, in fact, present in the lumbar cistern (cauda equina). That nervous tissue is not injured in a lumbar puncture depends on the level at which the lumbar puncture needle is introduced (i.e., below the L2–L3 intervertebral disc). (**B**) Spinal nerves do, indeed, exit the vertebral column below L2, so this does not explain why they are not injured in this procedure. (**D**) The vertebral column grows *longer*, rather than shorter, relative to the spinal cord. (**E**) The spinal cord is present in the lumbar region as far inferior as the conus medullaris at the L1–L2 intervertebral

disc. Thus, injury of the spinal cord would be likely only if the lumbar puncture needle is introduced at, or above, the level of the conus medullaris (i.e., the L2–L3 intervertebral disc). It is also possible that the spinal cord can be injured if the conus is located atypically low (i.e., at L3), although this is mitigated to some extent by the use of fluoroscopy or ultrasound to guide the lumbar puncture procedure.

75. Correct: C5–C6 (B)

(**B**) Shoulder dystocia is a complication of a vaginal delivery that occurs after the head is delivered and one or both shoulders is/are impeded by bones of the maternal pelvis. Traction on the head during delivery widens the angle between the head and the impeded shoulder, thereby stretching the neck to injure the C5 and/or C6 (sometimes C7) ventral rami (i.e., the roots of the brachial plexus). Known as an Erb's (or Erb–Duchenne) palsy, the most common complication of shoulder dystocia, this results in a characteristic posture of the upper limb: arm adduction due to paralysis of the supraspinatus (suprascapular nerve, C5–C6) and deltoid (axillary nerve, C5–C6), medial shoulder rotation due to paralysis of the infraspinatus (suprascapular nerve, C5–C6) and teres minor (axillary nerve, C5–C6), elbow extension due to paralysis of the biceps brachii and brachialis (musculocutaneous nerve, C5–C7), forearm pronation due to paralysis of the supinator (C5–C7 contributions to radial nerve), and finger flexion due to partial paralysis of finger extensors (C6–C7 contributions to radial nerve). (**A**) The C2–C4 ventral rami do not contribute to the brachial plexus and are not involved in Erb's palsy. (**C**) While the C5–T1 ventral rami form the brachial plexus, the C8–T1 rami are not involved in Erb's palsy. Their injury would result in other clinical signs and symptoms not characteristic of Erb's palsy (e.g., paralysis of intrinsic hand muscles). (**D**) Isolated injury of the C7 ventral ramus is not typical of Erb's palsy, and would not result in the signs and symptoms characteristic of this condition. (**E**) The C8–T1 ventral rami are not involved in Erb's palsy. Their injury, known as Klumpke's palsy (a lower brachial plexus injury), results in other clinical signs and symptoms not characteristic of Erb's palsy (e.g., paralysis of intrinsic hand muscles).

76. Correct: Hypogastric (B)

(**B**) Visceral afferents that innervate the uterine tubes follow sympathetic fibers that arise from the T10–L2 spinal cord levels. These fibers pass from each tube into the inferior hypogastric plexus, the hypogastric nerves, and then to the superior mesenteric plexus. (**A**) The greater splanchnic nerves arise from the T5–T9 spinal cord and most of their preganglionic sympathetic fibers synapse in the celiac ganglia. Postganglionic sympathetic fibers from this ganglion do not supply pelvic organs. (**B**) Pelvic splanchnic nerves carry preganglionic parasympathetic fibers from the S2–S4 spinal cord. Visceral afferent fibers that convey pain from organs below the pelvic pain line (i.e., uterine cervix and upper vagina) travel with these parasympathetic fibers. (**C–E**) The pelvic splanchnic and sacral splanchnic nerves, as well as the sacral sympathetic trunk are not involved in transmitting pain from the uterine tubes.

Refer to the following image for answer 76:

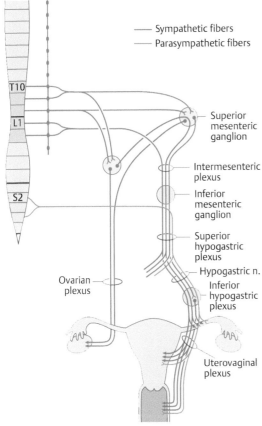

Source: Gilroy AM et al. Atlas of Anatomy. 3rd ed. 2016. Based on: Schuenke M, Schulte E, Schumacher U. THIEME Atlas of Anatomy. Volumes 1-3. Illustrations by Voll M and Wesker K. 2nd ed. New York: Thieme Medical Publishers; 2016

---

77. Correct: Carotid sinus (B)

(**B**) The carotid sinus is a dilation near the carotid bifurcation, either in the distal common carotid or the proximal internal carotid artery. The bifurcation is most commonly found at the C3 vertebral level. The sinus contains baroreceptors that are sensitive to changes in blood pressure (afferent fibers are provided by the glossopharyngeal nerve). Carotid sinus syncope in this patient likely occurred as a result of pressure on, and stimulation of, the sinus that caused bradycardia and the development of hypotension. (**A**) The carotid body, also located at the carotid bifurcation, contains chemoreceptors that are sensitive the changes in blood pO_2, pCO_2, and pH. (**C**) The otic ganglion, which is located in the infratemporal fossa, is a

parasympathetic ganglion whose postganglionic fibers supply the parotid salivary gland. (**D**) The stellate ganglion is a sympathetic ganglion located anterior to the C7 transverse process and is formed by the fusion of the inferior cervical and first thoracic ganglia. It is not involved with receptors located in the carotid sinus or carotid body. (**E**) The superior cervical ganglion typically lies along the anterior aspect of the C2 and C3 transverse processes. As such, it lies superior to the tumor and would unlikely be directly affected.

Refer to the following image for answer 77:

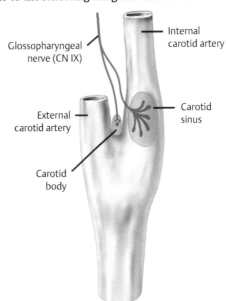

Source: Schuenke M, Schulte E, Schumacher U. THIEME Atlas of Anatomy. Head, Neck, and Neuroanatomy. Illustrations by Voll M and Wesker K. 2nd ed. New York: Thieme Medical Publishers; 2016

---

78. Correct: Maxillary (B)

(**B**) The bilateral maxillary sinuses are located lateral to the nasal cavity in the body of the maxilla, inferior to the orbit. Their surface projection is deep to the cheeks. The mucous membranes of the maxillary sinuses are innervated by the maxillary nerves (CN V2). Each maxillary sinus is drained through an ostium located in the superior aspect of its medial wall that empties into the semilunar hiatus underneath the middle nasal concha. The location of the maxillary ostium combined with the impaired effective clearing of secretions by the cilia predisposes the sinuses to bacterial growth and resulting infection and sinusitis. (**A**) The mandibular nerve (CN V3) does not innervate any of the paranasal sinuses. (**C**) The olfactory nerve (CN I) innervates the olfactory mucosa located in the superior portion of the nasal cavity. It does not innervate any of the paranasal sinuses. (**D**) The ophthalmic nerve (CN V1) innervates paranasal sinuses except the maxillary sinus (i.e., frontal ethmoidal air cells, and sphenoidal sinuses). (**E**) The vagus nerve does not innervate any of the paranasal sinuses.

Chapter 2

Musculoskeletal System

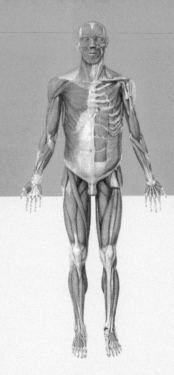

ANATOMICAL LEARNING OBJECTIVES

Upper and Lower Limbs

► Describe and identify the bones and joints of the upper and lower limbs, including their characteristic features, their range of motion, clinically significant anatomical relationships, and surface landmarks.

► Describe the fascial compartments of the upper and lower limbs, including the functional muscle groups contained within each and their action(s) and neurovasculature.

► Describe the stages of gait, including the skeletal structures and muscles involved.

► Describe the course and anatomical relationships of the neurovascular structures that pass between the root of the neck, thorax and upper limb, and between the pelvis, perineum, and lower limb. Identify the surface locations at which arterial pulses may be palpated in the limbs.

► Describe the origin, course, and distribution of the brachial and lumbosacral plexuses. List the innervation of upper and lower limb muscles, and differentiate between the dermatomal pattern and the cutaneous distribution of named nerves.

► Explain the anatomical basis for the tendon reflexes and identify the location of those commonly assessed in a physical examination.

► Describe the boundaries and contents of the anatomical spaces and passages of the upper and lower limbs.

► Explain the changes in the bones of the lower limb during infancy and early childhood.

► Explain the anatomical bases for, and characteristics of, hernias in the groin region.

► Recognize normal and pathological anatomy in standard diagnostic imaging of the upper and lower limbs.

Back and Vertebral Column

► Describe and identify the bones and joints of the vertebral column, including their characteristic features, their range of movement, clinically significant anatomical relationships, and surface landmarks.

► Describe the normal curvatures of the vertebral column.

► Identify the principal muscle groups of the vertebral column, including their action(s) and neurovasculature.

► Describe the course and anatomical relationships of the neurovascular structures associated with the back and vertebral column.

► Describe the anatomy of the spinal meninges, and the continuation of the ventricular system in the spinal cord that contains cerebrospinal fluid.

► Recognize normal and pathological anatomy in standard diagnostic imaging of the back and vertebral column.

Head and Neck

► Describe and identify the bone and joints of the cervical region and skull, including their characteristic features, their range of movement, clinically significant anatomical relationships, and surface landmarks.

► Describe the anatomy of the fontanelles in the neonate and infant, including the timeframe for their closure the formation of the cranial sutures.

► Describe the principal muscles and ligaments that contribute to stability and movement of the joints of the head and neck, including their attachments, action(s) and innervation.

► Describe the anatomy of the cervical triangles, including their fasciae, contents, and anatomical relationships.

► Describe the course and anatomical relationships of the neurovascular structures in the head and neck. Identify the surface locations at which arterial pulses may be palpated in the head and neck.

- Describe the anatomy of each cranial nerve, including their functional composition, origin, course, and distribution to structures in the head and neck.
- Describe the anatomy of the somatic cervical and brachial nerve plexuses, including their contributing nerve roots and the distribution of their branches to structures in the head and neck.
- Describe the distribution of somatic sensory nerve distribution in dermatomes on the head and neck, and the trigeminal nerve in the face.
- Describe the anatomical basis of the gag reflex.
- Describe the anatomy of the orbit, including its skeleton, neurovasculature, and the extra-ocular muscles and their attachments, actions, and innervation.
- Describe the anatomy of the nasal cavity and paranasal sinuses, including and their characteristic features, neurovasculature and anatomical relationships.
- Describe the anatomy of the tongue and soft palate, including their muscles, neurovasculature, and anatomical relationships.
- Describe the anatomy of the pharynx, larynx, and esophagus, including their neurovasculature and anatomical relationships.
- Describe the stages of swallowing, including the skeletal structures and muscles involved.
- Describe the developmental anatomy of the pharyngeal arches and list structures derived from each pharyngeal arch, pouch, and cleft.
- Recognize normal and pathological anatomy in standard diagnostic imaging of the head and neck.

Thorax

- Describe and identify the bones and joints of the thoracic skeleton, including their characteristic features, their range of motion, clinically significant anatomical relationships, and surface landmarks.
- Describe the typical intercostal space, including its muscles, neurovasculature, and clinically significant anatomical relationships.
- Describe the anatomy of the thoracic inlet, including the anatomical relationships of structures that pass through it.
- Recognize normal and pathological anatomy in standard diagnostic imaging of the thorax.

Abdomen

- Describe the anatomy of the abdominal walls, including their skeleton, muscles, fascial layers, and neurovasculature. Describe the umbilical folds and ligaments, and inguinal fossae on the internal aspect of the anterior abdominal wall.
- Describe the anatomy of the inguinal canal in the male and female, including its contents and anatomical relationships. Describe the role of the processus vaginalis in the development of the inguinal region.
- Describe the spermatic cord, including the derivation of its investing layers.
- Explain the anatomical basis for, and characteristics of, hernias in the abdomen and groin region.
- Describe the diaphragm, including its attachments, action(s), innervation, and anatomical relationships. Explain anatomical basis for, and characteristics of diaphragmatic hernias.
- Describe the sensory innervation of the anterior and lateral abdominal walls and identify dermatomes commonly assessed in a physical examination.
- Recognize normal and pathological anatomy in standard diagnostic imaging of the abdomen.

Pelvis and Perineum

- Describe the sex differences for the bony pelvis, including the palpable anatomical landmarks of the ilium, ischium, and pubis. Describe the pelvic inlet and outlet, their normal orientation, and their important obstetrical dimensions.
- Describe the anatomy of the perineum, including its muscles, erectile bodies, and neurovasculature.
- Describe the anatomy of the pelvic floor and walls, including its muscles and neurovasculature.
- Describe the anatomy of the organs of the pelvic cavity, including associated fasciae, peritoneum, muscles, neurovasculature, and anatomical relationships.
- Describe the sensory innervation of the pelvic and perineal regions, and identify dermatomes commonly assessed in a physical examination.
- Recognize normal and pathological anatomy in standard diagnostic imaging of the pelvis and perineum.

2.1 Questions

Easy	Medium	Hard

Upper Limb

Consider the following case for questions 1 to 3:

A 39-year-old medical illustrator presents to the orthopaedic clinic with pain, paresthesia, and anesthesia in the lateral three and a half digits of her right hand. She states that the pain increases during the night. Physical examination reveals difficulty in opposition of her right thumb.

1. Which of the following nerves is most likely affected in this patient?

A. Anterior interosseous
B. Median
C. Posterior interosseous
D. Superficial branch of the radial
E. Ulnar

2. The physician orders an MRI to assess the integrity of neurovascular structures at the wrist. Which structure is indicated by the *arrows* (refer to the accompanying image)?

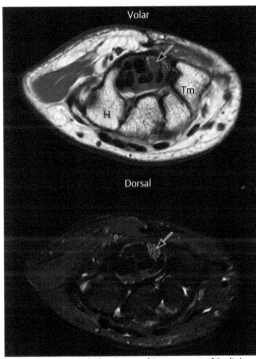

Source: Image provided courtesy of Department of Radiology, William Beaumont Hospital

A. Median nerve
B. Tendon of flexor carpi radialis
C. Tendon of flexor pollicis longus
D. Tendon of palmaris longus
E. Ulnar nerve

3. Which clinical condition most likely explains the symptoms in this patient?

A. Carpal tunnel syndrome
B. Dupuytren contracture
C. Hamate hook fracture
D. Scaphoid fracture
E. Ulnar canal syndrome

Consider the following case for questions 4 and 5:

A 37-year-old man presents to the primary care clinic with a 3-month history of worsening tingling, numbness, and weakness of the left hand, which is beginning to affect his work. Physical examination reveals wasting of the hypothenar eminence and reduced sensation in the ring and little fingers.

4. Which nerve is most likely affected in this patient?

A. Anterior interosseous
B. Median
C. Posterior interosseous
D. Superficial branch of radial
E. Ulnar

5. Physical examination of this patient reveals a positive Tinel's sign (distal tingling sensation on percussion of a damaged nerve) on percussion between the medial epicondyle of the humerus and the olecranon. Which of the following muscles is located at this position?

A. Flexor carpi radialis
B. Flexor carpi ulnaris
C. Flexor digitorum profundus
D. Pronator teres
E. Supinator

Consider the following case for questions 6 and 7:

A 47-year-old woman with breast cancer undergoes a mastectomy with the removal of axillary lymph nodes. Postoperatively, she experiences weakness in extension, medial rotation, and adduction of her arm on the same side.

6. Paralysis of which single muscle most likely accounts for the patient's diagnosed weakness in arm movements?

A. Latissimus dorsi
B. Serratus anterior
C. Subscapularis
D. Supraspinatus
E. Teres minor

7. Which nerve was most likely injured iatrogenically in this patient?

A. Dorsal scapular
B. Long thoracic
C. Suprascapular
D. Thoracodorsal
E. Upper subscapular

41

Consider the following case for questions 8 and 9:

A 27-year-old man is admitted to the emergency department with severe shoulder pain and inability to mobilize the glenohumeral joint. Radiologic imaging confirms an anterior shoulder dislocation and the joint was reduced without difficulty. During a follow-up visit to the orthopaedic clinic, physical examination reveals weakness of arm abduction.

8. Which of the following nerves is most likely injured in this patient?

A. Axillary
B. Dorsal scapular
C. Long thoracic
D. Lower subscapular
E. Suprascapular

9. Which of the following anatomical spaces is most likely affected in this patient?

A. Cubital tunnel
B. Quadrangular space
C. Suprascapular notch
D. Triangular space
E. Triceps hiatus

Consider the following case for questions 10 and 11:

A 62-year-old woman presents with pain and numbness of 1-month duration on the medial aspect of her right forearm and hand.

10. Which of the following portions of the brachial plexus gives rise to the sensory nerve(s) that account for her symptoms?

A. Lateral cord
B. Medial cord
C. Middle trunk
D. Posterior cord
E. Superior trunk

11. Which dermatome(s) are affected in this patient?

A. C5
B. C6
C. C7
D. C7 and C8
E. C8 and T1

Consider the following case for questions 12 and 13:

A 54-year-old woman presents to the orthopaedic clinic with left shoulder pain localized in the scapular region. A history reveals that her job involves repeated lifting of packages over her head. Over the past 6 months she has noticed progressive weakness and pain in the left upper extremity, which is exacerbated when lifting her arms over her head. Physical examination reveals significant weakness in lateral rotation and initiating abduction of her left arm.

12. Which muscle(s) most likely account(s) for the patient's weakness in arm movements?

A. Infraspinatus and supraspinatus
B. Infraspinatus and teres minor
C. Rhomboid major and rhomboid minor
D. Supraspinatus
E. Teres major and teres minor

13. Which of the following nerves is most likely affected in this patient?

A. Dorsal scapular
B. Lower subscapular
C. Suprascapular
D. Thoracodorsal
E. Upper subscapular

Consider the following case for questions 14 to 16:

A 28-year-old woman presents to the orthopaedic clinic with weakness, diffuse numbness, and severe pain in her left upper extremity. Positive clinical tests for neural and vascular compression are consistent with thoracic outlet syndrome. Surgical exploration reveals a large supraclavicular neuroma compressing the brachial plexus and subclavian artery. After removal of the neuroma and surgical decompression of these structures, the patient develops the deformity shown by *arrows* in the accompanying image.

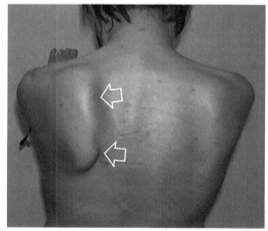

Source: Martinoli C, Gandolfo N, Perez MM, et al. Brachial plexus and nerves about the shoulder. Semin Musculoskelet Radiol. 2010 Nov;14(5):523–46

14. Which of the following muscles is most likely affected in this patient?

A. Levator scapulae
B. Serratus anterior
C. Serratus posterior superior
D. Subscapularis
E. Supraspinatus

15. Which of the following actions would most likely also be weakened in this patient?

A. Elevation of the scapula
B. Initiation of arm abduction
C. Medial rotation of the arm
D. Protraction of the scapula
E. Retraction of the scapula

16. Which of the following nerves was most likely injured iatrogenically during the surgery?

A. Dorsal scapular
B. Long thoracic
C. Suprascapular
D. Thoracodorsal
E. Upper subscapular

Consider the following case for questions 17 to 19:

A 43-year-old man with shoulder pain and limited ability to move his arm visits the orthopaedic clinic. Physical examination reveals difficulty abducting his shoulder. An MRI (refer to the accompanying images) reveals a complete muscle tear with proximal retraction of its tendon. Surgery is recommended to reattach the torn muscle.

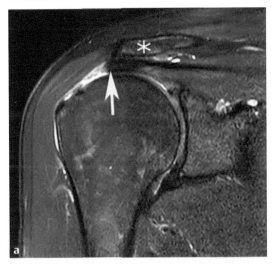

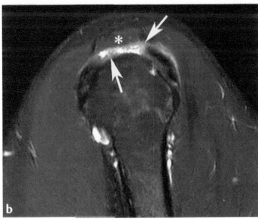

Source: Yablon C, Jacobson J. Rotator cuff and subacromial pathology. Semin Musculoskelet Radiol. 2015; 19(03): 231–242.

17. Which of the following structures is indicated by the *asterisks* in the images?

A. Acromion
B. Coracoacromial ligament
C. Coracoid process
D. Subscapular bursa
E. Supraglenoid tubercle

18. Which of the following muscles is most likely torn in this patient (refer to the *arrow* in image a)?

A. Deltoid
B. Infraspinatus
C. Supraspinatus
D. Teres major
E. Teres minor

19. At which of the following sites (A–E) does the torn muscle attach (refer to the accompanying image)?

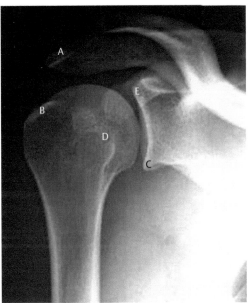

Source: Konermann W, Gruber G. Ultraschalldiagnostik der Bewegungsorgane. 2nd ed. Stuttgart: Thieme; 2006.

A. Acromion
B. Greater tubercle of the humerus
C. Infraglenoid tubercle
D. Lesser tubercle of the humerus
E. Supraglenoid tubercle

20. A 23-year-old college quarterback is admitted to the emergency department after being tackled. Physical examination reveals he is unable to move his right (throwing) arm and must support it with his left hand. Radiographic examination of his shoulder is performed to diagnose the patient (refer to the accompanying images). Which of the following clinical conditions best describes the patient's symptoms?

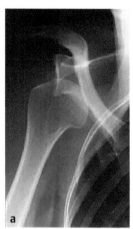
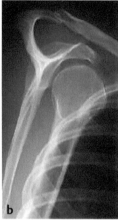

Source: Reiser M, Baur-Melnyk A, Glaser C. Direct Diagnosis in Radiology. Musculoskeletal Imaging. 1st Edition. Thieme; 2008.

A. Clavicle fracture
B. Colles' fracture
C. Shoulder dislocation
D. Shoulder separation
E. Smith's fracture

21. A 32-year-old man is admitted to the emergency department following a fall directly on his right shoulder with the arm abducted. He experienced pain and swelling of his shoulder immediately after the fall. Physical examination shows a "step deformity" (refer to the *asterisk* in the following image). Which of the following clinical conditions has occurred in this patient?

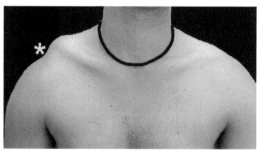

Source: Image provided courtesy of William Beaumont Hospital

A. Clavicle fracture
B. Colles' fracture
C. Shoulder dislocation
D. Shoulder separation
E. Smith's fracture

22. A 3-year-old girl presents to the emergency department with her mother after a visit to the park. The patient holds her right arm close to her side, with the elbow slightly flexed and the forearm pronated. Her mother states that she was holding her daughter's hands while swinging her and lifting her up and down, and her daughter began to scream and cry. The attending physician diagnoses nursemaid's elbow (radial head subluxation). Which of the following structures is most likely affected in this patient (refer to the accompanying image)?

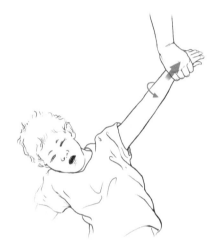

Source: Schuenke M, Schulte E, Schumacher U. THIEME Atlas of Anatomy. General Anatomy and Musculoskeletal System. Illustrations by Voll M and Wesker K. 2nd ed. New York: Thieme Medical Publishers; 2016

A. Anular ligament
B. Biceps tendon
C. Bicipital aponeurosis
D. Radial (lateral) collateral ligament
E. Ulnar (medial) collateral ligament

23. A 56-year-old man presents in the orthopaedic clinic with decreased mobility of his right ring and little fingers, which are in a flexed position and he cannot extend them. He reports that his hands began to feel stiff about 1 year ago, and he is seeking medical attention now because he cannot straighten the fingers and hold his woodworking tools. Physical examination reveals palpable, fixed nodules near the distal palmar skin crease of the ring and little fingers. Thumb movements are normal. He denies feeling any pain in his hands and sensory deficits in the hand are not detectable. Which of the following conditions best describes this patient's symptoms (refer to the accompanying image)?

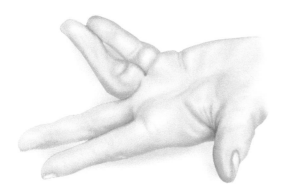

A. Dupuytren's contracture
B. Ganglion cyst
C. Mallet finger
D. Ulnar nerve entrapment
E. Volkmann's ischemic contracture

Consider the following case for questions 24 and 25:

A 54-year-old man is admitted to the emergency department after landing on the lateral aspect of his right shoulder in a bicycling accident. He is in significant pain and discomfort, and uses his left hand to support and hold his right arm close to his body. Physical examination reveals a deformity over the middle third of his clavicle, which is shown by radiological examination to be a midshaft clavicular fracture.

24. Which of the following neurovascular structures is at greatest risk in this patient?

A. Axillary artery
B. Brachiocephalic vein
C. Common carotid artery
D. Internal jugular vein
E. Subclavian vein

25. Which of the following muscles is most likely to protect the neurovascular structures that lie immediately posterior to the fractured portion of the clavicle in this patient?

A. Pectoralis major
B. Pectoralis minor
C. Sternocleidomastoid
D. Subclavius
E. Trapezius

Consider the following case for questions 26 and 27:

A 68-year-old woman with pain, deformity, and swelling of her right arm presents to the emergency department after she slipped and fell on ice. Radiological examination reveals a fracture in the middle one-third of the humerus.

26. An inability of which action would most likely be seen in this patient?

A. Arm abduction
B. Elbow extension
C. Forearm pronation
D. Forearm supination
E. Wrist extension

27. Which of the following areas on the dorsum of the hand (A–E; refer to the accompanying image) would most likely be affected in this patient?

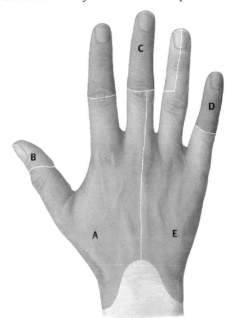

Source: Schuenke M, Schulte E, Schumacher U. THIEME Atlas of Anatomy. General Anatomy and Musculoskeletal System. Illustrations by Voll M and Wesker K. 2nd ed. New York: Thieme Medical Publishers; 2016

A. Lateral palm and proximal fingers 1 to 3
B. Tip of thumb
C. Distal ends of the fingers 2 to 4
D. Distal ends of the fingers 4 and 5
E. Medial palm and proximal fingers 3 to 5

28. A 48-year-old woman with a 3-week history of forearm pain, with numbness in her lateral palm, thumb, index, and middle fingers, and hand weakness presents to the orthopaedic clinic. Physical examination reveals a lack of thumb flexion and that the forearm pain is aggravated by resisted pronation. Which of the following nerves is most likely affected in this patient?

A. Deep branch of ulnar
B. Median
C. Radial
D. Recurrent branch of median
E. Ulnar

Consider the following case for questions 29 to 31:

A 54-year-old man presents to the orthopaedic clinic with weakness of elbow flexion and numbness along the lateral side of his right forearm. The patient reports that he spent much of the preceding weekend working in his backyard, lifting heavy loads with a shovel.

29. Which of the following nerves is most likely injured?

A. Axillary
B. Musculocutaneous
C. Median
D. Superficial branch of the radial
E. Ulnar

30. Which of the following dermatomes would be affected in this patient?

A. C4
B. C5
C. C6
D. C7
E. C8

31. Which of the following actions would you also expect to be weakened in this patient?

A. Abduction of the arm
B. Extension of the arm
C. Extension of the forearm
D. Flexion of the arm
E. Pronation

32. A 48-year-old construction worker with bilateral cubital fossa pain is admitted to the emergency department. A patient history reveals that he was lifting several sheets of drywall when he felt a "pop" in his right arm and then, almost immediately, felt another in his left arm after the weight shifted to that arm. During physical examination, the biceps tendon is not palpable and its muscle belly is retracted proximally. On this basis, a diagnosis of biceps brachii tendon rupture is made. Which of the following action(s) would be weakened in this patient?

A. Flexion of the elbow joint only
B. Flexion of the elbow joint and forearm pronation
C. Flexion of the elbow joint and forearm supination
D. Pronation only
E. Supination only

Consider the following case for questions 33 and 34:

During their internal medicine clerkship, a third-year medical student is asked to obtain a sample of venous blood.

33. Which vein is commonly used for this procedure?

A. Axillary
B. Basilic
C. Brachial
D. Cephalic
E. Median cubital

34. Which of the following nerves is most at risk of injury in venipuncture at the preferred site?

A. Axillary
B. Median
C. Musculocutaneous
D. Radial
E. Ulnar

35. A 19-year-old collegiate football player presents to the emergency department after falling hard on the wrist of his outstretched left arm during practice. He reports experiencing sudden pain when he fell. Physical examination of his wrist elicits sharp pain with palpation of the anatomical snuff box. Which bone is fractured in the radiographic image (as seen in the accompanying image) of his wrist?

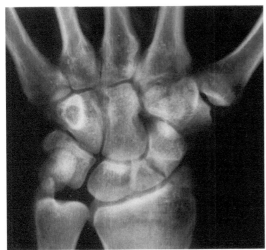

Source: Matzen P. Praktische Orthopädie. 3rd Edition. Stuttgart: J. A. Barth Verlag; Thieme; 2002

A. Lunate

B. Pisiform

C. Scaphoid

D. Trapezium

E. Trapezoid

Consider the following case for questions 36 and 37:

A 35-year-old man is admitted to the emergency department while suffering an asthma attack. Arterial blood is withdrawn from the left radial artery for arterial blood gas analysis.

36. The radial artery typically lies immediately lateral and adjacent to which of the following muscle tendons at the wrist?

A. Brachioradialis

B. Flexor carpi radialis

C. Flexor carpi ulnaris

D. Flexor digitorum superficialis

E. Palmaris longus

37. Prior to performing a radial puncture for arterial blood gas analysis, which of the following clinical tests would most likely be used to assess arterial patency in the hand?

A. Allen's test

B. Catheter angiography

C. CT angiography

D. MR angiography

E. Tinel's test

38. A 32-year-old woman with a 5-month history of difficulty using her right hand to perform daily tasks presents to the orthopaedic clinic. Physical examination reveals a positive Froment's sign (weakness in holding a piece of paper between the thumb and index finger when the examiner pulls the paper away). In addition, the interphalangeal joint of the thumb flexes on the affected side during this maneuver. Which of the following muscles was most likely weakened in this patient?

A. Abductor pollicis brevis

B. Abductor pollicis longus

C. Adductor pollicis

D. Flexor pollicis brevis

E. Flexor pollicis longus

39. A 58-year-old man visits his primary care physician for his annual physical examination. During the visit, the primary care physician determines that the brachioradialis tendon reflex is diminished. Which of the following spinal cord levels may be affected in this individual?

A. C4–C5

B. C5–C6

C. C6–C7

D. C7–C8

E. C8–T1

40. A 22-year-old man with a neck injury after being tackled during a collegiate football game is admitted to the emergency department. Radiologic examination reveals significant narrowing of the C6–C7 intervertebral foramen and herniation of the associated intervertebral disc. The patient reports radiculopathic pain in his hand, notably from his middle finger. Which of the following tendon reflexes would most likely be diminished in this patient?

A. Biceps brachii

B. Brachioradialis

C. Flexor carpi radialis

D. Pronator teres

E. Triceps brachii

Consider the following case for questions 41 and 42:

A 69-year-old woman, who had a prior left lung lower lobectomy for cancer, is scheduled for a left total shoulder arthroplasty (replacement) for degenerative disease and pain. Based on this previous history and current pulmonary function testing, the surgeon recommends using regional anesthesia and light sedation.

41. The target of the anesthetic injection in this patient would be between which of the following two muscles?

A. Anterior scalene and middle scalene

B. Anterior scalene and sternocleidomastoid

C. Middle scalene and posterior scalene

D. Posterior scalene and longus colli

E. Sternocleidomastoid and omohyoid

42. Following the nerve block, the patient demonstrates mild dyspnea (difficulty in breathing). Which of the following nerves is most likely affected?

A. Long thoracic

B. Phrenic

C. Recurrent laryngeal

D. Sympathetic chain

E. Vagus

Consider the following case for questions 43 and 44:

A 25-year-old woman is admitted to the emergency department with acute pain and swelling of her distal forearm and hand after falling from her horse onto her outstretched hand. Radiographic imaging confirms a fracture (refer to the accompanying image), which is subsequently reduced and casted.

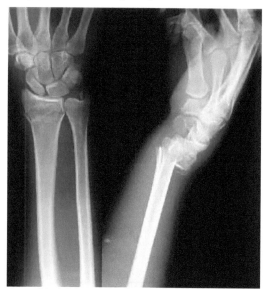

Source: Munk P, Ryan A. Teaching Atlas of Musculoskeletal Imaging. 1st Edition. Thieme; 2007

43. Based on the patient history and radiographic studies, which of the following bones is fractured in this patient?

A. Lunate

B. Pisiform

C. Radius

D. Scaphoid

E. Ulna

44. Which of the following types of fracture in shown in this patient?

A. Barton's

B. Chauffeur's

C. Colles'

D. Scaphoid

E. Smith's

Consider the following case for questions 45 and 46:

A 25-year-old woman with aching in her right anterior forearm and weakness in her wrist and hand visits her primary care physician. She reports having difficulty sewing and knitting, picking up coins, and fastening buttons. Her history reveals she often carries her child in a baby carrier on her right forearm. Physical examination reveals an inability to make the "OK" sign with her thumb and index finger.

45. Which of the following muscles are most likely affected in this patient?

A. Flexor carpi radialis and flexor digitorum superficialis

B. Flexor digitorum profundus and flexor pollicis longus

C. Flexor digitorum superficialis and flexor digitorum profundus

D. Flexor digitorum superficialis and flexor pollicis longus

E. Flexor pollicis longus and pronator teres

46. Would you expect sensory deficits from the upper limb in this patient?

A. No

B. Yes

47. An 18-year-old collegiate volleyball player with progressive pain over her anterior shoulder is examined by the team physician. The patient exhibits positive Yergason's test (pain over bicipital groove during resisted supination with the elbow flexed to 90 degrees) and Speed's test (pain over bicipital groove during resistance to shoulder flexion with the elbow extended and forearm supinated). Which of the following structures is being tested in this patient?

A. Coracobrachialis muscle

B. Pectoralis minor muscle

C. Subscapularis muscle

D. Tendon of the long head of biceps brachii

E. Tendon of the short head of biceps brachii

48. A 74-year-old man is admitted to the emergency department after slipping on ice and falling on his outstretched hand. Radiographic examination reveals a displaced fracture of the radial neck. Which of the following structures would most likely be injured by this fracture?

A. Anterior interosseous nerve

B. Deep artery of the arm

C. Median nerve

D. Posterior interosseous nerve

E. Ulnar artery

49. A 50-year-old woman presents with a 1-year history of pain in her left posterior forearm and the inability to extend her fingers. A soft tumor in the left proximal posterior forearm is palpable immediately distal to the elbow joint. Which of the following clinical symptoms would also be likely?

A. Loss of sensation from the little finger

B. Loss of sensation from the tip of the index finger

C. Paralysis of radial deviation of the wrist

D. Paralysis of thumb adduction

E. Weakened thumb abduction

50. A 49-year-old man with right elbow pain of 3-month duration visits his primary care physician. A patient history reveals he is a recreational tennis player and that the pain has worsened progressively over the previous three months and is notably aggravated when he hits a backhand tennis stroke. Physical examination elicits pain around the lateral epicondyle that is aggravated by resisted wrist extension. Which of the following muscles is most likely inflamed in this patient?

A. Brachioradialis

B. Flexor carpi ulnaris

C. Extensor carpi radialis brevis

D. Extensor pollicis longus

E. Pronator teres

51. A 39-year-old woman with shoulder pain and diminished ability to perform tasks that involve arm abduction or bearing weight on the shoulders presents to the orthopaedic clinic. Her history reveals she recently underwent parotidectomy. Physical examination reveals limited shoulder abduction and pain that radiates from the neck into the back. There is no winging of the scapula. Which of the following muscles is most likely impaired in this patient?

A. Deltoid

B. Rhomboid major

C. Serratus anterior

D. Supraspinatus

E. Trapezius

Consider the following case for questions 52 and 53:

A 55-year-old man with bruises over his left shoulder and a flail left upper limb is admitted to the emergency department after he was thrown from his motorcycle in a collision with a car. Physical examination reveals a weakness on the left of arm abduction and elbow flexion. There is diminished sensation from lateral portions of the shoulder, arm, forearm, and hand. Movement of the wrist and hand are normal and pulses are intact in the left arm.

52. Which of the following portions of the brachial plexus is most likely injured in this patient?

A. Axillary nerve

B. Inferior trunk

C. Musculocutaneous nerve

D. Posterior divisions

E. Superior trunk

53. With time, this patient develops chronic medial rotation of the arm. Which of the following muscles most likely medially rotates the arm in this patient?

A. Infraspinatus

B. Pectoralis major

C. Supraspinatus

D. Teres minor

E. Trapezius

54. A 46-year-old man presents to the orthopaedic clinic with a 6-month history of progressive hand weakness, numbness, and tingling. Physical examination reveals a weakness in grasping objects, atrophy of the thenar muscles, and anesthesia and paresthesia from the palmar aspect of the left thumb, index finger, and thenar eminence. When asked to make a fist, the patient's hand takes the "hand of benediction" position (refer to the accompanying image). Tinel's signs over the carpal and cubital tunnels are negative, although the patient cannot make the "OK" sign. Which of the following is the most likely diagnosis in this patient?

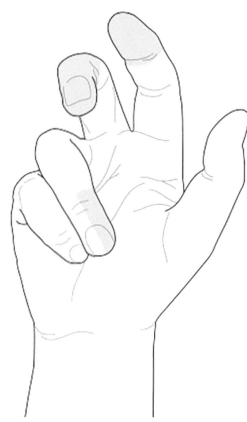

Source: Schuenke M, Schulte E, Schumacher U. THIEME Atlas of Anatomy. General Anatomy and Musculoskeletal System. Illustrations by Voll M and Wesker K. 2nd ed. New York: Thieme Medical Publishers; 2016

A. Anterior interosseous nerve lesion
B. Carpal tunnel syndrome
C. Cubital tunnel syndrome
D. Dupuytren's contracture
E. Pronator syndrome

Consider the following case for questions 55 and 56:

A 34-year-old woman with pain, deformity, and swelling of her left arm is brought to the emergency department after falling off her bicycle. Radiographic evaluation reveals a displaced, midshaft humeral fracture.

55. Which of the following nerves would most likely be affected by this injury?

A. Axillary
B. Median
C. Musculocutaneous
D. Radial
E. Ulnar

56. Which of the following movements would most likely be weakened in this patient?

A. Adduction of the thumb
B. Extension of the arm
C. Flexion of the wrist
D. Pronation of the forearm
E. Supination of the forearm

57. A 25-year-old man is brought to the emergency department with pain and swelling of his right forearm and wrist after falling off his motorcycle. Radiographic evaluation reveals a fracture (refer to the accompanying image). Which of the following bones (indicated by the *short arrow*) is fractured in this patient?

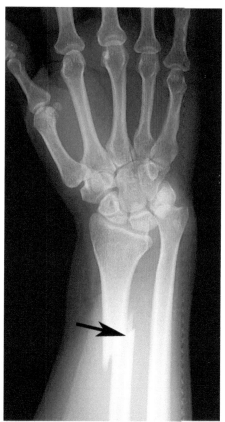

Source: Garcia G. RadCases: Musculoskeletal Radiology. 1st Edition. Thieme; 2010.

A. Hamate
B. Lunate
C. Radius
D. Scaphoid
E. Ulna

58. A 45-year-old secretary presents with weakness and pain in his right hand. Physical examination reveals paresthesia and anesthesia in the little finger of his right hand. Which of the following actions would most likely also be affected?

A. Abduction of the index finger

B. Extension of the middle finger

C. Flexion of the distal interphalangeal joint of the index finger

D. Flexion of the interphalangeal joint of the thumb

E. Opposition of the thumb

59. A 38-year-old woman with pain along the radial side of her right wrist presents to her family physician. A history reveals that the patient has a 5-month-old child. Physical examination reveals that the pain radiates to the radial side of the distal forearm and is exacerbated with abduction and/ or extension movements of the thumb, especially when picking up her child and when opening bottles with her dominant right hand. Tenderness over the first dorsal compartment and a tender nodule over the radial styloid are noted. A positive Finkelstein's test (with the thumb flexed across the palm and covered by the other fingers, the patient bends the wrist toward ulna as seen in the accompanying images) is elicited. Which of the following conditions is most consistent with the symptoms in this patient?

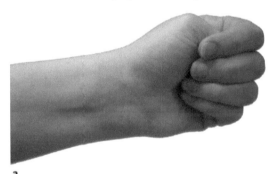

a

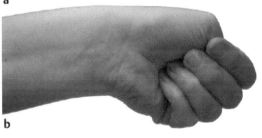

b

A. Carpal tunnel syndrome

B. Colles' fracture

C. De Quervain tenosynovitis

D. Dupuytren's contracture

E. Scaphoid fracture

Vertebral Column

60. A 65-year-old man with obvious thoracic hyperkyphosis presents to the orthopaedic clinic. The patient reports that his condition has progressed over 3 years and that it has been accompanied with lower back pain and diminished range of motion. His neurological examination is normal. The patient is diagnosed with diffuse idiopathic skeletal hyperostosis. Which of the following ligaments (indicated by the *arrows* in the accompanying image) was ossified in the section of this patient?

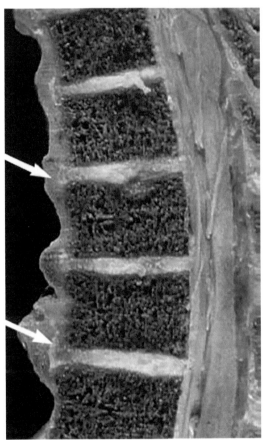

Source: Bohndorf K, Imhof H, Pope T. Musculoskeletal Imaging. A Concise Multimodality Approach. 1st Edition. Thieme; 2001.

A. Anterior longitudinal

B. Denticulate

C. Interspinous

D. Ligamenta flava

E. Posterior longitudinal

61. A 16-year-old girl with upper back pain is brought to the orthopaedic clinic. She reports that the pain began about 6 weeks previously and has increased in severity over the last 3 weeks, with gradual weakening and loss of sensation in both the lower limbs. The girl's mother notes that the girl has had occasional episodes of low grade fever and a minor cough with expectoration. Physical examination reveals a stiff spine that is painful with movement, and a gibbus deformity (short segment of spinal column with sharp angulation) at the T4 vertebral level that is tender on percussion. Laboratory tests are positive for tuberculosis disease. Which of the following conditions of the spine would most likely be present in this patient?

A. Kyphosis

B. Lordosis

C. Scoliosis

D. Spina bifida occulta

E. Spondylolisthesis

62. A 33-year-old man with a 3-month history of progressive, severe lower back pain that radiates along the posterior aspect of his right leg (sciatica) presents to the orthopaedic clinic. The patient reports that recently he "catches" his big toe as he walks. Physical examination reveals a "high step-page" gait and sensory loss from the dorsum of the foot and lateral side of the great toe. Radiologic imaging reveals a herniated intervertebral disc. Which of the following dermatomes is most likely affected by the herniation?

A. L3

B. L4

C. L5

D. S1

E. S2

63. A 42-year-old woman with severe lower back pain that radiates along the posterior aspect of her left leg (sciatica) comes to the orthopaedic clinic. Her history reveals that her job requires work at a computer, and physical examination reveals poor posture, as well as motor and sensory deficits in her lower limb. An MRI reveals a herniated intervertebral disc (refer to the accompanying image) impinging on a nerve root. Which of the following nerve roots is most likely compressed by the herniated disc?

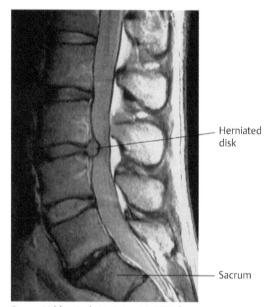

Source: Vahlensieck M, Reiser M. MRT des Bewegungsapparates. 2. Aufl. Stuttgart: Thieme; 2001

A. L3

B. L4

C. L5

D. S1

E. S2

64. A 34-year-old woman is admitted for labor and delivery at 36-weeks of gestation. At 4 to 5 cm of cervical dilation, a lumbar epidural is proposed for management of her labor pain. The procedure is performed at the L4–L5 intervertebral space using a paramedian approach. After passing through skin and subcutaneous tissue, which of the following is the correct sequence of structures through and into which the epidural needle passes to administer the anesthetic?

A. Interspinous ligament > subarachnoid space

B. Ligamentum flavum > epidural space

C. Ligamentum flavum > posterior longitudinal ligament > epidural space

D. Supraspinous ligament > epidural space > arachnoid mater > subarachnoid space

E. Supraspinous ligament > epidural space > conus medullaris

65. A 10-year-old boy is admitted to the hospital with headache and an upper respiratory infection. A lumbar puncture is performed to rule out central nervous system infection. Which of the following vertebral levels is most appropriate for insertion of the spinal needle?

A. L1–L2

B. L2–L3

C. L3–L4

D. L4–L5

E. L5–S1

Consider the following case for questions 66 and 67:

A 19-year-old woman with neck and limb pain is admitted to the emergency department following a front-end motor vehicle collision. A history reveals she was not wearing her seatbelt and that she hit her head on the dashboard during the collision. Physical examination reveals extensive soft-tissue swelling of the neck that causes her difficulty speaking and breathing. Preliminary neurological examination reveals extensive tetraparesis with sensory loss in the trunk and limbs. Radiological examination shows a cervical fracture-dislocation consistent with traumatic hyperextension of the cervical spine (refer to the accompanying image).

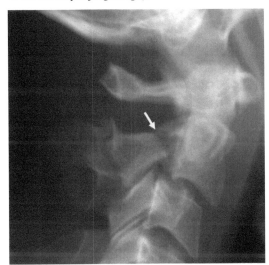

Source: Garcia G. RadCases: Musculoskeletal Radiology. 1st Edition. Thieme; 2010.

66. Which of her vertebra is fractured?

A. C1

B. C2

C. C3

D. C4

E. C5

67. Which of the following fractured structures is indicated by the *arrow* in the presented image?

A. Inferior articular facet

B. Lamina

C. Pedicle

D. Spinous process

E. Transverse process

68. A 27-year-old man presents with neck stiffness after falling on the top of his head while using a trampoline. Radiological examination reveals a cervical fracture. Which of the following fractured structures is indicated by the *arrows* in the accompanying image?

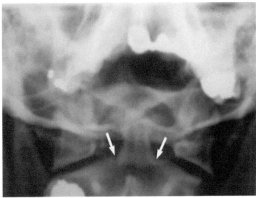

Source: Garcia G. RadCases: Musculoskeletal Radiology. 1st Edition. Thieme; 2010.

A. Dens

B. Lamina

C. Pedicle

D. Posterior arch of the atlas

E. Spinous process

69. A 27-year-old woman is brought to the emergency department after a motor vehicle collision in which her car was hit from behind. Her history reveals that she experienced neck pain and stiffness immediately after the accident. Which of the following ligaments is most likely injured in this patient?

A. Anterior longitudinal

B. Interspinous

C. Ligamentum flavum

D. Posterior longitudinal

E. Supraspinous

70. A 54-year-old man presents with left lumbar radiculopathy. Radiologic examination reveals a degenerative condition of his vertebral column (refer to the accompanying image). Which of the following conditions is present in this patient?

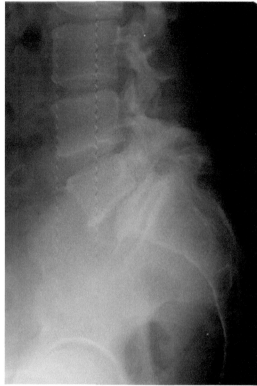

Source: Garcia G. RadCases: Musculoskeletal Radiology. 1st Edition. Thieme; 2010.

A. Kyphosis
B. Scoliosis
C. Spina bifida
D. Spondylolisthesis
E. Spondylolysis

71. A 34-year-old woman with vertigo that occurs upon rotation of her head to the left side (Bow hunter's syndrome) presents to the neurology clinic. CT angiography reveals that the C1 transverse foramen on the left is partially occluded. Which of the following structures in the transverse foramen was likely to be affected in this patient?

A. Ascending cervical artery
B. Internal carotid artery
C. Internal jugular vein
D. Vagus nerve
E. Vertebral artery

72. A 26-year-old man involved in an unrestrained motor vehicle collision is brought to the emergency department. Radiological examination reveals a transverse fracture of the vertebral column, immediately inferior to one of the intervertebral discs (see the *arrow* in the MRI; refer to the accompanying image). In which region of the vertebral column is the fracture?

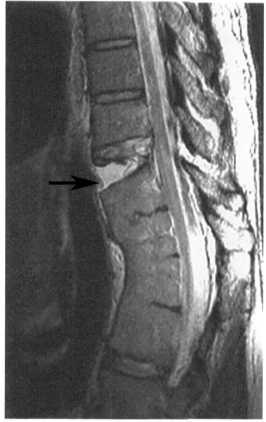

Source: Cassar-Pullicino V, Imhof H. Spinal Trauma: An Imaging Approach. Thieme; 2006.

A. Cervical
B. Thoracic
C. Lumbar
D. Sacral

73. A 37-year-old woman is admitted to the emergency department after being thrown from her horse and trampled by other horses during a steeplechase event. Radiologic examination shows a crush injury extending from the T8–L2 vertebral levels. In which of the following anatomical locations would cutaneous sensation most likely *remain intact*?

A. Great toe
B. Medial thigh
C. Nipple
D. Pubic symphysis
E. Umbilicus

74. A 5-month-old girl with a lumbosacral dimple is brought to the pediatrician. Physical examination reveals a small, midline tuft of hair over the lower lumbar region. MRI reveals discontinuity of posterior lumbar vertebral elements and communication of the epidural and subcutaneous fat. A diagnosis of spina bifida occulta is made. Which of the following structures most likely failed to form in this patient?

A. Inferior articular process

B. Lamina

C. Posterior longitudinal ligament

D. Transverse process

E. Vertebral body

75. On her way to the anatomy lab to study, a medical student finds a $20 dollar bill on the floor. As she bends forward to pick up the cash, she falls head-first to the floor. Which of the following muscles should have maintained her flexed vertebral column and prevented her from falling?

A. Anterolateral abdominal muscles

B. Erector spinae

C. Latissimus dorsi

D. Rhomboids

E. Serratus posterior superior

76. A 58-year-old man with a stiff neck visits his primary care physician (PCP). During physical examination, the PCP determines that the patient exhibits limited rotation of the head to the right. Which of the following muscles on the right side is most likely impaired?

A. Iliocostalis

B. Obliquus capitis

C. Semispinalis capitis

D. Splenius capitis

E. Trapezius

Consider the following case for questions 77 to 79:

A 24-year-old man is admitted to the emergency department after being involved in a head-on collision at home plate during a baseball game. He is experiencing neck and head pain and a radiologic examination of his cervical spine is performed.

77. As a medical student participating in an elective rotation in emergency medicine, you review the lateral C-spine radiograph (refer to the accompanying image). Which of the following structures is indicated by the *arrow*?

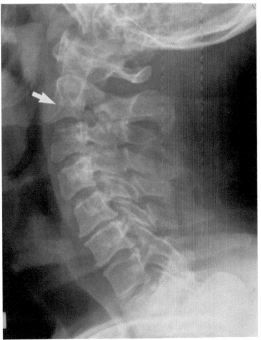

Source: Garcia G. RadCases: Musculoskeletal Radiology. 1st Edition. Thieme; 2010.

A. Anterior arch of the atlas

B. Dens

C. Posterior arch of the atlas

D. Spinous process of C2 vertebra

E. Vertebral body of C2 vertebra

78. The physician suspects injury of the spinal nerve that emerges at the position indicated by the "X" in the radiograph (refer to the accompanying image). Which of the following deficits would you expect?

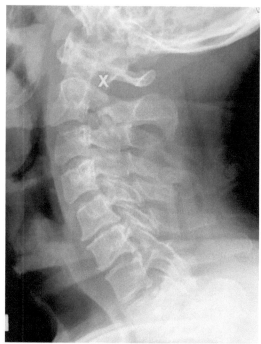

Source: Garcia G. RadCases: Musculoskeletal Radiology. 1st Edition. Thieme; 2010.

A. Sensory loss from the skin over the anterior cervical triangle

B. Sensory loss from the skin on the back of the head

C. Sensory loss from the skin over the frontal bone

D. Weakness of the deltoid muscle

E. Weakness of the trapezius muscle

79. A follow-up MRI is done to assess soft-tissue damage. Which of the following structures is indicated by the *arrow* in the accompanying MRI image?

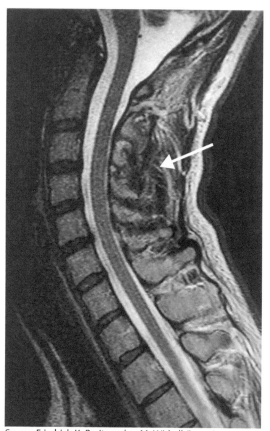

Source: Friedrich K, Breitenseher M. Wirbelbögen. In: Vahlensieck M, Reiser M. MRT des Bewegungsapparates. 2. Aufl. Stuttgart: Thieme; 2001

A. Facet joint capsule

B. Ligamentum flavum

C. Nuchal ligament

D. Posterior longitudinal ligament

E. Transverse ligament of the atlas

Lower Limb

80. The quarterback for State U. will not play in this Saturday's title game as he is suffering from "turf toe," a severe pain in the great toe that is exacerbated by toe extension during locomotion. Which of the following structures is most likely injured in this athlete?

A. Abductor hallucis muscle

B. Ligaments of the metatarsophalangeal joint

C. Sesamoid bones in tendons of flexor hallucis brevis

D. Tendon of extensor hallucis longus

E. Tendon of flexor hallucis longus

81. A 61-year-old man comes to the family clinic with a smooth, hard area on the sole of his foot that is painful when he walks. Physical examination confirms a plantar wart over the head of the third metatarsal. Which of the following nerves conducts afferent pain impulses from the area of the plantar wart?

A. Medial plantar

B. Obturator

C. Posterior ramus of S1

D. Saphenous

E. Superficial fibular

82. A 36-year-old man suffers a fracture of his right tibia during a downhill skiing accident. Physical examination reveals notable weakness (compared to the left side) in dorsiflexion and inversion. Sensation over the dorsum of the tarsal bones is normal. Which of the following nerves has been traumatized?

A. Common fibular

B. Deep fibular

C. Saphenous

D. Superficial fibular

E. Tibial

83. A 39-year-old woman with pain and tenderness at her right ankle visits the orthopaedics clinic. She has just returned from a 5-day holiday of downhill skiing, during which she used rented boots that, she admits, did not fit properly. Physical examination reveals touch tenderness over the medial-most tendon crossing the anterior aspect of the right ankle, and a pain reflex that results when the foot is inverted. Which of the following tendons is most likely inflamed?

A. Extensor digitorum brevis

B. Extensor digitorum longus

C. Extensor hallucis longus

D. Quadratus plantae

E. Tibialis anterior

84. A 38-year-old woman is brought to the emergency department by her partner. They were operating a log-splitter when a portion of a log broke free and struck the patient. There is a 15-cm-long splinter of wood piercing her right medial midthigh. Blood is flowing profusely from the wound. Which of the following arteries has most likely been injured in this accident?

A. Femoral

B. First perforating

C. Medial circumflex artery of the thigh

D. Obturator

E. Popliteal

85. A 58-year-old male victim of polio reports for his semiannual health check. Physical examination shows that, while walking, the right side of his pelvis tips downward during the swing phase of locomotion on that side. He is diagnosed with Trendelenburg gait due to post-polio syndrome. Paralysis of which of the following muscles accounts for most of the altered gait?

A. Left gluteus maximus

B. Left gluteus medius

C. Left tensor fasciae latae

D. Right gluteus maximus

E. Right gluteus medius

86. During her annual health evaluation, a 45-year-old elementary school teacher complains of severe right foot pain of 3-month duration. She states the pain is on the "bottom of my foot" and most severe on the heel. The symptoms are worse during her first steps after getting out of bed or walking after being seated for an extended period. Her previous health evaluation established a body mass index (BMI) of 31, adjusted for height and weight. Inflammation of which of the following structures is responsible for the pain at the heel?

A. Flexor digitorum brevis muscle

B. Long plantar ligament

C. Plantar calcaneonavicular ligament

D. Plantar aponeurosis

E. Quadratus plantae muscle

87. A 15-year-old junior varsity volleyball player is brought to the emergency department. During play, she assumed a deep squat to retrieve a hard-hit ball and immediately experienced severe pain in her right knee. Physical examination localizes the pain to the medial side of her right knee and MRI reveals damage to the medial meniscus (refer to the *arrows* in the accompanying image). Which of the following best describes the damaged structure in this patient?

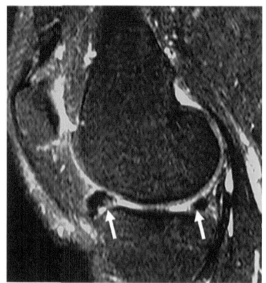

Source: Garcia G. RadCases: Musculoskeletal Radiology. 1st Edition. Thieme; 2010.

A. It can be palpated with the knee in full extension.
B. It is avascular.
C. It is bathed in synovial fluid.
D. It is composed of hyaline cartilage.
E. It is fused to the tendon of semimembranosus along its outer margin.

88. A 28-year-old man is brought to the emergency department after he experienced excruciating pain in his left calf region during a basketball game. Examination reveals his left foot is dorsiflexed and the calf has a conspicuous bulge. He is diagnosed with a rupture of the calcaneal (Achilles) tendon. Which of the following action(s) are produced by muscles that contribute to the ruptured tendon?

A. Eversion and plantar flexion
B. Inversion and plantar flexion
C. Knee flexion and plantar flexion
D. Knee rotation and plantar flexion
E. Plantar flexion only

89. A 16-year-old boy with pain in his right posterior heel is brought to his pediatrician. A history reveals that the boy is a member of the cross-country team at his school. Physical examination elicits pain when the foot is plantar flexed or dorsiflexed, and with deep pressure over the Achilles tendon at its attachment to the calcaneus. A diagnosis of subtendinous calcaneal bursitis is made. Which of the following spinal cord segments receives most of the afferent impulses from the area of pain?

A. L4
B. L3
C. S1
D. S3
E. S2

90. A 20-year-old scholarship soccer player with pain in the left upper medial thigh of 10-day duration visits the orthopaedic clinic. She has stopped playing because the pain increases while running or changing direction suddenly. Physical examination leads to a diagnosis of a groin muscle strain. Which of the following muscles is likely causing most of the symptoms?

A. Adductor longus
B. Gracilis
C. Iliopsoas
D. Obturator externus
E. Pectineus

91. A 28-year-old woman undergoes a gracilis harvest for reconstructive surgery in her upper limb. Which of the following nerves provide motor innervation for the harvested muscle?

A. Femoral
B. Ilioinguinal
C. Medial cutaneous nerve of the thigh
D. Obturator
E. Saphenous

92. Two days after being fitted with a cast for a fractured right tibia and fibula, a 16-year-old boy presents with burning, numbness, and tingling along the anterolateral leg and the entire dorsum of the foot on the casted side. Following removal of the cast, dorsiflexion and extension of the toes is also weaker than on the non-casted side. None of these symptoms was present during initial treatment. The original cast extended from 3 cm below the knee joint line to the metatarsal-phalangeal joints. Which of the following best explains the cause for the current presentation?

A. The deep fibular nerve is involved in the callus formation as part of bone healing at a fracture site.

B. The rim of the cast at the metatarsal-phalangeal joints is compressing the terminal branches of superficial and deep fibular nerves.

C. The rim edge of the cast is compressing the common fibular nerve at the neck of the fibula.

D. The upper rim of the cast is compressing the tibial nerve in the popliteal fossa.

E. There is a vascular compromise involving the anterior tibial artery.

93. A 33-year-old woman is brought to the emergency department by ambulance from an automobile accident. She is complaining of severe pain in her right hip. Imaging reveals a comminuted fracture of the right acetabulum, including its posterior acetabular wall (refer to the accompanying image). Which of the following pelvic arteries is most vulnerable to bone fragments from the posterior wall fracture?

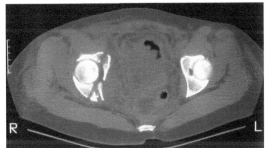

Source: Munk P, Ryan A. Teaching Atlas of Musculoskeletal Imaging. 1st Edition. Thieme; 2007

A. Common iliac

B. Internal pudendal

C. Superior gluteal

D. Superior vesical

E. Uterine

94. A 17-year-old varsity basketball player fell hard to her knees in a struggle for a rebound. She felt immediate pain in her right knee. The team physician administered the "drawer tests" at the sideline The "posterior drawer" test was positive with posterior displacement of the tibia with a soft endpoint. The test result suggests injury to which of the following knee structures?

A. Anterior cruciate ligament

B. Lateral collateral ligament

C. Medial collateral ligament

D. Medial meniscus

E. Posterior cruciate ligament

95. A college fraternity member jumped from the frat house portico to the ground. He landed on his feet and immediately experienced severe pain in his left foot. He walked with a limp and continued to experience pain. The next morning, he had a hematoma on the plantar surface of the foot. A radiograph of his left foot taken in the emergency department is shown in the following image. Which of the following tarsal bones (refer to the *arrow* in accompanying image) has been fractured in this patient?

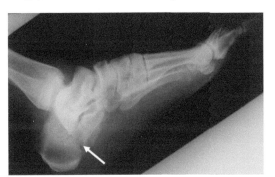

Source: Garcia G. RadCases: Musculoskeletal Radiology. 1st Edition. Thieme; 2010.

A. Calcaneus

B. Cuboid

C. Intermediate cuneiform

D. Medial cuneiform

E. Navicular

96. A 38-year-old multiparous woman describes to the physician a subcutaneous bulge in her left medial thigh. Physical examination reveals subcutaneous venous congestion in the area of the bulge. CT imaging reveals the neck of a hernia (refer to the accompanying image) lies medial to femoral vessels, posterior to the inguinal ligament, and anterior to the pubic bone. Which type of hernia is most likely present in this patient?

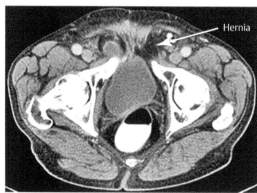

Source: Burgener F, Zaunbauer W, Meyers S et al. Differential Diagnosis in Computed Tomography. 2nd edition. Thieme; 2011.

A. Direct inguinal

B. Epigastric

C. Femoral

D. Indirect inguinal

E. Umbilical

97. A femoral arterial cannula is placed in a 58-year-old man. Adequate exposure requires that the surgeon incise an opaque fascial layer superficial to the artery. Which of the following is the fascial layer the surgeon incised?

A. Fascia lata

B. Lateral crus of inguinal ligament

C. Medial intermuscular septum of the thigh

D. Superficial fascia of the thigh

E. Transversalis fascia

98. An Army recruit in basic training experiences bilateral shin pain during marching and running. Muscles of the anterior legs are painful on palpation and dorsiflexion is weak bilaterally during the episodes. Venous congestion is one of the precipitating factors in this condition. Which of the following veins is compromised?

A. Anterior tibial

B. Great saphenous

C. Popliteal

D. Posterior tibial

E. Small saphenous

99. During a sandlot game of baseball, a 28-year-old man stepped on a stone and "twisted" his right ankle. He has difficulty walking without severe pain in his right foot. A teammate physical therapist performs the anterior drawer test of the ankle on the player's right ankle and found anterior displacement of the hindfoot with a soft endpoint. Injury to which of the following ligaments accounts for the test results?

A. Anterior talofibular

B. Anterior tibiofibular

C. Calcaneofibular

D. Posterior talofibular

E. Posterior tibiofibular

100. One month ago, an 87-year-old patient tripped over a bathmat, fell, and suffered an intracapsular fracture of her right femoral neck. At the time of the accident, the family elected to not have a surgical repair. She has had limited mobility since the accident. The accompanying image, showing necrosis in the femoral head, was taken yesterday. Which of the following is the parent artery that provides most blood to the area of necrosis?

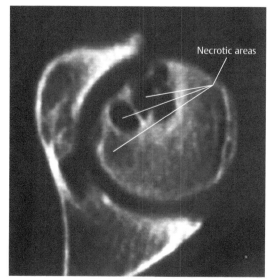

Source: Bohndorf K, Imhof H, Pope T. Musculoskeletal Imaging. A Concise Multimodality Approach. 1st Edition. Thieme; 2001.

A. Iliolumbar

B. Inferior gluteal

C. Internal iliac

D. Lateral circumflex femoral artery

E. Medial circumflex femoral artery

Consider the following case for questions 101 and 102:

A 10-year-old girl with cerebral palsy who has progressive difficulty with locomotion presents to the physician. Imaging reveals an angle of 115 degrees at the junction of the femoral neck with the shaft of her right femur.

101. Which of the following is the diagnosis from these results?

A. Hip dislocation

B. Coxa valga

C. Coxa vara

D. Genu valga

E. Genu vara

102. Which of the following knee ligaments is placed under most stress in the condition presented?

A. Anterior cruciate

B. Lateral collateral

C. Medial collateral

D. Patellofemoral

E. Posterior cruciate

103. One of Jayne's favorite pieces of equipment at the health club is the StairMaster which allows the user to climb an escalator-type stairway at variable speeds. Which of the following muscles is primarily responsible for hip extension during this activity?

A. Gluteus maximus

B. Gluteus medius

C. Piriformis

D. Psoas major

E. Tensor fasciae latae

104. During a scheduled annual physical examination of a 68-year-old man the physician cannot detect a pulse in the dorsalis pedis artery (dorsal artery of the foot). Which of the following tendons lies parallel and just medial to this artery?

A. Abductor hallucis

B. Extensor digitorum brevis

C. Extensor digitorum longus

D. Extensor hallucis longus

E. Tibialis anterior

105. The punter for a professional football team is writhing in pain on-field following a fourth down punt. Sideline evaluation by the team physician indicates palpation tenderness to the ischial tuberosity and proximal hamstring muscles. Which of the following muscles is most likely involved in this injury?

A. Adductor longus

B. Biceps femoris, long head

C. Biceps femoris, short head

D. Gluteus maximus

E. Gracilis

Consider the following case for questions 106 and 107:

A 53-year-old man with a history of latent tuberculosis is diagnosed with lumbar tuberculous osteomyelitis. Imaging reveals numerous abscesses in lumbar paraspinal tissues (refer to the *arrows* in the accompanying image). Musculoskeletal evaluation detects bilateral weak hip flexion, and neurological evaluation reveals a diminished patellar tendon reflex.

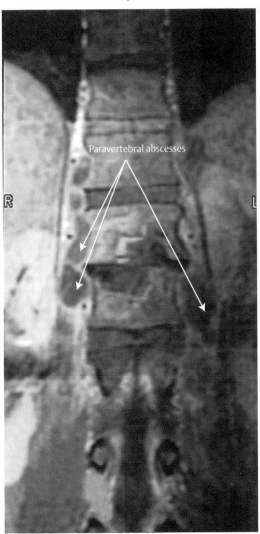

Source: Meyers S. MRI of Bone and Soft Tissue Tumors and Tumorlike Lesions. 1st Edition. Stuttgart: Thieme; 2007

106. Which of the following muscles would be involved as revealed by the musculoskeletal evaluation and accompanying image?

A. Diaphragm

B. Iliacus

C. Obturator internus

D. Piriformis

E. Psoas major

107. Which of the following spinal cord segments receives afferent impulses for the diminished tendon reflex observed in the patient?

A. L1

B. L4

C. L5

D. S1

E. T12

108. A surgery clerk observes that, during preparation for surgery, a patient is given an intramuscular injection to the buttocks. The needle is placed in the upper lateral quadrant (ventrogluteal) of the buttocks, with the patient lying on their side. Into which of the following muscles is the medication injected?

A. Gluteus maximus

B. Gluteus medius

C. Gluteus minimus

D. Sartorius

E. Tensor fasciae latae

109. A saphenous cutdown is performed on a hospitalized obese patient in order to administer electrolytes. Which of the following bony landmarks is reliable for identifying the location of the vein for this procedure?

A. Adductor tubercle

B. Medial border of patella

C. Medial malleolus

D. Sustentaculum tali

E. Tibial tuberosity

110. In preparation for coronary artery angiography on a 61-year-old man, a catheter is inserted in the femoral artery in the femoral triangle. The surface projection of a pulse in this artery can be located equidistant between which bony landmarks?

A. Anterior inferior iliac spine and anterior superior iliac spine

B. Anterior inferior iliac spine and pubic symphysis

C. Anterior inferior iliac spine and pubic tubercle

D. Anterior superior iliac spine and pubic symphysis

E. Anterior superior iliac spine and pubic tubercle

111. A 57-year-old woman with swelling and tenderness on the posteromedial aspect of her right knee visits her family physician. An axial MRI, with T2 weighting of the affected knee reveals a synovial popliteal (Baker's) cyst (refer to the accompanying image). Which of the following muscles is the cystic bursa most likely associated with?

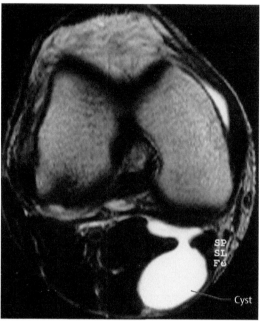

Source: Vahlensieck M, Reiser M. MRT des Bewegungsapparates. 3rd edition. Stuttgart: Thieme; 2006

A. Biceps femoris, long head

B. Biceps femoris, short head

C. Popliteus

D. Semimembranosus

E. Soleus

112. A 36-year-old man with a BMI of 35+ (adjusted for height and weight) and symptoms of numbness and tingling sensations along his right lateral thigh comes to the physician. The nerve causing the symptoms is a branch of which of the following?

A. Femoral

B. Inferior gluteal

C. Lumbar plexus

D. Obturator

E. Subcostal

113. A 43-year-old multiparous woman with pain, numbness, and muscle weakness in her left thigh comes to the physician. She weighs 45 kg (99 lb) with a BMI of 18 (adjusted for height and weight). During the physical examination, she exhibits a positive Howship–Romberg sign (pain while supine with the thigh flexed, adducted, and laterally [externally] rotated). In this position, a mass can be palpated in her left, proximal, medial thigh. The examination also reveals the pain and paraesthesia extends along the inner aspect of the thigh, down to the knee. Which of the following nerves is being compressed by the mass to give the clinical signs?

A. Femoral

B. Genitofemoral

C. Ilioinguinal

D. Medial femoral cutaneous

E. Obturator

114. A 29-year-old man with pain in his left buttock and posterior thigh, radiating as far as the knee comes to the physician. He is an investment broker and spends most of his day at his desk, but competes in trail races two or three times each month. Deep pressure to the left buttock produces a pain reflex. Radiographic imaging of his lower spine shows no pathology. Based on the evidence available, which of the following conditions does this man most likely have?

A. Compression of L5 spinal nerve by a herniated intervertebral disk

B. Compression of L4 spinal nerve by a herniated intervertebral disk

C. Compression of sciatic nerve by piriformis muscle in the greater sciatic foramen

D. Compression of superior gluteal nerve by piriformis muscle in greater sciatic foramen

E. Intrapelvic separation of the components of sciatic nerve (tibial and common fibular)

115. A 72-year-old man indicates for the physician that he has for years walked daily in his neighborhood. Recently, he has begun to experience severe pain in his right posterior calf region during the walks. If he stops walking for a few minutes, the pain subsides until he resumes walking. MRI of his right leg shows sclerotic buildup in the popliteal artery. Which of the following muscles is most likely involved in the pain this patient is experiencing?

A. Adductor magnus, hamstring part

B. Extensor digitorum longus

C. Fibularis tertius

D. Popliteus

E. Soleus

116. A 27-year-old man with symptoms of numbness and tingling in his right medial thigh comes to the physician. Which of the following dermatomes are represented in the area of symptoms (outlined in *red* and indicated by the *arrow* in the accompanying image)?

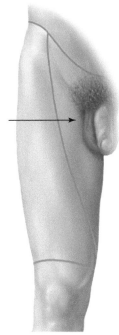

Source: Gilroy AM et al. Atlas of Anatomy. 3rd ed. 2016. Based on: Schuenke M, Schulte E, Schumacher U. THIEME Atlas of Anatomy. Volumes 1-3. Illustrations by Voll M and Wesker K. 2nd ed. New York: Thieme Medical Publishers; 2016

A. L1–L3

B. L3–L5

C. T11–L1

D. T10–T12

E. T12–L2

117. A 44-year-old woman has undergone internal iliac lymph node resection related to carcinoma of the uterine cervix. At her 1-month postoperative appointment she relates that she has stopped driving her car as she has difficulty moving her right foot from the accelerator pedal to the brake. Which of the following nerves was most likely injured iatrogenically during the lymph node resection?

A. Femoral

B. Genitofemoral

C. Ilioinguinal

D. Lumbosacral trunk

E. Obturator

63

118. The parents of a 3-year-old girl bring her to the physician with concern that she has bilateral flat feet (pes planus). Physical examination confirms that a longitudinal arch is not well formed. All other aspects of the child's musculoskeletal evaluation are within normal ranges. Which of the following is the diagnosis for this patient?

A. Normal; the longitudinal arches are not fully formed until age 5

B. Pes planus due to improper footwear

C. Pes planus due to malformed tarsal bones

D. Pes planus due to weak ligaments in the foot

E. Pes planus due to weak muscles of the anterior and posterior leg

119. An 18-year-old woman who plays soccer is brought to the emergency department with a laterally dislocated right patella. A medical history reveals that she has chronic pain in this knee and the patella has subluxed previously. Her medical records indicate that 6 months ago her Q-angle (quadriceps femoris muscle angle) for the right limb was determined to be 190 degrees. The patellofemoral articulation is restored and, as an alternative to surgical intervention for permanent resolution, the patient is referred for physical therapy. Which of the following muscles will the physician prescribe the physical therapist to target in this patient?

A. Rectus femoris

B. The entire quadriceps femoris complex

C. Vastus intermedius

D. Vastus lateralis

E. Vastus medialis

120. A 58-year-old woman is brought to the emergency department with her left knee locked at 30 degrees of flexion. She relates that she was descending a set of stairs at her home when she suddenly experienced sharp pain in the knee which quickly progressed to the presenting condition. She has no history of joint disease. During the physical examination, attempts to flex or extend the left knee produced intense pain. Imaging reveals a small foreign body lodged between the articular surface of the left medial femoral condyle and the corresponding tibial articular surface. Which of the following is the most likely source of the foreign body in this patient?

A. Anterior cruciate ligament

B. Medial collateral ligament

C. Medial meniscus

D. Posterior cruciate ligament

121. A 65-year-old man with a history of blunt trauma to his left gluteal region in a motorcycle accident presents to his primary care provider. He reports persistent pain of almost 2-year duration from his sacrum to his left hip that also radiates down his posterior thigh. On physical examination, pain is elicited with passive internal rotation of the hip (Freiburg's sign) and piriformis syndrome is suspected. Which of the following nerves is most likely entrapped in this individual?

A. Nerve to obturator internus

B. Nerve to piriformis

C. Pudendal

D. Sciatic

E. Superior gluteal

Head and Neck

122. A 49-year-old woman presents to the dental clinic with a painful click in her left jaw when she opens her mouth. Which of the following muscles is primarily responsible for moving the jaw into the position that causes the pain?

A. Digastric

B. Lateral pterygoid

C. Masseter

D. Medial pterygoid

E. Temporalis

123. A 38-year-old man comes to the emergency department with his mandible protracted and mouth open. Attempts to close his mouth produce severe pain in his jaw. Imaging reveals the head of the mandible is anterior to the articular tubercle bilaterally. The tubercle observed in the imaging belongs to which of the following bones?

A. Maxilla

B. Occipital

C. Sphenoid

D. Temporal

E. Zygomatic

124. Two days following a minor automobile accident, a 43-year-old woman is brought to the emergency department with pain on the left side of her neck. Her head is tilted to the left and her face is directed slightly in the opposite direction (refer to the accompanying image). Attempts to return the head to the neutral position produce pain. Imaging shows no skeletal pathology. Which of the following provides innervation for the muscle that has placed the patient's head in this position?

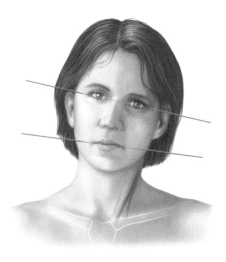

Source: Schuenke M, Schulte E, Schumacher U. THIEME Atlas of Anatomy. Head, Neck, and Neuroanatomy. Illustrations by Voll M and Wesker K. 2nd ed. New York: Thieme Medical Publishers; 2016

A. Accessory (CN XI)

B. Ansa cervicalis

C. Lesser occipital

D. Transverse cervical

E. Vagus (CN X)

125. It is determined that a tracheostomy is needed on a hospitalized patient with breathing difficulty. The senior resident retracts the infrahyoid muscles laterally to expose the thyroid isthmus and trachea. Which of the following muscles is most superficial in the area of the operation?

A. Cricothyroid

B. Mylohyoid

C. Sternohyoid

D. Sternothyroid

E. Thyrohyoid

126. While stopped for a traffic signal in his classic vehicle, a 34-year-old driver is hit from behind by another vehicle. Eighteen hours later, he presents with neck and upper back pain to the physician. Imaging shows no skeletal pathology. Which of the following ligaments is most vulnerable to injury in accidents of this type?

A. Alar ligaments

B. Anterior longitudinal ligament

C. Ligamenta flava

D. Posterior longitudinal ligament

E. Transverse ligament of atlas

127. A 61-year-old man with a long history of cigarette smoking is diagnosed with carcinoma in the left main bronchus. Which of the following muscles on the left side is most likely to have its nerve supply compromised?

A. Cricothyroid

B. Lateral cricoarytenoid

C. Omohyoid

D. Sternothyroid

E. Thyrohyoid

128. A 39-year-old woman presents with the following visual pattern (refer to the accompanying image). Which of the following extraocular muscles is not functioning properly in her right eye?

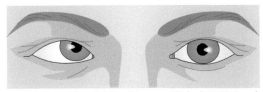

Source: Gilroy AM et al. Atlas of Anatomy. 3rd ed. 2016. Based on: Schuenke M, Schulte E, Schumacher U. THIEME Atlas of Anatomy. Volumes 1-3. Illustrations by Voll M and Wesker K. 2nd ed. New York: Thieme Medical Publishers; 2016

A. Inferior oblique

B. Inferior rectus

C. Medial rectus

D. Lateral rectus

E. Superior oblique

129. A 79-year-old woman comes to the physician for a scheduled annual checkup. As part of the neurological evaluation, the woman is asked to protrude her tongue. The tongue deviates to the patient's left side. Which of the following muscles is not functioning properly in this patient?

A. Left genioglossus

B. Left hyoglossus

C. Right genioglossus

D. Right hyoglossus

E. Right styloglossus

130. In preparation for surgery to remove an impacted right mandibular third molar, anesthetic is injected in the area of the mandibular foramen. Which of the following muscles may have its motor innervation compromised by anesthetic injected in this area?

A. Digastric, anterior belly

B. Genioglossus

C. Geniohyoid

D. Lateral pterygoid

E. Stylohyoid

131. A 19-year-old woman was playing softball with friends when she was struck in her left eye by a thrown ball. The accompanying coronal CT image was taken on arrival at the emergency department. Which of the following bones has been compromised in the area of trauma?

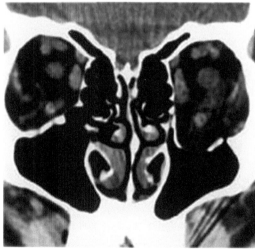

Source: Valvassori G, Mafee M, Becker M. Imaging of the Head and Neck. 2nd Edition. Thieme; 2004.

A. Ethmoid

B. Frontal

C. Lacrimal

D. Maxilla

E. Sphenoid

132. A 51-year-old man with complaints of chronic sinus infections and headaches presents to the physician. A coronal CT image from this patient is shown (refer to the accompanying image). Which of the following is indicated by the arrow numbered "6"?

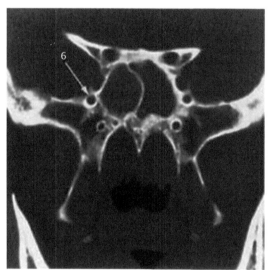

Source: Valvassori G, Mafee M, Becker M. Imaging of the Head and Neck. 2nd Edition. Thieme; 2004.

A. Infraorbital foramen

B. Foramen ovale

C. Foramen rotundum

D. Foramen spinosum

E. Pterygoid canal

133. During the routine 1-month evaluation of an infant, the physician notes in the patient's chart that the anterior fontanelle is normal. Which of the following represents the age by which this fontanelle would be expected to be closed?

A. Eight months

B. Eighteen months

C. Four months

D. Six months

E. Two years

134. A 7-year-old boy enjoys entertaining his younger siblings by rolling his tongue into a tube. Which of the following muscles dominate to allow the boy to exhibit this tongue movement?

A. Genioglossus

B. Hyoglossus

C. Intrinsic tongue muscles

D. Palatoglossus

E. Styloglossus

135. An 81-year-old man with progressive difficulty swallowing presents to his physician. The man's wife tells the physician that her husband has foul breath. A radiograph following a barium swallow reveals a pharyngoesophageal diverticulum (see the *asterisk* in the accompanying image). Which of the following represents the most likely vertebral level for the diverticulum in this patient?

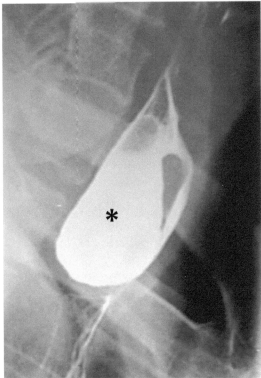

Source: Mukherji S, Chong V. Atlas of Head and Neck Imaging: The Extracranial Head and Neck. 1st Edition. Thieme; 2003.

A. C3

B. C4

C. C5

D. C6

E. C7

136. A 54-year-old woman, a chronic smoker, presents with sudden-onset voice hoarseness to her physician. She is referred for bronchoscopy and the examiner observes that the right vocal cord is midline and the left one is abducted. Which of the following muscles accounts for the observation made on the left side?

A. Arytenoid, transverse fibers

B. Lateral cricoarytenoid

C. Posterior cricoarytenoid

D. Thyroarytenoid

E. Vocalis

137. A 26-year-old man is brought to the emergency department with difficulty swallowing and pain when he rotates his head. One hour prior, he received a kick to the anterior neck during a mixed martial arts competition. Imaging reveals a fracture to the right greater cornu of the hyoid. Trauma to which of the following muscles could account for difficulty swallowing in this patient?

A. Geniohyoid

B. Middle pharyngeal constrictor

C. Omohyoid

D. Sternohyoid

E. Thyrohyoid

138. A 38-year-old woman with chronic throat discomfort when swallowing presents to an otolaryngologist. CT imaging shows considerable ossification of the stylohyoid ligament, causing elongation of the styloid process (refer to the accompanying image). Which of the following is the developmental origin for the ossified ligament seen in this patient?

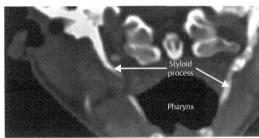

Source: Freyschmidt J, Wiens J, Brossmann J et al. Borderlands of Normal and Early Pathological Findings in Skeletal Radiography. 5th revised Edition. Thieme; 2002.

A. Fourth through sixth pharyngeal arches

B. Mandibular division of first pharyngeal arch

C. Maxillary division of second pharyngeal arch

D. Second pharyngeal arch

E. Third pharyngeal arch

139. A 38-year-old man with difficulty breathing through his right nostril presents to the family medicine clinic. He is aware that he snores and his phonation is somewhat muffled. Rhinologic examination reveals a deviated nasal septum. Which of the following bones forms the superior (upper) portion of the abnormal tissue in this patient?

A. Ethmoid

B. Maxilla

C. Nasal

D. Palatine

E. Vomer

140. A 22-year-old man is brought to the emergency department following an altercation at a bar. There is evidence of facial trauma, and his chin deviates downward when his mouth is closed. Imaging reveals bilateral fracture of the body of the mandible. Which of the following muscles is producing the deviation of the patient's chin?

A. Digastric

B. Lateral pterygoid

C. Masseter

D. Medial pterygoid

E. Temporalis

141. The 38-year-old man is brought to the emergency department after being rescued by companions after he dived from a dock into shallow water. He complains of severe neck pain. Axial CT imaging reveals a midline fracture of the anterior arch of the atlas vertebra (C1) and bilateral fractures to the posterior arch (refer to the accompaying image). Which of the following is the structure labeled "1" in the patient's CT?

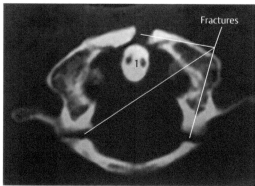

Source: Freyschmidt J, Wiens J, Brossmann J et al. Borderlands of Normal and Early Pathological Findings in Skeletal Radiography. 5th revised Edition. Thieme; 2002.

A. Displaced body of atlas vertebra (C1)

B. External occipital protuberance

C. Odontoid process

D. Part of the right occipital condyle

E. Vertebral arteries joining to form basilar artery

142. During the routine neurological evaluation of a 48-year-old woman, the physician observes that the soft palate and uvula deviate to the right when the gag reflex is stimulated. Follow-up CT imaging reveals a mass at the base of the skull near the left jugular foramen. Compression of which of the following cranial nerves could account for the deviation observed in this patient?

A. Accessory (CN XI)

B. Facial (CN VII)

C. Glossopharyngeal (CN IX)

D. Hypoglossal (CN XII)

E. Vagus (CN X)

143. A 17-year-old male comes to the emergency department with bilateral posterior neck pain after a weekend of playing video games on a wall-mounted monitor. Palpation of the upper neck and superior nuchal line, as well as asking the patient to look at the ceiling, all produce pain reflexes. Rotation of the head produces pain on the same side as the direction of rotation. Which of the following muscles has been strained in this patient?

A. Longus capitis

B. Occipitofrontalis

C. Splenius capitis

D. Sternocleidomastoid

E. Trapezius

Thorax

144. As a surgeon supervises a resident's placement of a drain tube in the posterior axillary line in the eighth intercostal space, he asks the resident to describe the layers of the thoracic wall that will be pierced. Between which of the following layers will vessels and nerves be located at the point of placement of the drain tube?

A. Endothoracic fascia and parietal pleura

B. Endothoracic fascia and visceral pleura

C. External intercostal and internal intercostal

D. Innermost intercostal and endothoracic fascia

E. Internal intercostal and innermost intercostal

145. A 38-year-old man is admitted to the emergency department with recent onset of numbness and tingling of his right upper limb. Imaging reveals a constriction in the right subclavian artery as it crosses rib 1. Which of the following represents the order, anterior to posterior, of structures in the area of vascular constriction?

A. Anterior scalene muscle, subclavian vein, middle scalene muscle, subclavian artery

B. Anterior scalene muscle, subclavian vein, subclavian artery, middle scalene muscle

C. Subclavian artery, anterior scalene muscle, subclavian vein, middle scalene muscle

D. Subclavian vein, anterior scalene muscle, subclavian artery, middle scalene muscle

E. Subclavian vein, subclavian artery, anterior scalene, middle scalene artery

146. A 44-year-old man tells the physician of the recent self-discovery of a hard lump "over my stomach." Physical examination reveals a hard but painless, midline, subcutaneous mass just distal to the body of the sternum. Which of the following is the most likely explanation for the palpable mass?

A. A mass on the lesser curvature of the stomach

B. A pleural adhesion to the distal sternum

C. Dislocation of a 7th costal cartilage from the sternum

D. Inflammation of the xiphisternal joint

E. Partial ossification of the xiphoid process

Abdomen

147. A 61-year-old man undergoes surgical repair for a direct inguinal hernia. The surgeon confirms the patient's hernia passes inferior to the conjoint tendon. Which of the following aponeurotic layers contribute to this tendon?

A. External abdominal oblique and internal abdominal oblique

B. External abdominal oblique and transversus abdominis

C. Internal abdominal oblique and transversus abdominis

D. Transversus abdominis and pyramidalis

E. Transversus abdominis and rectus abdominis

148. A 29-year-old female in the 41st week of pregnancy is scheduled for a cesarean delivery. During the procedure, a low transverse abdominal incision is made 1 to 2 cm superior to the mons pubis (incision known as a Phannenstiel or bikini line incision). Once the incision has passed through deepest layer of muscle, which of the following would be the next layer encountered?

A. Aponeurosis of transversus abdominis muscle

B. Broad ligament of the uterus

C. Parietal peritoneum

D. Transversalis fascia

E. Visceral peritoneum

149. A 44-year-old woman presents with frequent episodes of heartburn and abdominal discomfort to her primary care physician. Imaging with a barium swallow is shown in the following image. A diagnosis of paraesophageal hiatal hernia is made. Which of the following parts of the diaphragm did the hernia pass through to enter the thoracic cavity?

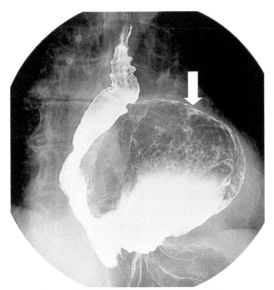

Source: Lorenz J. RadCases. Gastrointestinal Imaging. 1st Edition. Thieme; 2010.

A. Central tendon

B. Left crus

C. Muscular part of the left dome

D. Muscular part of the right dome

E. Right crus

150. A 47-year-old woman is prepared for a laparoscopic cholecystectomy (gallbladder removal). The paraumbilical region is anesthetized. Which of the following dermatomes is involved in the area of anesthesia?

A. L1

B. L2

C. T8

D. T10

E. T12

151. During vasectomy on a 39-year-old, the surgeon notes longitudinal fascicles of cremaster muscle in the spermatic cord. Which of the following muscles is the original source of the fibers observed?

A. Dartos

B. External abdominal oblique

C. Internal abdominal oblique

D. Rectus abdominis

E. Transversus abdominis

152. Following resection of the large intestine, an ileostomy is performed on a 51-year-old woman. While making the incision in the lower right quadrant of the anterior abdominal wall, the surgeon notes that the muscle fibers of one of the layers being incised are oriented in an inferomedial direction. Which of the following muscles has the surgeon observed?

A. External abdominal oblique

B. Internal abdominal oblique

C. Latissimus dorsi

D. Quadratus lumborum

E. Transversus abdominis

Consider the following case for questions 153 and 154:

A 23-year-old man presents with pain in the right inguinal region when he bends over (forwards) or lifts heavy items. Physical examination in the area of pain detects a bulge that extends into the scrotum. The patient's age and physical examination result in a diagnosis of an indirect inguinal hernia on the right side. The patient is scheduled for herniorrhaphy (surgical repair of the hernia).

153. At which of the following locations will the surgeon locate the extraperitoneal fat layer?

A. Between the internal and external oblique muscles

B. Deep to the parietal peritoneum

C. Deep to the transversalis fascia

D. Superficial to Camper's fascia

E. Superficial to Scarpa's' fascia

154. After surgery, the patient complains of severe right inguinal pain radiating to the medial and lateral aspect of his right thigh. Walking and hyperextension of the hip increases the pain. Ilioinguinal nerve entrapment is suspected and a second surgery is performed. During the second surgery, at which of the following locations would the surgeon locate the involved nerve?

A. Between the internal oblique and transversus abdominis muscles

B. Between the parietal peritoneum and extraperitoneal fat

C. Between the parietal peritoneum and visceral peritoneum

D. Deep to the parietal peritoneum

E. Deep to the transversalis fascia

155. A 54-year-old man with a bulge in his right groin, which is painful when he bends over, presents to a primary care physician. The swelling was first discovered several months ago when he attempted to lift a heavy object and it has progressively increased in size since. Physical examination reveals a swelling in the right inguinal region medial to the pubic tubercle, and ultrasound confirms a diagnosis of a direct inguinal hernia. Which of the following fossae is the hernia passing through in this patient?

A. Iliac

B. Ischioanal

C. Lateral inguinal

D. Medial inguinal

E. Supravesical

156. A 25-year-old man presents with a bulge in his right groin that is subsequently diagnosed as an indirect inguinal hernia associated with a patent processus vaginalis. The lumen of the patent structure in this patient has open communication with which of the following?

A. Cecum

B. Peritoneal cavity

C. Retroperitoneal space

D. Sigmoid colon

E. Urinary bladder

157. During a pre-participation physical examination of a 15-year-old boy, the physician involutes the skin of the scrotum with an index finger in an upward direction along the spermatic cord. The tip of the finger is placed just lateral to the pubic tubercle. At this stage, the physician asks the boy to cough. What structure did the physician palpate during this procedure to assess for a potential hernia?

A. Conjoint tendon

B. Normal testicle

C. Penis

D. Superficial inguinal ring

E. Suspensory ligament of penis

158. A 32-year-old woman presents with a swelling on the anterior abdominal wall. The patient history shows that she had previous abdominal surgery. Physical examination reveals a swelling between the two rectus abdominis muscles, superior to the umbilicus. A diagnosis of incisional hernia is made. Weakness in which of the following structures is most likely responsible for this hernia?

A. Arcuate line

B. Linea alba

C. Linea nigra

D. Semilunar line

E. Tendinous intersection

159. A 41-year-old man with a fever is diagnosed with a right-side psoas abscess. CT-guided percutaneous drainage is performed and culture of the fluid obtained from the abscess detects several species of *Peptostreptococcus*. After the procedure, the patient complains of numbness over the right femoral triangle. Stroking the medial side of the right thigh fails to elicit elevation of the testes. Which of the following nerves was most likely iatrogenically injured in this patient?

A. Femoral
B. Genitofemoral
C. Lateral cutaneous nerve of the thigh
D. Obturator
E. Subcostal

Pelvis and Perineum

160. A 49-year-old woman with recent onset of perianal pain that becomes intense during a bowel movement visits her gynecologist. She relates feeling tired the past few days and her current body temperature is 37.5°C. The perianal skin on the right side is reddened and tender to the touch. Ultrasound indicates an abscess in the ischioanal fossa on the right. During surgical treatment for the abscess the surgeon notes several small nerves. These nerves will be derived from which of the following spinal cord segments?

A. L3–L5
B. S1–S3
C. S2–S4
D. S3–S5
E. S5 only

161. A 41-year-old man with a spinal cord transection has an inflatable penile prosthesis surgically implanted. During the surgery the physician partially retracts a muscle on each crus of the penis. Which of the following muscles did the surgeon retract?

A. Bulbospongiosus
B. External urethral sphincter
C. Ischiocavernosus
D. Pubococcygeus part of levator ani
E. Superficial transverse perinei

162. A 48-year-old multiparous woman who experiences leakage of urine during physical activity visits the urology clinic. The uncontrollable urine loss also may occur when she sneezes or laughs. Compromise to which of the following muscles is primarily responsible for the patient's symptoms?

A. Bulbospongiosus
B. External urethral sphincter
C. Internal urethral sphincter
D. Ischiococcygeus
E. Levator ani

163. A 32-year-old woman comes to her obstetrician believing she is in the early weeks of pregnancy. Her suspicions are confirmed by a positive test for human chorionic gonadotropin. During physical examination, the obstetrician determines the diagonal conjugate dimension of her pelvis. This pelvic dimension is measured between which of the following bony features?

A. Ischial spine to the opposite ischial spine
B. Sacral promontory to inferior edge of the pubic symphysis
C. Sacral promontory to pubic tubercle
D. Tip of coccyx to ischial spine
E. Tip of coccyx to pubic tubercle

164. Rapid onset of labor in a term pregnancy of a 28-year-old results in delivery at home without medical personnel present. Evaluation of the woman later at hospital reveals some tearing of perineal tissues. Which of the following muscles is most vulnerable to damage in this patient?

A. Internal anal sphincter
B. Ischiococcygeus
C. Obturator internus
D. Piriformis
E. Pubococcygeus

165. A 27-year-old is planning her first pregnancy and the accompanying plain radiograph was recorded to establish her obstetrical conjugate diameter. Which of the following bone(s) border the foramen labelled "1" on the following image?

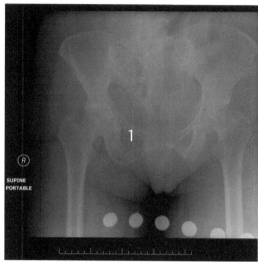

Source: Yu E, Jaffer N, Chung T et al. RadCases. Emergency Radiology. 1st Edition. Thieme; 2015.

A. Ilium

B. Ischium

C. Pubis

D. Pubis and ischium

E. Pubis, ischium, and ilium

166. A hunter discovered human skeletal remains in a remote wooded area. After examining the pelvic bones, the forensic pathologist determined that the deceased was female. Which of the following most closely represents angle of the pubic arch found on this skeleton?

A. 45 degrees

B. 65 degrees

C. 75 degrees

D. 90 degrees

E. 120 degrees

2.2 Answers and Explanations

Easy	Medium	Hard

Upper Limb

1.   Correct: Median (B)

Refer to the following image for answer 1:

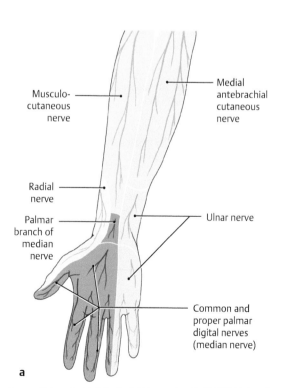

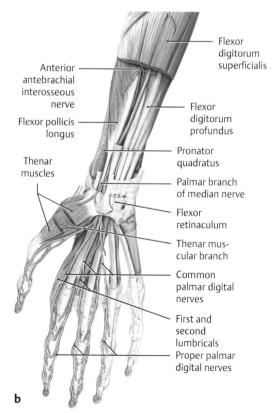

Source: Schuenke M, Schulte E, Schumacher U. THIEME Atlas of Anatomy. General Anatomy and Musculoskeletal System. Illustrations by Voll M and Wesker K. 2nd ed. New York: Thiem

(**B**) The median nerve supplies skin on the lateral (radial) palmar aspect of the hand, including the lateral three and a half digits (including the posterior aspects of the fingertips). It also innervates the thenar muscles and the first and second lumbricals. The opponens pollicis, one of the thenar muscles, is the only muscle that produces thumb opposition. (**A**) The anterior interosseous nerve supplies muscles in the deep anterior forearm: flexor pollicis longus, the lateral portion of flexor digitorum profundus, and pronator quadratus. It does not have a cutaneous distribution. (**C**) The posterior interosseous nerve supplies muscles in the posterior forearm: extensor carpi ulnaris, extensor digitorum, extensor digiti minimi, extensor indicis, and the snuff box muscles (abductor pollicis longus, extensor pollicis longus, extensor pollicis brevis). It does not have a cutaneous distribution. (**D**) The superficial branch of the radial nerve supplies skin on the dorsolateral aspect of the hand and lateral three and a half digits. (**E**) The ulnar nerve supplies most of the intrinsic hand muscles (hypothenar muscles, adductor pollicis, lumbricals 3 and 4, and all interossei) and skin on the medial hand, including the medial one and a half fingers.

2. Correct: Median nerve (A)

(**A**) The MRI shows the median nerve in the anterolateral aspect of the carpal tunnel, just deep to the flexor retinaculum (transverse carpal ligament). In this case, the nerve's increased signal and appearance as distinct fascicles indicates edema. (**B, D, E**) The tendons of flexor carpi radialis and palmaris longus, as well as the ulnar nerve, do not pass through the carpal tunnel. (**C**) The tendon of flexor pollicis longus is located medially within the carpal tunnel, but posterior to the median nerve. Because of collagen and water content, normal tendons appear with a low signal intensity (i.e., black).

Refer to the following images for answer 2:

Image key: H, hamate; Tm, trapezium.

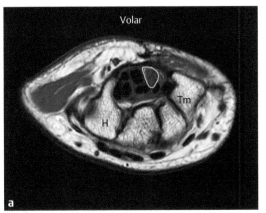

Source: Image provided courtesy of Department of Radiology, William Beaumont Hospital.

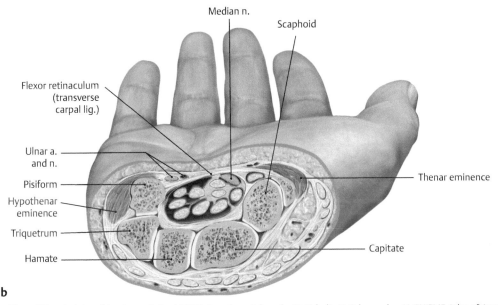

Source: Gilroy AM et al. Atlas of Anatomy. 3rd ed. 2016. Based on: Schuenke M, Schulte E, Schumacher U. THIEME Atlas of Anatomy. Volumes 1-3. Illustrations by Voll M and Wesker K. 2nd ed. New York: Thieme Medical Publishers; 2016

3. Correct: Carpal tunnel syndrome (A)

(**A**) Carpal tunnel syndrome results from compression of structures that pass through the carpal tunnel, with the median nerve most vulnerable. Carpal tunnel syndrome, a distal median nerve lesion, is the most common compression syndrome affecting the median nerve. Distal median nerve lesions present with sensory disturbances (anesthesia, hypesthesia, and/or paresthesia) from the lateral three and a half fingers and weakness of the thenar muscles and lateral two lumbricals, which can atrophy with time. (**B**) Dupuytren contracture is caused by thickening of the palmar fascia, which results in partial flexion of the metacarpophalangeal and proximal phalangeal joints of the 4th and 5th fingers. (**C**) Fracture of the hook of the hamate is generally associated with palmar pain that is aggravated by hand gripping and with flexion of the ring and little fingers. (**D**) Scaphoid fracture is typically associated with pain over the anatomical snuff box. (**E**) Ulnar (Guyon's) canal syndrome affects the ulnar nerve as it passes through a superficial passage in the flexor retinaculum. Distal to this point, the nerve affects only structures in the hand: sensory to the medial one and a half fingers and motor to most intrinsic hand muscles.

4. Correct: Ulnar (E)

(**E**) The ulnar nerve supplies most intrinsic hand muscles (hypothenar muscles, adductor pollicis, third and fourth lumbricals, and all interossei) and skin on the medial hand, including the medial one and a half fingers. (**A**) The anterior interosseous nerve supplies muscles in the deep anterior forearm: flexor pollicis longus, lateral half of flexor digitorum profundus, and pronator quadratus. It does not have a cutaneous distribution. (**B**) The median nerve supplies skin on the lateral palmar aspect of the hand, including the lateral three and a half digits (including the posterior aspects of the fingertips), and innervates the thenar muscles and the 1st and 2nd lumbricals. (**C**) The posterior interosseous nerve supplies muscles in the posterior forearm: extensor carpi ulnaris, extensor digitorum, extensor digiti minimi, extensor indicis, and the snuff box muscles (abductor pollicis longus, extensor pollicis longus, extensor pollicis brevis). It does not have a cutaneous distribution. (**D**) The superficial branch of the radial nerve supplies skin on the dorsolateral aspect of the hand and lateral three and a half fingers.

Refer to the following image for answer 4:

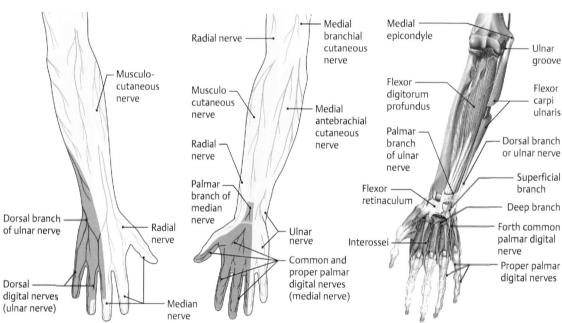

Source: Schuenke M, Schulte E, Schumacher U. THIEME Atlas of Anatomy. General Anatomy and Musculoskeletal System. Illustrations by Voll M and Wesker K. 2nd ed. New York: Thieme Medical Publishers; 2016

5. Correct: Flexor carpi ulnaris (B)

Refer to the following image for answer 5:

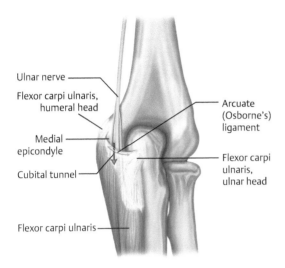

(**B**) The cubital tunnel is a passage for the ulnar nerve posterior to the elbow. It is formed by the medial epicondyle and an arching, fibrous band referred to as the arcuate (Osborne's) ligament between the humeral and ulnar heads of flexor carpi ulnaris. It is a proximal site of compression of the ulnar nerve. A positive Tinel's sign (light percussion over a compressed nerve that elicits paresthesia) at this location is typically observed. (**A, C–E**) The flexor carpi radialis, flexor digitorum profundus, pronator teres and supinator muscles do not contribute to the cubital tunnel.

6. Correct: Latissimus dorsi (A)

(**A**) The patient experiences a combination of weakness in extension, medial rotation, and adduction of her arm. Assuming damage to a single nerve, only paralysis of the latissimus dorsi would affect all of the involved actions. (**B**) The serratus anterior protracts (abducts) the scapula and rotates the scapula superiorly to assist in raising the arm above 90 degrees. (**C**) The subscapularis rotates the arm medially. (**D**) The supraspinatus abducts the arm. It is innervated by the suprascapular nerve, which originates from the superior trunk of the brachial plexus and, as such, would not be affected by an axillary surgical procedure. (**E**) The teres minor acts primarily to rotate the arm laterally. It is also a weak adductor of the arm.

7. Correct: Thoracodorsal (D)

Refer to the following image for answer 7:

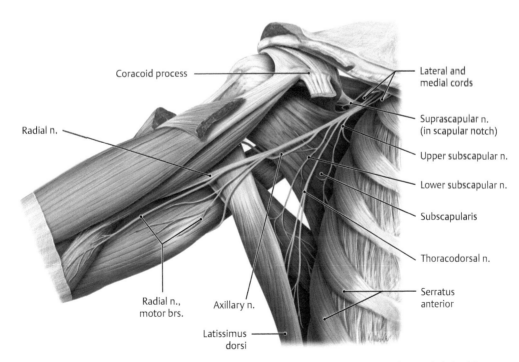

Source: Schuenke M, Schulte E, Schumacher U. THIEME Atlas of Anatomy. General Anatomy and Musculoskeletal System. Illustrations by Voll M and Wesker K. 2nd ed. New York: Thieme Medical Publishers; 2016

(**D**) The thoracodorsal nerve originates in the axilla from the posterior cord of the brachial plexus and passes inferiorly to latissimus dorsi, which produces extension, medial rotation, and adduction of the arm—all actions that are weak in this patient. Dissection of axillary lymph nodes may result in iatrogenic injury of the thoracodorsal nerve. (**A**) The dorsal scapular nerve, a supraclavicular branch of the brachial plexus that arises from the C5 trunk, does not pass through the axilla. Therefore, it is not susceptible to injury with axillary surgery. (**B**) The long thoracic nerve may also be injured during the surgery, which could result in weakened scapular abduction (protraction) and superior rotation (e.g., when raising the arm over the head). The typical clinical presentation known as "winged scapula" may be elicited with injury of the long thoracic nerve. (**C**) The suprascapular nerve, a supraclavicular branch of the brachial plexus that arises from the superior trunk, does not pass through the axilla. Therefore, it is not susceptible to injury with axillary surgery. (**E**) The upper subscapular nerve arises from the posterior cord, just proximal to the thoracodorsal nerve. Although susceptible to injury with axillary surgery, it would affect medial rotation of the arm only (subscapularis muscle).

8. Correct: Axillary (A)

(**A**) Although axillary nerve injury following anterior shoulder dislocation is rare, injury of this nerve is possible because of its relationship to the antero-inferior aspect of the glenohumeral joint capsule as it passes through the quadrangular space. Weakness of arm abduction following this type of dislocation is, therefore, consistent with involvement of the deltoid muscle, especially between 30 and 90 degrees of abduction where it becomes active after initiation of abduction by supraspinatus (innervated by the suprascapular nerve). (**B**) The dorsal scapular nerve innervates the rhomboids and levator scapulae, whose main actions are retraction (adduction) and elevation of the scapula. It would not be injured by anterior dislocation of the glenohumeral joint. (**C**) The long thoracic nerve innervates serratus anterior. This muscle protracts (abducts) the scapula and rotates it superiorly to assist in raising the arm above 90 degrees from the horizontal. It would not be injured by anterior dislocation of the glenohumeral joint. (**D**) The lower subscapular nerve innervates subscapularis and teres major. Subscapularis adducts and rotates the arm medially, whereas teres major acts to medially rotate, adduct, and extend the arm. It would not be injured by anterior dislocation of the glenohumeral joint. (**E**) It is highly unlikely that anterior shoulder dislocation would injure the suprascapular nerve because it passes through the suprascapular notch, proximal to the glenohumeral joint. Consequently, there would be no mechanism for the displacement of the proximal humerus to impact this nerve. If this nerve were injured, initiation of abduction would be apparent.

9. Correct: Quadrangular space (B)

Refer to the following image for answer 9:

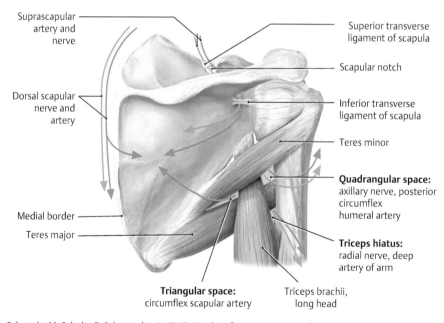

Source: Schuenke M, Schulte E, Schumacher U. THIEME Atlas of Anatomy. General Anatomy and Musculoskeletal System. Illustrations by Voll M and Wesker K. 2nd ed. New York: Thieme Medical Publishers; 2016

(**B**) The quadrangular space lies medial to the surgical neck of the humerus. The axillary nerve and posterior circumflex humeral vessels pass through this space to supply the deltoid and teres minor muscles. Inferior dislocation (referred to clinically as an anterior dislocation) of the glenohumeral joint of sufficient severity may impact this space and injure the axillary nerve. (**A, C–E**) The cubital tunnel, suprascapular notch, triangular space, and triceps hiatus would likely not be involved directly in anterior dislocation of the glenohumeral joint, nor do they transmit the neurovascular structures related to the clinical presentation.

10. Correct: Medial cord (B)

Refer to the following image for answer 10:

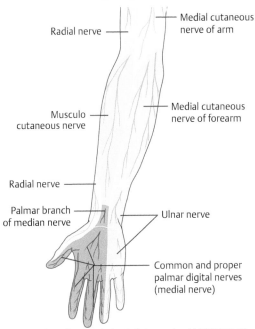

Source: Schuenke M, Schulte E, Schumacher U. THIEME Atlas of Anatomy. General Anatomy and Musculoskeletal System. Illustrations by Voll M and Wesker K. 2nd ed. New York: Thieme Medical Publishers; 2016

(**B**) The nerves that provide sensory innervation to the medial forearm, the medial cutaneous nerve of the forearm and the ulnar nerve, arise from the medial cord. (**A, C–E**) The lateral and posterior cords and the middle and superior trunks do not give rise to nerves that provide sensory innervation to the medial forearm.

11. Correct: C8 and T1 (E)

(**E**) Sensory innervation to the proximal medial forearm is provided primarily by the medial cutaneous nerve of the forearm (T1), whereas the distal forearm and medial hand is innervated by branches of the ulnar nerve (C8–T1).

Refer to the following images for answer 11:

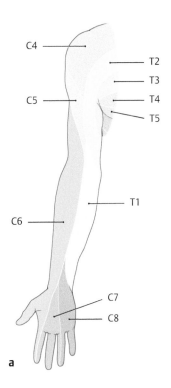

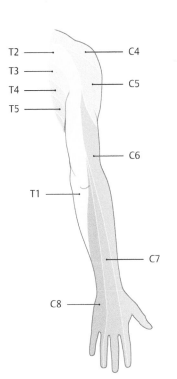

Source: Schuenke M, Schulte E, Schumacher U. THIEME Atlas of Anatomy. General Anatomy and Musculoskeletal System. Illustrations by Voll M and Wesker K. 2nd ed. New York: Thieme Medical Publishers; 2016

12. Correct: Infraspinatus and supraspinatus (A)

(**A**) Muscles involved in lateral rotation of the arm include the posterior portion of the deltoid, infraspinatus, and teres minor. Muscles involved in abducting the arm include the central portion of the deltoid and supraspinatus (which initiates abduction). Thus, only involvement of infraspinatus and supraspinatus accounts for the clinical presentation (i.e., weakness in lateral rotation and initiating abduction). (**B**) While both infraspinatus and teres minor are involved in lateral rotation of the arm, they do not produce arm abduction. (**C**) The rhomboids act on the scapula, primarily as retractors (adductors), but also as weak elevators. (**D**) The supraspinatus muscle initiates abduction of the arm. It is not, however, involved in rotational movements and cannot, by itself, account for the functional deficits in this patient. (**E**) Teres minor is a lateral rotator of the arm, whereas teres major is a medial rotator. Both muscles are also involved in adduction of the arm.

13. Correct: Suprascapular (C)

(**C**) The muscles that account for the clinical presentation, infraspinatus and supraspinatus, are both innervated by the suprascapular nerve. (**A**) The dorsal scapular nerve innervates levator scapulae and rhomboids. (**B**) The lower subscapular nerve innervates subscapularis and teres major. (**D**) The thoracodorsal nerve innervates latissimus dorsi. (**E**) The upper subscapular nerve innervates subscapularis.

Refer to the following image for answer 13:

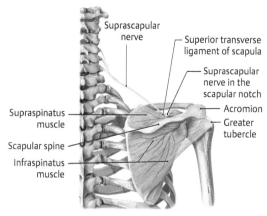

Source: Schuenke M, Schulte E, Schumacher U. THIEME Atlas of Anatomy. General Anatomy and Musculoskeletal System. Illustrations by Voll M and Wesker K. 2nd ed. New York: Thieme Medical Publishers; 2016

14. Correct: Serratus anterior (B)

(**B**) The serratus anterior is responsible for maintaining the position of the scapula against the posterior thoracic wall. Paralysis of this muscle (serratus anterior palsy) can result in winging of the scapula in which its medial (vertebral) border may "lift off" the posterior thoracic wall. This condition is known more specifically as "medial winging," in contrast with "lateral winging" caused by paralysis of trapezius and the rhomboids in which lateral parts of the scapula may be displaced from the thoracic wall. (**A, C–E**) The levator scapulae, serratus posterior superior, and subscapularis muscles are not responsible for maintaining the position of the scapula against the posterior thoracic wall.

15. Correct: Protraction of the scapula (D)

(**D**) The serratus anterior functions to protract the scapula (i.e., move it laterally and anteriorly). (**A–C, E**) None of these actions (scapular elevation or retraction, and arm rotation or abduction) are likely to be affected in this patient.

16. Correct: Long thoracic (B)

(**B**) The clinical presentation (medial scapular winging) supports the involvement of serratus anterior, which is innervated by the long thoracic nerve. Injury of the long thoracic nerve may occur from traumatic, iatrogenic, or idiopathic injury, which can result in paralysis or paresis of serratus anterior. (**A, C–E**) The dorsal scapular, suprascapular, thoracodorsal, and upper subscapular do not innervate the serratus anterior.

Refer to the following image for answer 16:

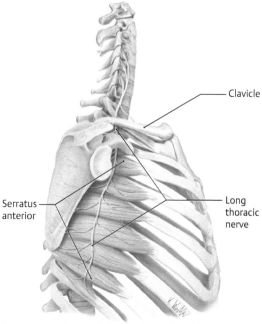

Source: Schuenke M, Schulte E, Schumacher U. THIEME Atlas of Anatomy. General Anatomy and Musculoskeletal System. Illustrations by Voll M and Wesker K. 2nd ed. New York: Thieme Medical Publishers; 2016

17. Correct: Acromion (A)

(**A**) The *asterisk* indicates the acromion. (**B–E**) The coracoacromial ligament, coracoid process, subscapular bursa, and supraglenoid tubercle are not indicated in the MRI.

Refer to the following images for answer 17:

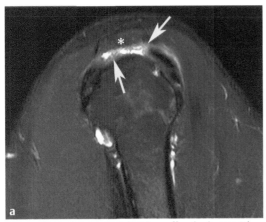

Source: Yablon C, Jacobson J. Rotator cuff and subacromial pathology. Semin Musculoskelet Radiol. 2015; 19(03): 231–242.

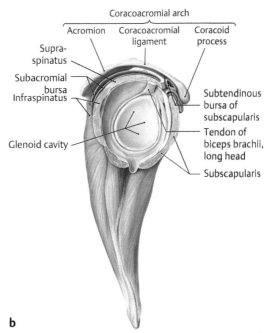

b

Source: Schuenke M, Schulte E, Schumacher U. THIEME Atlas of Anatomy. General Anatomy and Musculoskeletal System. Illustrations by Voll M and Wesker K. 2nd ed. New York: Thieme Medical Publishers; 2016

18. Correct: Supraspinatus (C)

(**C**) The *arrow* in the MRI indicates the supraspinatus tendon as it passes inferior to the acromion and superior to the humeral head before it attaches to the greater tubercle of the humerus.

Refer to the following image for answer 18:

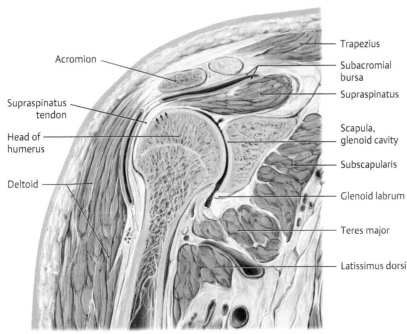

Source: Schuenke M, Schulte E, Schumacher U. THIEME Atlas of Anatomy. General Anatomy and Musculoskeletal System. Illustrations by Voll M and Wesker K. 2nd ed. New York: Thieme Medical Publishers; 2016

19. Correct: Greater tubercle of the humerus (B)

Refer to the following images for answer 19:

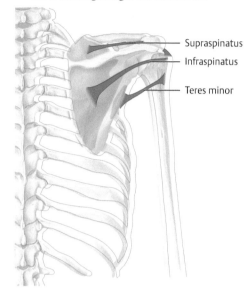

a

Source: Schuenke M, Schulte E, Schumacher U. THIEME Atlas of Anatomy. General Anatomy and Musculoskeletal System. Illustrations by Voll M and Wesker K. 2nd ed. New York: Thieme Medical Publishers; 2016

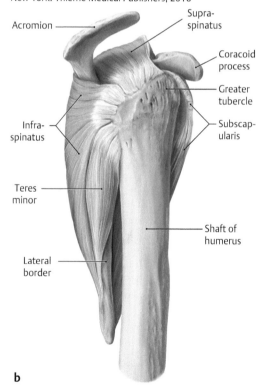

b

Source: Schuenke M, Schulte E, Schumacher U. THIEME Atlas of Anatomy. General Anatomy and Musculoskeletal System. Illustrations by Voll M and Wesker K. 2nd ed. New York: Thieme Medical Publishers; 2016

(**B**) The superior facet of the greater tubercle of the humerus is the location for the distal attachment (insertion) of the supraspinatus muscle. (**A**) The deltoid muscle attaches to the acromion at the greater

tubercle of the humerus. (**C**) The infraglenoid tubercle is the location for the proximal attachment (origin) of the long head of triceps brachii muscle. (**D**) The lesser tubercle of the humerus is the location for the distal attachment (insertion) of the subscapularis muscle. (**E**) The supraglenoid tubercle is the location for the proximal attachment (origin) of the long head of biceps brachii muscle.

20. Correct: Shoulder dislocation (C)

(**C**) The radiographs show an anterior shoulder dislocation of the glenohumeral joint. Most shoulder dislocations are caused by excessive forceful extension and lateral rotation of the humerus. In an anterior shoulder dislocation, the humeral head is usually forced anteriorly and inferiorly from the glenoid cavity. (**A**) Clavicle fractures occur most commonly in the middle one-third of the bone; no disruption of the clavicle is evident in the radiograph. (**B**) A Colles' fracture, often caused by a fall on an outstretched hand (FOOSH) with the hand and wrist in the flexed position, refers to any complete fracture of the distal end of the radius. This type of fracture is associated with dorsal displacement of the hand on the forearm ("dinner fork" deformity). (**D**) Shoulder separation involves disruption of the acromioclavicular joint, between the acromion and the lateral end of the clavicle. (**E**) A Smith's fracture is caused by a FOOSH with the hand and wrist in the flexed position. In contrast to a Colles' fracture, complete fracture of the distal end of the radius with a Smith's fracture is associated with volar displacement of the hand on the forearm. Thus, it is sometimes considered a "reverse" Colles' fracture.

21. Correct: Shoulder separation (D)

Refer to the following image for answer 21:

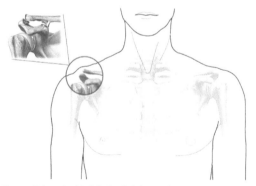

Source: Schuenke M, Schulte E, Schumacher U. THIEME Atlas of Anatomy. General Anatomy and Musculoskeletal System. Illustrations by Voll M and Wesker K. 2nd ed. New York: Thieme Medical Publishers; 2016

(**D**) Shoulder separation involves disruption of the acromioclavicular (AC) joint, between the acromion and the lateral end of the clavicle. A fall on the shoulder with the arm outstretched transfers force to the joint, forcing the proximal humerus into the acromion, and thereby disrupting the AC joint. Mild shoulder separation results in AC ligament sprain and the clavicle will be in its normal position relative to the acromion. More severe acromioclavicular injury tears the coracoclavicular ligament complex, resulting in the clavicle being displaced superiorly relative to the acromion. In the upright position, patients with severe shoulder dislocations (e.g., grades III–V) present with a noticeable "shelf" ("step deformity") due to the effect of gravity pulling the affected arm and acromion inferiorly with respect to the disrupted acromioclavicular joint and lateral end of the clavicle. (**A**) Clavicle fractures occur most commonly in the middle one-third of the bone. Patients may hear a snapping or sense a cracking at the time of the injury. These fractures are often easily recognized and diagnosed due to the subcutaneous position of the clavicle. Pain, swelling, and deformity over the clavicle may be observed. (**B**) A Colles' fracture, which is usually caused by a FOOSH with the wrist extended, refers to any complete fracture of the distal end of the radius. It is associated with dorsal displacement of the hand on the forearm (the so-called "dinner fork" deformity). (**C**) Shoulder dislocation refers to dislocations of the glenohumeral joint, most often caused by excessive, forceful extension and lateral rotation of the humerus. An anterior dislocation, with the humeral head forced inferiorly and anteriorly from the glenoid fossa, is most common. (**E**) A Smith's fracture is also caused by a FOOSH with the wrist flexed. In contrast to a Colles' fracture, complete fracture of the distal end of the radius with a Smith's fracture is associated ventral (anterior) displacement of the hand on the forearm.

22. Correct: Anular ligament (A)

Refer to the following image for answer 22:

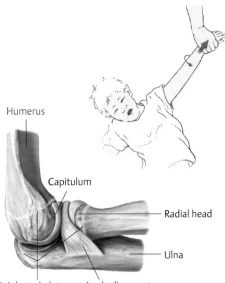

Humerus

Capitulum

Radial head

Ulna

Epiphyseal plates   Anular ligament

Source: Schuenke M, Schulte E, Schumacher U. THIEME Atlas of Anatomy. General Anatomy and Musculoskeletal System. Illustrations by Voll M and Wesker K. 2nd ed. New York: Thieme Medical Publishers; 2016

(**A**) Nursemaid's elbow ("pulled elbow") refers to traumatic dislocation of the radial head at the proximal radio-ulnar joint, which is normally maintained by the anular ligament. This condition occurs commonly in children younger than 6 years of age when they are picked up or pulled by the wrists or hands while the elbow joint is extended and the forearm is pronated. With increasing age, ligaments generally become stronger, reducing the risk of such injuries. (**B–E**) The biceps tendon, bicipital aponeurosis, and radial (lateral) and ulnar (medial) collateral ligaments are not responsible for maintaining the radial head in its anatomical position.

23. Correct: Dupuytren's contracture (A)

(**A**) Dupuytren's contracture results from thickened cords of palmar fascia that causes flexion contracture of the metacarpophalangeal and proximal interphalangeal joints to varying degrees. It usually affects the ring and little fingers, and most commonly affects men 40 to 60 years-of-age of northern European descent. Diagnosis is made by identifying a nodule in the palm caused by increased collagen deposition along the palmar fascia, usually at the distal palmar crease of the affected finger(s). Sensory deficits and other motor deficits are generally not present. (**B**) Ganglion cysts are small, benign, soft tissue sacs that typically contain air or fluid that present as movable nodules tender to palpation. They are slightly more common in women 20 to 40 years of age and are most often located on the dorsal wrist, although they may occur along the digital sheaths. They are not associated with contracture of the fingers. (**C**) Mallet finger is caused by evulsion of the flexor digitorum profundus tendon from the distal phalanx, resulting in the inability to extend the distal interphalangeal joint of the affected finger. (**D**) Ulnar nerve entrapment occurs most commonly at the elbow but may also occur distally at the ulnar tunnel (Guyon's canal) at the wrist. This results in sensory deficits (e.g., tingling or numbness) in the medial palm and dorsum of the hand, and the ring and little fingers. Since the ulnar nerve supplies most intrinsic hand muscles, patients may also report hand or grip weakness. The lack of sensory deficits in this patient's hand indicates that ulnar, median, and radial nerves are not involved. The ability to move his thumb indicates that the median and ulnar nerves are intact. (**E**) Volkmann's ischemic contracture results from contraction of the long flexor muscles resulting in a flexed wrist and fingers. The lack of adhesions along the sheath or palmar fascia (e.g., as occurs in Dupuytren's contracture) permits some passive extension, although this manipulation may elicit forearm pain. Because this is a late finding in forearm compartment syndrome, the fingers may be cyanotic and are often edematous.

24. Correct: Subclavian vein (E)

(**E**) From anterior-to-posterior, neurovascular structures that lie in close proximity to the posterior aspect of the middle third of the clavicle are: subclavian vein, subclavian artery, and brachial plexus. All are at risk of injury with midclavicular fracture, although the subclavian vein is closest and, therefore, most vulnerable. (**A**) The axillary artery begins at the lateral border of rib 1. It is inferior and lateral to the clavicle and is, therefore, unlikely to be injured with midshaft clavicle fracture. (**B**) The brachiocephalic vein lies posterior to the medial end of the clavicle and would not likely be injured by the midshaft fracture. (**C**) The right common carotid artery branches from the brachiocephalic trunk, which lies posterior to the sternoclavicular joint and is not as likely to be injured by the midshaft fracture. (**D**) The internal jugular vein joins the subclavian vein posterior to the medial end of the clavicle to form the brachiocephalic vein. It is unlikely likely to be injured by the midshaft fracture.

Refer to the following image for answer 24:

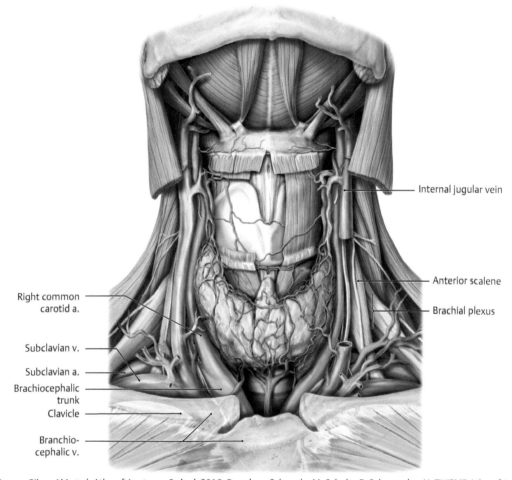

Source: Gilroy AM et al. Atlas of Anatomy. 3rd ed. 2016. Based on: Schuenke M, Schulte E, Schumacher U. THIEME Atlas of Anatomy. Volumes 1-3. Illustrations by Voll M and Wesker K. 2nd ed. New York: Thieme Medical Publishers; 2016

25. Correct: Subclavius (D)

(**D**) The subclavius muscle lies along the inferior aspect of the clavicle. In the middle portion of the clavicle, it lies anterior to the subclavian vein and may prevent damage to the neurovascular structures (subclavian vein, subclavian artery, brachial plexus) that lie posterior to the clavicle. The anterior scalene, near its attachment to the first rib, protects a limited portion of the subclavian artery and brachial plexus, which pass posterior to the muscle. (**A–C, E**) The pectoralis major and minor, sternocleidomastoid and trapezius muscles do not lie between the clavicle and the neurovascular structures (subclavian vein, subclavian artery, brachial plexus) that lie posterior to the clavicle.

26. Correct: Wrist extension (E)

Refer to the following image for answer 26:

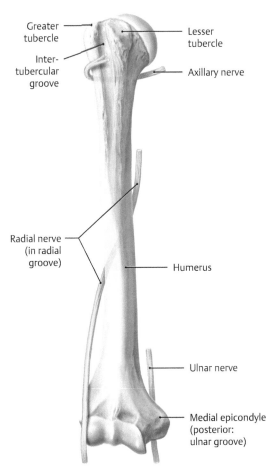

Greater tubercle
Lesser tubercle
Inter-tubercular groove
Axillary nerve
Radial nerve (in radial groove)
Humerus
Ulnar nerve
Medial epicondyle (posterior: ulnar groove)

Source: Schuenke M, Schulte E, Schumacher U. THIEME Atlas of Anatomy. General Anatomy and Musculoskeletal System. Illustrations by Voll M and Wesker K. 2nd ed. New York: Thieme Medical Publishers; 2016

(**E**) "Wrist drop" is the characteristic clinical sign of radial nerve injury. In the middle third of the humerus, the radial nerve courses in the radial (spiral) groove. Because its lies close to the humeral shaft, the nerve is at risk of injury in fractures of this portion of the bone. Distal to this, the radial nerve innervates muscles of the posterior forearm (extensor-supinator), including those that extend the wrist. (**A**) The radial nerve does not innervate muscles that act to abduct the arm. (**B**) Injury to the radial nerve in the middle one-third of the arm does not paralyze the triceps brachii completely because its lateral and long heads receive their radial innervation in the proximal arm. Thus, elbow extension is only weakened. (**C**) The radial nerve does not innervate muscles that act to pronate the forearm. (**D**) While injury to the radial nerve will affect the supinator muscle, supination is only weakened because the musculocutaneous nerve is intact and the supination action of biceps brachii remains functional.

27. Correct: Lateral palm and proximal fingers 1 to 3 (A)

Refer to the following image for answer 27:

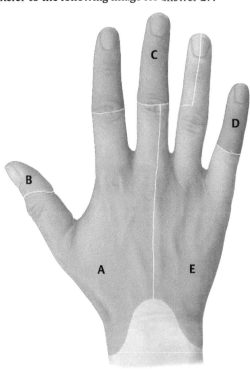

Source: Schuenke M, Schulte E, Schumacher U. THIEME Atlas of Anatomy. General Anatomy and Musculoskeletal System. Illustrations by Voll M and Wesker K. 2nd ed. New York: Thieme Medical Publishers; 2016

(**A**) The superficial branch of the radial nerve is a cutaneous nerve that supplies skin on the dorsolateral aspect of the hand and fingers. (**B, C**) The indicated areas are innervated by the median nerve. (**D, E**) The indicated areas are innervated by the ulnar nerve.

28. Correct: Median (B)

Refer to the following images for answer 28:

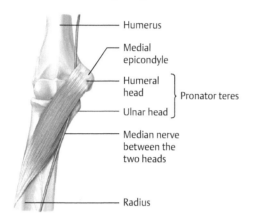

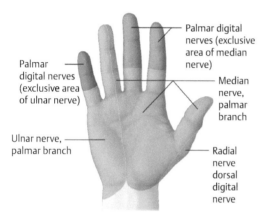

Source: Schuenke M, Schulte E, Schumacher U. THIEME Atlas of Anatomy. General Anatomy and Musculoskeletal System. Illustrations by Voll M and Wesker K. 2nd ed. New York: Thieme Medical Publishers; 2016

(**B**) This patient has pronator syndrome due to compression of the median nerve in the proximal forearm as it passes between the humeral (superficial) and ulnar (deep) heads of the pronator teres. Involvement of the median nerve is indicated by the sensory deficits and the loss of thumb flexion due to involvement of both flexor pollicis brevis and longus. Median nerve compression can also account for the forearm pain and the ability of provocative tests (e.g., resisted pronation) to aggravate the pain and tenderness over the pronator teres. This condition is distinguished from carpal tunnel syndrome, the most common entrapment syndrome of the median nerve, by sensory deficits in the proximal palm, which is innervated by the palmar cutaneous branch of the median nerve that does not pass through the carpal tunnel. (**A**) The deep branch of the ulnar nerve supplies most intrinsic hand muscles, including the deep head of flexor pollicis brevis. However, this muscle cannot compensate for loss of action of

the flexor pollicis longus and superficial head of the flexor pollicis brevis, both of which are innervated by the median nerve. (**C**) The radial nerve does not supply thumb flexors, the lateral fingers, or the lateral palm. (**D**) The recurrent branch of the median nerve innervates the thenar muscles and two lateral lumbricals. (**E**) The deep branch of the ulnar nerve supplies most intrinsic muscles of the hand except the thenar muscles and two lateral lumbricals. The superficial branch of the ulnar nerve supplies cutaneous innervation to the medial hand.

29. Correct: Musculocutaneous (B)

Refer to the following image for answer 29:

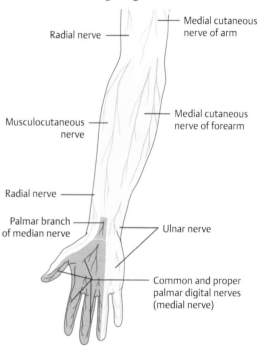

Source: Schuenke M, Schulte E, Schumacher U. THIEME Atlas of Anatomy. General Anatomy and Musculoskeletal System. Illustrations by Voll M and Wesker K. 2nd ed. New York: Thieme Medical Publishers; 2016

(**B**) The musculocutaneous nerve innervates muscles in the anterior (flexor) compartment of the arm, including coracobrachialis, biceps brachii, and brachialis. Since biceps brachii and brachialis are the primary flexor muscles of the forearm, a musculocutaneous mononeuropathy would lead to weakened elbow (forearm) flexion. The musculocutaneous nerve terminates as the lateral cutaneous nerve of the forearm; injury of this nerve leads to sensory deficits from this area of the upper limb. (**A**) The axillary nerve supplies the deltoid and teres minor muscles, as well as the skin over the deltoid (i.e., lateral upper arm). Axillary nerve injury would not affect forearm flexion or sensation from the lateral forearm. (**C**) The median nerve innervates most muscles in the anterior (flexor) compartment of the arm (except flexor carpi ulnaris and the medial aspect of the flexor digitorum profundus), as well as several intrinsic hand muscles (thenar and two lumbricals). It also innervates the skin on the anterolateral aspect of the hand. Median neuropathy would not affect forearm flexion or sensation from the lateral forearm. (**D**) The superficial branch of the radial nerve is a cutaneous nerve that innervates skin on the posterolateral aspect of the hand. Radial neuropathy would not affect forearm flexion or sensation from the lateral forearm. (**E**) The ulnar nerve innervates muscles in the anterior (flexor) compartment of the arm (flexor carpi ulnaris and the medial aspect of the flexor digitorum profundus) and the most intrinsic hand muscles. It also innervates skin on the medial aspect (anteriorly and posteriorly) of the hand. Ulnar neuropathy would not affect forearm flexion or sensation from the lateral forearm.

---

30.   Correct: C6 (C)

(**C**) Sensory fibers (all from the C6 spinal cord level) carried in the musculocutaneous nerve enter its terminal branch, the lateral cutaneous nerve of the forearm. Thus, the C6 dermatome is served by the lateral cutaneous nerve of the forearm. (**A, B, D, E**) See dermatome map.

Refer to the following images for answer 30:

---

31.   Correct: Flexion of the arm (D)

(**D**) The coracobrachialis and short head of the biceps, both innervated by the musculocutaneous nerve, produce flexion of the arm (glenohumeral joint). Weak forearm flexion would be possible due to action of the brachioradialis muscle, the lateral portion of which is innervated by the radial nerve. (**A–C, E**) Arm abduction and extension, forearm extension, and pronation are actions of muscles that are not innervated by the musculocutaneous nerve.

---

32.   Correct: Flexion of the elbow joint and forearm supination (C)

(**C**) The biceps brachii muscle flexes the elbow joint. With the elbow joint flexed, it is the major supinator of the forearm. (**A**) The muscle whose sole action is to flex the elbow joint is the brachialis. Injury of the musculocutaneous nerve would greatly impair the elbow flexion action of the brachialis and biceps brachii muscles. (**B**) Injury of the biceps brachii muscle would affect elbow flexion, but not pronation (the secondary action of this muscle is supination, not pronation). (**D**) The main forearm pronators are the pronator teres and pronator quadratus muscles. (**E**) Injury of the biceps brachii muscle through rupture of its tendon would impair supination, but the supinator muscle would remain functional.

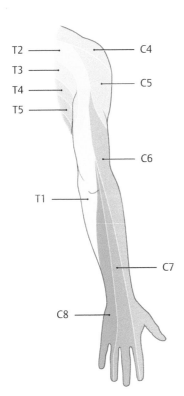

a

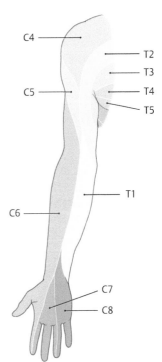

b

Source: Source: Schuenke M, Schulte E, Schumacher U. THIEME Atlas of Anatomy. General Anatomy and Musculoskeletal System. Illustrations by Voll M and Wesker K. 2nd ed. New York: Thieme Medical Publishers; 2016

33. Correct: Medial cubital (E)

(**E**) The median cubital vein, which connects the cephalic and basilic veins in the superficial fascia over the cubital fossa, is most commonly used for venipuncture. Venipuncture using this vein is least likely to cause damage to nearby cutaneous nerves (i.e., lateral and medial cutaneous nerves of the forearm). (**A, C**) The brachial and axillary veins are deep veins of the arm and axilla, respectively. They are not typically used for venipuncture. (**B, D**) The basilic and cephalic veins are superficial veins of the upper limb. They arise from the dorsal venous network on the hand. Near the elbow, they are superficial and may be used for venipuncture, although their proximity to the lateral and medial cutaneous nerves of the forearm, make them less suitable.

Refer to the following image for answer 33:

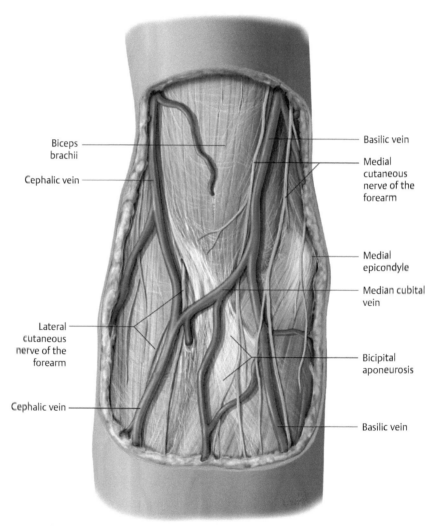

Source: Schuenke M, Schulte E, Schumacher U. THIEME Atlas of Anatomy. General Anatomy and Musculoskeletal System. Illustrations by Voll M and Wesker K. 2nd ed. New York: Thieme Medical Publishers; 2016

34. Median (B)

(B) The median nerve and the terminal portion of the brachial artery pass through the cubital fossa. The bicipital aponeurosis forms the roof of the fossa and, to some extent, protects the median nerve and brachial artery at this location. Nevertheless, these structures may be injured during venipuncture if the needle is inserted too steeply and deeply. (A) The axillary nerve is located in the shoulder. (C) The terminal branch of the musculocutaneous nerve (lateral cutaneous nerve of the forearm) crosses the elbow lateral to the cubital fossa. It is more likely to be injured if the cephalic vein is used for venipuncture. (D) The radial nerve at the elbow crosses the lateral portion of the cubital fossa. It is protected to some extent by the brachioradialis muscle and is more likely to be injured if the cephalic vein is used. (E) The ulnar nerve at the elbow is posterior to the medial epicondyle. It is unlikely to be injured during venipuncture.

Refer to the following image for answer 34:

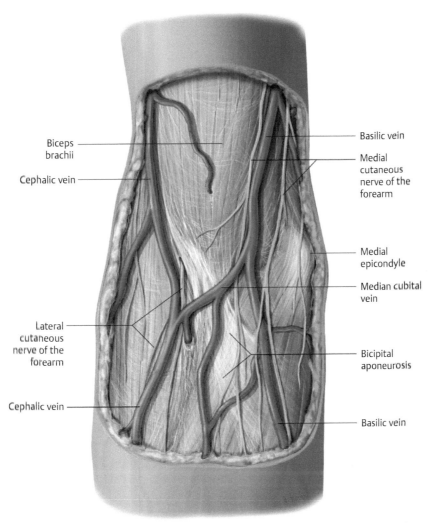

Source: Schuenke M, Schulte E, Schumacher U. THIEME Atlas of Anatomy. General Anatomy and Musculoskeletal System. Illustrations by Voll M and Wesker K. 2nd ed. New York: Thieme Medical Publishers; 2016

35. Correct: Scaphoid (C)

Refer to the following image for answer 35:

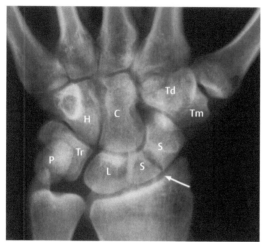

Source: Matzen P. Praktische Orthopädie. 3rd Edition. Stuttgart: J. A. Barth Verlag; Thieme; 2002

(**C**) The X-ray shows a fracture of the scaphoid waist (*arrow*), the most common location for fracture of this bone. Fracture of the scaphoid may occur essentially at any age, but occurs most commonly in adolescents and young adults where it accounts for 70 to 80% of all carpal bone fractures. A fall on an outstretched hand in older individuals is more likely to result in a distal radial fracture (especially a Colles' fracture). (**A, B, D, E**) The lunate, pisiform, trapezium, and trapezoid appear normal in the radiograph. Image key: Proximal row of carpal bones: S, scaphoid; L, lunate; Tr, triquetrum; P, pisiform. Distal row of carpal bones: Tm, trapezium; Td, trapezoid; C, capitate, H, hamate.

36. Correct: Flexor carpi radialis (B)

(**B**) At the wrist, the radial artery typically lies immediately lateral and adjacent to the tendon of flexor carpi radialis. (**A**) At the wrist, the radial artery typically lies medial to the tendon of brachioradialis. (**C–E**) The tendons of flexor carpi ulnaris, flexor digitorum superficialis, and palmaris longus lie further medial to the radial artery at the wrist than does the tendon of flexor carpi radialis.

Refer to the following image for answer 36:

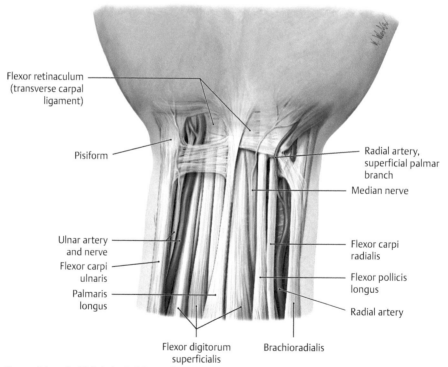

Source: Schuenke M, Schulte E, Schumacher U. THIEME Atlas of Anatomy. General Anatomy and Musculoskeletal System. Illustrations by Voll M and Wesker K. 2nd ed. New York: Thieme Medical Publishers; 2016

37. Correct: Allen's test (A)

(**A**) The Allen's test is a noninvasive, nonimaging method to assess blood flow through the radial and ulnar arteries from the wrist into the palmar arterial arches. This test assesses the suitability of the radial artery for arterial blood gas sampling or cannulation by determining whether the ulnar artery is capable of sufficient collateral circulation to prevent ischemia should the radial artery become unavailable due to complication of the arterial puncture procedure (e.g., local hematoma, arterial vasospasm, infection at the puncture site). First, the examiner's fingers are used to firmly occlude both the radial and ulnar arteries at the wrist. Then, the occlusive pressure is released to permit blood to flow individually through the radial and ulnar arteries, thereby assessing whether each artery is capable of full collateral circulation of the hand via the palmar arterial arches. (**B–D**) These imaging methods are either more expensive, invasive (application of contrast dyes), or utilize ionizing radiation, and are not commonly used to assess arterial patency of the hand. (**E**) The Tinel's test is used to detect whether a nerve is irritated. It involves light percussion over the nerve in order to elicit paresthesia (tingling) from its cutaneous distribution.

38. Correct: Adductor pollicis (C)

(**C**) Froment's sign tests the strength of the adductor pollicis muscle in cases of suspected ulnar nerve injury. This muscle is used to adduct the thumb to hold a piece of paper between the thumb and adjacent index finger. A patient with ulnar nerve palsy cannot activate adductor pollicis and, consequently, will flex the affected thumb at the interphalangeal joint to try to hold on to the paper. (**A, D, E**) The abductor and flexor pollicis brevis muscles are innervated by the median nerve and are not involved in the muscle weakness evident in this patient. Flexor pollicis longus, also innervated by the median nerve, is responsible for flexion of the interphalangeal joint of the thumb to compensate for weakness of the adductor pollicis. (**B**) Abductor pollicis longus is innervated by the radial nerve and is not involved in the muscle weakness evident in this patient.

39. Correct: C5–C6 (B)

(**B**) The biceps brachii and brachioradialis reflexes are mediated by the C5–C6 nerve roots: C5 is predominant for the biceps brachii and C6 for brachioradialis. (**C**) The triceps reflex is mediated by the C6–C7 spinal nerve roots, with C7 predominating. (**A, D, E**) These nerve root pairs do not typically predominate in deep tendon reflexes of the upper limb.

40. Correct: Triceps brachii (E)

(**E**) The C7 spinal nerve passes through the C6–C7 intervertebral foramen and would likely be affected by the disc herniation. The triceps reflex, which is mediated by the C6 and C7 spinal nerve roots (with C7 predominating) would most likely be affected. (**A, B**) The biceps brachii (and brachioradialis) reflexes are mediated by the C5 and C6 nerve roots; C5 predominating for the biceps brachii and C6 predominating for brachioradialis. (**C, D**) The flexor carpi radialis and pronator teres muscles are not associated with a tendon reflex.

41. Correct: Anterior scalene and middle scalene (A)

(**A**) The proximal portion of the brachial plexus, primarily the superior roots and part of the trunks, is typically targeted for regional anesthesia using an interscalene approach, between the anterior and middle scalene muscles. Branches from the brachial plexus innervate the glenohumeral (shoulder) joint, as well as the skin over the deltoid muscle and the medial side of the arm and axilla. (**B–E**) The brachial plexus does not pass between any of these pairs of muscles.

42. Correct: Phrenic (B)

(**B**) The postoperative dyspnea (difficulty breathing) indicates involvement of the diaphragm, which is innervated by the phrenic nerve. The roots of the phrenic nerve (C3–C5) are located in the interscalene interval, and are affected by the anesthetic injected for the brachial plexus block. Alternatively, the anesthetic may have spread to the phrenic nerve itself, located along the anterior aspect of the anterior scalene muscle. (**A, C–E**) The long thoracic, recurrent laryngeal, and vagus nerves, and the sympathetic chain would not be expected to affect the diaphragm and lead to dyspnea. Injury of the recurrent laryngeal, unlikely in this patient, could result in dyspnea due to paralysis of the vocal cord.

43. Correct: Radius (C)

(**C**) The distal radius was fractured in this patient as shown in the radiographs. (**A, B, D, E**) The lunate, pisiform, scaphoid, and ulna appear normal in the radiograph.

44. Correct: Colles' (C)

(**C**) This patient sustained a Colles' fracture (image A) that was caused by a fall on the outstretched hand (FOOSH) with the hand and wrist in the extended position. This type of fracture refers to any complete fracture of the distal end of the radius and is associated with dorsal displacement of the hand on the forearm due to the pull of brachioradialis (this displacement creates the characteristic "dinner fork" deformity). Colles' fracture is most common in post-menopausal women (osteoporosis being a predisposing factor), although it can also occur in younger individuals, especially those who participate in ice hockey, football, wrestling, riding, and skiing. (**A**) A Barton's fracture is an intra-articular fracture of the dorsal aspect of the distal radius with radiocarpal dislocation. (**B**) A chauffeur's fracture ("backfire" or Hutchinson's fracture) is an intra-articular fracture of the radial styloid process that is typically caused by direct trauma to the posterior side of the wrist. (**D**) Fracture of the scaphoid occurs most commonly in adolescents and young adults who fall on their outstretched hand (older patients falling in a similar manner usually sustain a Colles' fracture). A scaphoid fracture is classically associated with pain in the anatomical snuffbox. It is not associated with deformity of the distal forearm and hand. (**E**) A Smith's fracture (image a) is caused by a FOOSH with the hand and wrist in the flexed position. In contrast to a Colles' fracture, complete fracture of the distal end of the radius with a Smith's fracture is associated volar displacement of the hand on the forearm. Thus, it is sometimes considered a "reverse" Colles' fracture.

Refer to the following image for answer 44:

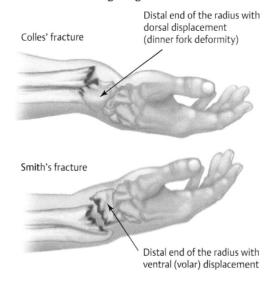

Colles' fracture

Distal end of the radius with dorsal displacement (dinner fork deformity)

Smith's fracture

Distal end of the radius with ventral (volar) displacement

45. Correct: Flexor digitorum profundus and flexor pollicis longus (B)

(**B**) An inability to make the "OK" sign (made with the thumb and index finger) is pathognomic for an anterior interosseous nerve lesion: the "OK" sign would flatten due to loss of flexion at the interphalangeal joints of the thumb and index finger. An anterior interosseous nerve lesion affects three deep anterior forearm muscles: flexor pollicis longus, the lateral (radial) part of flexor digitorum profundus, and pronator quadratus. The first two muscles flex the interphalangeal joint of the thumb and the interphalangeal joints of the index finger, respectively. The anterior interosseous nerve in this patient was most likely compressed in the proximal forearm by repeated pressure of the baby carrier handle. (**A, C–E**) None of the other pairs of muscles listed account for flexion of both the interphalangeal joint of the thumb and the distal interphalangeal joint of the index finger.

46. Correct: No (A)

(**A**) Sensation from the upper limb would not be affected because the anterior interosseous nerve is primarily a motor nerve. Its small, sensory component has no cutaneous distribution and supplies branches only to joints of the wrist.

47. Correct: Tendon of the long head of biceps brachii (D)

(**D**) The tendon of the long head of biceps brachii passes through the bicipital groove (intertubercular sulcus). The anterior shoulder pain and pain elicited over the groove indicates inflammation of this tendon. Each of the tests elicits pain from the bicipital groove during resisted movement of the arm involving action(s) of the biceps brachii muscle, that is, forearm supination (Yergason's test) and shoulder flexion (Speed's test). (**A–C, E**) None of these structures (coracobrachialis, pectoralis minor, subscapularis muscles, and the tendon of the short head of biceps brachii) pass through the bicipital groove and, therefore, would not elicit this type of pain.

48. Correct: Posterior interosseous nerve (D)

(**D**) The deep branch of the radial nerve passes between the two heads of the supinator muscle and along the radial neck, which places the nerve at risk with fracture and can affect its distal targets. The deep branch of the radial nerve under cover of supinator is sometimes referred to as the posterior interosseous nerve, although some sources consider the posterior interosseous nerve only after it emerges from the distal edge of supinator to enter the posterior (extensor-supinator) compartment of the forearm. (**A–C, E**) The anterior interosseous and median nerves, deep artery of the arm, and ulnar artery do not course along the radial neck and, therefore, are not likely to be injured in this patient.

Refer to the following image for answer 48:

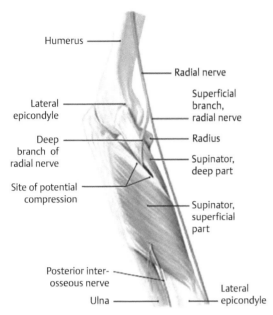

- Humerus
- Radial nerve
- Lateral epicondyle
- Superficial branch, radial nerve
- Deep branch of radial nerve
- Radius
- Supinator, deep part
- Site of potential compression
- Supinator, superficial part
- Posterior inter-osseous nerve
- Ulna
- Lateral epicondyle

Source: Schuenke M, Schulte E, Schumacher U. THIEME Atlas of Anatomy. General Anatomy and Musculoskeletal System. Illustrations by Voll M and Wesker K. 2nd ed. New York: Thieme Medical Publishers; 2016

49. Correct: Weakened thumb abduction (E)

(**E**) The inability to extend the fingers indicates injury of the posterior interosseous nerve and paralysis of long digital extensor muscles (extensor digitorum, extensor digiti minimi, extensor indicis, extensor pollicis brevis and longus). Abductor pollicis longus, a snuff box muscle, is also innervated by the posterior interosseous nerve, and its paralysis would result in weakened thumb abduction (abductor pollicis brevis, a thenar muscle, would retain function since it is innervated by the recurrent branch of the median nerve). (**A**) Loss of sensation from the little finger would involve the ulnar nerve. (**B**) Loss of sensation from the tip of the index finger would involve the median nerve. (**C**) Radial deviation of the wrist would be weakened, but not abolished: while the deep branch of the radial nerve innervates extensor carpi radialis brevis is affected by the tumor, the median nerve innervation of flexor carpi radialis is not. (**D**) Paralysis of thumb adduction (adductor pollicis) would involve the deep branch of the ulnar nerve.

50. Correct: Extensor carpi radialis brevis (C)

(**C**) This patient has lateral epicondylitis ("tennis elbow"), an overuse syndrome that can occur with repetitive, forceful wrist extension. With the tennis backhand stroke, the elbow and wrist are extended and, with overuse and/or weakness, the extensor carpi radialis brevis and longus muscles of the forearm may become inflamed at or near their attachment to the lateral epicondyle of the humerus. This condition is distinguished from medial epicondylitis ("golfer's elbow"), which affects the attachment of flexor carpi radialis at the medial epicondyle. (**A, B, D, E**) The brachioradialis, flexor carpi ulnaris, extensor pollicis longus, and pronator teres muscles do not attach to the lateral epicondyle and are, therefore, not involved in lateral epicondylitis.

51. Correct: Trapezius (E)

(**E**) The trapezius muscle (with levator scapulae) elevates the scapula. Acting isometrically, trapezius plays a role in counteracting weight-load on the shoulder. Acting synergistically with serratus anterior, it also rotates the glenoid cavity superiorly and, thus, also plays a role in abduction of the arm. Iatrogenic injury of the accessory nerve (CN XI) may result from surgeries, such as parotidectomy, that involve regions of the neck traversed by this nerve. (**A**) The deltoid muscle has multiple actions: the middle (acromial) part retracts (adducts) the arm; the anterior (clavicular) part flexes and medially rotates the arm; and the posterior (spinal) part extends and laterally rotates the arm. Neither the deltoid muscle nor its innervation (axillary nerve) is likely to be injured during a parotidectomy. (**B**) Rhomboid major retracts (adducts) the scapula and rotates the glenoid cavity inferiorly. Neither the rhomboid major muscle nor its innervation (dorsal scapular nerve) is likely to be injured during a parotidectomy. (**C**) The serratus anterior muscle protracts (abducts) the scapula and rotates the glenoid cavity superiorly. It also plays an important role in holding the scapula against the thoracic wall. The absence of scapular winging indicates that this muscle is not affected in this patient. Neither the serratus anterior muscle nor its innervation (long thoracic nerve) is likely to be injured during a parotidectomy. (**D**) Supraspinatus plays an important role in initiating abduction of the arm. It is innervated by the suprascapular nerve, which arises in the neck from the superior trunk of the brachial plexus and traverses the root of the neck to reach the scapula. It is, therefore, distant from the parotid gland and unlikely to be injured during a parotidectomy.

52. Correct: Superior trunk (E)

(**E**) The signs and symptoms in this patient are best explained by an injury of the upper part of the brachial plexus, as might occur with avulsion of the C5 and C6 ventral rami. This type of injury, an upper brachial plexus (Erb's or Erb–Duchenne) palsy, would affect branches of the ventral rami, as well as the superior trunk and its branches. This injury may result from excessive traction that increases the angle between the neck and shoulder (e.g., traumatic injury with excessive lateral flexion of the neck; shoulder dystocia during delivery). The signs and symptoms associated with this injury may be explained as follows:

- Weakened glenohumeral abduction indicates involvement of the supraspinatus (suprascapular nerve, C4–C6), deltoid (axillary nerve, C5–C6), and/or serratus anterior (long thoracic nerve, C5–C7) muscles.
- Weakened elbow flexion indicates involvement of the biceps brachii and brachialis muscles (musculocutaneous nerve, C5–C7).
- The sensory deficits indicate involvement of the axillary (skin over the deltoid, C5 dermatome), radial and musculocutaneous (skin over lateral arm and forearm, C6 dermatome), and median (skin over lateral hand, C6 dermatome) nerves.
- The neural structures common to all these nerves are the C5 and C6 ventral rami and the superior trunk of the brachial plexus.

(**A–D**) The axillary and musculocutaneous nerves, nor the inferior trunk or posterior divisions of the brachial plexus offer a common, proximal pathway that would explain the clinical signs and symptoms.

Refer to the following image for answer 52:

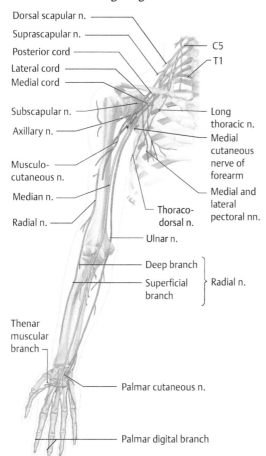

Dorsal scapular n.
Suprascapular n.
Posterior cord
Lateral cord
Medial cord
C5
T1
Subscapular n.
Axillary n.
Long thoracic n.
Medial cutaneous nerve of forearm
Musculo-cutaneous n.
Median n.
Radial n.
Thoraco-dorsal n.
Medial and lateral pectoral nn.
Ulnar n.
Deep branch
Superficial branch
Radial n.
Thenar muscular branch
Palmar cutaneous n.
Palmar digital branch

Source: Gilroy AM et al. Atlas of Anatomy. 3rd ed. 2016. Based on: Schuenke M, Schulte E, Schumacher U. THIEME Atlas of Anatomy. Volumes 1-3. Illustrations by Voll M and Wesker K. 2nd ed. New York: Thieme Medical Publishers; 2016

53. Correct: Pectoralis major (B)

(**B**) This patient has an upper brachial plexus injury that affects the C5 and C6 ventral rami and their branches, as well as the superior trunk and its branches. The sternocostal portion of pectoralis major is innervated by the medial pectoral nerve (C7–T1) and is not affected by the injury. As a result, it can still medially rotate the arm. Subscapularis (subscapular nerve, C5–C6) and the anterior deltoid muscle (axillary nerve, C5–C6) would likely be paralyzed by the injury, but the teres major (lower subscapular nerve, C5–C7) and latissimus dorsi muscles (thoracodorsal nerve, C6–C8) would be only partially affected by the injury and could contribute to medial rotation of the arm. (**A, D**) Infraspinatus and teres minor laterally rotate the arm. Their actions would be affected by the injury because their nerves (suprascapular and axillary, respectively) carry C5 and C6 axons. (**C**) Supraspinatus abducts the arm. Its action would be affected by the injury because its nerve (suprascapular) carries C5 and C6 axons. (**E**) Trapezius acts on the scapula, not on the arm, and its actions would not be affected by the injury because its nerve (accessory; CN XI) does not carry C5 or C6 axons.

54. Correct: Pronator syndrome (E)

Refer to the following image for answer 54:

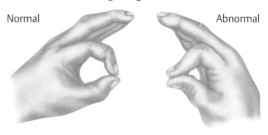

Normal   Abnormal

(**E**) Proximal median nerve lesions can be caused by nerve compression in the distal arm (e.g., due to an anomalous supracondylar process), at the cubital fossa by a tight bicipital aponeurosis, or by entrapment within pronator teres muscle. Typical clinical features include impaired grasping, loss of thumb opposition, atrophy of the thenar muscles, and sensory disturbances from the lateral palm and three and a half fingers. The patient's hand will take a "hand of benediction" position when attempting to make a fist: the thumb, index, and middle fingers will exhibit minimal or no flexion (loss of median nerve innervation to flexor pollicis longus, flexor digitorum superficialis, and the lateral portion of flexor digitorum profundus); the ring and little fingers are capable of greater flexion due to unaffected ulnar innervation to the medial portion of flexor digitorum profundus. In addition, weakened forearm pronation against resistance may be observed if the lesion is proximal to the innervation of pronator teres. The inability of the patient to make an "OK" sign on the affected side indicates involvement of the anterior interosseous nerve, a branch of the median nerve that would likely also be affected in pronator syndrome as this branch is distal to the point of compression in the pronator teres. (**A**) An isolated anterior interosseous nerve (AIN) lesion affects three deep muscles in the anterior forearm: flexor pollicis longus, the lateral part of flexor digitorum profundus, and pronator quadratus. The first two muscles flex the interphalangeal joint of the thumb and the interphalangeal joints of the index finger, respectively. An inability to make the "OK" sign is pathognomic for an AIN lesion: the "OK" sign would flatten due to loss of flexion at the interphalangeal joints of the thumb and index finger. This condition is not associated with sensory deficits since the AIN does not have a cutaneous distribution. (**B**) Carpal tunnel syndrome results in sensory deficits from loss of the median nerve function in the hand. Unlike more proximal median nerve lesions, sensation from the thenar eminence would be spared because the palmar cutaneous branch of the median nerve does not pass through the carpal tunnel. Tinel's sign over the carpal tunnel and the Phalen test would likely be positive. If advanced, carpal tunnel syndrome can affect thenar muscles leading to atrophy and weakness in thumb movements. (**C**) Cubital tunnel syndrome results from compression of the ulnar nerve as it passes from the arm, posterior to the medial epicondyle, and then into the medial forearm compartment. The ulnar nerve supplies several forearm muscles and all other intrinsic hand muscles not supplied by the median nerve; it is also sensory to the medial one and one half digits. This syndrome is most often associated with sensory disturbances (paresthesia and sensory loss) from the ring and little fingers. (**D**) Dupuytren's contracture is a disease caused by thickening of the palmar fascia. It results in partial flexion of the metacarpophalangeal and proximal phalangeal joints of the fourth and fifth fingers. Although the hand in Dupuytren's contracture is similar in appearance to the "hand of benediction," it is static and not formed by the patient when asked to make a fist.

55. Correct: Radial (D)

(**D**) The radial nerve passes obliquely and inferolaterally posterior to the humeral shaft in the radial (spiral) groove. The displaced edges of the fractured midshaft of the humerus can stretch or lacerate the nerve in the groove. (**A–C, E**) The axillary, median, musculocutaneous, and ulnar nerves do not lie in close proximity to the middle portion of the humeral shaft and are not at risk for injury from a displaced fracture.

56. Correct: Supination of the forearm (E)

(**E**) Distal to a midshaft humeral fracture, the radial nerve innervates muscles in the posterior forearm that contribute to supination, including the supinator and brachioradialis muscles. Biceps brachii, which also contributes to supination, is innervated by the musculocutaneous nerve and would not be affected by the lesion. Consequently, the patient would exhibit paresis in supination. (**A**) Adduction of the thumb is controlled by adductor pollicis, which is innervated by the deep branch of the ulnar nerve. (**B**) Extension of the arm, to which the long head of triceps contributes, is not likely to be affected since the branches of the radial nerve that supply this muscle leave the radial nerve proximal to the radial (spiral) groove. (**C**) Flexion of the wrist joint is not affected in this patient because the wrist flexors are innervated by the median and ulnar nerves. (**D**) The primary forearm pronators (pronators teres and quadratus) are innervated by the median nerve and would, therefore, not be affected in this patient.

57. Correct: Radius (C)

(**C**) The radiograph shows an overriding spiral fracture of the distal radius (*arrow*). (**A, B, D, E**) The hamate, lunate, scaphoid, and ulna are not fractured (the ulna is, however, dislocated).

58. Correct: Abduction of the index finger (A)

(**A**) Loss of abduction of the index finger indicates involvement of the first dorsal interosseous muscle, which is innervated by the deep branch of the ulnar nerve. This is consistent with the sensory deficits in the little finger. Since there are both sensory and motor deficits, this suggests a lesion of the ulnar nerve proximal to its division into its superficial (sensory) and deep (motor) branches. (**B**) Loss of finger extension indicates involvement of the forearm extensor muscles, which are innervated by the radial nerve. (**C**) Loss of flexion of the distal interphalangeal joint of the index finger indicates involvement of the lateral portion of the flexor digitorum superficialis muscle, which is innervated by the median nerve. (**D**) Loss of flexion of the interphalangeal joint of the thumb indicates involvement of the flexor pollicis longus muscle, which is innervated by the median nerve. (**E**) Loss of thumb opposition indicates involvement of the opponens pollicis muscle, which is innervated by the recurrent median nerve.

59. Correct: De Quervain tenosynovitis (C)

Refer to the following images for answer 59:

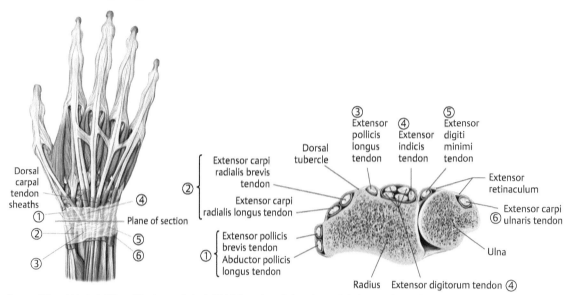

Source: Gilroy AM et al. Atlas of Anatomy. 3rd ed. 2016. Based on: Schuenke M, Schulte E, Schumacher U. THIEME Atlas of Anatomy. Volumes 1-3. Illustrations by Voll M and Wesker K. 2nd ed. New York: Thieme Medical Publishers; 2016

(**C**) De Quervain tenosynovitis (or tendonitis) is an inflammation of the tendons of the extensor pollicis brevis and abductor pollicis longus muscles as they pass through the first dorsal compartment at the radial (thumb) side of the wrist. This condition is usually caused by repetitive movements or overuse, especially in activities that involve abduction and/or extension of the thumb (e.g., gripping or squeezing objects, and moving the wrist in the opposite direction of the thumb). The condition is seen in assembly-line workers and secretaries, and it is more common in women 30 to 50 years of age (picking up children is a noted problem in new mothers). In a Finkelstein test (which has good sensitivity and specificity for de Quervain tenosynovitis), pain is elicited along the radial side of the wrist as the inflamed tendons of extensor pollicis brevis and abductor pollicis longus are compressed in the first dorsal compartment when the wrist is placed into ulnar deviation. (**A**) Carpal tunnel syndrome, which results from compression of the median nerve in the carpal tunnel, results in sensory disturbances from the lateral three and a half fingers and selective thenar weakness (due to involvement of the thenar muscles and the lateral two lumbricals). (**B**) A Colles' fracture, often caused by a FOOSH with the wrist extended, refers to any complete fracture of the distal end of the radius; it is associated with dorsal displacement of the hand on the forearm (the so-called "dinner fork" deformity). (**D**) Dupuytren contracture is a disease caused by thickening of the palmar fascia, which results in partial flexion of the metacarpophalangeal and proximal phalangeal joints of the fourth and fifth fingers. (**E**) Scaphoid fracture, typically associated with pain over the anatomical snuff box, results from a FOOSH.

Vertebral Column

60. Correct: Anterior longitudinal (A)

(**A**) The anterior longitudinal ligament, located along the anterior aspect of the vertebral column and evident by its location on the concave (anterior) side of the column, was ossified in this patient. Calcification and ossification of the anterior longitudinal ligament, accompanied by spondylosis deformans and fibro-ostosis at sites of attachment of the ligament to the vertebral bodies, is part of the pathology associated with diffuse idiopathic skeletal hyperostosis, a disease that occurs primarily in men over 50 years of age. (**B–E**) The denticulate, interspinous, and posterior longitudinal ligaments and ligamenta flava are not located along the anterior aspect of the vertebral column.

61. Correct: Kyphosis (A)

(**A**) The spine is the most common site for skeletal tuberculosis. Infection usually starts in the anterior part of a disc, and spreads to the adjacent surface of the body of a vertebra, or to two adjacent ones. The result is that, as the vertebral bodies collapse, the spine become kyphotic (kyphosis is a normal posteriorly convex curvature of the thoracic and sacral vertebral regions; exaggeration of these curvatures is perhaps more correctly referred to as hyperkyphosis). Commonly, as this deformity gets worse, a sharp angle (gibbus) appears. (**B**) Lordosis is the normal anteriorly convex curvature of the lumbar and cervical vertebral regions. Exaggeration of these curvatures (hyperlordosis) is not a consequence of tuberculosis of the thoracic spine. (**C**) Scoliosis is an abnormal lateral curvature of the spine and is not usually a consequence of tuberculosis. (**D**) Spina bifida occulta is a congenital defect wherein the vertebral arches fail to form. It is unrelated to tuberculosis. (**E**) Spondylolisthesis is a condition in which one of the bones of the vertebral column slips anteriorly out of alignment with the adjacent, inferior vertebra. This occurs most commonly between the L5 and S1 vertebrae, but it may occur at higher vertebral levels. Radicular pain can occur if the nerve root is impinged as a result of the misaligned vertebrae.

62. Correct: L5 (C)

(**C**) The dorsum of the foot includes the L5 dermatome. The "catching" of the patient's great toe when walking and the compensatory "high steppage" gait (using flexion of the hip and knee to raise the foot high enough to prevent the toes from striking the ground) indicate a weakness in dorsiflexion. The dorsiflexor muscles (tibialis anterior, extensor hallucis longus and extensor digitorum longus) are all innervated by the deep fibular nerve (L4-L5). (**A, B, D, E**) Fibers from other spinal nerve roots do not supply the affected dermatome, nor do they dominate the dorsiflexor muscles.

63. Correct: L4 (B)

(**B**) Posterolateral herniation of an intervertebral disc in the lumbar region usually does not compress the spinal nerve roots at the *same* level because they exit the vertebral canal superior to the herniation. The herniated disc does, however, compresses the spinal nerve of the *next lower* level as it passes inferiorly to exit the spinal column. Thus, the L3-L4 disc impinges on the L4 spinal nerve.

Refer to the following image for answer 63:

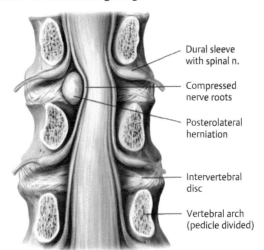

Source: Source: Schuenke M, Schulte E, Schumacher U. THIEME Atlas of Anatomy. General Anatomy and Musculoskeletal System. Illustrations by Voll M and Wesker K. 2nd ed. New York: Thieme Medical Publishers; 2016

64. Correct: Ligamentum flavum > epidural space (B)

Refer to the following image for answer 64:

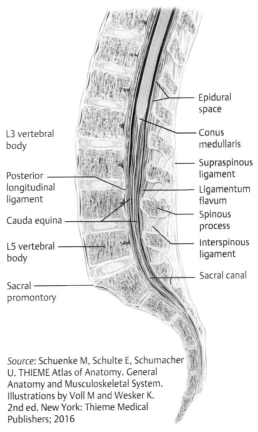

Source: Schuenke M, Schulte E, Schumacher U. THIEME Atlas of Anatomy. General Anatomy and Musculoskeletal System. Illustrations by Voll M and Wesker K. 2nd ed. New York: Thieme Medical Publishers; 2016

(**B**) In a paramedian approach, the epidural needle would not pass through the supra- or interspinous ligaments. Instead, the needle would encounter a ligamentum flavum, which connects adjacent laminae, before it entering the epidural space to administer anesthetic. (**A, D, E**) Since this is a paramedian approach, and the supra- or interspinous ligaments lie in the median plane, neither of these ligaments would be encountered by the epidural needle. In addition, administration of an epidural targets the epidural space, so any space deep to this (e.g., the subarachnoid space) would not be appropriate. (**B**) The denticulate ligament is located laterally and would not be involved in a median approach. (**C**) After passing through the ligamentum flavum, the needle would be in the epidural space. In order to encounter the posterior longitudinal ligament, the needle would have to continue anteriorly through arachnoid mater, subarachnoid space, cauda equina, and then again through arachnoid and dura mater before encountering the posterior longitudinal ligament (which lies within the vertebral canal along the posterior aspect of the vertebral bodies).

65. Correct: L4–L5 (D)

(**D**) The goal of a lumbar puncture is to obtain a sample of cerebrospinal fluid from the subarachnoid space in the region of the lumbar cistern. To perform this procedure safely, it is essential that the spinal needle be inserted inferior to conus medullaris (the inferior end of the spinal cord), which is usually located between the L1 and L2 vertebrae. The L3–L4 interspace can be palpated at the level of the supracristal plane (the highest points of the iliac crests) and then moving inferiorly to the L4–L5 interspace. The L4–L5 interspace is usually the widest space and is safely inferior to conus medullaris.

66. Correct: C2 (B)

(**B**) A "hangman's" fracture, caused by forceful, traumatic hyperextension of the cervical spine fractures the C2 vertebra (axis).

67. Correct: Pedicle (C)

(**C**) A "hangman's" fracture, which is caused by forceful, traumatic hyperextension of the cervical spine, causes a fracture that extends through the pedicle(s) of the C2 vertebra (axis). The *arrow* in radiograph in the question indicates a fracture of the pedicle of the C2 vertebra.

68. Correct: Dens (A)

(**A**) The *arrows* in radiograph in the question indicate a fracture at the base of the dens of the C2 vertebra.

69. Correct: Anterior longitudinal (A)

(**A**) Motor vehicle collisions that involve an impact from the rear commonly result in sudden, forceful hyperextension of the neck ("whiplash"), which

can cause a strain injury of the anterior longitudinal ligament. (**B–E**) The interspinous, posterior longitudinal, supraspinous ligaments, and ligamenta flava are located posterior to the vertebral bodies and, as a result, would not be stretched or injured in a cervical hyperextension injury.

70. Correct: Spondylolisthesis (D)

(**D**) Spondylolisthesis is a condition in which one of the bones of the vertebral column slips anteriorly out of alignment with the adjacent inferior vertebra (in this case, the L5 vertebral has "slipped" anteriorly from the sacrum). Radicular pain can occur if a nerve root is impinged as a result of the misaligned vertebrae. (**A**) Kyphosis (hyperkyphosis) is an accentuation of the normal thoracic kyphotic curvature. (**B**) Scoliosis is an abnormal lateral curvature of the vertebral column. (**C**) Spina bifida is a spinal congenital defect in which the vertebral arch fails to close properly. (**E**) Spondylolysis refers to a fracture or congenital defect of the pars interarticularis, most often relating to the L5 vertebra. Spondylolysis of sufficient severity can result in spondylolisthesis.

71. Correct: Vertebral artery (E)

(**E**) The vertebral artery passes through the transverse foramina of the C1–C6 vertebrae. This patient is experiencing symptomatic vertebrobasilar insufficiency due to occlusion of the vertebral artery, which is provoked by head rotation (also known as Bow hunter's syndrome). (**A–D**) The ascending cervical and internal carotid arteries, internal jugular vein, and vagus nerve do not pass through transverse foramina and would, therefore, not be affected by the provoked by head rotation to produce vertigo.

72. Correct: Thoracic (B)

(**B**) The image shows a transverse fracture of the body of the T9 vertebral body, immediately inferior to the T8–T9 disc. The inferiorly directed, overlapping spinous processes are characteristic of thoracic vertebrae, especially in the mid-thoracic levels. The tapering, inferior end of the spinal cord is apparent in the lower thoracic region (in the normal spinal cord, the inferior end includes the lumbosacral enlargement. (**A**) Spinous processes of cervical vertebrae generally do not angle inferiorly and their bodies are not as large as those in more inferior vertebral regions. (**C**) Lumbar vertebrae have short, robust spinous processes and relatively large vertebral bodies. (**D**) The shape of the sacrum is concave anteriorly (kyphotic) and it tapers inferiorly to meet the coccyx.

73. Correct: Nipple (C)

(**C**) Injury of the spinal cord at the T8 vertebral level would be expected to affect all spinal cord levels *inferior* to the T8 or T9 levels. Therefore, any nerve that arises superior to T8 would not be affected by this injury. Since the nipple is generally considered to be innervated by the T4 intercostal nerve, cutaneous sensation would remain intact. (**A, B, D, E**) Cutaneous innervation to all of these structures arise from spinal cord levels inferior to T8–T9: L5 (via the superficial fibular nerve) for the skin over the great toe; L2–L3 (via the obturator nerve) for the skin over the medial thigh; L1 (via the iliohypogastric and/or ilioinguinal nerves) for the skin over the pubic symphysis; and T10 (via the T10 thoracoabdominal nerve) for the skin over the umbilicus.

74. Correct: Lamina (B)

(**B**) Spina bifida is a developmental defect that affects the vertebral canal, with partial or complete absence of the vertebral arch (laminae and pedicles). The mildest form (spina bifida occulta) may not be associated with clinical signs or symptoms other than the presence of a small tuft of hair or subcutaneous "dimple" overlying the presumed vertebral defect. (**A, C–E**) The inferior articular process, posterior longitudinal ligament, transverse process, and vertebral body do not contribute to the vertebral arch.

75. Correct: Erector spinae (B)

(**B**) Acting concentrically, the erector spinae muscles function to extend the vertebral column. In addition, they can act isometrically to maintain the posture of the flexed vertebral column. (**A**) The vertebral flexor muscles (abdominal obliques and rectus abdominis) cannot extend the vertebral column or act isometrically to maintain a flexed position. (**C**) Latissimus dorsi acts on the arm, not the vertebral column. (**D**) Rhomboid muscles act on the scapulae, not the vertebral column. (**E**) Serratus posterior superior is an accessory muscle of respiration. It does not act on the vertebral column.

76. Correct: Splenius capitis (D)

(**D**) Acting unilaterally, the splenius muscles (capitis and cervicis) rotate the head to the same side (acting bilaterally, they extend the head and neck). Thus, the right splenius muscles rotate the head to the right side and could be affected in this patient. (**A**) The iliocostalis muscles do not rotate the vertebral column or head. (**B**) Acting unilaterally, obliquus capitis (a suboccipital muscle) rotates the head to the contralateral side. Thus, the right obliquus capitis rotates the head to the left side and would not likely be affected in this patient. (**C**) Acting unilaterally, semispinalis capitis (a transversospinal muscle) rotates the head to the contralateral side. Thus, the right semispinalis capitis rotates the head to the left side. (**E**) Trapezius (an extrinsic back muscle) rotates the head to the contralateral side. Thus, the right trapezius rotates the head to the left side.

77. Correct: Vertebral body of C2 vertebra (E)

(**E**) The *arrow* in the radiograph indicates the C2 vertebral body.

78. Correct: Sensory loss from the skin on the back of the head (B)

(**B**) The "X" indicates the location at which the C2 spinal nerve exits the vertebral column. This nerve (greater occipital nerve) provides sensory innervation to most of the skin on the back of the head. (**A**) Skin over the anterior cervical triangle is innervated by the transverse cervical nerve (C3). (**C**) Skin over the frontal bone is innervated by the ophthalmic division of the trigeminal nerve (CN V1). (**D, E**) Neither the deltoid nor the trapezius muscle would be affected as they are innervated by the axillary nerve (C5–C6) and the accessory nerve (CN XI), respectively.

Refer to the following image for answer 78:

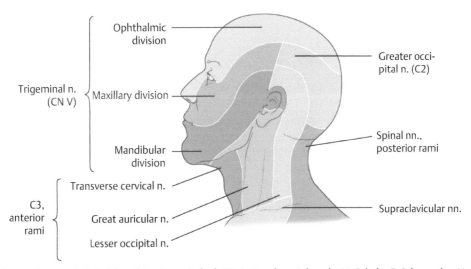

Source: Gilroy AM et al. Atlas of Anatomy. 3rd ed. 2016. Based on: Schuenke M, Schulte E, Schumacher U. THIEME Atlas of Anatomy. Volumes 1-3. Illustrations by Voll M and Wesker K. 2nd ed. New York: Thieme Medical Publishers; 2016

79.   Correct: Nuchal ligament (C)

Refer to the following images for answer 79:

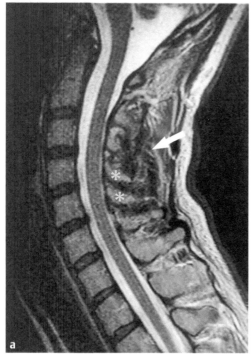

a

Source: Friedrich K, Breitenseher M. Wirbelbögen. In: Vahlensieck M, Reiser M. MRT des Bewegungsapparates. 2. Aufl. Stuttgart: Thieme; 2001

(C) The *arrow* indicates the nuchal ligament. It attaches to the cervical spinous processes (*asterisks*) and represents the supraspinous ligament in the cervical region. (**A, B, D, E**) None of these structures (facet joint capsule, ligamentum flavum, posterior longitudinal ligament, transverse ligament of the atlas) are indicated by the *arrow*.

Lower Limb

80.   Correct: Ligaments of the metatarsophalangeal joint (B)

(B) Turf toe usually involves structures crossing the metatarsophalangeal joint of the great toe, causing pain during locomotion. The condition is commonly described as a sprain to this joint due to hyperextension. By definition, a sprain involves ligamentous structures. (**A, C–E**) The abductor hallucis muscle, sesamoid bones (in the tendons of flexor hallucis brevis), and the tendons of extensor hallucis longus and flexor hallucis longus are not involved in a sprain of the metatarsophalangeal joint of the great toe.

81.   Medial plantar (A)

(A) Cutaneous branches of medial plantar nerve carry sensory impulses from the medial plantar aspect of the foot, including the toes 1 to 3 and the medial half of toe 4. The head of the third metatarsal would lie within the field of distribution for medial plantar nerve (L4–L5). (**B**) Obturator nerve does not distribute to the foot. (**C**) The S1 spinal cord segment

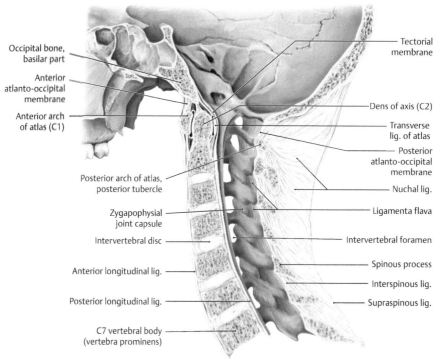

b

Source: Gilroy AM et al. Atlas of Anatomy. 3rd ed. 2016. Based on: Schuenke M, Schulte E, Schumacher U. THIEME Atlas of Anatomy. Volumes 1-3. Illustrations by Voll M and Wesker K. 2nd ed. New York: Thieme Medical Publishers; 2016

receives sensory input conveyed via the sural nerve from the lateral foot. (**D, E**) The saphenous and superficial fibular nerves supply skin of the medial margin and dorsum, respectively, of the foot.

Refer to the following images for answer 82:

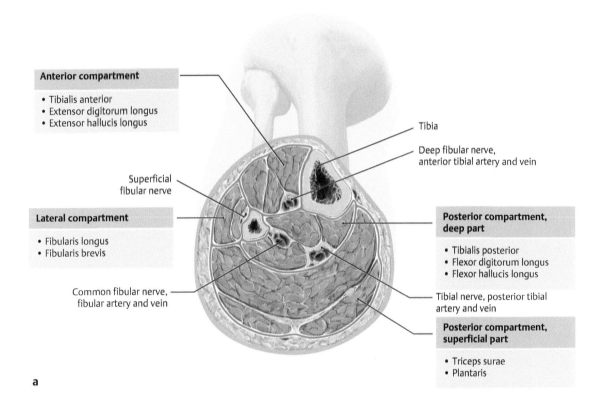

a

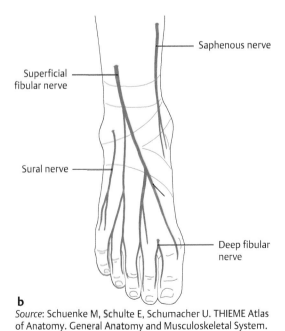

b

Source: Schuenke M, Schulte E, Schumacher U. THIEME Atlas of Anatomy. General Anatomy and Musculoskeletal System. Illustrations by Voll M and Wesker K. 2nd ed. New York: Thieme Medical Publishers; 2016

(**B**) The deep fibular nerve is closely associated with the tibia and innervates all muscles in the anterior compartment of the leg (image a). These muscles (tibialis anterior, extensor digitorum longus, extensor hallucis longus) are involved primarily in dorsiflexion (talocrural joint) and inversion (subtalar joints) of the foot. The sensory distribution for this nerve is limited to the dorsum of the foot, between adjacent sides of the great and second toes (image b). (**A**) The common fibular nerve contains fibers that distribute motor and sensory innervation for both the anterior and lateral compartments of the leg and sensory fibers to the skin on the dorsum of the foot. (**C**) The saphenous nerve is a sensory branch of the femoral nerve that conducts impulses from skin over the medial malleolus. (**D**) The superficial fibular nerve conducts sensory impulses from the skin over the dorsal aspect of the tarsal bones, but not between adjacent sides of the great and second toes. (**E**) The tibial nerve distributes to the posterior leg and plantar foot (medial and lateral plantar nerves).

83. Correct: Tibialis anterior (E)

Refer to the following image for answer 83:

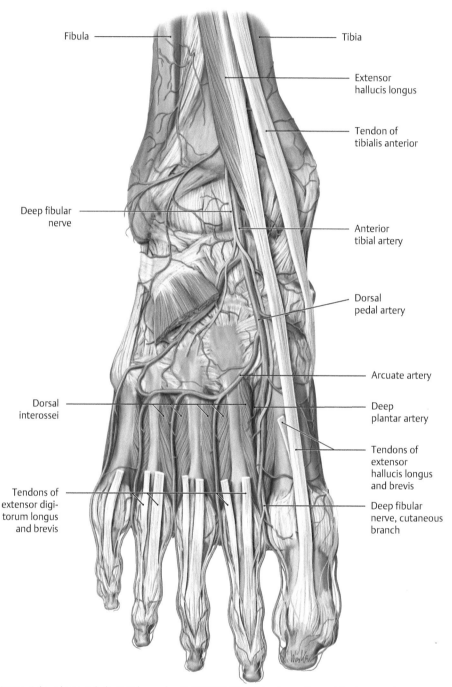

Fibula

Tibia

Extensor hallucis longus

Tendon of tibialis anterior

Deep fibular nerve

Anterior tibial artery

Dorsal pedal artery

Arcuate artery

Dorsal interossei

Deep plantar artery

Tendons of extensor hallucis longus and brevis

Tendons of extensor digitorum longus and brevis

Deep fibular nerve, cutaneous branch

Source: Schuenke M, Schulte E, Schumacher U. THIEME Atlas of Anatomy. General Anatomy and Musculoskeletal System. Illustrations by Voll M and Wesker K. 2nd ed. New York: Thieme Medical Publishers; 2016

(**E**) The tibialis anterior muscle is the largest and most medial muscle of the anterior leg compartment. Its tendon crosses the anterior aspect of the ankle, medial to the tendons of extensor hallucis longus and extensor digitorum longus, before it attaches to the medial cuneiform and first metatarsal. While it assists in dorsiflexion at the ankle, it is the most effective muscle for inversion (subtalar joint). Activities such as hiking, skiing, or running up or downhill may "overuse" the tibialis anterior muscle and cause inflammation of its tendon at the ankle. The risk of this increases if improper (too tight) footwear is used. (**A**) The extensor digitorum brevis muscle does not act on the ankle or subtalar joints. (**B, C**) The extensor digitorum longus and extensor hallucis longus muscles have only minimal involvement in inversion. (**D**) The quadratus plantae is an intrinsic muscle of the plantar aspect of the foot and is not involved in inversion.

---

84. Correct: Femoral (A)

Refer to the following image for answer 84:

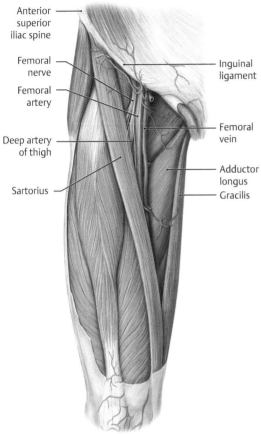

Anterior superior iliac spine

Femoral nerve

Femoral artery

Deep artery of thigh

Sartorius

Inguinal ligament

Femoral vein

Adductor longus

Gracilis

Source: Schuenke M, Schulte E, Schumacher U. THIEME Atlas of Anatomy. General Anatomy and Musculoskeletal System. Illustrations by Voll M and Wesker K. 2nd ed. New York: Thieme Medical Publishers; 2016

(**A**) The femoral artery is the major artery found in the midportion of the medial thigh. It lies in the adductor canal (subsartorial canal; Hunter's canal) with its companion vein, the saphenous nerve, and the nerve to the vastus medialis muscle. Some authors consider the femoral artery to end at the branch point of the deep artery of the thigh (profunda femoris) and the continuing vessel is, therefore, termed the superficial femoral artery. (**B, C**) The perforating arteries branch from the deep artery of the thigh (profunda femoris) in the proximal thigh and would not likely to be injured by the wound in the medial midthigh. (**D**) The obturator artery branches from the internal iliac and distributes to the medial (adductor) muscles of the thigh. At the midthigh, it is typically present as a series of small muscular branches. (**E**) The popliteal artery represents the continuation of the femoral artery in the posterior distal thigh. The femoral artery becomes popliteal as it enters the popliteal region in the posterior knee.

---

85. Correct: Left gluteus medius (B)

(**B**) Normal function of the gluteus medius muscle (and to a lesser degree gluteus minimus) is essential for normal locomotion. During locomotion, these muscles contract on the weight-bearing limb to stabilize the hip joint and prevent the pelvis from tipping downward on the non–weight-bearing side. This allows the non–weight-bearing limb to enter the swing phase of the gait cycle (image a). Injury to the deep gluteal muscles (or the superior gluteal nerve), compromises their ability to prevent the hip from tipping downward on the non–weight-bearing side. This results in a characteristic pelvic dipping on the non–weight bearing side when that limb is in the swing phase of gait. To compensate for the pelvic dipping, the individual will lean away from the non–weight-bearing limb and raise the foot higher to allow the foot to clear; this is known as a Trendelenburg, or gluteus medius gait (images b and c). Since spinal polio preferentially affects the lower lumbar and upper sacral levels of the spinal cord, the superior gluteal nerve (L4–S1) that supplies gluteus medius can be affected. Post-polio syndrome is a second attack of by the polio virus on average 35 years after the initial symptoms. It leads to increased muscle weakness in the same, or additional, muscles that are involved in the first bout. (**A**) Quadratus femoris is the collective term for a major muscle group (rectus femoris, vastus lateralis, vastus intermedius, vastus medialis) involved in extension of the knee joint and would not be involved in producing Trendelenburg gait. (**C**) Tensor fasciae latae acts as a flexor muscle of the hip joint and would not be involved in producing a Trendelenburg gait. (**D**) Piriformis is involved in lateral rotation of the hip and is not a significant muscle in walking. (**E**) Gluteus maximus does not have a major function during walking. Rather, its role in hip extension is significant during running, climbing stairs, and rising from the seated position.

Refer to the following image for answer 85:

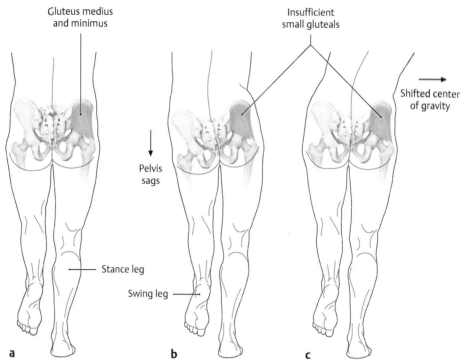

Gluteus medius and minimus

Insufficient small gluteals

Shifted center of gravity

Pelvis sags

Stance leg

Swing leg

a   b   c

Source: Schuenke M, Schulte E, Schumacher U. THIEME Atlas of Anatomy. General Anatomy and Musculoskeletal System. Illustrations by Voll M and Wesker K. 2nd ed. New York: Thieme Medical Publishers; 2016

86. Correct: Plantar aponeurosis (D)

(**D**) The plantar aponeurosis is the thick central band of plantar deep fascia that extends from the plantar aspect of the calcaneus to the toes and acts as a superficial ligament. It lies superficial to the intrinsic muscle layers of the plantar aspect of foot and acts as a major support for the arches of the foot. Excessive and repetitive stretching of the plantar aponeurosis by exercise on hard surfaces, long periods of standing, improper footwear, obesity, and foot malformations can cause this fascia to develop small tears and to become inflamed (plantar fasciitis). Classic symptoms are heel and foot pain when standing, especially when the foot has not been bearing weight for some time (first steps out of bed or after sitting for extended periods). (**A, E**) Individually, these intrinsic muscles of the plantar foot would rarely account for foot pain. (**B, C**) Individually, these ligaments of the foot would rarely account for foot pain. The plantar calcaneonavicular ("spring") ligament is a primary support for the head of the talus and its failure allows the head of the talus to sag, leading to a flat foot. Plantar fasciitis may develop secondary to flat feet (pes planus).

Refer to the following image for answer 86:

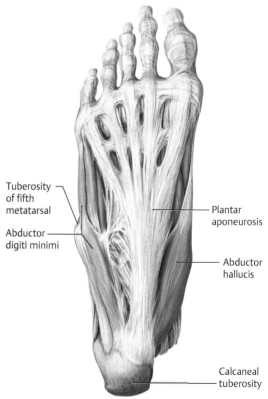

Tuberosity of fifth metatarsal

Abductor digiti minimi

Plantar aponeurosis

Abductor hallucis

Calcaneal tuberosity

Source: Schuenke M, Schulte E, Schumacher U. THIEME Atlas of Anatomy. General Anatomy and Musculoskeletal System. Illustrations by Voll M and Wesker K. 2nd ed. New York: Thieme Medical Publishers; 2016

87. Correct: It is bathed in synovial fluid. (C)

Refer to the following image for answer 87:

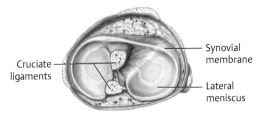

Source: Schuenke M, Schulte E, Schumacher U. THIEME Atlas of Anatomy. Internal Organs. Illustrations by Voll M and Wesker K. 2nd ed. New York: Thieme Medical Publishers; 2016

(**C**) The synovial membrane attaches to the outer margin of the menisci, placing them within the synovial cavity of the knee. (**A**) The menisci cannot be distinguished on palpation due to the collateral ligaments that lie superficial to them. (**B**) The outer, thicker region of the menisci receives small blood vessels from the genicular arteries. The central portion of the menisci is less vascularized. (**D**) The menisci are composed of fibrocartilage. (**E**) The medial meniscus is less mobile than the lateral meniscus because it is fused with the medial collateral ligament along its outer margin.

88. Correct: Knee flexion and plantar flexion (C)

(**C**) The calcaneal (Achilles) tendon, which attaches to the posterior calcaneus, is formed by the union of the tendons from gastrocnemius and soleus (triceps surae). The gastrocnemius muscle has medial and lateral heads of origin from the respective condyles of the femur, whereas soleus has bony origin from the tibia and fibula. The gastrocnemius can flex the knee and the combined muscles are powerful plantar flexors. (**A, B, D**) Gastrocnemius is not involved in rotation at the knee, and neither gastrocnemius nor soleus produces inversion or eversion. (**E**) Gastrocnemius and soleus produce plantar flexion but, because gastrocnemius crosses the knee joint, it is also involved in knee flexion.

Refer to the following image for answer 88:

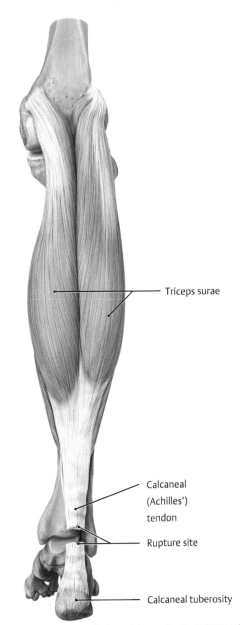

Source: Schuenke M, Schulte E, Schumacher U. THIEME Atlas of Anatomy. Head, Neck, and Neuroanatomy. Illustrations by Voll M and Wesker K. 2nd ed. New York: Thieme Medical Publishers; 2016

89. Correct: S1 (C)

Refer to the following images for answer 89:

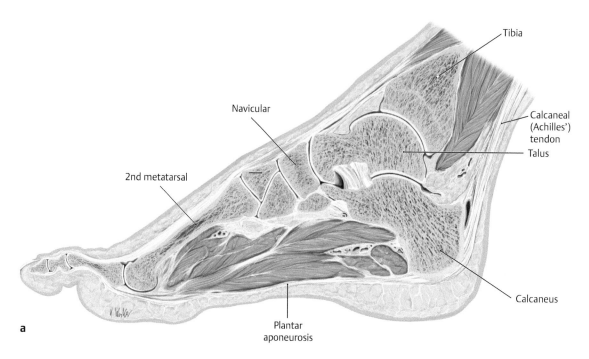

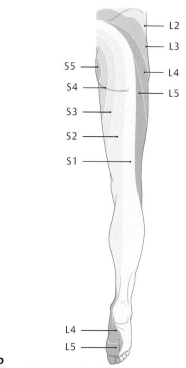

b

Source: Gilroy AM et al. Atlas of Anatomy. 3rd ed. 2016.
Based on: Schuenke M, Schulte E, Schumacher U.
THIEME Atlas of Anatomy. Volumes 1-3. Illustrations by
Voll M and Wesker K. 2nd ed. New York:
Thieme Medical Publishers; 2016

(C) Most afferent impulses from the distal calcaneal (Achilles) tendon (image a) and posterior heel region enter the S1 spinal cord segment (image b). (A, B, D, E) The L3, L4, S2, and S3 spinal cord levels are not represented in the posterior heel region (image b).

90. Correct: Adductor longus (A)

(A) The more powerful adductor muscles of the hip are the adductor longus muscle and the adductor portion of adductor magnus (fibers with origin from ischial tuberosity). Adductor longus is frequently injured in athletes and the strain is usually at the musculotendinous junction. It is known that the sarcomeres near this transition zone are less elastic, that the area has a poorer blood supply, and a rich nerve supply, all of which help explain why the adductor longus is vulnerable to strain, why the healing is prolonged, and why the pain is severe. An example is the soccer player who is attempting to kick a ball (which activates the adductor muscles) when an opposing player tries to kick the ball at the same time in the opposite direction. This eccentric action on the contracting adductor muscles may cause tearing at the musculotendinous junctions. (B, D, E) While the gracilis, obturator externus, and pectineus muscles are involved in hip adduction, their role is minor. Obturator externus and pectineus are more associated with stabilization at the hip joint. (C) Iliopsoas is the most powerful hip flexor and is not involved in hip adduction.

91. Correct: Obturator (D)

Refer to the following image for answer 91:

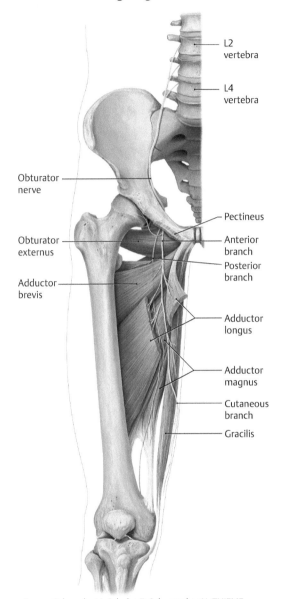

Source: Schuenke M, Schulte E, Schumacher U. THIEME Atlas of Anatomy. General Anatomy and Musculoskeletal System. Illustrations by Voll M and Wesker K. 2nd ed. New York: Thieme Medical Publishers; 2016

(**D**) Obturator nerve provides the motor supply for the gracilis muscle. (**A**) The femoral nerve does not supply the gracilis muscle. (**B, C, E**) The ilioinguinal, saphenous and medial femoral cutaneous nerves have only sensory distribution in the thigh.

92. Correct: The rim edge of the cast is compressing the common fibular nerve at the neck of the fibula. (C)

(**C**) When the leg is placed in a cast, it is common for the upper edge of the cast to lie at the level of the neck of the fibula. This corresponds to the subcutaneous position of the common fibular nerve. Therefore, a cast that is initially too tight or one that does not allow for post-trauma swelling may lead to the common fibular nerve being compressed between the cast and the fibula. (**A**) Two-days postfracture is too soon for callus formation to have impacted function of the deep fibular nerve. (**B**) Diminished sensation to the anterolateral leg and weak toe extension indicates that the nerve trauma is proximal to the metatarsophalangeal region. (**D**) The tibial nerve is surrounded by soft tissues in the popliteal fossa and compression by a cast is unlikely. In addition, the neurological symptoms do not suggest involvement of the tibial nerve. (**E**) The symptoms are all neurological and do not suggest a vascular compromise.

Refer to the following image for answer 92:

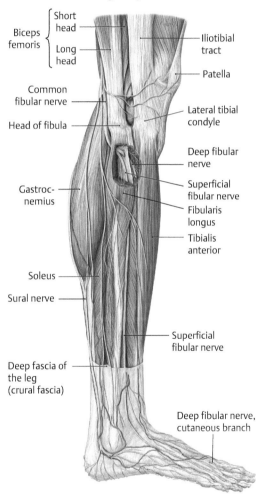

Source: Schuenke M, Schulte E, Schumacher U. THIEME Atlas of Anatomy. General Anatomy and Musculoskeletal System. Illustrations by Voll M and Wesker K. 2nd ed. New York: Thieme Medical Publishers; 2016

93. Internal pudendal (B)

(**B**) The greater sciatic notch borders the posterior wall of the acetabulum. The internal pudendal artery, a branch of the internal iliac artery within the true (lesser) pelvis, leaves the pelvic cavity via the inferior portion of the greater sciatic notch. This portion of the greater sciatic notch is located opposite the posterior acetabular wall. (**A**) The common iliac artery does not enter the true pelvis and is not closely associated with the acetabulum. (**C–E**) The superior gluteal, superior vesical, and uterine arteries are not closely associated with the acetabulum.

94. Posterior cruciate ligament (E)

(**E**) A primary function of the posterior cruciate ligament is to check posterior displacement of the tibia on the femur when the knee is flexed. Falling on the flexed knees results in the tibial tuberosities receiving the brunt of the fall, being displaced posteriorly on the femoral condyles, and spraining or tearing the posterior cruciate ligament. The posterior drawer test is assessed with the limb non-weight bearing and the knee flexed. If the examiner can slide the tibia posteriorly with a soft endpoint, the test is considered positive. The test should be applied to both knees to establish a basis for comparison. (**A**) The anterior drawer (Lachman) test is reliable in assessing the integrity of the anterior cruciate ligament. The test should be applied to both knees to establish a basis for comparison. If, in the injured knee, the tibia can be displaced anteriorly on the femoral condyles with a soft endpoint, the anterior cruciate ligament is failing in its function to limit this movement. Injury to the anterior cruciate ligament is 10 times more frequent than to the posterior cruciate ligament. (**B, C**) The collateral ligaments of the knee are only taut during knee extension and falling on the flexed knee typically will not affect these ligaments. (**D**) Medial meniscus tears typically occur during sudden rotation or blows to the lateral knee with the knee in extension and the foot planted. This injury may also involve the anterior cruciate and medial collateral ligaments (unhappy triad).

95. Correct: Calcaneus (A)

(**A**) The calcaneus is one of the primary contact points when the foot is planted on a flat surface. It is the first part of the foot to contact the ground at the end of the swing phase of locomotion (heel strike). When falling from a height and landing on the heel or flat foot, the calcaneus receives a majority of the force and can be fractured. Subsequent formation of a hematoma on the plantar foot is diagnostic for calcaneal fracture. (**B–E**) The cuboid, intermediate cuneiform, medial cuneiform, and navicular bones do not have significant contact with the ground and are less vulnerable in blunt trauma to the plantar foot. They are most often injured in crushing injuries and frequently are involved in fractures of multiple tarsal bones.

96. Correct: Femoral (C)

(**C**) The femoral ring is a weak point in the abdominal wall. The ring opens into the femoral canal, which lies medial to the femoral vein and inferolateral to the pubic tubercle. Since the canal contains only fat, lymphatic vessels, and lymph nodes, a loop of small intestine may enter the femoral canal and progress into the femoral triangle of the anterior thigh. The hernia sac may eventually present as a subcutaneous elevation by passing through the saphenous opening in the fascia lata. The presence of the hernia in the femoral triangle compromises venous flow in the region and causes vein distension. The opening of the femoral ring is wider in females due to a greater transverse dimension of the bony pelvis, thus femoral hernias are more common in women (approximately 70%). (**A, B, D, E**) Direct inguinal, epigastric, indirect inguinal, and umbilical hernias will not enter the thigh. Indirect The inguinal hernias can extend into the labia majora/scrotum.

Refer to the following image for answer 96:

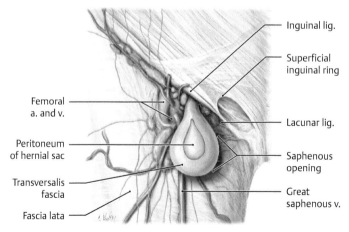

Source: Gilroy AM et al. Atlas of Anatomy. 3rd ed. 2016. Based on: Schuenke M, Schulte E, Schumacher U. THIEME Atlas of Anatomy. Volumes 1-3. Illustrations by Voll M and Wesker K. 2nd ed. New York: Thieme Medical Publishers; 2016

97. Correct: Fascia lata (A)

Refer to the following image for answer 97:

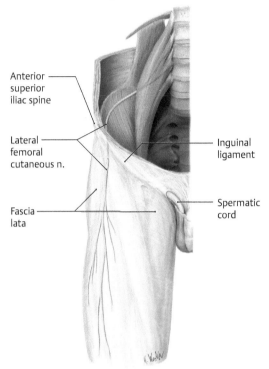

Source: Gilroy AM et al. Atlas of Anatomy. 3rd ed. 2016. Based on: Schuenke M, Schulte E, Schumacher U. THIEME Atlas of Anatomy, Volumes 1-3. Illustrations by Voll M and Wesker K. 2nd ed. New York: Thieme Medical Publishers; 2016

(**A**) The arterial cannula must pass through the deep fascia of the thigh, termed the fascia lata. This fascia is thick and opaque and surrounds the thigh, separating subcutaneous from deep structures. Extensions of the fascia lata (intermuscular septae) pass deep and attach to the femur, creating the anatomical compartmentalization. (**B**) The inguinal ligament is not fascia. (**C**) The intermuscular septa of the thigh are extensions of the fascia lata from its deep side. They attach to the femur and compartmentalize the structures of the thigh. (**D**) The superficial fascia of the thigh lies just deep to the skin, between the skin and fascia lata. It contains variable amounts of fat. (**E**) Transversalis fascia is extraperitoneal fascia of the anterior abdominal wall.

98. Correct: Anterior tibial (A)

(**A**) Chronic exertional compartment syndrome involves structures of the anterior compartment of the leg. Structures in this compartment are tightly bound by crural fascia and the shaft of the tibia. The anterior tibial vein is the major vein of this compartment. Its deep position renders it vulnerable to compression in cases of edema and swelling of muscles in the compartment. The vein is usually paired, with each member of the pair closely applied to either side of the accompanying artery (venae comitantes). (**B, E**) The great and small saphenous veins are subcutaneous veins and would not be affected directly in compartment syndrome. They do communicate with deep veins and may eventually show some distension. (**C**) The popliteal vein is formed in the knee region with the union of anterior and posterior tibial veins. Its course in the leg is very short. (**D**) The posterior tibial vein is resident to the deep posterior compartment of the leg.

Refer to the following image for answer 98:

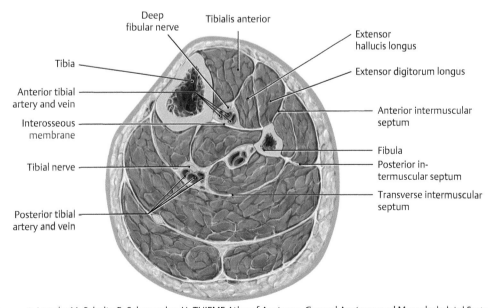

Source: Schuenke M, Schulte E, Schumacher U. THIEME Atlas of Anatomy. General Anatomy and Musculoskeletal System. Illustrations by Voll M and Wesker K. 2nd ed. New York: Thieme Medical Publishers; 2016

99. Correct: Anterior talofibular (A)

Refer to the following image for answer 99:

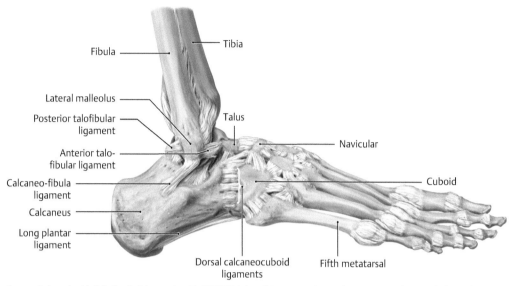

Source: Schuenke M, Schulte E, Schumacher U. THIEME Atlas of Anatomy. General Anatomy and Musculoskeletal System. Illustrations by Voll M and Wesker K. 2nd ed. New York: Thieme Medical Publishers; 2016

(**A**) Anterior talofibular ligament is part of the lateral complex of ankle ligaments. It is the weakest of the three (anterior talofibular, posterior talofibular, calcaneofibular) and is responsible for preventing anterior displacement of the talus. It is most vulnerable when the foot is plantar flexed and inverted. Anterior displacement of the hindfoot (anterior drawer test for ankle) is diagnostic for anterior talofibular ligament damage. (**B, E**) The tibiofibular ligaments are typically not injured in ankle sprains. (**C, D**) The calcaneofibular and posterior talofibular ligaments of the lateral complex are strong bands that are most often injured in subluxation of the talus.

100. Medial circumflex femoral artery (E)

(**E**) Three vessels contribute to the blood supply for the intracapsular portion of the proximal femur: the medial and lateral circumflex femoral arteries, and the artery of the head of femur (foveal artery). The medial femoral circumflex artery provides more retinacular branches to the neck and head of the femur than does the lateral femoral circumflex. The artery of the head of the femur is relatively small; it passes within the ligament of the head of the femur and cannot itself support the head and neck of the femur. (**A–C**) The iliolumbar, inferior gluteal, and internal iliac vessels do not supply the intracapsular portion of the hip joint. (**D**) The lateral circumflex femoral artery does provide retinacular arteries to the neck and head of the femur, but significantly fewer than the medial circumflex femoral artery.

Refer to the following image for answer 100:

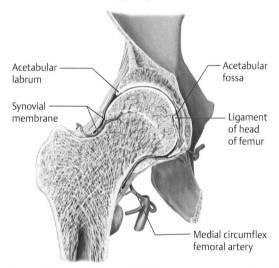

Source: Schuenke M, Schulte E, Schumacher U. THIEME Atlas of Anatomy. General Anatomy and Musculoskeletal System. Illustrations by Voll M and Wesker K. 2nd ed. New York: Thieme Medical Publishers; 2016

101. Correct: Coxa vara (C)

Refer to the following image for answer 101:

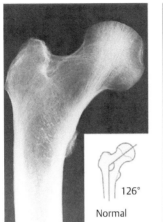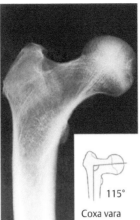

126°
Normal

115°
Coxa vara

Source: Source: Schuenke M, Schulte E, Schumacher U. THIEME Atlas of Anatomy. General Anatomy and Musculoskeletal System. Illustrations by Voll M and Wesker K. 2nd ed. New York: Thieme Medical Publishers; 2016

(**C**) The normal angle between the neck and shaft of the femur should be in the 125 to 135 degrees range. Measurements outside this range result in an abnormal junction of the femur and tibia. Angles less than 125 degrees produce coxa vara (commonly called "knock-knee"), whereas angles above the range of normalcy result in coxa valga (commonly called "bow-legged"). (**A**) A dislocated hip would not, necessarily, exhibit abnormal angulation between the neck and shaft of the femur. (**B**) Coxa valga would involve neck/shaft angulation greater than 135 degrees. (**D, E**) Genu vara and valga are malalignments of the femur and tibia independent of the angle of the femoral neck and shaft. Determinations for genu vara and valga are based on the Q-angle, which is the angle between a vertical line through the patella and a line connecting the patella and the anterior superior iliac spine (ASIS).

102. Correct: Medial collateral (C)

(**C**) The medial deviation of the femur in coxa vara as it articulates with the tibia will tend to force the two bones apart at their medial sides, "opening" the joint and placing increased tension on the medial collateral ligament. (**B**) The lateral collateral ligament will tend to be slackened in coxa vara. (**A, D, E**) The cruciate and patellofemoral ligaments will not have significantly increased stress in coxa vara.

103. Correct: Gluteus maximus (A)

(**A**) Gluteus maximus is the primary muscle involved in hip extension while climbing or rising from the seated position. During walking on a flat surface, the hamstring muscles (semitendinosus, semimembranosus, and long head of biceps femoris) act as the primary hip extensors. (**B, C**) The gluteus medius and piriformis muscles are not significant in producing hip extension: gluteus medius (abduction of the non–weight-bearing limb) and piriformis (external rotation). (**D, E**) The psoas major and tensor fasciae latae muscles are involved in hip flexion.

104. Correct: Extensor hallucis longus (D)

(**D**) The tendon of extensor hallucis longus is subcutaneous on the dorsum of the foot and courses medial and parallel to the dorsal artery of the foot (dorsalis pedis artery). (**A, E**) Abductor hallucis and tibialis anterior lie along the medial margin of the foot and are not related to the dorsal artery of the foot. (**B**) The tendons of extensor digitorum brevis lie deep to the dorsal artery of the foot. (**C**) The tendons of extensor digitorum longus are lateral to the dorsal artery of the foot.

Refer to the following image for answer 104:

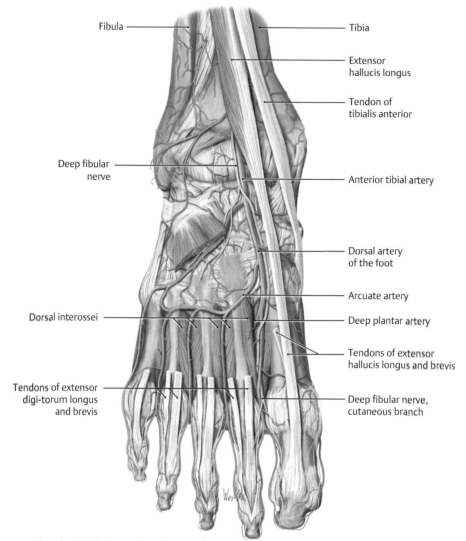

Fibula

Tibia

Extensor hallucis longus

Tendon of tibialis anterior

Deep fibular nerve

Anterior tibial artery

Dorsal artery of the foot

Arcuate artery

Dorsal interossei

Deep plantar artery

Tendons of extensor hallucis longus and brevis

Tendons of extensor digi-torum longus and brevis

Deep fibular nerve, cutaneous branch

Source: Schuenke M, Schulte E, Schumacher U. Atlas of Anatomy. General Anatomy and Musculoskeletal System. 2nd Edition. New York, NY: Thieme Medical Publishers; 2014. Illustration by Karl Wesker/Markus Voll.

105. Correct: Biceps femoris, long head (B)

(**B**) The long head of biceps femoris is one of the hamstring group of muscles (long head of biceps femoris, semimembranosus, semitendinosus, hamstring portion of adductor magnus), all of which have their proximal attachment on the ischial tuberosity.

These muscles are vulnerable to injury when the hip is strongly flexed with the knee in full extension (punting a football; high kick in dancing). (**A, C–E**) The adductor longus, short head of biceps femoris, gluteus maximus, and gracilis do not attach to the ischial tuberosity.

Refer to the following image for answer 105:

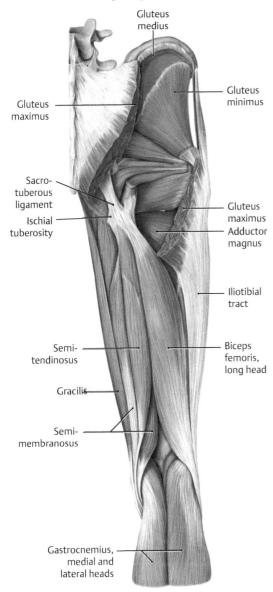

Source: Schuenke M, Schulte E, Schumacher U. THIEME Atlas of Anatomy. General Anatomy and Musculoskeletal System. Illustrations by Voll M and Wesker K. 2nd ed. New York: Thieme Medical Publishers; 2016

---

106. Correct: Psoas major (E)

(E) Psoas major, the most effective flexor of the hip joint, has origin from the transverse processes of all

five lumbar vertebrae—the location of the lumbar paraspinal abscesses—and the intervening intervertebral discs. The lumbar nerve plexus passes through the belly of the muscle, and is also likely affected by the abscesses and accounts for the diminished patellar tendon reflexes (L4). (**A**) The crura of the diaphragm are attached to the upper lumbar vertebra but do not act on the hip joint. (**B–D**) The iliacus, obturator internus, and piriformis muscles are not attached to lumbar vertebrae, nor do any of them flex the hip joint.

---

107. Correct: L4 (B)

Refer to the following image for answer 107:

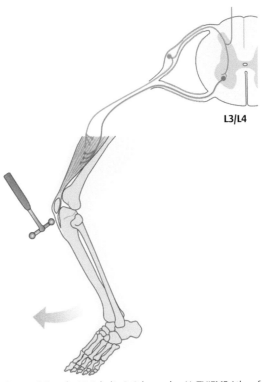

L3/L4

Source: Schuenke M, Schulte E, Schumacher U. THIEME Atlas of Anatomy. General Anatomy and Musculoskeletal System. Illustrations by Voll M and Wesker K. 2nd ed. New York: Thieme Medical Publishers; 2016

(**B**) Afferent impulses from deep tendon receptors in the patellar ligament will enter the spinal cord at L3-L4 levels, with most of the fibers entering at L4. (**A, C–E**) Reflex impulses from the patellar ligament do not enter the T12, L1, L5, or S1 spinal cord levels.

108. Correct: Gluteus medius (B)

(**B**) A properly placed intramuscular injection to the gluteal region will have the needle inserted in the anterior-most portion of the gluteus medius muscle. This so-called ventrogluteal placement site is located in the upper lateral quadrant of the gluteal region, far from the sciatic and superior gluteal nerves. This quadrant overlies the origin of gluteus medius from the ilium. (**A**) Injections into gluteus maximus are high risk because the sciatic nerve and large branches of the superior and inferior gluteal vessels lie immediately deep to the muscle. (**C**) Gluteus minimus is very deep in the gluteal region and reliable surface landmarks for its location are lacking. (**D, E**) The sartorius and tensor fasciae latae muscles are not located in the buttocks.

Refer to the following image for answer 108:

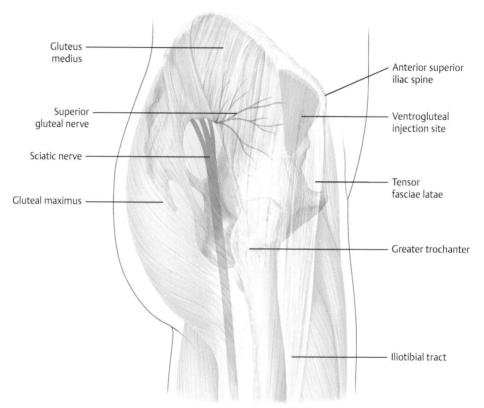

Source: Schuenke M, Schulte E, Schumacher U. THIEME Atlas of Anatomy. General Anatomy and Musculoskeletal System. Illustrations by Voll M and Wesker K. 2nd ed. New York: Thieme Medical Publishers; 2016

109. Correct: Medial malleolus (C)

Refer to the following image for answer 109:

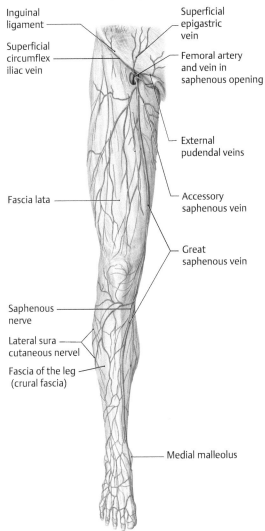

Source: Schuenke M, Schulte E, Schumacher U. THIEME Atlas of Anatomy. General Anatomy and Musculoskeletal System. Illustrations by Voll M and Wesker K. 2nd ed. New York: Thieme Medical Publishers; 2016

(**C**) The great saphenous vein can be found reliably just *anterior* to the medial malleolus. (**A, B, D, E**) The adductor tubercle, medial border of the patella, sustentaculum tali, and tibial tuberosity are not reliable landmarks for the location of the great saphenous vein.

110. Correct: Anterior superior iliac spine and pubic symphysis (D)

(**D**) The femoral artery is superficial in the femoral triangle. Pressure just inferior to the inguinal ligament at the midpoint between the anterior superior iliac spine and pubic symphysis is the proper point to assess a femoral pulse. (**A–C**) The anterior inferior iliac spine is not palpable as it is deep to sartorius muscle. (**E**) The midpoint between the anterior superior iliac spine and pubic tubercle would be lateral to femoral artery.

111. Correct: Semimembranosus (D)

(**D**) Subtendinous bursae are found on semimembranosus and the medial head of gastrocnemius. These bursae frequently communicate with the synovial cavity of the knee joint and effusion of synovial fluid may produce a painful swelling in the medial part of the popliteal fossa. This type of cyst has several names, including: synovial popliteal cyst, gastrocnemio-semimembranosus cyst, and Baker's cyst. (**A, B**) Both heads of biceps femoris border the lateral aspect of the popliteal fossa. The patient's symptoms and the imaging indicate the cyst is on the medial side of the popliteal fossa. (**C**) The popliteus muscle lies in the floor of the popliteal fossa. The patient's symptoms and the imaging indicate the cyst is on the medial side of the popliteal fossa. (**E**) Soleus is not associated with the popliteal fossa.

112. Correct: Lumbar plexus (C)

Refer to the following images for answer 112:

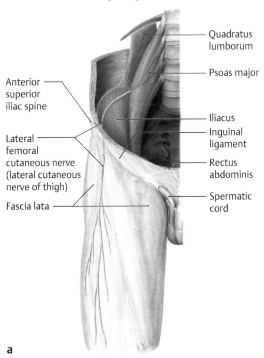

a

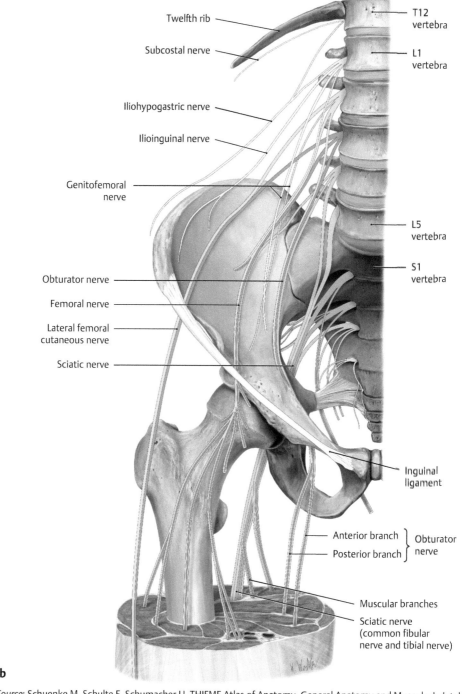

Twelfth rib

Subcostal nerve

Iliohypogastric nerve

Ilioinguinal nerve

Genitofemoral
nerve

Obturator nerve

Femoral nerve

Lateral femoral
cutaneous nerve

Sciatic nerve

T12
vertebra

L1
vertebra

L5
vertebra

S1
vertebra

Inguinal
ligament

Anterior branch ⎫ Obturator
Posterior branch ⎰ nerve

Muscular branches

Sciatic nerve
(common fibular
nerve and tibial nerve)

b

Source: Schuenke M, Schulte E, Schumacher U. THIEME Atlas of Anatomy. General Anatomy and Musculoskeletal System. Illustrations by Voll M and Wesker K. 2nd ed. New York: Thieme Medical Publishers; 2016

(**C**) Meralgia paresthetica is a burning, tingling, and/ or numbness along the lateral thigh due to compression of the lateral femoral cutaneous nerve (L2–L3) (image A). This nerve, a direct branch from the lumbar plexus on the posterior abdominal wall (image B), enters the thigh deep to the inguinal ligament and just medial to the anterior superior iliac spine. In obese individuals, the weight of a pendulous abdomen may compress the nerve against the inguinal ligament or anterior superior iliac spine, leading to

meralgia paresthetica. (**A, B, D, E**) The femoral, inferior gluteal, obturator, and subcostal nerves do not distribute to the lateral thigh.

113.   Correct: Obturator (E)

(**E**) This patient has an obturator hernia that is compressing the obturator nerve as it lies in the obturator canal. Compression of this nerve affects the motor supply to the muscles of the medial compartment of the thigh (gracilis, obturator externus, adductor longus and brevis, part of adductor magnus), as well as the sensory distribution of obturator nerve to the medial thigh. Obturator hernias, while not common, tend to occur in women who are multiparous and have low body fat. (**A**) A femoral hernia may project to a similar region of the medial thigh. However, this type of hernia will affect the femoral nerve and its branches and would not account for the signs and symptoms in this patient. (**B–D**) The genitofemoral, ilioinguinal, and medial femoral cutaneous nerves are only sensory in their distribution to the thigh, and their compression cannot account for the positive Howship–Romberg sign.

114. Correct: Compression of sciatic nerve by piriformis muscle in the greater sciatic foramen (C)

Refer to the following image for answer 114:

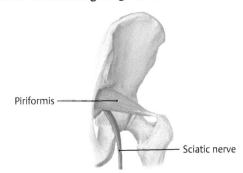

Source: Schuenke M, Schulte E, Schumacher U. THIEME Atlas of Anatomy. General Anatomy and Musculoskeletal System. Illustrations by Voll M and Wesker K. 2nd ed. New York: Thieme Medical Publishers; 2016

(**C**) Based on his profession (and the likelihood that he sits at desk for long periods), personal activities (trail runner), and pain on deep compression to the buttock, this man most likely has piriformis syndrome. In this syndrome, a hypertrophied piriformis compresses the sciatic and posterior femoral cutaneous nerves as they exit the pelvis through the greater sciatic foramen. Symptoms may mimic those of a herniated disk, especially pain in the buttock and posterior thigh (sciatica). (**A, B**) Although some of the symptoms are similar to those elicited by a herniated (e.g., posterior thigh pain suggestive of involvement of the S1 or S2 spinal nerves), the MRI does not support a diagnosis of this pathology (e.g., disc herniation compressing either the L4 or L5 spinal nerve would likely have sensory deficits in the anterior thigh. (**D**) Compression of the superior gluteal nerve would likely result in weakness of the gluteus medius and minimus (i.e., hip abduction) or tensor fasciae latae muscles. (**E**) In some individuals the sciatic nerve, or its common fibular part, may pass through, or superior to, the piriformis muscle. These variations would not necessarily predispose for piriformis syndrome.

115. Correct: Soleus (E)

Refer to the following image for answer 115:

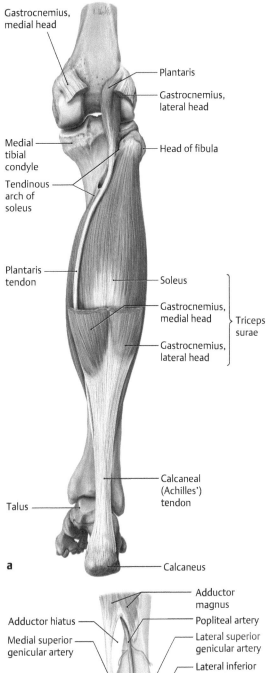

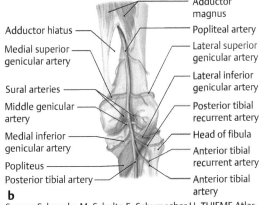

Source: Schuenke M, Schulte E, Schumacher U. THIEME Atlas of Anatomy. General Anatomy and Musculoskeletal System. Illustrations by Voll M and Wesker K. 2nd ed. New York: Thieme Medical Publishers; 2016

(E) The initial stages of locomotion involve lifting the heel from the ground (plantar flexion). Since this involves lifting the body weight from the surface, it requires powerful muscles. The muscles most important in plantar flexion are those in the superficial division of the posterior leg, the gastrocnemius and soleus (image a). Soleus is considered the "workhorse" of plantar flexion. Reduced blood flow due to peripheral vascular disease will cause these muscles to exhibit transitory pain during exercise (intermittent claudication). Branches from the popliteal artery (sural arteries) supply most of the blood to soleus and gastrocnemius (image b). (A–D) These muscles are not involved in plantar flexion: adductor magnus, hamstring part (hip extension); extensor digitorum longus (dorsiflexion and extension of toes); fibularis tertius (dorsiflexion and eversion); and popliteus (rotation of femur on tibia).

116. Correct: L1–L3 (A)

(A) While there is considerable overlap of adjacent dermatomes, and a lack of consensus among authors regarding dermatome mapping, the best answer is L1–L3 as the area indicated has representation from these three spinal cord levels. The sensory fibers for these dermatomes are conveyed by the ilioinguinal (L1), femoral branch of the genitofemoral (L1–L2), femoral (L2–L4), and obturator (L2–L4) nerves. (B–E) See the dermatome map in the accompanying image.

Refer to the following image for answer 116:

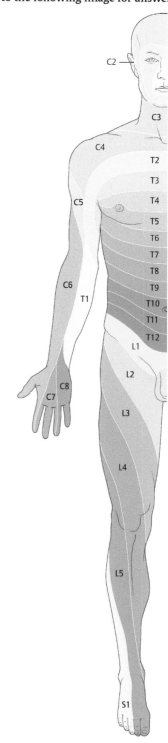

Source: Schuenke M, Schulte E, Schumacher U. THIEME Atlas of Anatomy. General Anatomy and Musculoskeletal System. Illustrations by Voll M and Wesker K. 2nd ed. New York: Thieme Medical Publishers; 2016

117. Correct: Obturator (E)

(**E**) This patient has difficulty moving her right foot from the accelerator to brake pedal, an action involving adduction of the thigh. The muscles of the medial (adductor) compartment of the thigh (adductor longus, adductor brevis, adductor part of adductor magnus, gracilis, obturator externus, pectineus) are the primary muscles for thigh adduction, and are innervated by the obturator nerve (L2–L4; image a). The nerve is closely associated with the internal iliac vessels and branches along the lateral pelvic wall before the nerve exits the pelvis via the obturator canal to enter the medial thigh. As such, the nerve is at some risk of injury during resection of the internal iliac lymph nodes. The internal and external iliac nodes, superficial and deep inguinal nodes, and sacral nodes all receive lymph from female pelvic organs (image b). (**A**) Other than pectineus (which commonly receives dual nerve supply from obturator and femoral), the femoral nerve does not innervate any muscles with a primary action of thigh adduction. (**B, C**) The distribution of the genitofemoral and ilioinguinal nerves and in the thigh is only sensory. (**D**) The lumbosacral trunk (L4–L5) does not innervate any muscles as such. Rather, it joins the sacral plexus and its fibers are distributed with branches of that plexus to the posterior thigh, leg, and foot.

Refer to the following images for answer 117:

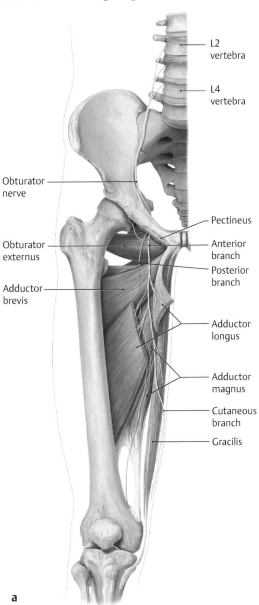

a

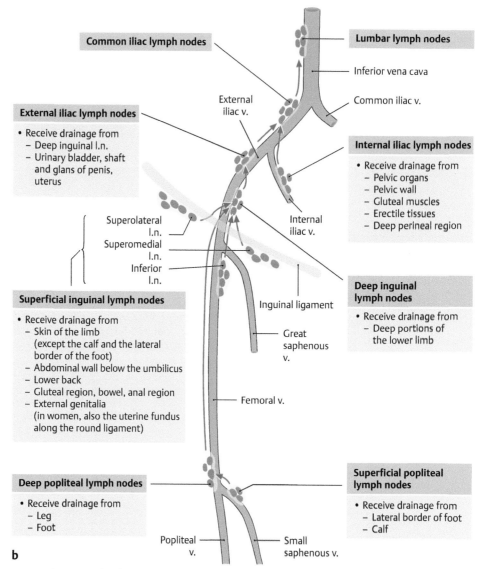

Common iliac lymph nodes

Lumbar lymph nodes

Inferior vena cava

External iliac v.

Common iliac v.

External iliac lymph nodes

- Receive drainage from
  - Deep inguinal l.n.
  - Urinary bladder, shaft and glans of penis, uterus

Internal iliac lymph nodes

- Receive drainage from
  - Pelvic organs
  - Pelvic wall
  - Gluteal muscles
  - Erectile tissues
  - Deep perineal region

Superolateral l.n.
Superomedial l.n.
Inferior l.n.

Internal iliac v.

Superficial inguinal lymph nodes

- Receive drainage from
  - Skin of the limb (except the calf and the lateral border of the foot)
  - Abdominal wall below the umbilicus
  - Lower back
  - Gluteal region, bowel, anal region
  - External genitalia (in women, also the uterine fundus along the round ligament)

Inguinal ligament

Great saphenous v.

Deep inguinal lymph nodes

- Receive drainage from
  - Deep portions of the lower limb

Femoral v.

Deep popliteal lymph nodes

- Receive drainage from
  - Leg
  - Foot

Superficial popliteal lymph nodes

- Receive drainage from
  - Lateral border of foot
  - Calf

Popliteal v.

Small saphenous v.

b

Source: Gilroy AM et al. Atlas of Anatomy. 3rd ed. 2016. Based on: Schuenke M, Schulte E, Schumacher U. THIEME Atlas of Anatomy. Volumes 1-3. Illustrations by Voll M and Wesker K. 2nd ed. New York: Thieme Medical Publishers; 2016

118. Correct: Normal; the longitudinal arches are not fully formed until age 5 (A)

(**A**) The longitudinal arches of the foot are not present at birth. They begin to develop at approximately age 3 and are typically not fully formed until age 5. Pes planus in a 3-year-old would be considered normal, lacking other physical evidence. (**B–E**) Physical evaluation of this child did not provide evidence for any malformations of her feet.

119. Correct: Vastus medialis (E)

(**E**) The physical therapist would prescribe exercises that strengthen the vastus medialis muscle since a part of this muscle inserts on the medial border of the patella. A strong vastus medialis helps reduce

the chance of lateral dislocation of the patella. This patient has patellofemoral syndrome, a condition in which the patellofemoral joint is painful and the patella is prone to subluxation, almost always laterally. It is most common in female athletes with an increased Q-angle. The normal Q-angle for an adult female is approximately 170 degrees. The greater transverse dimension for the female bony pelvis accounts for the Q-angle being higher in females (normal male Q-angle is approximately 140 degrees). An increased Q-angle places more stress on the joints of the knee (patellofemoral and tibiofemoral). (**A–D**) Neither the quadriceps femoris complex as a whole nor the vastus intermedius or vastus lateralis separately attach to the medial aspect of the patella. Therefore, they would not be effective in reducing the lateral displacement of the patella.

Refer to the following image for answer 119:

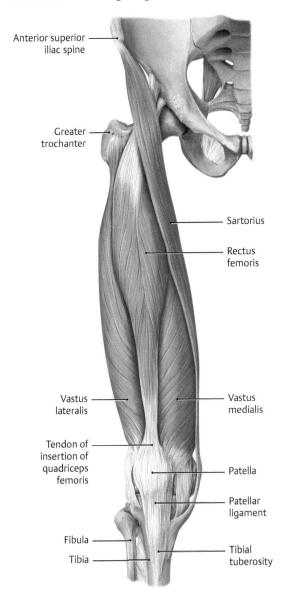

Anterior superior iliac spine

Greater trochanter

Sartorius

Rectus femoris

Vastus lateralis

Vastus medialis

Tendon of insertion of quadriceps femoris

Patella

Patellar ligament

Fibula

Tibia

Tibial tuberosity

Source: Schuenke M, Schulte E, Schumacher U. THIEME Atlas of Anatomy. General Anatomy and Musculoskeletal System. Illustrations by Voll M and Wesker K. 2nd ed. New York: Thieme Medical Publishers; 2016

---

120. Medial meniscus (C)

(**C**) Free, floating pieces of tissue in the synovial cavity ("joint mice") are usually either cartilage or bone fragments. In the knee joint, the most common source is the cartilaginous menisci. If these fragments become trapped between articular surfaces, they stimulate pain receptors and often cause the joint to lock as a defense mechanism to prevent further damage to articular surfaces. (**A, B, D**) Neither the cruciate ligaments nor the medial collateral ligament is intrasynovial and, therefore, they would not release fragments into the synovial cavity.

---

121. Correct: Sciatic (D)

(**D**) The sciatic nerve (L4–S3) exits the greater sciatic foramen inferior to the piriformis muscle. Piriformis syndrome occurs when the piriformis muscle spasms and causes buttock pain. The piriformis muscle can also irritate the nearby sciatic nerve and cause pain, numbness, and tingling along the posterior leg and into the foot, causing sciatica. (**A**) The nerve to obturator internus (L5–S2) exits the pelvis via the greater sciatic foramen inferior to the piriformis muscle, typically between the posterior cutaneous nerve of the thigh and the pudendal nerve. While it might be affected in piriformis syndrome, the symptoms are not consistent with it being involved in this individual. (**B**) The nerve to the piriformis pierces the anterior surface of the piriformis muscle within the pelvis and is, therefore, unlikely to be affected in this individual. (**C**) The pudendal nerve, derived from S2 to S4 ventral rami, also exits the pelvis through the greater sciatic foramen. Involvement of the pudendal nerve would lead to symptoms affecting perineal structures and these symptoms are not evident in this patient. (**E**) The superior gluteal nerve (L4–S1) leaves the pelvis superior to the piriformis muscle and is distributed to the gluteus medius and minimus and tensor fascia lata muscles. Compromised innervation to these muscles would lead to weak abduction in the affected hip joint and disturbances in gait.

Refer to the following image for answer 121:

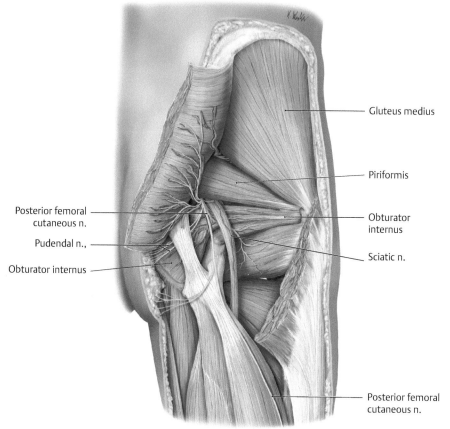

Gluteus medius

Piriformis

Posterior femoral cutaneous n.

Obturator internus

Pudendal n.,

Sciatic n.

Obturator internus

Posterior femoral cutaneous n.

Source: Source: Schuenke M, Schulte E, Schumacher U. THIEME Atlas of Anatomy. General Anatomy and Musculoskeletal System. Illustrations by Voll M and Wesker K. 2nd ed. New York: Thieme Medical Publishers; 2016

Head and Neck

122.   Correct: Lateral pterygoid (B)

Refer to the following image for answer 122:

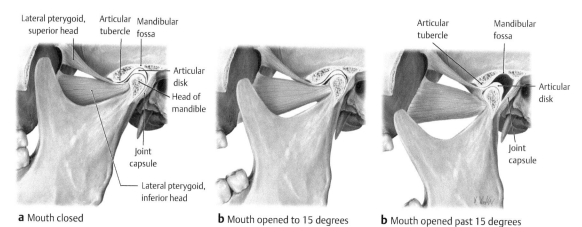

Lateral pterygoid, superior head

Articular tubercle

Mandibular fossa

Articular disk

Head of mandible

Joint capsule

Lateral pterygoid, inferior head

Articular tubercle

Mandibular fossa

Articular disk

Joint capsule

a Mouth closed   **b** Mouth opened to 15 degrees   **b** Mouth opened past 15 degrees

Source: Gilroy AM et al. Atlas of Anatomy. 3rd ed. 2016. Based on: Schuenke M, Schulte E, Schumacher U. THIEME Atlas of Anatomy. Volumes 1-3. Illustrations by Voll M and Wesker K. 2nd ed. New York: Thieme Medical Publishers; 2016

(**B**) The lateral pterygoid muscle with its orientation on the anterior-posterior plane has the greatest mechanical advantage to draw the head of the mandible out of the mandibular fossa onto the articular tubercle (protraction). (**A, C–E**) Subdivisions of the digastric, masseter, medial pterygoid, and temporalis muscles may be recruited to assist in protraction, but that is not their primary action.

123. Correct: Temporal (D)

(**D**) The articular tubercle belongs to the petrous part of the temporal bone. (**A–C, E**) The maxilla, and occipital, sphenoid, and zygomatic bones do not contribute to the temporomandibular joint.

124. Correct: Accessory (CN XI) (A)

(**A**) The unilateral action of sternocleidomastoid muscle is to tilt the head to the same side and rotate it so the face is turned superiorly and toward the opposite side. The accessory nerve (CN XI) is the motor supply for this muscle. This patient is experiencing a condition known as cervical dystonia, commonly termed torticollis or wry neck. Because of trauma or strain, possibly caused by the seatbelt in the auto accident, sternocleidomastoid will become spasmodic. Unilateral spasms of the sternocleidomastoid will pull the head into the position seen in this patient. (**B**) Ansa cervicalis provides innervation to infrahyoid muscles. (**C, D**) The lesser occipital and transverse cervical nerves are sensory branches of the cervical plexus. (**E**) Somatic motor branches of the vagus nerve in the neck are distributed to the pharynx and larynx.

125. Correct: Sternohyoid (C)

(**C**) The sternohyoid muscle is the most superficial of the infrahyoid muscles in the area of a tracheostomy, usually extending across tracheal cartilages 2 to 4. (**A**) The cricothyroid muscle is an intrinsic muscle of the larynx extending between the cricoid and thyroid cartilages. It lies superior to the tracheostomy. (**B**) The mylohyoid muscle extends from the mylohyoid line of the mandible to the hyoid bone. It lies superior to the tracheostomy. (**D**) The sternothyroid muscle lies immediately deep to sternohyoid. (**E**) The thyrohyoid extends from the lamina of the thyroid cartilage to the hyoid bone and lies superior to the tracheostomy.

Refer to the following image for answer 125:

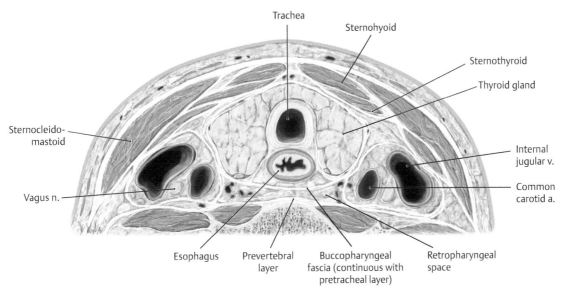

Source: Gilroy AM et al. Atlas of Anatomy. 3rd ed. 2016. Based on: Schuenke M, Schulte E, Schumacher U. THIEME Atlas of Anatomy. Volumes 1-3. Illustrations by Voll M and Wesker K. 2nd ed. New York: Thieme Medical Publishers; 2016

126. Correct: Anterior longitudinal ligament (B)

Refer to the following image for answer 126:

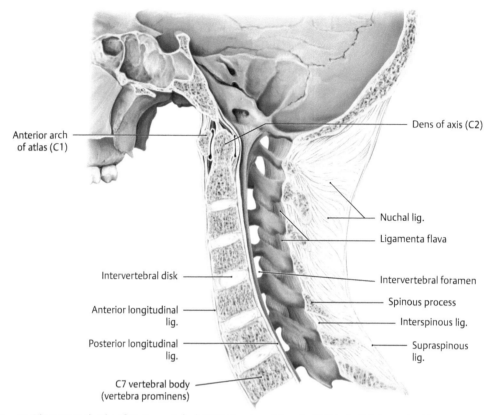

Anterior arch of atlas (C1)

Dens of axis (C2)

Nuchal lig.

Ligamenta flava

Intervertebral disk

Intervertebral foramen

Anterior longitudinal lig.

Spinous process

Interspinous lig.

Posterior longitudinal lig.

Supraspinous lig.

C7 vertebral body (vertebra prominens)

Source: Gilroy AM et al. Atlas of Anatomy. 3rd ed. 2016. Based on: Schuenke M, Schulte E, Schumacher U. THIEME Atlas of Anatomy. Volumes 1-3. Illustrations by Voll M and Wesker K. 2nd ed. New York: Thieme Medical Publishers; 2016

(**B**) The anterior longitudinal ligament courses the length of the vertebral column on the anterior surface of vertebral bodies. It provides the primary resistance to cervical hyperextension. Forced hyperextension of the neck, as in this "whiplash" injury, often produces a strain to this ligament, resulting in neck pain. (**A, E**) Ligaments supporting the atlanto-occipital (alar) and atlantoaxial (transverse ligament of atlas) are usually not strained or torn unless there are cervical fractures or dislocations. (**C**) These ligaments connect the lamina of adjacent vertebrae. They resist separation of laminae during cervical hyperflexion. (**D**) The posterior longitudinal ligament, which is much weaker than the anterior longitudinal ligament, courses within the vertebral canal along the posterior surface of vertebral bodies. In the neck it provides the primary resistance to cervical hyperflexion.

127. Correct: Lateral cricoarytenoid (B)

(**B**) The left recurrent laryngeal nerve is a branch of vagus. After it branches from the vagus, as it loops under the aortic arch, it comes to associate closely with the left main bronchus as it ascends toward the neck. It distributes to the esophageal and pharyngeal muscles in the neck and ends by supplying intrinsic muscles of the larynx (except cricothyroid). Bronchial carcinoma may involve the recurrent laryngeal nerve in the thorax near its origin from the vagus nerve, as it courses under the aorta and along the trachea, and thereby impacting its innervation of laryngeal musculature. (**A**) The paired cricothyroid muscles are the only intrinsic muscles of the larynx not innervated by the vagus nerves and would not be directly affected by the carcinoma. (**C, D**) The omohyoid and sternohyoid muscles receive innervation from the ansa cervicalis, which is not related to the bronchial carcinoma. (**E**) The thyrohyoid muscle is innervated by the nerve to thyrohyoid, which carries fibers from the C1 ventral ramus.

Refer to the following image for answer 127:

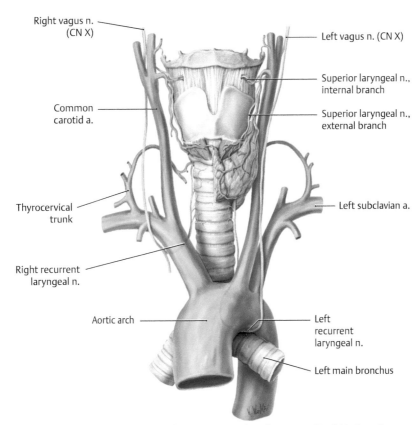

Right vagus n. (CN X)

Left vagus n. (CN X)

Superior laryngeal n., internal branch

Common carotid a.

Superior laryngeal n., external branch

Thyrocervical trunk

Left subclavian a.

Right recurrent laryngeal n.

Aortic arch

Left recurrent laryngeal n.

Left main bronchus

Source: Schuenke M, Schulte E, Schumacher U. THIEME Atlas of Anatomy. Head, Neck, and Neuroanatomy. Illustrations by Voll M and Wesker K. 2nd ed. New York: Thieme Medical Publishers; 2016

128. Correct: Superior oblique (E)

(**E**) The superior oblique muscle, which intorts, depresses, and abducts the eye, is innervated by the trochlear nerve (CN IV). With a trochlear nerve lesion (refer to accompanying image b), the affected eye will be hypertropic (i.e., deviated upward relative to the unaffected eye). This is especially notable with attempted *abduction* of the eye because the upward pull of the inferior oblique muscle is not compensated by the normal *abduction* action of superior oblique. Most patients report that double vision when looking downwards and inwards (vertical diplopia), as would happen when looking down to go down a flight of stairs. (**A–C**) The inferior oblique and most rectus muscles (except lateral rectus) are innervated by the oculomotor nerve (CN III). With unilateral oculomotor palsy, the affected eye is typically exotropic (deviated laterally) and hypotropic (deviated downward) (refer to accompanying image c). There may also be partial or complete ptosis (depending on involvement of levator labii superioris) and the pupil may be mydriatic (dilated) due to involvement of the parasympathetic pupillary constrictor fibers that travel in the third nerve. (**D**) The lateral rectus muscle, the primary abductor of the eye, is innervated by the abducens nerve (CN VI). A palsy of CN VI would result in esotropia (medial deviation) of the affected eye (image a), a distinction that would be exacerbated when asking the patient to look away from the affected eye. A palsy of the abducens nerve, therefore, results in hypertropia and extorsion. The torsion seldom is noticed by patients. Instead, they complain of vertical diplopia, especially on reading or looking down.

Refer to the following image for answer 128:

Oculomotor palsies

Oculomotor palsies may result from a lesion involving an eye muscle or its associated cranial nerve (at the nucleus or along the course of the nerve). If one extraocular muscle is weak or paralyzed, deviation of the eye will be noted.

Impairment of the coordinated actions of the extraocular muscles may cause the visual axis of one eye to deviate from its normal osition.The patient will therefore perceive a double image (diplopia).

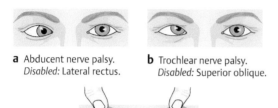

a Abducent nerve palsy.
Disabled: Lateral rectus.

b Trochlear nerve palsy.
Disabled: Superior oblique.

c Complete oculomotor palsy. *Disabled:* Superior, inferior, and medial recti and inferior oblique.

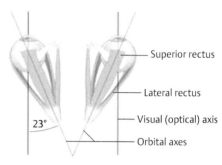

d Normal visual and orbital axes.

Source: Schuenke M, Schulte E, Schumacher U. THIEME Atlas of Anatomy. Head, Neck, and Neuroanatomy. Illustrations by Voll M and Wesker K. 2nd ed. New York: Thieme Medical Publishers; 2016

---

129.   Correct: Left genioglossus (A)

Refer to the following images for answer 129:

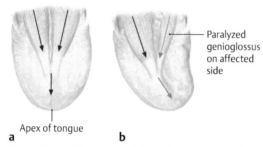

a   **b**

Source: Source: Gilroy AM et al. Atlas of Anatomy. 3rd ed. 2016. Based on: Schuenke M, Schulte E, Schumacher U. THIEME Atlas of Anatomy. Volumes 1-3. Illustrations by Voll M and Wesker K. 2nd ed. New York: Thieme Medical Publishers; 2016

(**A**) Protruding the tongue in the midline depends on the bilateral action of the genioglossus muscles (image a). The hypoglossal nerve (CN XII) innervates the extrinsic tongue muscles (except palatoglossus) on the same side. With unilateral palsy of a hypoglossal nerve, the protruded tongue will deviate from midline, toward the side of the lesion (image b). This results from the intact genioglossus muscle forcing the tongue to deviate toward the side of the lesion. (**B, D, E**) These muscles are not involved in protrusion of the tongue: hyoglossus muscles depress the tongue; styloglossus muscles retract the tongue. (**C**) A lesion involving the right genioglossus muscle would cause the protruded tongue to deviate toward the right.

130.   Correct: Digastric, anterior belly (A)

(**A**) The nerve to mylohyoid is a motor branch of the inferior alveolar nerve (from the mandibular division of CN V), branching from the latter within the infratemporal fossa near the mandibular foramen. The inferior alveolar nerve enters the mandibular foramen and canal to distribute to mandibular teeth on the respective side. The mylohyoid nerve continues along the medial side of the mandibular ramus to reach the mylohyoid and anterior digastric muscles. (**B**) Genioglossus is innervated by CN XII (hypoglossal). (**C**) Geniohyoid is innervated by nerve to geniohyoid (C1–C2). (**D**) As a muscle of mastication, the lateral pterygoid is innervated by a direct branch of the mandibular nerve (CN V3). (**E**) Stylohyoid is innervated by CN VII (facial).

Refer to the following image for answer 130:

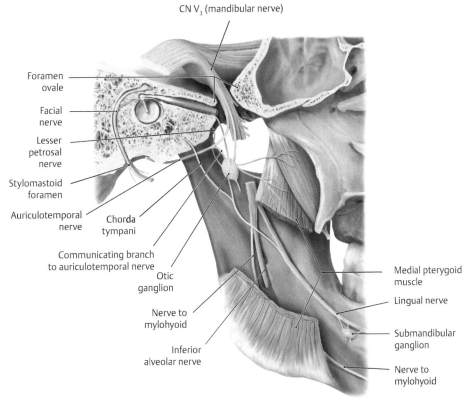

CN V₃ (mandibular nerve)

Foramen
ovale

Facial
nerve

Lesser
petrosal
nerve

Stylomastoid
foramen

Auriculotemporal
nerve

Chorda
tympani

Communicating branch
to auriculotemporal nerve

Otic
ganglion

Nerve to
mylohyoid

Inferior
alveolar nerve

Medial pterygoid
muscle

Lingual nerve

Submandibular
ganglion

Nerve to
mylohyoid

Source: Gilroy AM et al. Atlas of Anatomy. 3rd ed. 2016. Based on: Schuenke M, Schulte E, Schumacher U. THIEME Atlas of Anatomy. Volumes 1-3. Illustrations by Voll M and Wesker K. 2nd ed. New York: Thieme Medical Publishers; 2016

131. Correct: Maxilla (D)

(**D**) The orbital floor is formed primarily by the maxilla, with additional small contributions from the orbital processes of the palatine and zygomatic bones. The orbital portion of the maxilla is thin and sudden increased pressure (an anterior blow) makes it vulnerable to fracture. It is the most commonly fractured bone with orbital blowout fractures. (**A–C, E**) the ethmoid, frontal and lacrimal and sphenoid bones do not contribute to the floor of the orbit.

Refer to the following image for answer 131:

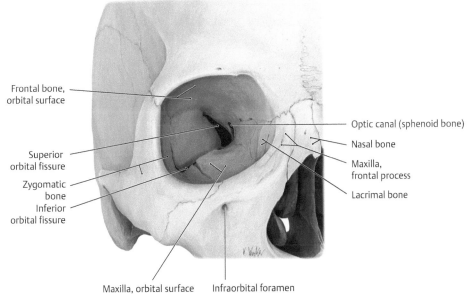

Frontal bone,
orbital surface

Superior
orbital fissure

Zygomatic
bone

Inferior
orbital fissure

Optic canal (sphenoid bone)

Nasal bone

Maxilla,
frontal process

Lacrimal bone

Maxilla, orbital surface   Infraorbital foramen

Source: Gilroy AM et al. Atlas of Anatomy. 3rd ed. 2016. Based on: Schuenke M, Schulte E, Schumacher U. THIEME Atlas of Anatomy. Volumes 1-3. Illustrations by Voll M and Wesker K. 2nd ed. New York: Thieme Medical Publishers; 2016

132. Correct: Foramen rotundum (C)

(C) A series of foramina, canals, and fissures are associated with the sphenoid bone, all of them opening into the middle cranial fossa. The foramen rotundum lies on the anterior floor of the temporal region of the middle cranial fossa, just inferior to the medial end of the superior orbital fissure. It is in the lateral wall of the sphenoidal sinus. It conducts the maxillary division of the trigeminal nerve (CN V2). (A) The infraorbital foramen opens onto the face via the maxillary bone. It conducts the infraorbital nerve and vessels. (B, D) The foramen ovale and foramen spinosum lie in the floor of the middle cranial fossa. Foramen ovale conducts the mandibular division of the trigeminal nerve (CN V3) into the infratemporal fossa. Foramen spinosum conducts the middle meningeal artery from the infratemporal fossa into the middle cranial fossa. (E) The pterygoid canal traverses the body of the sphenoid bone at the base of the medial pterygoid plate. It conducts the nerve of the pterygoid canal (Vidian nerve) and companion vessels into the pterygopalatine fossa.

133. Correct: Eighteen months (B)

(B) The anterior fontanelle is located at the junction of the unpaired frontal and the paired parietal bones. It is present at birth and normally closes between 9 and 18 months of age. (A, C, D) The anterior fontanelle is normally present until at least 9 months of age. (E) The anterior fontanelle should be closed by 18 months of age.

134. Correct: Intrinsic tongue muscles (C)

(C) Changing the shape of the tongue is accomplished primarily by its intrinsic muscles (transverse, longitudinal, and oblique groups). The transverse fibers have the major role in curling the edges of the tongue. (A, B, D, E) The genioglossus, hyoglossus, palatoglossus, and styloglossus are all extrinsic tongue muscles and are involved primarily in movements of the tongue (protraction, retraction, elevation, depression).

135. Correct: C6 (D)

(D) The pharynx (laryngopharynx or hypopharynx) becomes continuous with the esophagus at the lower border of the cricoid cartilage, which typically lies at the C6 vertebral level. A diverticulum (Zenker's) may develop in the elderly at this level as it is considered the weakest point in the pharyngeal wall (between the inferior border of inferior constrictor and the superior border of cricopharyngeus). Dysphagia and halitosis are common symptoms of this malady. (A–C, E) The C3 to C5 vertebral levels are superior to the junction of the pharynx and esophagus. The C7 vertebral level is inferior to the junction of the pharynx and esophagus.

136. Correct: Posterior cricoarytenoid (C)

(C) The posterior cricoarytenoid muscle extends from the cricoid cartilage to the muscular process of the arytenoid cartilage. Contraction of this muscle causes external (lateral) rotation of the arytenoid cartilage, which abducts the vocal cord on that side and opens the rima glottidis. With injury of the ipsilateral recurrent laryngeal nerve, the muscle is paralyzed and the vocal cord cannot be abducted; consequently, it presents in a midline position. (A) The transverse fibers of the arytenoid muscle adduct the arytenoid cartilages and vocal cords. (B) The lateral cricoarytenoid muscle is the antagonist of posterior cricoarytenoid and produces medial rotation of the arytenoid cartilage, resulting in adduction of the vocal cord and narrowing the rima glottidis. (D, E) The thyroarytenoid and vocalis muscles parallel the vocal cord and their contraction will slacken the vocal cord, changing pitch. They will also assist in adduction of the vocal cord, narrowing the rima glottidis.

Refer to the following images and table for answer 136:

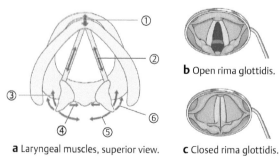

a Laryngeal muscles, superior view.
b Open rima glottidis.
c Closed rima glottidis.

Actions of the laryngeal muscles		
Muscle	Action	Effect on rima glottidis
① Cricothyroid m.*	Tightens the vocal folds	None
② Vocalis m.		
③ Thyroarytenoid m.	Adducts the vocal folds	Closes
④ Transverse arytenoida m.		
⑤ Posterior cricoarytenoid m.	Abducts the vocal folds	Opens
⑥ Lateral cricoarytenoid m.	Adducts the vocal folds	Closes

* The cricothyroid is innervated by the external laryngeal nerve. All other intrinsic laryngeal muscles are innervated by the recurrent laryngeal nerve.

Source: Gilroy AM et al. Atlas of Anatomy. 3rd ed. 2016. Based on: Schuenke M, Schulte E, Schumacher U. THIEME Atlas of Anatomy. Volumes 1-3. Illustrations by Voll M and Wesker K. 2nd ed. New York: Thieme Medical Publishers; 2016

137. Correct: Middle pharyngeal constrictor (B)

Refer to the following image for answer 137:

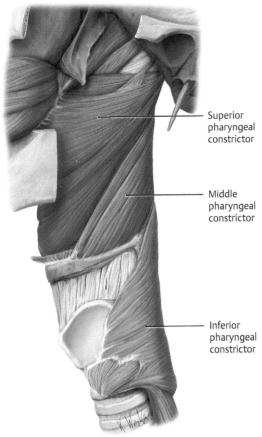

Source: Gilroy AM et al. Atlas of Anatomy. 3rd ed. 2016. Based on: Schuenke M, Schulte E, Schumacher U. THIEME Atlas of Anatomy. Volumes 1-3. Illustrations by Voll M and Wesker K. 2nd ed. New York: Thieme Medical Publishers; 2016

(**B**) The difficulty swallowing in this patient is related to function of the middle pharyngeal constrictor muscle, which takes its origin from the lesser and greater cornua of the hyoid. During swallowing, the pharyngeal constrictor muscles force the bolus of food inferiorly into the esophagus. (**A, C–E**) The geniohyoid, omohyoid, sternohyoid, and thyrohyoid muscles do not contribute to the pharyngeal wall, and their functions are related to fixation of the hyoid bone from above (geniohyoid) or below (omohyoid, sternohyoid, thyrohyoid).

138. Correct: Second pharyngeal arch (D)

(**D**) The styloid process, stylohyoid ligament, and lesser cornu of the hyoid bone are derived from the cartilaginous elements (Reichert's cartilage) of the second branchial arch. Together, they form the "stylohyoid chain." A styloid process greater than 3 cm in length is considered elongated. Calcification/ossification of the stylohyoid ligament may result in discomfort when swallowing due to the close association with the lateral pharyngeal wall. (**A–C, E**) The mandibular division of first pharyngeal arch, the maxillary division of second pharyngeal arch, and pharyngeal arches 3 to 6 do not contribute to the stylohyoid chain.

139. Correct: Ethmoid (A)

(**A**) The perpendicular plate of the ethmoid bone forms the superior portion of the bony nasal septum. (**B–D**) The maxilla and the nasal and palatine bones are minor contributors to the nasal septum. (**E**) The vomer forms the inferior portion of the bony nasal septum.

Refer to the following image for answer 139:

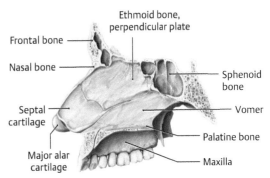

Source: Schuenke M, Schulte E, Schumacher U. THIEME Atlas of Anatomy. Head, Neck, and Neuroanatomy. Illustrations by Voll M and Wesker K. 2nd ed. New York: Thieme Medical Publishers; 2016

140. Correct: Digastric (A)

(**A**) The action of the digastric muscle (posterior and anterior bellies working together) on the temporomandibular joint is to depress the mandible. Since the anterior belly inserts at the symphysis of the mandible, the force is applied at the chin. With bilateral fracture of the body of the mandible, the action of digastric is unopposed by other muscles acting on the temporomandibular joint. Thus, the chin will be depressed even when the mouth is closed. (**B**) The main actions of the lateral pterygoid are protraction and rotation at the temporomandibular joint. While this muscle is not involved in rotation of the mandibular head, it would be involved in depressing the chin after the mandibular head translates onto the articular tubercle. (**C-E**) The masseter, medial pterygoid, and temporalis muscles do not depress the mandible.

141. Correct: Odontoid process (C)

Refer to the following image for answer 141:

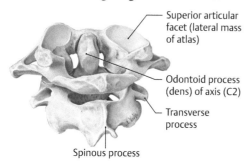

Source: Gilroy AM et al. Atlas of Anatomy. 3rd ed. 2016. Based on: Schuenke M, Schulte E, Schumacher U. THIEME Atlas of Anatomy. Volumes 1-3. Illustrations by Voll M and Wesker K. 2nd ed. New York: Thieme Medical Publishers; 2016

(**C**) The odontoid process (dens) projects superiorly from the body of the C2 vertebra (axis) to articulate with the anterior arch of the C1 vertebra (atlas). (**A**) The atlas does not have a body. (**B, D**) The external occipital protuberance and the occipital condyle do not project into the vertebral canal. (**E**) The vertebral arteries unite to form the basilar artery after they enter the cranial cavity.

142. Correct: Vagus (CN X) (E)

(**E**) The paired levator veli palatini muscles and musculus uvulae elevate the soft palate and uvula, respectively, as part of the gag reflex. Both are innervated by motor branches from the vagus nerve (CN X) via the pharyngeal plexus (sensory fibers for the gag reflex are provided by the glossopharyngeal nerve, CN IX). Unilateral injury of the vagus nerve, which exits the cranium via the jugular foramen (with CNs IX and XI, and the internal jugular vein) at the skull base, will cause the soft palate and uvula to deviate to the side opposite the lesion. (**A**) The accessory nerve (CN XI), as it exits the skull, is composed of its spinal contribution only. It will provide motor innervation to trapezius and sternocleidomastoid. (**B, D**) The facial (CN VII) and hypoglossal (CN XII) nerves do not traverse the jugular foramen. (**C**) The glossopharyngeal nerve provides the afferent limb of the gag reflex, but the efferent impulses are carried by the vagus nerve.

Refer to the following image for answer 142:

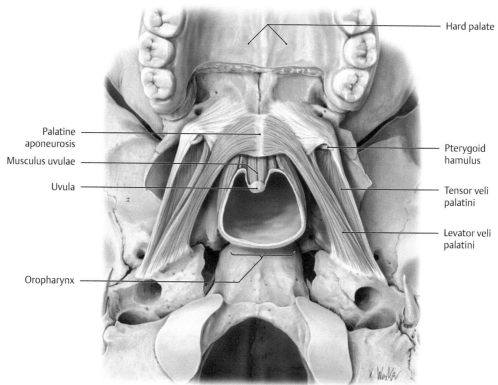

Source: Source: Gilroy AM et al. Atlas of Anatomy. 3rd ed. 2016. Based on: Schuenke M, Schulte E, Schumacher U. THIEME Atlas of Anatomy. Volumes 1-3. Illustrations by Voll M and Wesker K. 2nd ed. New York: Thieme Medical Publishers; 2016

143. Correct: Splenius capitis (C)

Refer to the following image for answer 143:

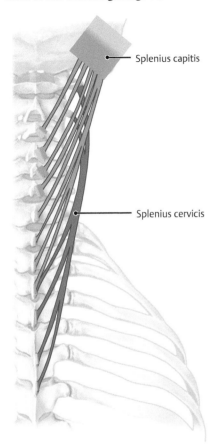

Splenius capitis

Splenius cervicis

Source: Gilroy AM et al. Atlas of Anatomy. 3rd ed. 2016. Based on: Schuenke M, Schulte E, Schumacher U. THIEME Atlas of Anatomy. Volumes 1-3. Illustrations by Voll M and Wesker K. 2nd ed. New York: Thieme Medical Publishers; 2016

(**C**) Bilateral contraction of the splenius capitis muscles produces extension of the cervical spinal column and the head. Unilateral contraction produces ipsilateral rotation of the neck and head. The muscle has origin from the ligamentum nuchae and spinous processes of C7 to T3 and it inserts along the lateral portion of the superior nuchal line and the mastoid process. Prolonged periods of neck extension may strain the splenius capitis muscles, producing posterior neck pain. (**A**) Longus capitis is a prevertebral muscle and would assist in flexion of the neck and head. (**B**) Occipitofrontalis is a muscle of facial expression and does not act on the atlanto-occipital or any cervical vertebral joints. (**D**) Sternocleidomastoid extends diagonally across the neck from the sternum and clavicle to the mastoid process. Its primary action is rotation of the neck and head to the contralateral side. Bilateral contraction produces flexion of the lower cervical vertebrae and extension at the upper cervical vertebrae and at the atlanto-occipital joint. (**E**) Trapezius is a muscle of the upper limb and its main actions involve the scapula (elevation, adduction, depression, rotation). While it does have origin from the skull, ligamentum nuchae, and spinous processes of vertebrae, its actions on the neck and head are secondary.

Thorax

144. Correct: Internal intercostal and innermost intercostal (E)

Refer to the following image for answer 144:

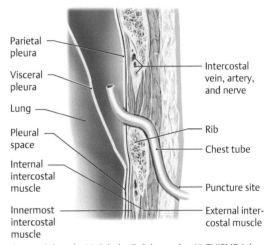

Parietal pleura

Visceral pleura

Lung

Pleural space

Internal intercostal muscle

Innermost intercostal muscle

Intercostal vein, artery, and nerve

Rib

Chest tube

Puncture site

External intercostal muscle

Source: Schuenke M, Schulte E, Schumacher U. THIEME Atlas of Anatomy. Head, Neck, and Neuroanatomy. Illustrations by Voll M and Wesker K. 2nd ed. New York: Thieme Medical Publishers; 2016

(**E**) The intercostal neurovascular bundle lies between the internal and innermost intercostal muscles at the posterior axillary line. (**A–D**) There are no major vessels or nerves located in the connective tissue separating any of these layers (endothoracic fascia and pleura, external and internal intercostal muscles, innermost intercostal muscle and endothoracic fascia).

145. Correct: Subclavian vein, anterior scalene muscle, subclavian artery, middle scalene muscle (D)

(**D**) As the subclavian vein and artery cross the superior surface of rib 1, they are separated by the anterior scalene muscle. Since the vein lies anterior to the muscle, this position is a favored site for placement of a central venous catheter. The subclavian artery passes between the anterior and middle scalene muscles (along with the trunks of the brachial plexus). (**A-C, E**) None of these combinations of structures represents anterior-to-posterior order of structures associated with rib 1.

Refer to the following image for answer 145:

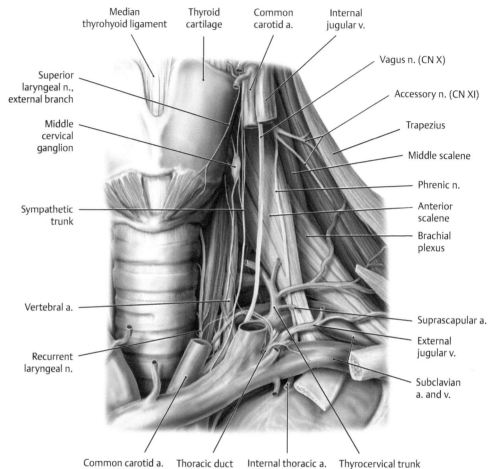

Source: Gilroy AM et al. Atlas of Anatomy. 3rd ed. 2016. Based on: Schuenke M, Schulte E, Schumacher U. THIEME Atlas of Anatomy. Volumes 1-3. Illustrations by Voll M and Wesker K. 2nd ed. New York: Thieme Medical Publishers; 2016

146. Correct: Partial ossification of the xiphoid process (E)

(**E**) In the first 3 to 4 decades, the xiphoid process of the sternum is cartilaginous and most people are unaware of its presence. By age 40, most individuals have at least partial calcification/ossification of the xiphoid process and may discover a hard midline "lump" and become concerned that it represents an abnormal growth. The subcutaneous location makes the diagnosis straightforward. (**A, B**) The mass in this patient is subcutaneous. (**C, D**) Dislocation of a seventh costal cartilage from the sternum, and inflammation of the xiphisternal joint would produce pain reflexes during breathing and palpation. They would not result in a hard, painless, midline, subcutaneous mass just distal to the body of the sternum that was discovered in this patient.

Abdomen

147. Correct: Internal abdominal oblique and transversus abdominis (C)

(**C**) The conjoint tendon (falx inguinalis), which lies on the deep side of the superficial inguinal ring, is formed through the union of the lower portions of the aponeurotic tendons of the internal abdominal oblique and transversus abdominis muscles. The conjoint tendon attaches to the superior pubic ramus. It is common for a direct inguinal hernia to project into the superficial inguinal ring by passing inferior to the lower (free) border of the conjoint tendon. (**A, B, D, E**) The external abdominal oblique, pyramidalis, nor the rectus abdominis contribute to the conjoint tendon.

Refer to the following image for answer 147:

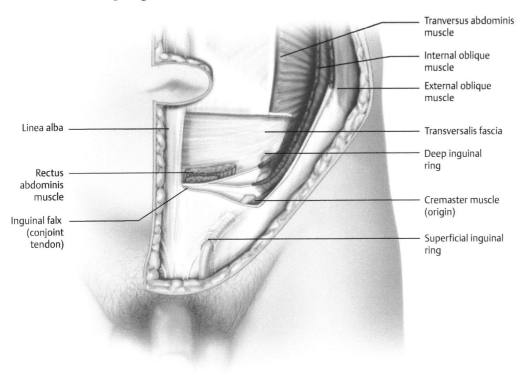

148. **Correct: Transversalis fascia (D)**

(**D**) The transversalis fascia is a layer of loose connective tissue separating the parietal peritoneum from the muscular and fibrous portions of the anterior abdominopelvic walls. The position of the incision slightly above the mons pubis is inferior to the arcuate line, at which point the posterior rectus sheath is not present and the transversalis fascia (and underlying peritoneum) lies immediately deep to the muscle. (**A**) The aponeurosis of the transversus abdominis muscle is the tendon of the transversus abdominis muscle and it is distinct from the transversalis fascia. (**B**) The broad ligament of the uterus is the mesentery of the uterus and would not be incised during a cesarean delivery. (**C**) The parietal peritoneum is separated from the deep muscle layer, and along linea alba, by the transversalis fascia. (**E**) The visceral peritoneum of the uterus (epimetrium) covers the outer surface of the body of the uterus. It would be encountered only after opening the peritoneal cavity.

Refer to the following image for answer 148:

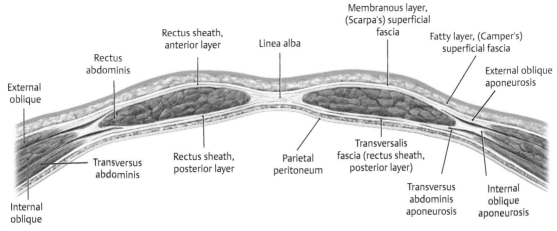

Source: Schuenke M, Schulte E, Schumacher U. THIEME Atlas of Anatomy. General Anatomy and Musculoskeletal System. Illustrations by Voll M and Wesker K. 2nd ed. New York: Thieme Medical Publishers; 2016

149. Correct: Right crus (E)

(**E**) The esophagus passes through esophageal hiatus in the right crus of the diaphragm to enter the abdominal cavity. If the gastroesophageal junction and part or all of the stomach is found in the thoracic cavity, a hiatal hernia exists. If the gastroesophageal junction is in its normal position in the abdomen and portions of the stomach are found in the thoracic cavity, a paraesophageal hernia exists in which the stomach passed through the esophageal hiatus alongside the esophagus. This type of hernia is of greater clinical relevance due to the higher risk of gastric ischemia. (**A**) The inferior vena cava passes through the caval hiatus in the central tendon of the diaphragm. (**B**) The left greater and lesser splanchnic nerves pierce the left crus. (**C, D**) No major structures pierce the muscular domes of the diaphragm.

150. Correct: T10 (D)

Refer to the following image for answer 150:

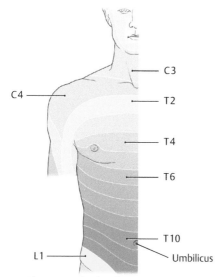

Source: Gilroy AM et al. Atlas of Anatomy. 3rd ed. 2016. Based on: Schuenke M, Schulte E, Schumacher U. THIEME Atlas of Anatomy. Volumes 1-3. Illustrations by Voll M and Wesker K. 2nd ed. New York: Thieme Medical Publishers; 2016

(**D**) The umbilicus is typically located in the T10 dermatome. (**A–C, E**) The L1, L2, T8, and T12 dermatomes do not include the paraumbilical region.

151. Correct: Internal abdominal oblique (C)

(**C**) As the testicle and associated structures pass through the anterior abdominal wall to their adult position in the scrotum, the internal abdominal oblique muscle contributes a fascial layer containing skeletal muscle fibers (cremaster) to the spermatic cord. This layer is termed the cremasteric fascia. (**A**) Dartos is smooth muscle located in the subcutaneous tissues of the scrotum. (**B**) External abdominal oblique contributes a fascial layer (external spermatic fascia) to the spermatic cord, but no muscle fibers. (**D**) Rectus abdominis does not contribute to the structure of the spermatic cord. (**E**) Transversus abdominis contributes a fascial layer (internal spermatic fascia) to the spermatic cord, but no muscle fibers.

Refer to the following image for answer 151:

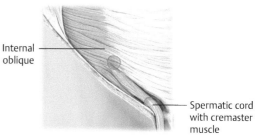

Source: Gilroy AM et al. Atlas of Anatomy. 3rd ed. 2016. Based on: Schuenke M, Schulte E, Schumacher U. THIEME Atlas of Anatomy. Volumes 1-3. Illustrations by Voll M and Wesker K. 2nd ed. New York: Thieme Medical Publishers; 2016

152. Correct: External abdominal oblique (A)

(**A**) The fibers of the external abdominal oblique are oriented in an inferomedial direction. The strength of the anterior and lateral abdominal walls is enhanced by the fibers of the external and internal abdominal oblique muscles being arranged at near-right angles to one another. (**B**) The internal abdominal oblique fibers are oriented in a superomedial direction. (**C, D**) The latissimus dorsi and quadratus lumborum muscles do not contribute to the anterior abdominal wall. (**E**) Transversus abdominis muscle fibers are oriented on the near-horizontal plane.

Refer to the following image for answer 152:

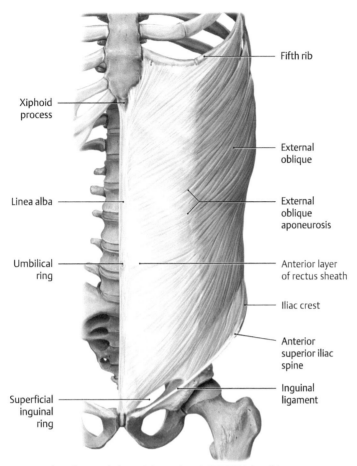

Source: Schuenke M, Schulte E, Schumacher U. THIEME Atlas of Anatomy. General Anatomy and Musculoskeletal System. Illustrations by Voll M and Wesker K. 2nd ed. New York: Thieme Medical Publishers; 2016

153. Correct: Deep to the transversalis fascia (C)

(**C**) Extraperitoneal fat lies between the transversalis fascia and parietal peritoneum. (**A, D, E**) The internal and external oblique muscles and Camper's and

Scarpa's fasciae are located superficial to the layer of extraperitoneal fat. (**B**) The parietal peritoneum is deep to the extraperitoneal fat.

Refer to the following image for answer 153:

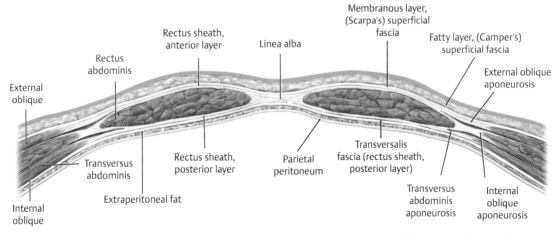

Source: Schuenke M, Schulte E, Schumacher U. THIEME Atlas of Anatomy. General Anatomy and Musculoskeletal System. Illustrations by Voll M and Wesker K. 2nd ed. New York: Thieme Medical Publishers; 2016

154.   Correct: Between the internal oblique and transversus abdominis muscles (A)

(**A**) The ilioinguinal nerve, a branch of the L1 ventral ramus, appears at the lateral border of the psoas major and courses anterior to quadratus lumborum and iliacus. Near the anterior part of the iliac crest, this nerve pierces transversus abdominis, passes between the transverse abdominus and internal oblique muscles (which it supplies), and then pierces the internal oblique near the deep inguinal ring to enter the inguinal canal. It exits the inguinal canal through the superficial inguinal ring to distribute to the skin of the medial thigh and upper part of the scrotum (male) or labium majus and mons pubis (females). In case of ilioinguinal nerve entrapment, walking and hyperextension of the hip increases the pain as this causes increased tension on the nerve. (**B–E**) The ilioinguinal nerve is always superficial to peritoneum and transversalis fascia.

155.   Correct: Medial inguinal (D)

(**D**) The medial inguinal fossa (inguinal or Hesselbach's triangle) is located between the medial and lateral umbilical folds. The inguinal fossae are shallow depressions on the anterior abdominal wall defined by the umbilical folds. The umbilical folds are ridges in the parietal peritoneum created by the underlying obliterated umbilical artery (medial fold) and the inferior epigastric artery (lateral fold). The medial umbilical fossa is a potential site for direct inguinal hernias. (**A**) The iliac fossa is not part of the groin or anterior abdominal wall, and is not related to direct inguinal hernia. (**B**) The ischioanal fossa is the space on either side of the anal canal and is bound by the levator ani on its lateral aspect. It is not part of the anterolateral abdominal wall, and it is not related to a direct inguinal hernia. (**E**) The supravesical fossa is located between the median and medial umbilical folds. A direct inguinal hernia does not pass through this fossa. (**C**) The lateral inguinal fossa is located lateral to the lateral umbilical fold. It is a potential site for the most common type of hernia in the anterior abdominal wall, an indirect inguinal hernia.

Refer to the following image for answer 155:

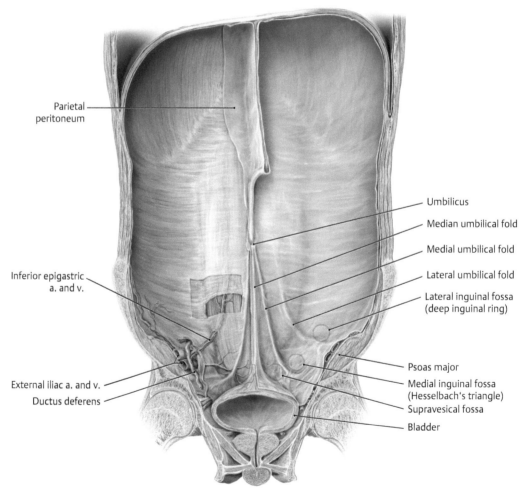

Parietal peritoneum

Inferior epigastric a. and v.

External iliac a. and v.

Ductus deferens

Umbilicus

Median umbilical fold

Medial umbilical fold

Lateral umbilical fold

Lateral inguinal fossa (deep inguinal ring)

Psoas major

Medial inguinal fossa (Hesselbach's triangle)

Supravesical fossa

Bladder

Source: Gilroy AM et al. Atlas of Anatomy. 3rd ed. 2016. Based on: Schuenke M, Schulte E, Schumacher U. THIEME Atlas of Anatomy. Volumes 1-3. Illustrations by Voll M and Wesker K. 2nd ed. New York: Thieme Medical Publishers; 2016

156. Correct: Peritoneal cavity (B)

Refer to the following image for answer 156:

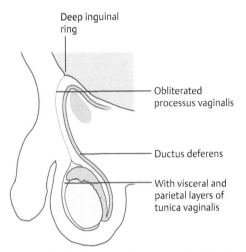

Source: Schuenke M, Schulte E, Schumacher U. THIEME Atlas of Anatomy. Internal Organs. Illustrations by Voll M and Wesker K. 2nd ed. New York: Thieme Medical Publishers; 2016

(**B**) The processus vaginalis is a diverticulum of parietal peritoneum that forms during the 12th week of development and extends through the inguinal region into the developing scrotum/labium majus. Its proximal portion normally degenerates completely, losing communication with the peritoneal cavity at the deep inguinal ring. In the male, the distal portion of the processus vaginalis does not degenerate. Instead, it forms the tunica vaginalis that envelops the testis. If the proximal portion of the processus vaginalis persists, the condition is termed a patent processus vaginalis. Because the lumen of a patent processus vaginalis would open into the greater sac of the peritoneal cavity, a patent processus vaginalis significantly increases the risk of developing an indirect inguinal hernia. (**A, C–E**) The lumen of a patent processus vaginalis would not communicate with the cecum, retroperitoneal space, sigmoid colon, or urinary bladder.

157. Correct: Superficial inguinal ring (D)

(**D**) An inguinal hernia is a protrusion of abdominal cavity contents into the inguinal region. There are two types of inguinal hernia, indirect and direct, and both of them eventually involve the superficial ring at the medial end of the inguinal ligament. An examination for evidence of an inguinal hernia involves palpation at the superficial inguinal ring. Having the patient cough during the examination increases intra-abdominal pressure and, if a hernia exists, it can be palpated at the superficial ring. (**A–C, E**) Palpation of conjoint tendon, suspensory ligament of the penis, penis, or a normal testicle will not help a physician with a diagnosis of an inguinal hernia.

Refer to the following image for answer 157:

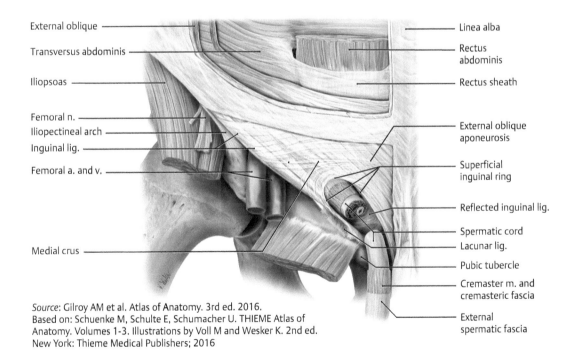

Source: Gilroy AM et al. Atlas of Anatomy. 3rd ed. 2016. Based on: Schuenke M, Schulte E, Schumacher U. THIEME Atlas of Anatomy. Volumes 1-3. Illustrations by Voll M and Wesker K. 2nd ed. New York: Thieme Medical Publishers; 2016

158. Correct: Linea alba (B)

(**B**) The linea alba (Latin, white line) is a fibrous, midline raphe between the pubic symphysis and the xiphoid process. It is formed by the aponeuroses of the external abdominal oblique, internal abdominal oblique, and transversus abdominis muscles. A weakness in linea alba, typically after a midline surgical incision, could result in a midline hernia. (**A**) The arcuate line, located approximately one-third of the distance from the pubic crest to the umbilicus, is formed by the inferior margin of the posterior layer of the rectus sheath. Inferior to the arcuate line, the aponeuroses from the external oblique, internal oblique, and transversus abdominis combine as they pass anterior to rectus abdominis to form the anterior rectus sheath. As a result, inferior to the arcuate line, the rectus abdominis muscle is in contact posteriorly with transversalis fascia. (**C**) The semilunar line (linea semilunaris) is the lateral edge of the rectus sheath. A Spigelian hernia may occur at this location. (**D**) The tendinous intersections are transversely oriented, fibrous bands in the rectus abdominis muscle. In physically fit individuals, this feature may help to create the appearance on the abdominal wall often referred to as a "six pack." (**E**) The linea nigra (also known as the "pregnancy line") is a vertical, pigmented line in the midline of the anterior abdominal wall seen in many pregnant women (it may be absent in women who have very fair skin). Formation of a linea nigra is thought to be due to increased melanocyte-stimulating hormone made by the placenta, which also causes darkening of the nipples and melasma (darkened skin patches). This line typically disappears a few months after delivery.

159. Correct: Genitofemoral (B)

(**B**) The genitofemoral nerve (L1, L2) is derived from the lumbar plexus and emerges from anterior aspect of the psoas major muscle. The genital (medial) branch has a motor and sensory component in men. It enters the inguinal canal via the deep inguinal ring and supplies motor innervation to cremaster muscle. Cutaneous branches emerge from the superficial inguinal ring to distribute to the skin of the anterolateral scrotum. In women, the genital branch is entirely sensory, with distribution to the labum majus and mons pubis. The femoral (lateral) branch passes deep to the inguinal ligament to distribute cutaneous branches to skin over the femoral triangle in both sexes. Injury to the genitofemoral nerve during percutaneous drainage will result in numbness over the femoral triangle and (in men) an absent cremasteric reflex (elevation of the testis on tactile stimulation of the skin of the anteromedial thigh). (**A**) The femoral nerve (L2–L4), a branch of the lumbar plexus, emerges from the lateral aspect of psoas major muscle and enters the thigh posterior to the inguinal ligament. Injury to the femoral nerve can result in weak thigh extension and paresthesia in the anteromedial thigh and medial leg and foot. (**C**) The lateral cutaneous nerve of the thigh (L2-L3), a branch of the lumbar plexus, emerges from the lateral aspect of the psoas major. Compression of this nerve as it exits the pelvis near the anterior superior iliac spine can result in meralgia paresthetica (pain in the lateral thigh). (**D**) The obturator nerve (L2–L4) passes through the psoas major muscle to reach its medial aspect and exit the pelvis via the obturator canal. The obturator nerve distributes to the medial thigh and its injury to can weaken hip adduction and lead to pain and sensory loss in the medial thigh and knee. (**E**) The subcostal nerve (T12) courses along the inferior border of the rib 12 and then anterior to quadratus lumborum muscle. It gives rise to anterior and lateral cutaneous branches to the abdominal wall, as well as muscular branches.

Pelvis and Perineum

160. **Correct: S2–S4 (C)**

Refer to the following image for answer 160:

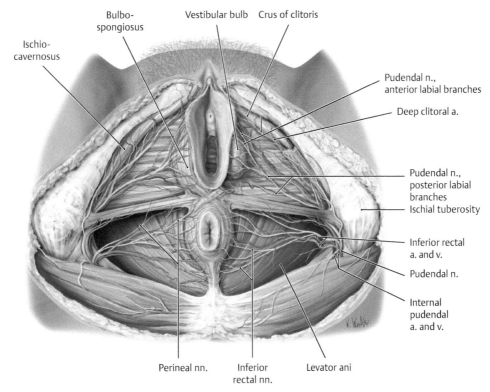

Source: Gilroy AM et al. Atlas of Anatomy. 3rd ed. 2016. Based on: Schuenke M, Schulte E, Schumacher U. THIEME Atlas of Anatomy. Volumes 1-3. Illustrations by Voll M and Wesker K. 2nd ed. New York: Thieme Medical Publishers; 2016

(**C**) The nerves are the inferior rectal and perineal nerves. These nerves are branches of the pudendal nerve, which contains nerve fibers from the S2-S4 ventral rami. (**A, B, D, E**) L4, L5, S1, and S5 do not contribute to nerves in the ischioanal fossa.

161. Correct: Ischiocavernosus (C)

Refer to the following image for answer 161:

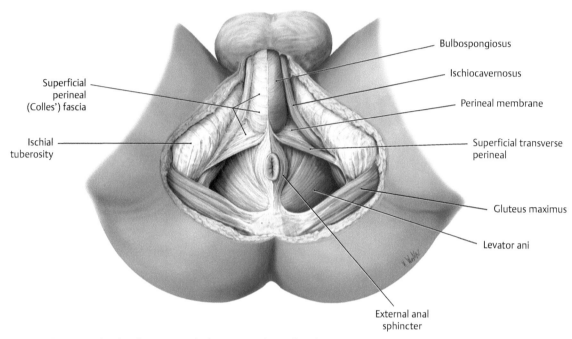

Source: Gilroy AM et al. Atlas of Anatomy. 3rd ed. 2016. Based on: Schuenke M, Schulte E, Schumacher U. THIEME Atlas of Anatomy. Volumes 1-3. Illustrations by Voll M and Wesker K. 2nd ed. New York: Thieme Medical Publishers; 2016

(**C**) Surgical implantation of an inflatable prosthesis into the crura requires retraction of the ischiocavernosus muscles. Each crus of the penis (erectile tissue) is covered on its inferior surface by an ischiocavernosus muscle. While the crura enter the shaft of the penis as the corpora cavernosa, these muscles do not extend beyond the root of the penis. (**A**) The bulbospongiosus muscles cover the inferior aspect of the bulb of the penis. (**B, D, E**) The external urethral sphincter, pubococcygeus, and superficial transverse perinei muscles are not associated with the erectile bodies of the penis.

162.   Correct: Levator ani (E)

Refer to the following images for answer 162:

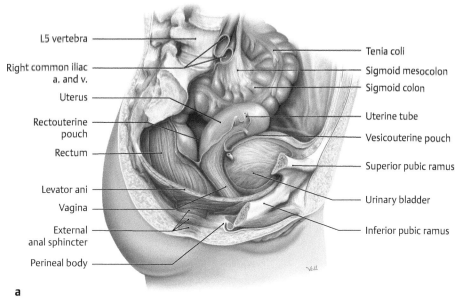

L5 vertebra

Right common iliac
a. and v.

Uterus

Rectouterine
pouch

Rectum

Levator ani

Vagina

External
anal sphincter

Perineal body

Tenia coli

Sigmoid mesocolon

Sigmoid colon

Uterine tube

Vesicouterine pouch

Superior pubic ramus

Urinary bladder

Inferior pubic ramus

a

Source: Gilroy AM et al. Atlas of Anatomy. 3rd ed. 2016. Based on: Schuenke M, Schulte E, Schumacher U. THIEME Atlas of Anatomy. Volumes 1-3. Illustrations by Voll M and Wesker K. 2nd ed. New York: Thieme Medical Publishers; 2016

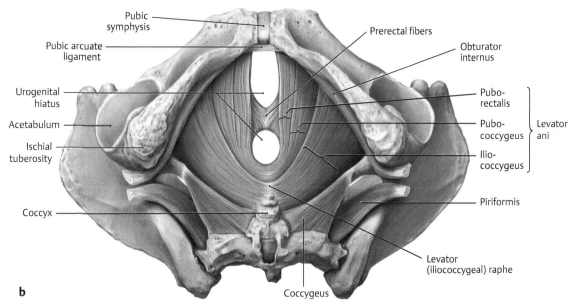

Pubic
symphysis

Pubic arcuate
ligament

Urogenital
hiatus

Acetabulum

Ischial
tuberosity

Coccyx

Prerectal fibers

Obturator
internus

Pubo-
rectalis

Pubo-
coccygeus

Ilio-
coccygeus

Levator
ani

Piriformis

Levator
(iliococcygeal) raphe

Coccygeus

b

Source: Schuenke M, Schulte E, Schumacher U. THIEME Atlas of Anatomy. General Anatomy and Musculoskeletal System. Illustrations by Voll M and Wesker K. 2nd ed. New York: Thieme Medical Publishers; 2016

(**E**) Adequate tone in levator ani (image a) and its subdivisions (puborectalis, pubococcygeus, iliococcygeus; image b) is considered the most important factor in maintaining the proper position of the pelvic viscera. A weak or damaged levator ani can lead to altered positions and functions of organs such as the urinary bladder, urethra, vagina, uterus, and rectum. A cardinal sign of compromised levator ani muscle is urine leakage during exercise or while laughing, sneezing, etc. This is known clinically as urinary stress incontinence. (**A–C**) The bulbospongiosus, external urethral sphincter, and internal urethral sphincter muscles do not provide significant support to the pelvic floor. (**D**) Ischiococcygeus (often termed coccygeus) contributes to the posterior portion of the pelvic diaphragm (consisting of the levator ani and ischiococcygeus muscles). However, it is frequently fibrous in nature and does not form a major part of the pelvic floor.

163.   Correct: Sacral promontory to inferior edge of the pubic symphysis (B)

Refer to the following image for answer 163:

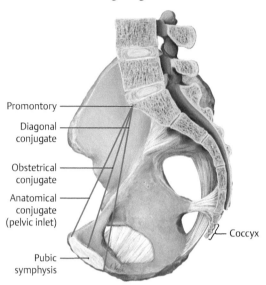

Source: Gilroy AM et al. Atlas of Anatomy. 3rd ed. 2016. Based on: Schuenke M, Schulte E, Schumacher U. THIEME Atlas of Anatomy. Volumes 1-3. Illustrations by Voll M and Wesker K. 2nd ed. New York: Thieme Medical Publishers; 2016

(**B**) There are two measurements of the anterior-posterior dimension of the female pelvic inlet useful to the obstetrician. The diagonal conjugate is determined by transvaginal palpation to approximate the distance, typically 12.5 cm or more, between the inferior edge of the pubic symphysis and the sacral promontory. Less commonly, the true (obstetrical) conjugate is determined radiographically and is the distance between the sacral promontory and the pelvic surface of the pubic symphysis. This distance is usually 11 cm or more. (**A**) This dimension establishes the transverse dimension at the pelvic outlet. (**C–E**) The measurements from the sacral promontory to the pubic tubercle, from the tip of coccyx to ischial spine, and from the tip of coccyx to pubic tubercle do not have any obstetric significance.

164.   Correct: Pubococcygeus (E)

(**E**) Fibers of pubococcygeus form a major portion of levator ani. During a vaginal delivery the pubococcygeus fibers near the midline of the pelvic floor are most vulnerable to strain and tearing, especially if there is tearing of the posterior vaginal wall and gynecological perineum. It is important to distinguish between the diamond-shaped, anatomical perineum limited by bony landmarks (tip of coccyx, ischial spines, pubic symphysis) and the gynecological perineum (area between vagina and rectum), which is occupied by the midline perineal body. (**A**) The internal anal sphincter (smooth muscle) is in the wall of the anal canal and would not typically be traumatized during childbirth. (**B**) Ischiococcygeus (often termed coccygeus) contributes to the posterior portion of the pelvic diaphragm (levator ani and ischiococcygeus). Although coccygeus is thin and contains few muscular fibers, its attachment to the underlying sacrospinous ligament reinforces the muscle and significantly strengthens the posterior portion of the pelvic diaphragm. (**C, D**) Obturator internus and piriformis have attachment to the lateral pelvic wall and exit the pelvis to act on the hip joint. They are insignificant during childbirth.

Refer to the following image for answer 164:

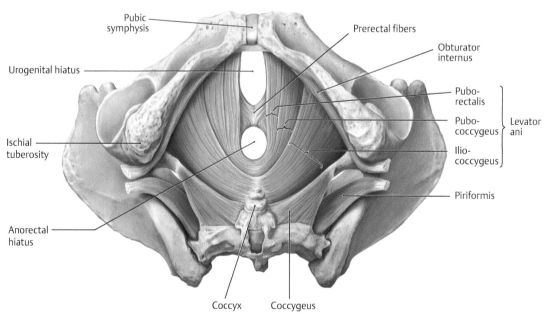

Source: Schuenke M, Schulte E, Schumacher U. THIEME Atlas of Anatomy. General Anatomy and Musculoskeletal System. Illustrations by Voll M and Wesker K. 2nd ed. New York: Thieme Medical Publishers; 2016

165. Correct: Pubis, ischium, and ilium (E)

Refer to the following image for answer 165:

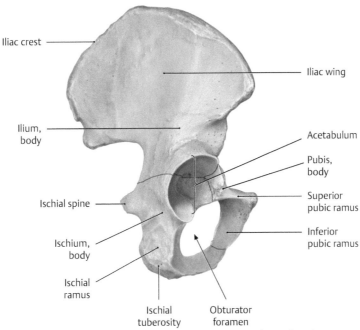

Iliac crest

Iliac wing

Ilium, body

Acetabulum

Pubis, body

Superior pubic ramus

Ischial spine

Ischium, body

Inferior pubic ramus

Ischial ramus

Ischial tuberosity

Obturator foramen

Source: Gilroy AM et al. Atlas of Anatomy. 3rd ed. 2016. Based on: Schuenke M, Schulte E, Schumacher U. THIEME Atlas of Anatomy. Volumes 1-3. Illustrations by Voll M and Wesker K. 2nd ed. New York: Thieme Medical Publishers; 2016

(**E**) The pubis (body, inferior ramus, and superior ramus) and the ischium (body and ramus) contribute to the margins of the obturator foramen. (**A, E**) The ilium does not border the obturator foramen. (**B**) Portions of the ischium border the obturator foramen, but the pubis also contributes to the margins. (**C**) The pubis borders the obturator, but the ischium also contributes to the margins.

166. Correct: 90 degrees (D)

(**D**) The bodies of the pubic bones meet anteriorly in the midline to contribute to the pubic symphysis. The inferior pubic rami diverge from the bodies of the pubic bones in a posterolateral direction, forming the inferior border of the obturator foramina. The angle formed by the divergent rami (pubic arch) approximates 90 degrees in the female. This angle is closer to 45 degrees in the male. (**A**) This represents the angle of the pubic arch in the male. (**B, C**) The angle of the pubic arch in the female usually exceeds 65 degrees. (**E**) The angle of the pubic arch in the female typically does not exceed 90 degrees.

Chapter 3

Cardiovascular System

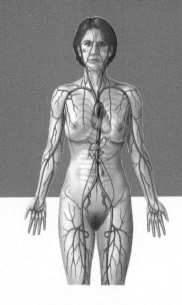

ANATOMICAL LEARNING OBJECTIVES

▶ Describe the blood supply to the brain and cranial meninges, including their arterial supply and venous drainage.

▶ Describe the blood supply for the eye.

▶ Describe the blood supply for the nasal cavity.

▶ Describe the anatomy of the infratemporal fossa, including the course of the maxillary artery and the distribution of its branches.

▶ Describe the blood supply for the palatine, pharyngeal, and lingual tonsils.

▶ Describe the anatomy of the common, internal and external carotid arteries, including their branches and distribution.

▶ Describe the anatomy of the anterior cervical triangle, including its subdivisions, contents, and anatomical relationships.

▶ Identify the points in the neck and head where an arterial pulse can be palpated.

▶ Describe the developmental anatomy of the pharyngeal apparatus.

▶ Describe the anatomy of the thoracic outlet.

▶ Describe the anatomy of the heart, including its membranes, chambers, blood supply, and conducting system

▶ Describe the surface projections and auscultation points for the heart valves.

▶ Describe the developmental anatomy of the heart, including prenatal circulation, and circulatory changes that occur at birth.

▶ Describe the blood supply for the posterior mediastinum.

▶ Describe the anatomy of the abdominal aorta, and its branches and their distribution

▶ Describe the anatomy of the hepatic portal system, including its anastomoses with systemic veins

▶ Describe the blood supply for the abdomen, including its walls and viscera.

▶ Describe the blood supply for the pelvic cavity.

▶ Describe the blood supply for the male external genitalia and explain the neurovascular mechanism for tumescence (erection) and detumescence.

▶ Describe the anatomy of the major blood vessels of the lower limb, including their branches, distribution, and pulse points.

▶ Describe the mechanisms involved in regulating plasma electrolytes and blood pressure.

▶ Recognize normal and pathological anatomy in standard diagnostic imaging of the cardiovascular system.

3.1 Questions

Easy	Medium	Hard

1. A 61-year-old man with complaints of progressively worsening headaches and concern that his vision is rapidly deteriorating visits his primary care physician. After an initial workup is unrevealing, the patient is referred for CT angiography that shows a saccular-type (berry) aneurysm on an artery on the ventral surface of the brain (refer to the *arrow* in the accompanying image). Which of the following arteries has the aneurysm in this patient?

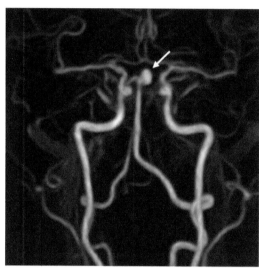

Source: Wolf K, Grozdanovic Z, Albrecht T et al. Direct Diagnosis in Radiology. Vascular Imaging. 1st Edition. Thieme; 2009.

A. Anterior cerebral

B. Basilar

C. Middle cerebral

D. Posterior cerebral

E. Posterior communicating

Consider the following case for questions 2 and 3:

A 14-year-old girl is struck on the right temporal region by a wildly thrown ball during a softball game. She collapsed and was transported by ambulance to the emergency department. Imaging reveals a hematoma with defined margins in the region of the injury (refer to the *arrows* in the accompanying image).

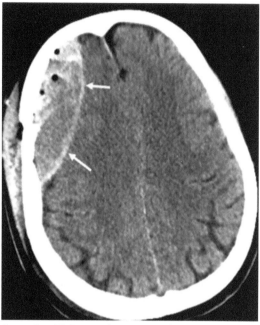

Source: Anzai Y, Tozer-Fink K. Imaging of Traumatic Brain Injury. 1st Edition. Thieme; 2015.

2. Which of the following hematoma types has developed in this patient?

A. Epicranial

B. Epidural

C. Subarachnoid

D. Subcutaneous

E. Subdural

3. The artery that has been ruptured in this patient is a branch of which of the following?

A. External carotid

B. Facial

C. Internal carotid

D. Maxillary

E. Superficial temporal

4. A 45-year-old woman describes to her primary care physician a persistent pain and clicking sound in her right temporomandibular joint. During physical examination, an arterial pulse is detected at the anterior edge of the masseter muscle, where the muscle attaches to the mandible. Which artery is most likely palpated in this patient?

A. External carotid

B. Facial

C. Lingual

D. Maxillary

E. Submental

F. Superficial temporal

5. A 27-year-old woman is brought to the emergency department. She describes left-side frontal headaches of increasing intensity over the past 2 days and indicates visual problems in her left eye. A history reveals that she has taken oral contraceptives since the birth of her 7-month-old daughter. MR venography reveals an intracranial thrombus (refer to *the arrows* in the accompanying image). In a normal flow pattern, blood in the dural sinus with the thrombus would next enter which of the following?

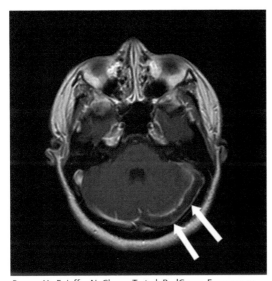

Source: Yu E, Jaffer N, Chung T et al. RadCases. Emergency Radiology. 1st Edition. Thieme; 2015.

A. Confluence of sinuses

B. Internal jugular vein

C. Occipital dural venous sinus

D. Sigmoid dural venous sinus

E. Straight dural venous sinus

6. A 17-year-old boy is brought to the emergency department with his left eye esotropic (adducted) during primary gaze. He has serious facial acne with some of the lesions showing signs of infection. MR venography discloses a thrombus in the left cavernous dural venous sinus. Which of the following vessels passes through the dural sinus with the thrombus?

A. Anterior cerebral vein

B. Internal carotid artery

C. Middle cerebral vein

D. Middle meningeal artery

E. Ophthalmic artery

7. A 46-year-old woman comes to the physician because she has recently noticed a swelling in the right side of her neck. Physical examination reveals a nodule on the right lobe of the thyroid gland. The pathology report for a fine needle biopsy classifies the nodule as malignant and the patient is referred for thyroidectomy. During surgery to remove the diseased lobe, an artery that descends in the neck to reach the gland is ligated. The ligated artery is a direct branch of which of the following?

A. Common carotid

B. External carotid

C. Internal carotid

D. Thyrocervical trunk

E. Vertebral

8. During a routine physical examination of a 48-year-old man, the physician detects a strong pulse on the left side at the level of the cricoid cartilage (C6 vertebral level). From which of the following arteries is the pulse recorded?

A. Common carotid

B. External carotid

C. Internal carotid

D. Superior thyroid

E. Vertebral

9. A 61-year-old man with a history of right atrioventricular valve disease meets with the cardiovascular surgeon to discuss a valve replacement procedure. During evaluation of the patient, the surgeon notes a visible distension of the superficial neck veins when the patient is sitting upright. Which of the following unite to form the distended veins?

A. Anterior division of retromandibular and facial

B. Anterior jugular and posterior auricular

C. Maxillary and facial

D. Occipital and facial

E. Posterior division of retromandibular and posterior auricular

145

10. A 12-year-old boy is brought to the physician because he is experiencing recurring episodes of sore throat and discomfort when swallowing. His parents indicate that he snores. Evaluation of the oral cavity reveals large palatine tonsils (refer to the accompanying image) that protrude medially well beyond the limits of the tonsillar sinuses (fossae or beds). Considering the options presented, the parents elect to schedule the boy for tonsillectomy. The primary artery to the enlarged gland is a branch of which of the following?

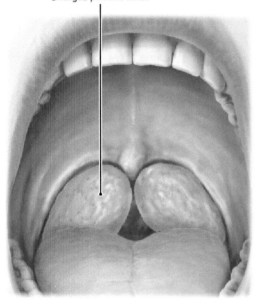

Enlarged palatine tonsil

Source: Gilroy AM et al. Atlas of Anatomy. 3rd ed. 2016. Based on: Schuenke M, Schulte E, Schumacher U. THIEME Atlas of Anatomy. Volumes 1-3. Illustrations by Voll M and Wesker K. 2nd ed. New York: Thieme Medical Publishers; 2016

A. Deep temporal
B. External carotid
C. Facial
D. Lingual
E. Maxillary

11. The parents of a 3-year-old girl bring her to the physician because they have noticed a persistent drainage from a small pore in her neck. An MRI confirms a branchial cleft sinus at the level of the superior horn of the thyroid cartilage. There is no evidence of infection and the child is scheduled for surgical removal of the sinus. Which of the following arteries is most vulnerable during the surgery?

A. Facial
B. Inferior thyroid
C. Lingual
D. Occipital
E. Superior thyroid

12. A 68-year-old woman with a lump just below her jaw on the left side comes to the physician. She indicates the lump is painless and has increased in size progressively over the past 4 weeks. Biopsy of the mass indicates an adenoid cystic carcinoma of the submandibular gland. During surgery to remove the diseased gland, care is taken to preserve a tortuous artery that grooves several surfaces of the gland. Which of the following arteries occupies "grooves" on the surface of the diseased gland?

A. External carotid
B. Facial
C. Internal carotid
D. Lingual
E. Superior thyroid

13. A 40-year-old man is admitted to the hospital for extraction of an impacted left mandibular third molar. He is administered anesthetic to the area of the mandibular foramen on the left side. Which of the following arteries is nearest to the point of anesthetic administration?

A. Deep temporal
B. Inferior alveolar
C. Masseteric
D. Mental
E. Posterior superior alveolar

14. During "horseplay" with a group of friends, a 9-year-old boy accidently has a small stick forced into his left nostril. He immediately experiences epistaxis (nose bleed) that cannot be controlled. He is brought to the emergency department by a parent where personnel pack the nostril with gauze and arrest the bleeding. Subsequent rhinologic examination indicates that an artery of the anterior nasal septum has been traumatized. Which of the following arteries directly provides most of the blood to the area of injury?

A. Descending palatine
B. Infraorbital
C. Maxillary
D. Posterior lateral nasal
E. Sphenopalatine

15. A 14-year-old girl lost her balance and falls from the beam during gymnastic practice. She strikes her posterior head on an adjacent piece of equipment and immediately experiences bleeding from an occipital scalp laceration. The vessel causing the bleeding is a branch of which of the following arteries?

A. Common carotid
B. External carotid
C. Facial
D. Posterior auricular
E. Superficial temporal

Consider the following case for questions 16 and 17:

A 71-year-old man comes to the physician because he has experienced two transitory episodes of left eye blindness over the last week. History reveals that he is diabetic, hypertensive, and a chronic cigarette smoker. After an initial workup is negative, an ophthalmology consult recommends angiography. Evaluation of the left retina shows a plaque embolism in a retinal vessel as well as plaque stenosis in a major artery of the neck (refer to the *arrow* in the accompanying image).

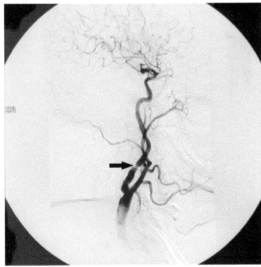

Source: Gunderman R. Essential Radiology. Clinical Presentation, Pathophysiology, Imaging. 3rd Edition. Thieme; 2014.

16. The stenosis seen in the arteriogram (*arrow*) is located in which of the following arteries?

A. Common carotid

B. External carotid

C. Internal carotid

D. Middle meningeal

E. Ophthalmic

17. The retinal embolus was undoubtedly derived from the plaque in the carotid system. Which of the following is the most likely explanation for why the embolus entered the ophthalmic artery?

A. It branches from the internal carotid outside the cranial cavity

B. It is the first branch of the internal carotid artery

C. It is the largest branch of the internal carotid artery

D. It is the least tortuous branch of the internal carotid artery

E. It is the shortest branch of the internal carotid artery

18. A 45-year-old homeless woman with an incomplete previous history presents to the emergency department in the middle of the night with chest pain over a period of 3 days. Coronary CT is performed to determine if there is a cardiac cause for the chest pain and, unexpectedly, the imaging reveals that the patient has had prior stenting (see the *arrow* in the accompanying image). A significant stenotic lesion is revealed within the same vessel with the stent (refer to the *arrowhead* in the accompanying image). Which of the following represents the diseased vessel in this patient?

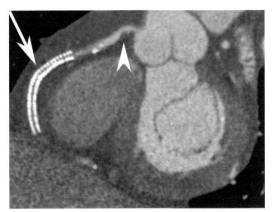

Source: Halpern E. ed. Clinical Cardiac CT: Anatomy and Function. 2nd Edition. Thieme; 2008.

A. Anterior interventricular

B. Circumflex

C. Left coronary

D. Posterior interventricular

E. Right coronary

19. A 29-year-old woman is brought to the emergency department by ambulance. She was driving her father's classic automobile when she rear-ended another vehicle. She was thrown into the steering wheel and the windshield. Physical examination reveals tachycardia (elevated heart rate), tachypnea (elevated respiratory rate), and jugular vein distension. A bedside transthoracic echocardiogram reveals a circumferential anechoic area surrounding the heart. Further evaluation reveals a pulsus paradoxus (greater than 10 mm Hg fall in blood pressure during inspiration) and cardiac tamponade (increased pressure in the pericardial sac caused by the accumulation of blood or fluids) secondary to the chest trauma. The anechoic area in echocardiogram is located between which of the following?

A. Myocardium and parietal serous pericardium

B. Myocardium and visceral serous pericardium

C. Parietal serous pericardium and fibrous pericardium

D. Visceral serous pericardium and endocardium

E. Visceral serous pericardium and parietal serous pericardium

20. At the scheduled 1-month evaluation of their infant son, the parents express concern that the boy seems to have constant "heavy breathing," even when sleeping. He also has a very poor appetite, taking only a few ounces of milk at each feeding. The pediatrician detects a heart murmur and refers the infant to a pediatric cardiologist. A CT with maximum intensity projection is performed. Which of the following represents the situation seen in this patient (refer to the *arrow* in the accompanying image)?
Image key: left subclavian artery (S), left common carotid (C) artery, ascending (AAo) and descending (DAo) aorta, right (R) and left (L) pulmonary arteries, confluence of the pulmonary veins (PV).

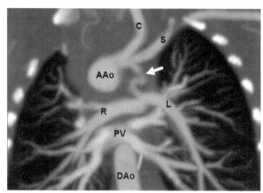

Source: Restrepo C, Bardo D. RadCases. Cardiac Imaging. 1st Edition. Thieme; 2010.

A. Anomalous origin of brachiocephalic artery

B. Anomalous origin for left coronary artery

C. Anomalous origin for right subclavian artery

D. Coarctation of aorta

E. Patent ductus arteriosus

21. A 67-year-old man experiences chest pain during a stress test following an outpatient visit for angina. Follow-up coronary angiography reveals a 95% occlusion at the proximal end of the anterior interventricular artery (left anterior descending). He is scheduled for arterio-arterial coronary graft bypass surgery. Postoperative imaging confirms patency at the graft site (refer to the accompanying image). Which of the following arteries was most likely used for the graft in this patient?

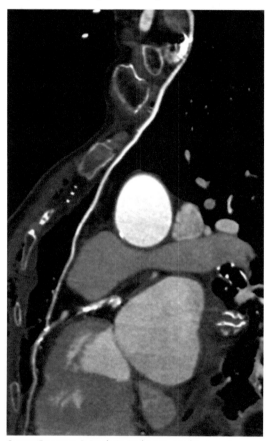

Source: Restrepo C, Bardo D. RadCases. Cardiac Imaging. 1st Edition. Thieme; 2010.

A. Fifth anterior intercostal

B. Fifth posterior intercostal

C. Internal thoracic

D. Pericardiacophrenic

E. Superior phrenic

22. A 32-year-old woman presents with progressive difficulty swallowing. She states that she has always had some discomfort in her chest when swallowing food and the problem has become more troublesome over the past several months. A contrast-enhanced CT shows an aberrant artery in the mediastinum (refer to the *arrow* in the accompanying image). The aberrant vessel in this patient is normally a branch of which of the following?

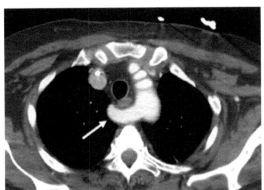

Source: Ferral H, Lorenz J. Radcases: Interventional Radiology. 2nd Edition. Thieme; 2018.

A. Ascending aorta

B. Brachiocephalic trunk

C. Postductal arch of aorta

D. Preductal arch of aorta

E. Right common carotid artery

23. The radiologist is reviewing sonograms of the thorax from a patient brought to the emergency department following an industrial accident. She observes the parasternal union of two large vessels at the level of the right first intercostal space. The union of the observed vessels will form which of the following?

A. Azygos vein

B. Brachiocephalic trunk

C. Coronary sinus

D. Right pulmonary vein

E. Superior vena cava

24. During the physical examination of a simulated patient the supervising physician helps a first-year medical student properly position the diaphragm of the stethoscope to best auscultate the sound that corresponds to the closure of the aortic valve and for murmurs generated by stenosis of this valve. The stethoscope diaphragm should be placed in which of the following positions to auscultate the desired heart sound?

A. Midclavicular line, left fifth intercostal space

B. Midclavicular line, right third intercostal space

C. Sternal border, left fourth intercostal space

D. Sternal border, left second intercostal space

E. Sternal border, right second intercostal space

Consider the following case for questions 25 and 26:

A 61-year-old man who is experiencing chest pain consistent with ischemic heart disease is brought to the emergency department. After cardiology consultation, a coronary arteriogram CT reveals several areas of plaque within a heart vessel (refer to the *arrow* in the accompanying image).

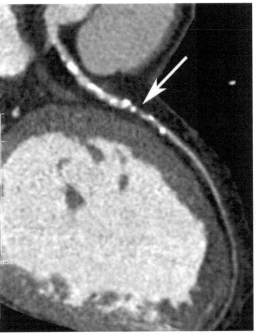

Source: Halpern E. ed. Clinical Cardiac CT: Anatomy and Function. 2nd Edition. Thieme; 2008.

25. The arteriogram indicates calcified and non-calcified (*arrow* in the accompanying image) areas of narrowing along which of the following arteries?

A. Anterior interventricular

B. Circumflex coronary

C. Left coronary

D. Left marginal

E. Right coronary

26. Which of the following veins is a companion to the diseased vessel in the arteriogram?

A. Coronary sinus

B. Great cardiac

C. Middle cardiac

D. Right marginal

E. Small cardiac

27. A 35-year-old woman with concerns about swelling of her ankles and feet comes to the physician. She describes chronic feelings of fatigue and shortness of breath after climbing stairs in her home. During the physical examination a systolic murmur is detected at the left sternal border in the fourth or fifth intercostal space. The murmur varies in intensity with quiet respiration. Which of the following valves is associated with this murmur?

A. Aortic

B. Left atrioventricular

C. Pulmonary

D. Right atrioventricular

28. A 16-year-old boy is brought to the physician by his parents. He is a high school varsity athlete and is experiencing episodes of fatigue and exhaustion during mild exertion. Physical examination suggests an enlarged right heart and echocardiography confirms an enlarged right atrium and right ventricle. Imaging also indicates that the right atrioventricular (tricuspid) valve is displaced toward the heart apex (Ebstein's anomaly) and is not functioning properly. Which of the following are the proper terms for the cusps of the involved valve?

A. Anterior, posterior, lateral

B. Anterior, posterior, septal

C. Right, left, anterior

D. Right, left, posterior

E. Right, left, septal

29. A 23-year-old man with concerns about shortness of breath, a rapid pulse, and chronic feelings of fatigue visits his primary care physician. Physical evaluation establishes a resting respiratory rate of 23 breaths per minute and a resting pulse rate of 112 beats per minute. After initial assessment by cardiology, he is sent for further evaluation by more advanced cardiac imaging. Which of the following is indicated by the *arrow* in the accompanying CT image of this patient's heart?

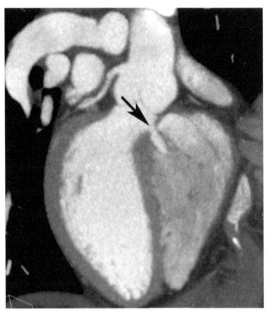

Source: Halpern E. ed. Clinical Cardiac CT: Anatomy and Function. 2nd Edition. Thieme; 2008.

A. Membranous interventricular septal defect

B. Muscular interventricular septal defect

C. Primum-type atrial septal defect

D. Secundum-type atrial septal defect

30. A 19-year-old woman with concerns about recent episodes of shortness of breath and chest pain comes to the physician. Physical examination reveals a systolic heart murmur and contrast-enhanced CT angiography shows a post-valvular narrowing of the aortic root (refer to the *arrow* in the accompanying image). Which of the following arteries might be expected to show aneurysmal distension in this patient?

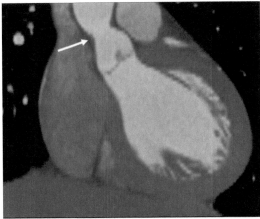

Source: Restrepo C, Bardo D. RadCases. Cardiac Imaging. 1st Edition. Thieme; 2010.

A. Brachiocephalic

B. Coronary

C. Left common carotid

D. Right bronchial

E. Right subclavian

31. The parents of a 3-week-old female bring her to the emergency department with concerns that she is breathing rapidly and has difficulty feeding. The infant was born at 36 weeks gestation. The physical examination detects a continuous heart murmur and echocardiography reveals a large patent ductus arteriosus. Which of the following would be expected in this infant as a result of the developmental anomaly?

A. Decreased blood flow to the lungs

B. Increased blood flow to the lungs

C. Left ventricular hypoplasia

D. Normal blood flow to the lungs

E. Right ventricular hypoplasia

32. The emergency medical services bring a 68-year-old man who is vomiting blood to the emergency department. The man's history reveals hepatic cirrhosis due to a chronic Hepatitis C infection. Endoscopy reveals bleeding varicose veins in the lower esophagus. The bleeding vessels normally drain blood preferentially into which of the following veins?

A. Azygos

B. Hepatic

C. Portal

D. Splenic

E. Superior mesenteric

33. A 23-year-old woman comes to the physician expressing concern that her right hand frequently has bouts of numbness and tingling. She also reports that her right hand is colder and often appears to have less "color" than her left hand. Physical examination reveals a weak brachial artery pulse and confirms the pallor of the right hand. Radiographic images show a cervical rib on the right side and she is diagnosed with arterial thoracic outlet syndrome. Which of the following arteries is being compressed in this patient?

A. Axillary

B. Brachial

C. Brachiocephalic

D. Deep Brachial

E. Subclavian

34. A 49-year-old man is brought to the emergency department because he has experienced two episodes of nonexertional chest pain during the past hour. History indicates that just prior to the first episode he had consumed a spicy meal. He is a smoker but does not have a history of heart disease. A coronary CT arteriogram is performed with curved maximum intensity projection for the left coronary artery and its branches. Which of the following arteries is indicated by the *arrowhead* in the accompanying arteriogram?

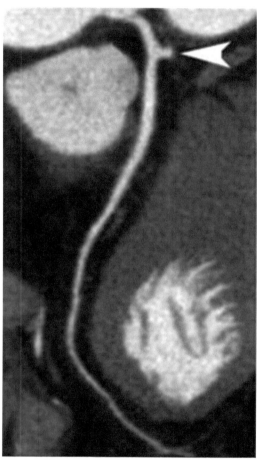

Source: Halpern E. ed. Clinical Cardiac CT: Anatomy and Function. 2nd Edition. Thieme; 2008.

A. Anterior interventricular (left anterior descending)

B. Atrial

C. Circumflex

D. Left coronary

E. Left marginal

35. A 47-year-old woman with concerns that she has recently experienced feelings of weakness and fatigue presents to her primary care physician. She also indicates that several times during the day her heart feels like it's "fluttering." An electrocardiogram indicates she has atrial fibrillation. The physician uses an MRI from another patient with artist-applied conduction system (refer to the accompanying image) to explain atrial fibrillation to her. Which of the following vessels usually provides blood to the region labelled "1" in the MRI?

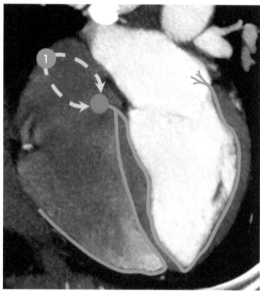

Source: Restrepo C, Bardo D. RadCases. Cardiac Imaging. 1st Edition. Thieme; 2010.

A. Anterior interventricular

B. Left coronary

C. Posterior interventricular

D. Right coronary

E. Right marginal

36. A 39-year-old woman is brought to the emergency department with sudden onset of chest pain, dyspnea (shortness of breath), and tachycardia (elevated heart rate). History indicates that she has smoked most of her adult life and she has used oral contraceptives for eight years. Chest CT with maximum intensity projection reveals thrombi in major vessels. Which of the following vessels contain the thrombus indicated by the *arrows* in the following image?

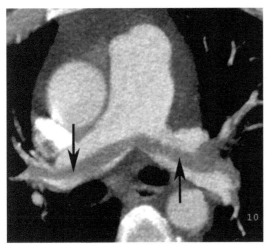

Source: Restrepo C, Bardo D. RadCases. Cardiac Imaging. 1st Edition. Thieme; 2010.

A. Aortic arch and brachiocephalic artery
B. Right and left brachiocephalic veins
C. Right and left lobar arteries
D. Right and left pulmonary arteries
E. Right and left pulmonary veins

37. A 48-year-old woman with upper right abdominal pain comes to her primary care physician. A patient history reveals the symptoms are worse following consumption of fatty foods. Imaging indicates gallbladder disease and her gallbladder is removed by laparoscopic surgery. While hospitalized, she developed symptoms of thrombotic obstruction of the hepatic veins (Budd–Chiari syndrome). Which of the following veins could be distended as a result of the thrombus?

A. Right inferior phrenic
B. Right ovarian
C. Right renal
D. Right suprarenal
E. Splenic

38. A 30-year-old woman is brought to the emergency department because she began having abdominal pain around her umbilicus 6 hours ago. The pain has subsequently moved to her lower right abdomen. She sits in an abdominal guarding position and describes feeling nauseous. Physical examination reveals a fever of 37.7°C (100°F) and she has rebound tenderness on the lower right abdominal wall. A diagnosis of acute appendicitis is made. The artery that supplies the diseased organ is a branch of which of the following?

A. Ileocolic
B. Marginal artery (of Drummond)
C. Right colic
D. Right renal
E. Superior mesenteric

39. During laparoscopic surgery for a pelvic pathology, a trocar injures a vessel in the wall of the lower left abdominal quadrant of a 43-year-old man. Postoperative examination reveals a palpable, tender mass on the anterior abdominal wall and imaging confirms a hematoma in the left rectus sheath. Which of the following arteries was traumatized during the procedure?

A. Deep circumflex iliac
B. Inferior epigastric
C. Superficial circumflex iliac
D. Superficial epigastric
E. Superior epigastric

40. A 70-year-old man with a four-decade history of tobacco use visits his primary care physician for an annual examination. During the physical examination of the abdomen, the physician detects a pulsating mass in the lower abdomen, near the midline. Ultrasound reveals an aortic aneurysm (see the *star* in the accompanying image) at the L3 and L4 vertebral level. Which of the following arteries is indicated by the *arrow* in the accompanying image?

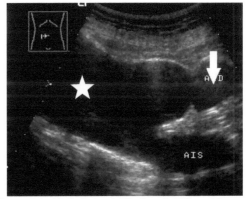

Source: Schmidt G, Greiner L, Nürnberg D. Differential Diagnosis in Ultrasound Imaging. 2nd Edition. Thieme; 2014.

A. Common iliac
B. Inferior mesenteric
C. Left colic
D. Renal
E. Testicular

153

41. A 63-year-old man with concerns about abdominal cramping after eating comes to the physician. The pain has become progressively worse over the past few weeks. He also relates that he has experienced unintended weight loss during this period. His history indicates long-term atherosclerosis exacerbated by tobacco use. Colonoscopy indicates ischemic colitis and angiography shows numerous areas of sclerotic buildup in the arteries to the descending colon. Which of the following arteries is the primary source of blood to the area of diseased bowel?

A. Ileocolic

B. Left colic

C. Middle colic

D. Sigmoid

E. Superior rectal

42. A 55-year-old man with concerns about chronic heartburn, especially after eating and when lying down, comes to the physician. He also describes difficulty swallowing food and has chronic belching. Physical examination reveals a weight of 124 kg (273 lbs). An esophagram (barium swallow) indicates a hiatal hernia with the fundus of the stomach in the thoracic cavity. Which of the following arteries provides the majority of blood to the portion of the organ that is herniated?

A. Left gastric

B. Left gastroepiploic

C. Right gastric

D. Right gastroepiploic

E. Short gastric

43. Following several years of progressive kidney failure and dialysis, a 46-year-old man is selected for a right kidney transplant. At which of the following vertebral levels does the main artery to the diseased organ usually branch from the aorta?

A. L1–L2

B. L2–L3

C. L3–L4

D. L4–L5

E. T12–L1

44. A 24-year-old woman comes to her primary care physician with episodes of pain and cramping in her left thigh. She indicates that sometimes the cramping also involves her leg and foot. She is a competitive cyclist and estimates that she trains by riding approximately 100 miles each week. Angiography indicates stenosis in a major abdominal artery (see the *arrowheads* in the accompanying image). With further evaluation she is diagnosed with exercise-induced arterial endofibrosis and stenosis caused by positional compression and stress to the artery while cycling. Which of the following arteries has been injured?

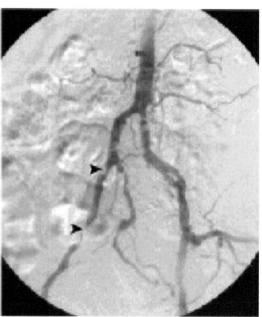

Source: Bakal C, Silberzweig J, Cynamon J et al. Vascular and Interventional Radiology. Principles and Practice. 1st Edition. Thieme; 2000.

A. Deep femoral

B. External iliac

C. Internal iliac

D. Obturator

E. Popliteal

45. A 59-year-old man is discovered to be hypertensive while in the emergency department for treatment following a minor automobile accident. He is referred to his primary care physician who confirms the hypertension and prescribes appropriate medications. After multiple follow-up visits with lack of blood pressure control on multidrug therapy, the patient is referred to nephrology for further evaluation. Renal artery stenosis is suspected and angiography is performed. Stenosis shown in the arteriogram (refer to the *arrow* in the accompanying image) will stimulate the organ it supplies to increase the release of which of the following?

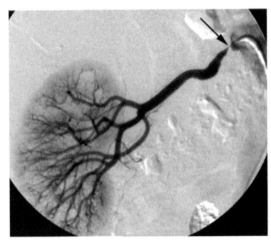

Source: Reiser M, Kuhn FP, Debus J. Duale Reihe Radiologie. Thieme, 2006

A. Aldosterone

B. Angiotensin I

C. Angiotensin II

D. Angiotensinogen

E. Renin

46. A 39-year-old woman returns to her physician 3 weeks after an elective vaginal hysterectomy. Her symptoms include a foul-smelling vaginal discharge and constant leakage of urine from her vagina. Physical examination of the vagina discloses a vesicovaginal fistula. Further evaluation determines that, during the hysterectomy, a major artery to the urinary bladder base was included in a closing suture of the upper vagina. The artery that supplies the area of the organ iatrogenically compromised in this patient is usually a branch of which of the following?

A. Common iliac

B. Inferior gluteal

C. Internal iliac

D. Middle rectal

E. Obturator

47. A 37-year-old man confides to his physician that he is experiencing erectile dysfunction. After a thorough evaluation the physician finds no organic basis for the symptoms and then prescribes tadalafil (CialisR). Tadalafil inhibits phosphodiesterase type 5 and causes tumescence. Venous blood exiting the tissues impacted by the prescribed medication will first enter which of the following?

A. Deep dorsal

B. External pudendal

C. Inferior rectal

D. Internal pudendal

E. Superficial dorsal

48. A 71-year-old man describes to his physician symptoms of a very weak urine stream and the feeling of urinary urgency. His laboratory results indicate a prostatic-specific antigen level of 12 ng/mL (normal: 4). Transrectal needle biopsy shows adenocarcinoma of the prostate. The venous plexus surrounding the diseased organ will directly receive blood from which of the following?

A. Abdominal part of ureter

B. Corpus spongiosum

C. Rectum

D. Sigmoid colon

E. Upper anal canal

49. A 12-year-old boy is brought to the emergency department with contusions to his perineum. He was on his bicycle, racing with friends, when his foot slipped from a pedal and he came down hard, straddling the bicycle's center bar. Physical examination reveals an area of hematoma over the bulb of the penis. Which of the following arteries supplies blood to the area of injury?

A. Dorsal artery of the penis

B. External pudendal

C. Inferior gluteal

D. Internal pudendal

E. Obturator

50. A 33-year-old woman comes to the physician during the seventh month of her third pregnancy. She indicates recent episodes of pain and intense itching around her anus. She states that, periodically, there is blood on the toilet tissue. Physical examination shows three subcutaneous, dark blue elevations at the anal aperture. Which of the following veins normally drains blood from the involved area?

A. Inferior gluteal

B. Inferior rectal

C. Femoral

D. Superficial dorsal vein of the clitoris

E. Superior rectal

Consider the following case for questions 51 and 52:

A 22-year-old man comes to the emergency department with concerns about pain in his left leg when he exercises. He is a member of the club rugby team at his university and indicates he can typically only play a few minutes before severe pain sets in below his left knee, especially in the calf region. Resting for a few minutes usually relieves the pain, but returning to the playing field results in the same symptoms. He is not experiencing leg pain now. His dorsalis pedis pulse is normal during dorsiflexion but weak during plantarflexion on the left side. CT with contrast imaging is ordered (refer to the accompanying images).

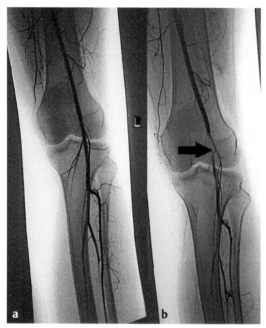

Source: Ferral H, Lorenz J. Radcases: Interventional Radiology. 2nd Edition. Thieme; 2018.

51. Which of the following arteries is occluded (indicated by *arrow* in arteriograph "b")?

A. Anterior tibial

B. Deep femoral

C. Femoral

D. Popliteal

E. Posterior tibial

52. During plantar flexion, which of the following muscles is most likely causing entrapment of the artery indicated by the *arrow* in arteriograph "b"?

A. Biceps femoris

B. Gastrocnemius

C. Popliteus

D. Semimembranosus

E. Soleus

53. A 67-year-old woman comes to the physician with concerns regarding right leg and foot pain during exertion. History indicates she is diabetic and a smoker. Physical examination reveals poor hair growth, objective coolness, and shiny skin on the right leg and foot. She is scheduled for ultrasonography to assess the vascular status in the right leg and foot. Which of the following arteries will be best visualized with the transducer in the position shown in the accompanying photograph?

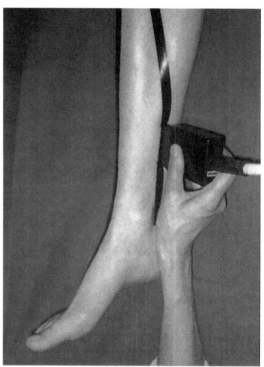

Source: Hennerici M, Neuerburg-Heusler D. Vascular Diagnosis with Ultrasound. 2. revised edition. Stuttgart: Thieme; 2005.

A. Anterior tibial

B. Dorsal artery of the foot

C. Lateral plantar

D. Medial plantar

E. Posterior tibial

54. A 54-year-old man comes to the physician with concerns about muscle cramping in his thigh and leg, especially when he walks. His history indicates he has smoked for several decades and 3 years ago had a stent placed in the proximal left coronary artery. He has an abnormal ankle-brachial index and is referred for ultrasonography to assess his lower limb vasculature. Which of the following arteries is labelled "B" in the sonogram (refer to the accompanying image)?

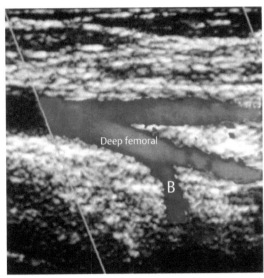

Source: Hennerici M, Neuerburg-Heusler D. Vascular Diagnosis with Ultrasound. 2. revised Edition. Stuttgart: Thieme; 2005.

A. Deep circumflex iliac

B. External pudendal

C. Lateral circumflex femoral

D. Obturator

E. Perforating

55. A 64-year-old man is brought to the emergency department with symptoms of pelvic pain. History indicates he had an open prostatectomy 8 weeks prior. Tests indicate he has pelvic hemorrhage and an internal iliac arteriogram is ordered. Which of the following arteries is represented by the number "3" in the accompanying arteriogram?

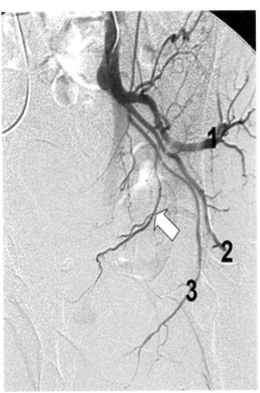

Source: Ferral H, Lorenz J. Radcases: Interventional Radiology. 2nd Edition. Thieme; 2018.

A. Inferior gluteal

B. Internal pudendal

C. Obturator

D. Superior gluteal

E. Superior vesical

56. A 19-year-old woman is brought to the emergency department by ambulance following an automobile accident. At the accident site she complained of severe bilateral hip pain. MRI does not reveal any injuries. Which of the following arteries provides the primary blood supply to the structure labelled "13" in the accompanying image?

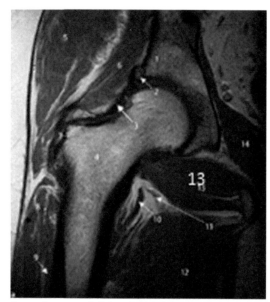

Source: Rummeny E, Reimer P, Heindel W. MR Imaging of the Body. 1st Edition. Thieme; 2008.

A. External iliac
B. Internal iliac
C. Obturator
D. Lateral circumflex femoral
E. Deep circumflex iliac

57. An Army recruit in basic training experiences bilateral shin pain during marching and running. Muscles of the anterior legs are painful on palpation and dorsiflexion is weak bilaterally during the episodes. Venous congestion is one of the precipitating factors in this condition. Which of the following veins is compromised?

A. Anterior tibial
B. Great saphenous
C. Popliteal
D. Posterior tibial
E. Small saphenous

58. A 38-year-old woman is brought to the emergency department by her partner. They were operating a log-splitter when a portion of a log broke free and struck the patient. There is a 15 cm-long splinter of wood piercing her right medial midthigh and blood is flowing from the wound. Which of the following arteries is most likely injured in this patient?

A. Femoral
B. First perforating
C. Medial circumflex artery of the thigh
D. Obturator
E. Popliteal

59. A 63-year-old man presents with angina and coronary angiography reveals 90% stenosis of his proximal anterior interventricular (left anterior descending) artery. A coronary artery bypass graft procedure is scheduled and the surgeon elects to use the left internal thoracic artery for the graft. Which of the following arteries that supply the diaphragm would be interrupted when harvesting the internal thoracic artery for this procedure?

A. Anterior intercostal and posterior intercostal
B. Musculophrenic and pericardiacophrenic
C. Musculophrenic and superior phrenic
D. Pericardiacophrenic and superior phrenic
E. Superior phrenic and anterior intercostal

3.2 Answers and Explanations

Easy	Medium	Hard

1. Correct: Posterior cerebral (D)

Refer to the following image for answer 1:

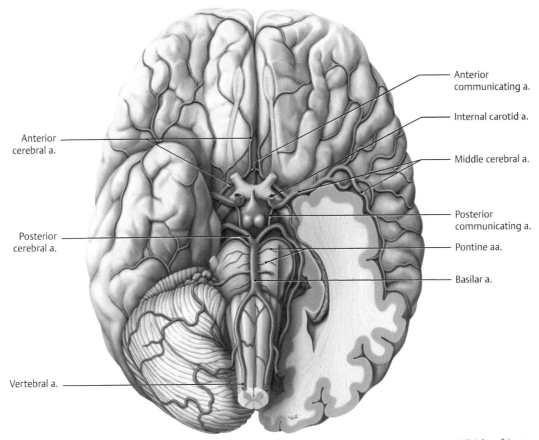

Source: Gilroy AM et al. Atlas of Anatomy. 3rd ed. 2016. Based on: Schuenke M, Schulte E, Schumacher U. THIEME Atlas of Anatomy. Volumes 1-3. Illustrations by Voll M and Wesker K. 2nd ed. New York: Thieme Medical Publishers; 2016

(**D**) This patient has a saccular (berry) aneurysm on the posterior cerebral artery. The paired posterior cerebral arteries are terminal branches of the basilar artery. Saccular aneurysms on the cerebral arterial circle are most common on the anterior communicating artery. (**A**) The anterior cerebral arteries (right and left) course parallel toward the frontal lobes of the brain after branching from the internal carotid arteries. They are united across the midline by the anterior communicating artery. (**B**) The single basilar artery, formed by the union of the right and left vertebral arteries, courses anteriorly in the midline along the surface of the pons and ends by dividing into the right and left posterior cerebral arteries. (**C**) The middle and anterior cerebral arteries are the terminal branches of the internal carotid artery. (**E**) The posterior communicating artery connects the posterior cerebral and middle cerebral arteries. The posterior communicating artery connects terminal branches of the internal carotid and basilar arteries. This connection completes the posterior portion of the cerebral arterial circle (of Willis).

2. Correct: Epidural (B)

Refer to the following image for answer 2:

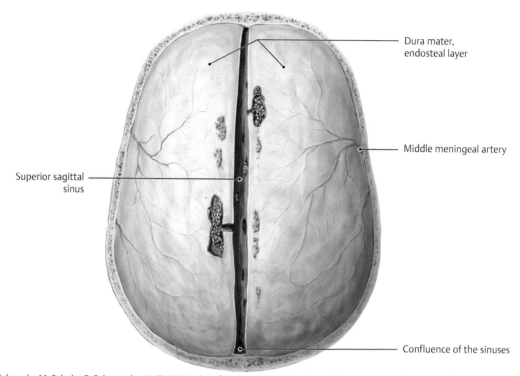

Source: Schuenke M, Schulte E, Schumacher U. THIEME Atlas of Anatomy. Head, Neck, and Neuroanatomy. Illustrations by Voll M and Wesker K. 2nd ed. New York: Thieme Medical Publishers; 2016

(**B**) This patient has an epidural hematoma due to trauma to the middle meningeal vessels. The middle meningeal artery, which is most often involved, enters the cranial vault via the foramen spinosum and its branches course in grooves on the inner surface of the relatively thin temporal bone. It lies between the bone and dura mater and is vulnerable with blunt force trauma/fracture to the temporal region. Hemorrhage from the middle meningeal vessels will collect in the potential space (epidural) between the bone and dura mater. The hemorrhage will have defined borders since the dura is firmly anchored to bone at suture lines, limiting the spread of the extravasated blood. Since these hematomas cannot cross sutures (unless there is diastasis or "opening up" of the suture secondary to fracture), the blood is more tightly contained and tends to assume a "biconvex" shape. (**A**) An epicranial hematoma would be present on the outer surface of the skull and would possibly be visible on physical examination. (**C**) Subarachnoid hemorrhages most often involve cerebral vessels coursing within the subarachnoid space. The subarachnoid space lies between the arachnoid and pia mater and contains cerebrospinal fluid. The hemorrhage may be caused by trauma, but the most frequent cause is rupture of an aneurysm on a cerebral artery. Since the escaping blood joins the cerebrospinal fluid in the subarachnoid space, imaging will show the blood to have a diffuse pattern of spread. (**D**) A subcutaneous hematoma, like the epicranial hematoma, would lie extracranial. It would be located in the loose connective tissue layers of the scalp and possibly be evident on physical examination. (**E**) A subdural hematoma involves the accumulation of extravasated blood into the potential space between the dura and arachnoid mater. Subdural hematomas are usually venous in origin. Cerebral veins cross the subdural potential space as they course from the subarachnoid space to empty into the dural venous sinuses, especially the superior sagittal sinus. Blunt force trauma that causes shearing forces at the dura–arachnoid interface may tear bridging veins, allowing blood to collect in the subdural "space." Since the subdural hematoma involves venous blood, the hematoma may take days, weeks, or longer to produce symptoms.

NOTE: All intracranial hemorrhages, if not stopped, will produce symptoms as the accumulating blood puts pressure on the brain. Symptoms may be acute, subacute, or chronic in presentation.

3. Correct: Maxillary (D)

Refer to the following images for answer 3:

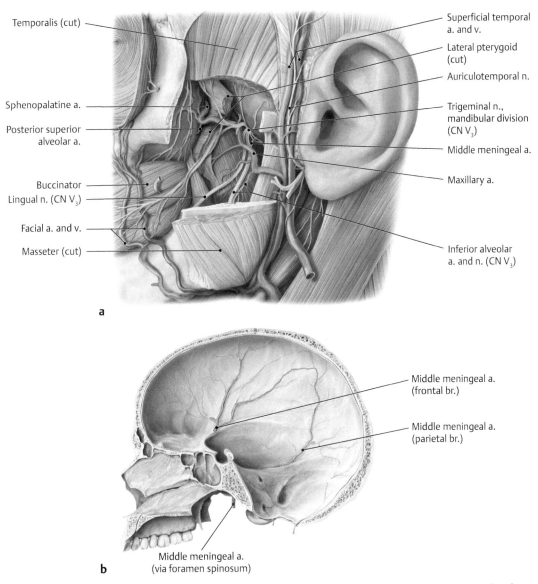

Temporalis (cut)

Sphenopalatine a.

Posterior superior alveolar a.

Buccinator

Lingual n. (CN V₃)

Facial a. and v.

Masseter (cut)

Superficial temporal a. and v.

Lateral pterygoid (cut)

Auriculotemporal n.

Trigeminal n., mandibular division (CN V₃)

Middle meningeal a.

Maxillary a.

Inferior alveolar a. and n. (CN V₃)

a

Middle meningeal a. (frontal br.)

Middle meningeal a. (parietal br.)

b   Middle meningeal a. (via foramen spinosum)

Source: Gilroy AM et al. Atlas of Anatomy. 3rd ed. 2016. Based on: Schuenke M, Schulte E, Schumacher U. THIEME Atlas of Anatomy. Volumes 1-3. Illustrations by Voll M and Wesker K. 2nd ed. New York: Thieme Medical Publishers; 2016

(**D**) The middle meningeal artery is a branch of the first part of the maxillary artery (between its origin and the lateral pterygoid muscle; see the accompanying image a). From its origin in the infratemporal fossa, the middle meningeal artery typically splits the roots of the auriculotemporal nerve before passing through the foramen spinosum of the sphenoid bone. It is accompanied through the foramen spinosum by the middle meningeal vein and the meningeal branch of the mandibular division of the trigeminal nerve (CN V). In the middle cranial fossa, the artery courses within distinct grooves in the temporal bone and usually divides into anterior (frontal) and posterior (parietal) branches (see the accompanying image b). (**A–C, E**) The middle meningeal artery does not branch from any of these vessels (external carotid, facial, internal carotid, superficial temporal).

4. Correct: Facial (B)

Refer to the following image for answer 4:

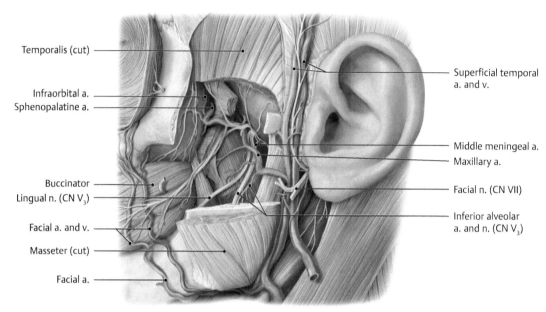

Temporalis (cut)

Infraorbital a.

Sphenopalatine a.

Buccinator

Lingual n. (CN V₃)

Facial a. and v.

Masseter (cut)

Facial a.

Superficial temporal a. and v.

Middle meningeal a.

Maxillary a.

Facial n. (CN VII)

Inferior alveolar a. and n. (CN V₃)

Source: Gilroy AM et al. Atlas of Anatomy. 3rd ed. 2016. Based on: Schuenke M, Schulte E, Schumacher U. THIEME Atlas of Anatomy. Volumes 1-3. Illustrations by Voll M and Wesker K. 2nd ed. New York: Thieme Medical Publishers; 2016

(**B**) The facial artery, a branch of the external carotid artery in the neck, enters the face by crossing the body of the mandible at the anterior edge of the insertion point for the masseter muscle. Here, the artery is in contact with the mandible and compression at this location provides a pulse for the examiner. (**A, C–F**) None of these vessels (external carotid, lingual, maxillary, submandibular, superficial temporal) cross the superficial surface of the body of the mandible.

5. Correct: Sigmoid dural venous sinus (D)

(**D**) Blood from the transverse dural venous sinus will next enter the sigmoid dural venous sinus. The transition occurs at the point where the transverse sinus reaches the petrous part of the temporal bone. (**A**) The transverse dural venous sinus arises from the confluence of sinuses. Blood in the transverse dural venous sinus is derived from the confluences of sinuses. (**B**) Blood from the sigmoid dural venous sinus will next enter the internal jugular vein at the

jugular foramen in the base of the skull. (**C, E**) The occipital and sigmoid dural venous sinuses join the confluence of sinuses.

Refer to the following image for answer 5:

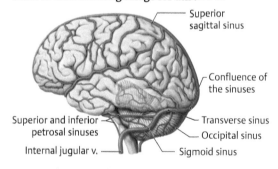

Superior sagittal sinus

Confluence of the sinuses

Superior and inferior petrosal sinuses

Internal jugular v.

Transverse sinus

Occipital sinus

Sigmoid sinus

Source: Gilroy AM et al. Atlas of Anatomy. 3rd ed. 2016. Based on: Schuenke M, Schulte E, Schumacher U. THIEME Atlas of Anatomy. Volumes 1-3. Illustrations by Voll M and Wesker K. 2nd ed. New York: Thieme Medical Publishers; 2016

6. Correct: Internal carotid artery (B)

Refer to the following image for answer 6:

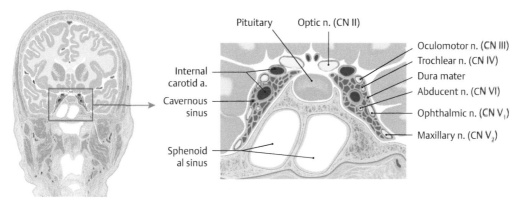

Source: Gilroy AM et al. Atlas of Anatomy. 3rd ed. 2016. Based on: Schuenke M, Schulte E, Schumacher U. THIEME Atlas of Anatomy. Volumes 1-3. Illustrations by Voll M and Wesker K. 2nd ed. New York: Thieme Medical Publishers; 2016

(**B**) The internal carotid artery (ICA) enters the cavernous dural venous sinus immediately upon entering the middle cranial fossa from the carotid canal. (**A, C–E**) As the ICA passes through the cavernous sinus, it comes to lie adjacent to the abducens nerve (CN VI), and an aneurysm at this point may lead to impairment of the lateral rectus muscle and a lateral gaze palsy (i.e., the affected eye will be adducted). The oculomotor (CN III), trochlear (CN IV), and ophthalmic (CN V1) nerves also lie nearby in the lateral wall of the sinus. None of these vessels (anterior cerebral vein, middle cerebral vein, middle meningeal artery, ophthalmic artery) are within the cavernous dural venous sinus. The ophthalmic artery is the first branch of the internal carotid artery, but this branching occurs after the internal carotid artery has exited the cavernous dural venous sinus.

7. Correct: External carotid (B)

(**B**) The superior thyroid artery is usually the first branch of the external carotid artery. (**A, C–E**) The superior thyroid artery is not a branch from any of these arteries (common carotid, internal carotid, thyrocervical trunk, vertebral).

Refer to the following image for answer 7:

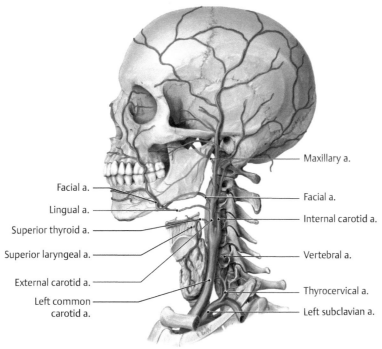

Source: Gilroy AM et al. Atlas of Anatomy. 3rd ed. 2016. Based on: Schuenke M, Schulte E, Schumacher U. THIEME Atlas of Anatomy. Volumes 1-3. Illustrations by Voll M and Wesker K. 2nd ed. New York: Thieme Medical Publishers; 2016

8. Correct: Common carotid (A)

(**A**) A pulse can be detected in the common carotid artery at the side of the cricoid cartilage (C6 vertebral level). The artery lies just deep to sternocleidomastoid muscle at this level. (**B, C**) The external and internal carotid arteries branch from the common carotid artery at the upper border of thyroid cartilage (C4 vertebral level). (**D**) The superior thyroid artery, which branches from the external carotid artery and descends to reach the thyroid gland, is relatively small and a pulse would not be detected in this vessel on palpation of the neck. (**E**) The vertebral artery is a branch of the subclavian artery. It lies deep in the root of the neck at its origin and courses cranially in the transverse foramina of the upper six cervical vertebrae. A pulse cannot be palpated in this artery.

Refer to the following image for answer 8:

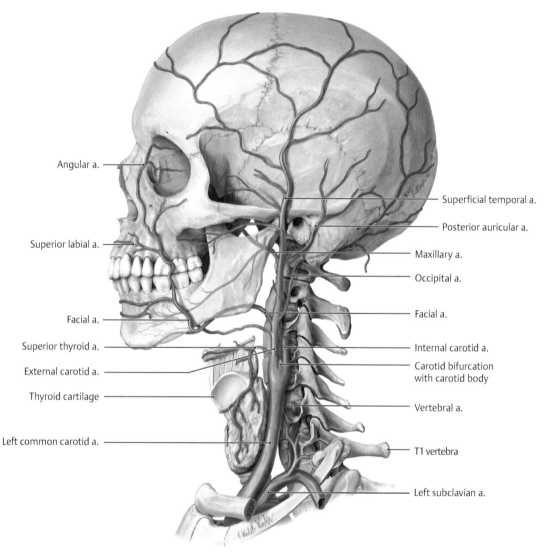

Angular a.

Superior labial a.

Facial a.

Superior thyroid a.

External carotid a.

Thyroid cartilage

Left common carotid a.

Superficial temporal a.

Posterior auricular a.

Maxillary a.

Occipital a.

Facial a.

Internal carotid a.

Carotid bifurcation with carotid body

Vertebral a.

T1 vertebra

Left subclavian a.

Source: Gilroy AM et al. Atlas of Anatomy. 3rd ed. 2016. Based on: Schuenke M, Schulte E, Schumacher U. THIEME Atlas of Anatomy. Volumes 1-3. Illustrations by Voll M and Wesker K. 2nd ed. New York: Thieme Medical Publishers; 2016

9. Correct: Posterior division of retromandibular and posterior auricular (E)

Refer to the following image for answer 9:

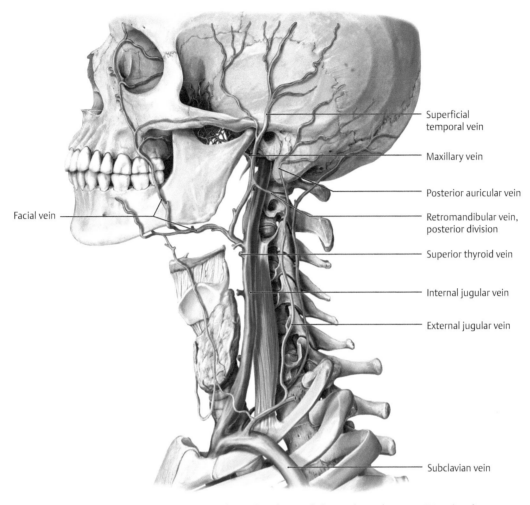

Facial vein

Superficial temporal vein

Maxillary vein

Posterior auricular vein

Retromandibular vein, posterior division

Superior thyroid vein

Internal jugular vein

External jugular vein

Subclavian vein

Source: Gilroy AM et al. Atlas of Anatomy. 3rd ed. 2016. Based on: Schuenke M, Schulte E, Schumacher U. THIEME Atlas of Anatomy. Volumes 1-3. Illustrations by Voll M and Wesker K. 2nd ed. New York: Thieme Medical Publishers; 2016

(**E**) Near the angle of the mandible the retromandibular vein splits into an anterior and posterior division. The posterior division joins the posterior auricular vein to form the external jugular vein, which is distended in this patient. The anterior division of the retromandibular vein joins the facial vein to form the common facial vein. (**A, C**) Neither of these pairs of veins (anterior division of retromandibular and facial; maxillary and facial) unite to form a common trunk. (**B**) The maxillary vein unites with the superficial temporal vein near the temporomandibular joint to form the retromandibular vein. The anterior division of the retromandibular vein joins the facial vein near the angle of the mandible to form the common facial vein. The common facial vein then joins the internal jugular vein. (**D**) The anterior division of the retromandibular vein joins the facial vein near the angle of the mandible to form the common facial vein. The common facial vein then joins the internal jugular vein.

10. Correct: Facial (C)

(**C**) The tonsillar artery, a cervical branch of the facial, is the primary source of blood for the palatine tonsil. (**A**) The deep temporal artery does not supply any blood to the palatine tonsil. (**B**) The external carotid does not give any direct branches to the palatine tonsil. (**D**) The lingual and maxillary arteries, both branches of the external carotid, have branches that provide small, variable branches to the palatine tonsil. For example, the dorsal lingual artery, a branch of the lingual artery, may distribute small branches to the palatine tonsil. (**E**) The maxillary artery does not provide any branches that supply the palatine tonsil.

11. Correct: Superior thyroid (E)

Refer to the following images for answer 11:

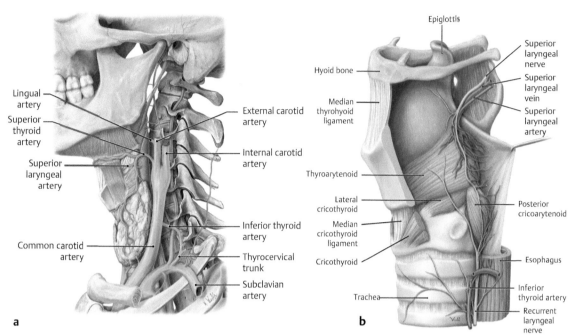

a

Source: Gilroy AM et al. Atlas of Anatomy. 3rd ed. 2016. Based on: Schuenke M, Schulte E, Schumacher U. THIEME Atlas of Anatomy. Volumes 1-3. Illustrations by Voll M and Wesker K. 2nd ed. New York: Thieme Medical Publishers; 2016

b

Source: Schuenke M, Schulte E, Schumacher U. THIEME Atlas of Anatomy. Head, Neck, and Neuroanatomy. Illustrations by Voll M and Wesker K. 2nd ed. New York: Thieme Medical Publishers; 2016

(**E**) The superior thyroid artery branches from the external carotid artery at the level of the thyrohyoid membrane and descends in the neck to distribute to the superior lobe of the thyroid gland The vessel has one major branch, the superior laryngeal, which pierces the thyrohyoid membrane with the internal laryngeal nerve. The superior thyroid artery is vulnerable during surgery in the anterior triangle of the neck. (**A, C**) The facial and lingual arteries are branches of the external carotid artery but they ascend from their point of origin to distribute in the head. (**B**) The inferior thyroid artery, a branch of the thyrocervical trunk, ascends from its origin in the root of the neck to distribute to the lower lobe of thyroid gland. (**D**) The occipital artery is a branch of the external carotid and it ascends along the posterior border of the sternocleidomastoid muscle to reach the occipital triangle.

12. Correct: Facial (B)

(**B**) The facial artery, a branch of the external carotid artery in the neck, ascends toward the mandibular margin. The artery grooves the superior surface of the submandibular gland before crossing the mandible at the anterior edge of masseter muscle to enter the face. (**A, C**) The external and internal carotid arteries lie posterior to the submandibular gland. (**D**) The lingual artery ascends medial to

the submandibular gland. (**E**) The superior thyroid artery branches from the external carotid artery inferior to the submandibular gland and descends in the neck to reach the thyroid gland.

Refer to the following image for answer 12:

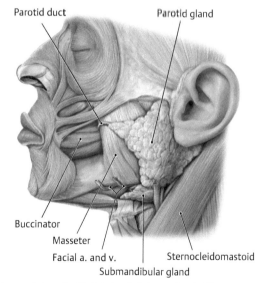

Source: Schuenke M, Schulte E, Schumacher U. THIEME Atlas of Anatomy. Head, Neck, and Neuroanatomy. Illustrations by Voll M and Wesker K. 2nd ed. New York: Thieme Medical Publishers; 2016

13. Correct: Inferior alveolar (B)

Refer to the following image for answer 13:

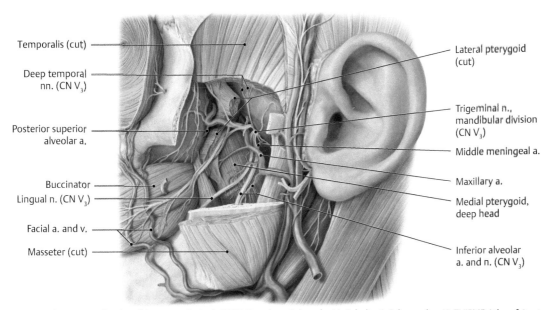

Temporalis (cut)

Deep temporal
nn. (CN V₃)

Posterior superior
alveolar a.

Buccinator

Lingual n. (CN V₃)

Facial a. and v.

Masseter (cut)

Lateral pterygoid
(cut)

Trigeminal n.,
mandibular division
(CN V₃)

Middle meningeal a.

Maxillary a.

Medial pterygoid,
deep head

Inferior alveolar
a. and n. (CN V₃)

Source: Gilroy AM et al. Atlas of Anatomy. 3rd ed. 2016. Based on: Schuenke M, Schulte E, Schumacher U. THIEME Atlas of Anatomy. Volumes 1-3. Illustrations by Voll M and Wesker K. 2nd ed. New York: Thieme Medical Publishers; 2016

(**B**) The inferior alveolar artery, a branch of the maxillary artery, accompanies the inferior alveolar nerve through the mandibular foramen to supply the mandibular teeth. (**A, C, E**) The deep temporal, masseteric, and posterior superior alveolar arteries, all branches of the maxillary artery, do not pass through the mandibular foramen to supply the mandibular teeth. (**D**) The mental artery, which branches from the inferior alveolar artery within the body of the mandible, exits the mental foramen to distribute to the skin of the chin.

14. Correct: Sphenopalatine (E)

(**E**) The dominant artery to the nasal septum is the sphenopalatine artery, a branch of the maxillary artery. The septal branch of the superior labial artery contributes to the septum near the nasal vestibule. (**A–D**) None of these vessels (descending palatine, infraorbital, maxillary, posterior lateral nasal)

distribute to the nasal septum. The sphenopalatine artery is a branch of the maxillary, but the maxillary artery does not directly supply the septum.

Refer to the following image for answer 14:

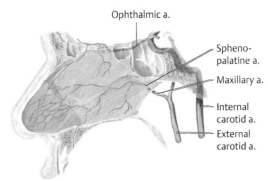

Ophthalmic a.

Spheno-
palatine a.

Maxillary a.

Internal
carotid a.

External
carotid a.

Source: Gilroy AM et al. Atlas of Anatomy. 3rd ed. 2016. Based on: Schuenke M, Schulte E, Schumacher U. THIEME Atlas of Anatomy. Volumes 1-3. Illustrations by Voll M and Wesker K. 2nd ed. New York: Thieme Medical Publishers; 2016

15. Correct: External carotid (B)

(**B**) The occipital artery distributes most of the blood to the occipital region of the scalp. It is a posterior branch of the cervical portion of the external carotid artery. (**A**) The common carotid artery usually gives no named branches prior to its bifurcation into the internal and external carotid arteries. (**C**) As its name implies, the facial artery distributes to the face with no branches reaching the scalp. (**D**) The posterior auricular artery is a posterior branch of the cervical portion of the external carotid. Most of its distribution is to the external ear and lateral side of the head, posterior to the ear. (**E**) The superficial temporal artery is a terminal branch of the external carotid with wide distribution to the lateral aspect of the scalp.

Refer to the following image for answer 15:

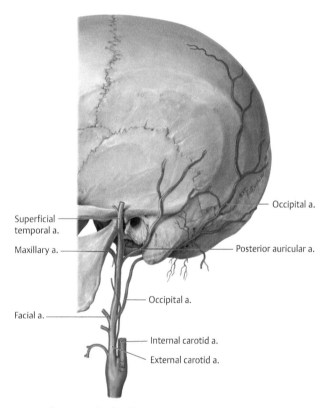

Source: Gilroy AM et al. Atlas of Anatomy. 3rd ed. 2016. Based on: Schuenke M, Schulte E, Schumacher U. THIEME Atlas of Anatomy. Volumes 1-3. Illustrations by Voll M and Wesker K. 2nd ed. New York: Thieme Medical Publishers; 2016

16. Correct: Internal carotid (C)

(**C**) The stenosis is located in the internal carotid artery near its branching from the common carotid artery. The internal carotid artery has no branches in the neck. (**A**) The common carotid artery gives rise to the internal and external carotid arteries. The stenosis is not in the common carotid. (**B**) The external carotid artery is a branch of the common carotid artery. It can be distinguished from the internal carotid artery by the presence of numerous branches in the neck. The stenosis is not in the external carotid artery. (**D**) The middle meningeal artery is a branch of the maxillary artery in the infratemporal fossa. The maxillary artery is a branch of the external carotid artery. (**E**) The ophthalmic artery is the first branch of the internal carotid artery. This does not occur until the internal carotid has entered the cranial cavity.

17. Correct: It is the first branch of the internal carotid artery (B)

(**B**) The ophthalmic artery is the first branch of the internal carotid artery, thus, increasing the likelihood that a thrombus originating in the internal carotid artery will enter the ophthalmic artery and become lodged in one of its small branches. (**A**) The ophthalmic artery branches from the internal carotid artery inside the cranial cavity. (**C**) The ophthalmic artery is usually the smallest branch of the internal carotid artery. (**D**) None of the branches of the internal carotid artery are tortuous. (**E**) The ophthalmic artery is the shortest branch of the internal carotid artery, but this is unrelated to why the embolus enters it. The embolus entered the ophthalmic artery because it is the first branch of the internal carotid artery.

18. Correct: Right coronary (E)

(**E**) The vessel with occlusion seen in the image is the right coronary artery as it lies in the atrioventricular groove. (**A–D**) None of these vessels (anterior interventricular, circumflex, left coronary, posterior interventricular) represent the occluded vessel shown in image in the question.

19. Correct: Visceral serous and parietal serous pericardium (E)

Refer to the following image for answer 19:

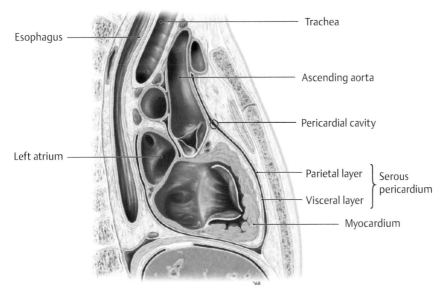

Source: Gilroy AM et al. Atlas of Anatomy. 3rd ed. 2016. Based on: Schuenke M, Schulte E, Schumacher U. THIEME Atlas of Anatomy. Volumes 1-3. Illustrations by Voll M and Wesker K. 2nd ed. New York: Thieme Medical Publishers; 2016

(E) The pericardial space (cavity), a potential space, lies between the visceral and parietal layers of the serous pericardium. (A) The parietal serous pericardium and the myocardium are not in contact. They are separated by the visceral serous pericardium and the pericardial space. (B) The visceral serous pericardium (also known as epicardium) is tightly adherent to the myocardium with no potential space separating them. (C) The parietal serous pericardium and the fibrous pericardium are tightly fused with no potential space separating them. (D) The visceral serous pericardium (also known as epicardium) and the endocardium are separated by the myocardium.

20. Correct: Patent ductus arteriosus (E)

(E) This infant has a patent ductus arteriosus. The patency extends between the arch of the aorta and the pulmonary trunk. This prenatal shunt normally closes soon after birth. (A–C) The are no anomalous vessel origins in the image in this question. (D) Coarctation of the aorta involves a narrowing (stenosis) of the aorta, usually somewhere near the ductus arteriosus. There is no evidence of aortic stenosis in the image with this question.

21. Correct: Internal thoracic (C)

(C) Over the past decade the internal thoracic (internal mammary) artery has become a common vessel used for grafts to diseased coronary arteries. In some cases, bilateral use of the internal thoracic arteries is necessary though there is risk of poor sternal wound healing. (A) The anterior intercostal arteries are too small in caliber for grafting to coronary arteries. (B) The posterior intercostal arteries are small and inaccessible for coronary grafts. (D) The pericardiacophrenic artery is a long slender branch of the internal thoracic artery and is companion to the phrenic nerve. It is too small for coronary grafts and dissecting it would put the phrenic nerve at risk. (E) The superior phrenic artery is the last branch of the thoracic aorta. It is a small artery that distributes onto the thoracic surface of the diaphragm. It is inaccessible for coronary grafts.

22. Correct: Brachiocephalic trunk (B)

(B) The right subclavian artery is normally a branch of the brachiocephalic trunk (artery). In the case of a retroesophageal (aberrant) right subclavian artery, this artery is a fourth (last) branch from the arch of the aorta, passing posterior to the esophagus to reach the right upper limb. In this case, there is no brachiocephalic trunk as the right common carotid branches directly from the arch of the aorta. This patient would be diagnosed with dysphagia lusoria—a condition in which the esophagus is compressed between the trachea anteriorly and aberrant right subclavian artery posteriorly. (A, C, D) The right subclavian artery does not normally branch from the aorta (ascending aorta, postductal arch of aorta, preductal arch of aorta). (E) The right common carotid artery and the right subclavian artery are branches of the brachiocephalic trunk.

Refer to the following image for answer 22:

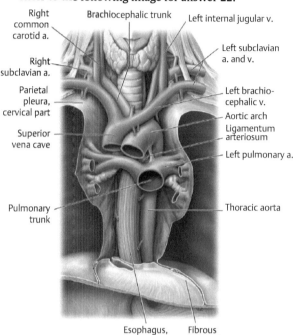

Right common carotid a.
Brachiocephalic trunk
Left internal jugular v.
Right subclavian a.
Left subclavian a. and v.
Parietal pleura, cervical part
Left brachio-cephalic v.
Aortic arch
Ligamentum arteriosum
Superior vena cave
Left pulmonary a.
Pulmonary trunk
Thoracic aorta
Esophagus, thoracic part
Fibrous pericardium

Source: Gilroy AM et al. Atlas of Anatomy. 3rd ed. 2016. Based on: Schuenke M, Schulte E, Schumacher U. THIEME Atlas of Anatomy. Volumes 1-3. Illustrations by Voll M and Wesker K. 2nd ed. New York: Thieme Medical Publishers; 2016

23. Superior vena cava (E)

(**E**) The superior vena cava is formed at the level of the right first intercostal space by the union of the right and left brachiocephalic veins. (**A, C, D**) All of these structures (azygos vein, coronary sinus, right pulmonary vein) lie inferior to the first intercostal space. (**B**) The brachiocephalic trunk divides into the right common carotid and right subclavian arteries at the thoracic outlet.

Refer to the following image for answer 23:

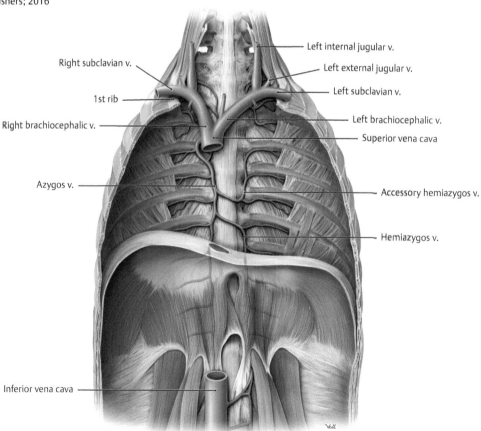

Right subclavian v.
1st rib
Right brachiocephalic v.
Azygos v.
Left internal jugular v.
Left external jugular v.
Left subclavian v.
Left brachiocephalic v.
Superior vena cava
Accessory hemiazygos v.
Hemiazygos v.
Inferior vena cava

Source: Gilroy AM et al. Atlas of Anatomy. 3rd ed. 2016. Based on: Schuenke M, Schulte E, Schumacher U. THIEME Atlas of Anatomy. Volumes 1-3. Illustrations by Voll M and Wesker K. 2nd ed. New York: Thieme Medical Publishers; 2016

24. Correct: Sternal border, right second intercostal space (E)

Refer to the following image for answer 24:

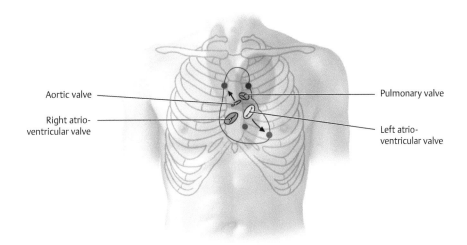

Source: Gilroy AM et al. Atlas of Anatomy. 3rd ed. 2016. Based on: Schuenke M, Schulte E, Schumacher U. THIEME Atlas of Anatomy. Volumes 1-3. Illustrations by Voll M and Wesker K. 2nd ed. New York: Thieme Medical Publishers; 2016

(**E**) The best position for auscultation of sounds related to the aortic valve is at the sternal border in the second right intercostal space. (**A**) The left atrioventricular (bicuspid or mitral) valve sound can be best heard in the left fifth intercostal space on the midclavicular line, moving toward the left axilla. (**B**) No heart valve sound will be clearly discerned on the midclavicular line of the right third intercostal space. (**C**) The left atrioventricular valve lies at the left sternal margin in the fourth intercostal space. However, the best position for auscultation of the sound produced by this valve is in the left fifth intercostal space on the midclavicular line. (**D**) The sound of the pulmonary valve can best be discerned with the stethoscope over the second intercostal space at the left sternal edge.

Refer to the following image for answers 25 and 26:

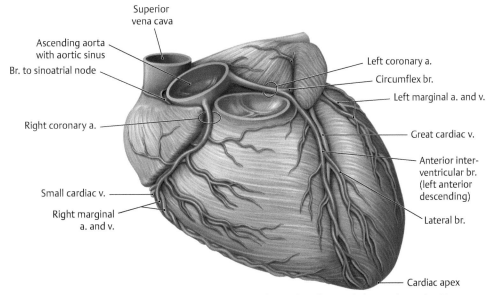

Source: Gilroy AM et al. Atlas of Anatomy. 3rd ed. 2016. Based on: Schuenke M, Schulte E, Schumacher U. THIEME Atlas of Anatomy. Volumes 1-3. Illustrations by Voll M and Wesker K. 2nd ed. New York: Thieme Medical Publishers; 2016

25. Correct: Anterior interventricular (A)

(**A**) The anterior interventricular artery (left anterior descending) branches from the left coronary artery and courses in the anterior interventricular groove toward the heart apex. (**B, C, E**) None of these vessels (circumflex, left coronary, right coronary) course onto the ventricles. Each of them lies in the atrioventricular sulcus. (**D**) The left marginal artery, a branch of the circumflex artery, courses along the left ventricular margin.

26. Correct: Great cardiac (B)

(**B**) The great cardiac vein is the companion to the anterior interventricular artery. (**A**) The coronary sinus lies in the atrioventricular sulcus, not the anterior interventricular sulcus. It receives the major veins (great, middle, and small cardiac) of the heart before emptying into the right atrium. (**C**) The middle cardiac vein accompanies the posterior interventricular artery. (**D**) The right marginal vessel is an artery. It is accompanied by the small cardiac vein. (**E**) The small cardiac vein accompanies the right marginal artery.

27. Correct: Right atrioventricular (D)

(**D**) The proper place to auscultate the sound of the right atrioventricular valve (tricuspid) is at the sternal edge in the left fifth intercostal space. (**A**) Auscultation of the aortic valve is best resolved in the right second intercostal space at the sternal edge. (**B**) Auscultation of the left atrioventricular valve is best resolved in the left fifth intercostal space on the midclavicular line. (**C**) Auscultation of the pulmonary valve is best resolved in the left second intercostal space at the sternal edge.

Refer to the following image for answer 27:

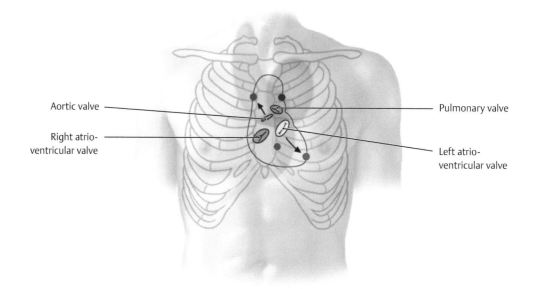

Aortic valve

Right atrio-
ventricular valve

Pulmonary valve

Left atrio-
ventricular valve

Source: Gilroy AM et al. Atlas of Anatomy. 3rd ed. 2016. Based on: Schuenke M, Schulte E, Schumacher U. THIEME Atlas of Anatomy. Volumes 1-3. Illustrations by Voll M and Wesker K. 2nd ed. New York: Thieme Medical Publishers; 2016

28. Correct: Anterior, posterior, septal (B)

Refer to the following image for answer 28:

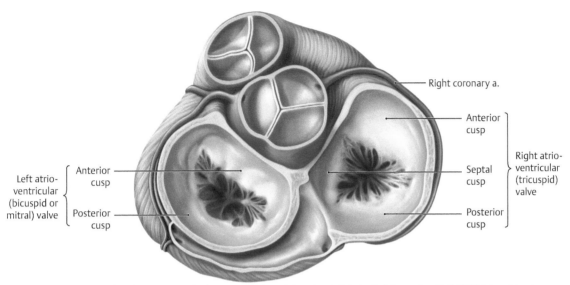

Source: Gilroy AM et al. Atlas of Anatomy. 3rd ed. 2016. Based on: Schuenke M, Schulte E, Schumacher U. THIEME Atlas of Anatomy. Volumes 1-3. Illustrations by Voll M and Wesker K. 2nd ed. New York: Thieme Medical Publishers; 2016

(**B**) The proper terms for the three cusps of the right atrioventricular valve are anterior, posterior, and septal. (**A, C–E**) None of these combinations (anterior, posterior, left; right, left, anterior; right, left, posterior; right, left, septal) are correct for naming the right atrioventricular valve cusps.

29. Correct: Membranous interventricular septal defect (A)

(**A**) The image in this question reveals leakage from the left to the right ventricle through a membranous interventricular septal defect. This defect causes oxygenated blood in the left ventricle to enter the right ventricle to be returned to the lungs. The left ventricular output into the aorta is decreased leading to symptoms of fatigue, shortness of breath, and increased heart rate. Shortness of breath is due to the increased blood flow to the lungs and the resultant pulmonary edema which compromises gas exchange. (**B**) The muscular portion of the interventricular septum is intact. (**C, D**) The defect is not in the atrial septum.

30. Correct: Coronary (B)

(**B**) The coronary arteries branch from the ascending aorta proximal to the stenosis. Increased pressure proximal to the stenosis may lead to distension of one or both coronary arteries. (**A, C–E**) All of these arteries (brachiocephalic, left common carotid, right bronchial, right subclavian) have their origin distal to the stenosis and would not be expected to show distension.

31. Correct: Increased blood flow to the lungs (B)

Refer to the following image for answer 31:

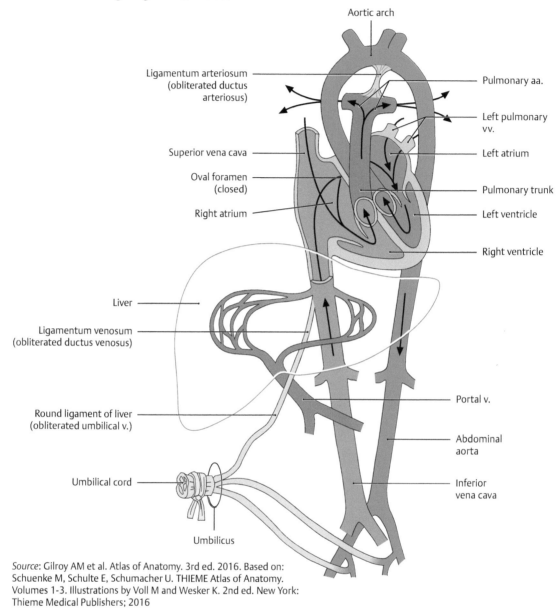

Source: Gilroy AM et al. Atlas of Anatomy. 3rd ed. 2016. Based on: Schuenke M, Schulte E, Schumacher U. THIEME Atlas of Anatomy. Volumes 1-3. Illustrations by Voll M and Wesker K. 2nd ed. New York: Thieme Medical Publishers; 2016

(**B**) Before birth, the ductus arteriosus connects the pulmonary trunk to the arch of the aorta, thereby permitting most blood ejected from the right side of the heart to bypass the lungs and enter the systemic circulation (a "right-to-left" shunt). After birth, the ductus arteriosus typically close as a result, in part, of increased pressure in the aorta, allowing the outflow from the right ventricle to enter the now functional lungs. Failure of the ductus arteriosus to close after birth, a condition termed a patent ductus arteriosus, maintains the fetal shunt but with the increased aortic pressure the shunt becomes a "left-to-right." This increased blood flow to the lungs, if not corrected, leads to pulmonary hypertension and potentially congestive heart failure and cardiac arrhythmias. (**A**) Blood flow to the lungs will not decrease, but will actually increase due to the higher pressure in the aorta, forcing an increased volume of blood into the pulmonary arteries. The pulmonary trunk will contain the right ventricular output together with the shunted blood from the aorta via the patent ductus arteriosus. (**C, E**) Both ventricles will hypertrophy as long as the patent ductus arteriosus exists. The shunting of blood out of the aorta and into the pulmonary arteries will cause the left ventricle to hypertrophy due to the increased demand to perfuse the body. The right ventricle will hypertrophy due to the overload on the pulmonary vasculature created by the patent ductus arteriosus. (**D**) The blood flow to the lungs will increase due to the added blood being shunted into the pulmonary arteries by the patent ductus arteriosus.

32. Correct: Portal (C)

(**C**) Veins of the lower esophagus drain preferentially into the portal vein via gastric veins. The veins of the lower esophagus form one of the portal–systemic anastomoses. The esophageal veins connect with both the portal system and with the systemic veins via the azygos veins. (**A**) Blood in the veins of the inferior esophagus may enter the azygos vein if the resistance to flow through the liver is increased. Normally, the veins of the lower esophagus drain into the gastric veins and then into the portal vein. (**B**) Blood in the veins of the lower esophagus do not drain directly into the hepatic veins. This blood will enter the hepatic veins only after the portal system takes the blood through the liver. (**D, E**) Blood in the lower esophageal veins does not enter the splenic or superior mesenteric veins. These two veins unite to form the portal vein.

Refer to the following image for answer 32:

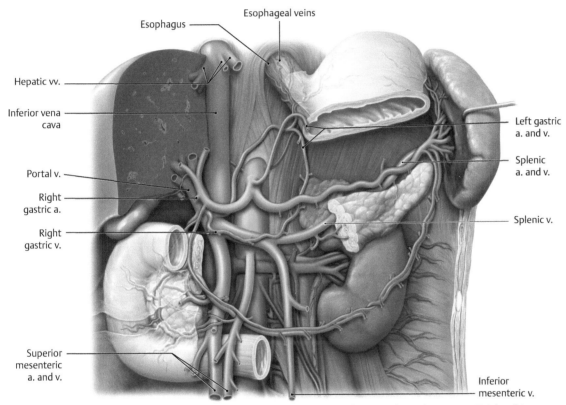

Source: Gilroy AM et al. Atlas of Anatomy. 3rd ed. 2016. Based on: Schuenke M, Schulte E, Schumacher U. THIEME Atlas of Anatomy. Volumes 1-3. Illustrations by Voll M and Wesker K. 2nd ed. New York: Thieme Medical Publishers; 2016

33. Correct: Subclavian (E)

Refer to the following image for answer 33:

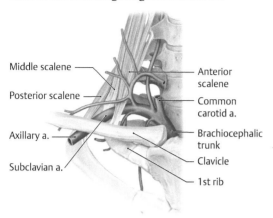

Source: Gilroy AM et al. Atlas of Anatomy. 3rd ed. 2016. Based on: Schuenke M, Schulte E, Schumacher U. THIEME Atlas of Anatomy. Volumes 1-3. Illustrations by Voll M and Wesker K. 2nd ed. New York: Thieme Medical Publishers; 2016

(**E**) The right subclavian artery exits the thoracic outlet and arches over rib 1 posterior to the anterior scalene muscle. The presence of a complete or partial rib attached to the seventh cervical vertebra (cervical rib) may (1) crimp the subclavian artery as it extends into the root of the neck to cross the aberrant rib or (2) compress the subclavian artery as it passes between rib 1 and the cervical rib. In either case, blood flow to the upper limb is compromised. (**A**) By definition, the axillary artery begins at the lateral border of rib 1 as a continuation of the subclavian artery. (**B**) By definition, the brachial artery begins at the lower border of the teres major muscle as a continuation of the axillary artery. (**C**) The brachiocephalic artery is the first branch of the arch of the aorta. It is a common trunk for the right common carotid and right subclavian arteries. The brachiocephalic artery is located entirely in the thoracic cavity. (**D**) The deep brachial artery is a branch of the brachial artery in the arm.

34. Correct: Circumflex (C)

(**C**) The *arrowhead* indicates the origin of the circumflex branch of the left coronary artery. The left coronary artery is relatively short, dividing into the circumflex and anterior interventricular (left anterior descending) arteries as it emerges between the left atrial appendage and the pulmonary trunk. The circumflex branch stays in the atrioventricular sulcus while the anterior interventricular courses in the interventricular groove. (**A, D**) The left coronary artery, as it branches from the aorta, is indicated by the *arrow* in the image. The left coronary artery divides into the circumflex and anterior interventricular arteries. (**B**) Atrial branches of the left coronary artery and its circumflex branch would be small and somewhat irregular. (**E**) The left marginal artery is usually a branch of the circumflex artery. It courses along the left margin of the left ventricle.

Refer to the following image for answer 34:

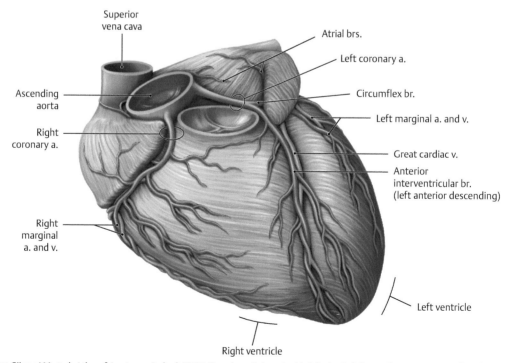

Source: Gilroy AM et al. Atlas of Anatomy. 3rd ed. 2016. Based on: Schuenke M, Schulte E, Schumacher U. THIEME Atlas of Anatomy. Volumes 1-3. Illustrations by Voll M and Wesker K. 2nd ed. New York: Thieme Medical Publishers; 2016

35. Correct: Right coronary (D)

(**D**) The structure indicated is the sinuatrial (SA) node of the cardiac conduction system. It predominantly receives its blood supply from a sinuatrial artery that branches from the right coronary artery. Less frequently, the sinuatrial artery is a branch of the circumflex artery and, in rarer cases, the SA node receives a dual arterial supply. (**A, C**) The anterior and posterior interventricular arteries do not supply nodal tissue of the conduction system. The anterior interventricular artery does supply blood to infranodal portions of the conduction system via septal branches. (**B**) The left coronary artery does not directly supply branches to nodal tissues (the left coronary artery branching from the aorta is indicated by the *arrow* in the image in this question). The left coronary artery divides into the circumflex and anterior interventricular arteries. Its circumflex branch may give branches to nodal tissue, especially in left coronary artery dominance. (**E**) The right marginal artery does not contribute to the vascularization of the conduction system.

36. Correct: Right and left pulmonary arteries (D)

(**D**) Thrombus formation is seen in the right and left pulmonary arteries (saddle thrombus). These vessels are seen as they branch from the pulmonary trunk. (**A**) The arch of the aorta and its branches are not seen in the image in this question. (**B**) The vessels seen in the image are arteries emerging from the ventricles of the heart. (**C**) The thrombus can be seen to extend into some lobar arteries, but the vessels indicated by the *arrows* are the right and left pulmonary arteries. (**E**) There are usually four pulmonary veins, two from each lung, that enter the left atrium. These vessels are not seen in this image.

37. Correct: Splenic (E)

(**E**) Blockage of venous outflow from the liver (hepatic veins) would cause increased pressure in veins bringing blood to the liver (hepatic portal system). The splenic vein could well show distension because it is a tributary to the portal vein. (**A–D**) None of these vessels (right inferior phrenic, right ovarian, right renal, right suprarenal) empty into the hepatic portal system.

Refer to the following image for answer 37:

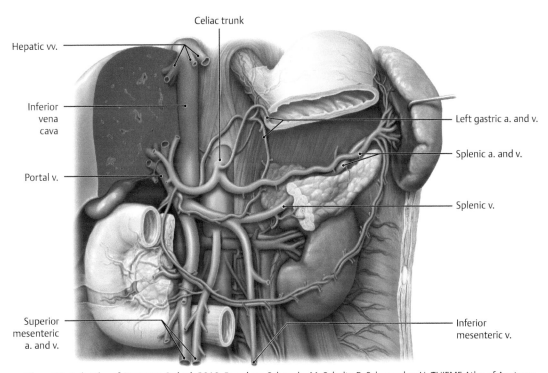

Celiac trunk

Hepatic vv.

Inferior vena cava

Portal v.

Superior mesenteric a. and v.

Left gastric a. and v.

Splenic a. and v.

Splenic v.

Inferior mesenteric v.

Source: Gilroy AM et al. Atlas of Anatomy. 3rd ed. 2016. Based on: Schuenke M, Schulte E, Schumacher U. THIEME Atlas of Anatomy. Volumes 1-3. Illustrations by Voll M and Wesker K. 2nd ed. New York: Thieme Medical Publishers; 2016

38. Correct: Ileocolic (A)

Refer to the following image for answer 38:

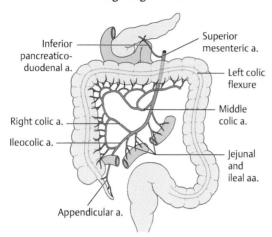

Source: Gilroy AM et al. Atlas of Anatomy. 3rd ed. 2016. Based on: Schuenke M, Schulte E, Schumacher U. THIEME Atlas of Anatomy. Volumes 1-3. Illustrations by Voll M and Wesker K. 2nd ed. New York: Thieme Medical Publishers; 2016

(**A**) The appendicular artery is a branch of the ileocolic artery. The ileocolic artery is derived from the superior mesenteric artery. (**B**) The marginal artery (of Drummond) courses along the margin of the colon. It receives contributions from the right, middle, and left colic arteries that anastomose to create an uninterrupted vessel. (**C**) The right colic artery does not give rise to the appendicular artery. The

ileocolic artery, a branch of the superior mesenteric artery, gives rise to the appendicular artery. (**D**) The right renal artery does not supply blood to the digestive tract. (**E**) The superior mesenteric artery is the parent artery for the right colic, middle colic, and ileocolic arteries.

39. Correct: Inferior epigastric (B)

(**B**) The inferior epigastric artery branches from the external iliac artery and courses superiorly and obliquely toward the midline. It creates a peritoneal ridge known as the lateral umbilical fold. At the arcuate line of the rectus sheath, the vessel enters the rectus sheath on the posterior side of rectus abdominis muscle and is a major source of blood for the muscle. Its position in the lower abdominal quadrant makes it vulnerable during interventional procedures in this area. (**A, C**) The deep and superficial circumflex iliac arteries do not cross the lower abdominal quadrant. (**D**) The superficial epigastric artery, a branch of the femoral artery, is a subcutaneous vessel. The vessel parallels the rectus abdominis muscle as it ascends toward the umbilicus. (**E**) The superior epigastric artery, a terminal branch of the internal thoracic artery, courses onto the anterior abdominal wall near the midline. It distributes to the upper rectus abdominis muscle. It does not extend into the lower abdominal quadrant.

Refer to the following image for answer 39:

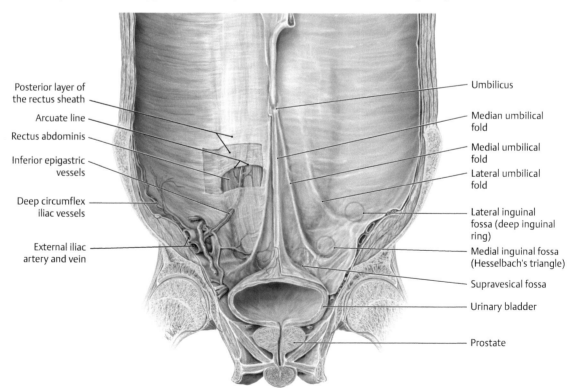

Source: Schuenke M, Schulte E, Schumacher U. THIEME Atlas of Anatomy. General Anatomy and Musculoskeletal System. Illustrations by Voll M and Wesker K. 2nd ed. New York: Thieme Medical Publishers; 2016

40. Correct: Common iliac (A)

Refer to the following image for answer 40:

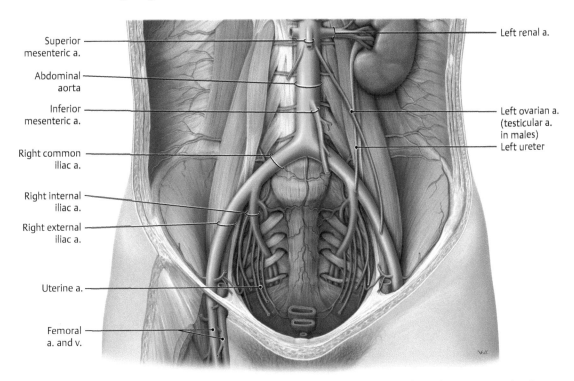

Source: Gilroy AM et al. Atlas of Anatomy. 3rd ed. 2016. Based on: Schuenke M, Schulte E, Schumacher U. THIEME Atlas of Anatomy. Volumes 1-3. Illustrations by Voll M and Wesker K. 2nd ed. New York: Thieme Medical Publishers; 2016

(**A**) The vessel indicated by the *arrow* in the question is the common iliac artery. The image shows the abdominal aorta dividing into its terminal branches, the right and left common iliac arteries. This occurs at the L4 level of the vertebral column. (**B**) The inferior mesenteric artery branches from the aorta at the L3 vertebral level. (**C**) The left colic artery is not a branch of the aorta. It branches from the inferior mesenteric artery. (**D**) The renal artery branches from the aorta at the L1 and L2 vertebral level. (**E**) The testicular artery branches from the aorta at the L2 vertebral level.

41. Correct: Left colic (B)

(**B**) The left colic artery, a branch of the inferior mesenteric artery, provides the majority of blood to the descending colon. (**A**) The ileocolic artery, a branch of the superior mesenteric artery distributes to the terminal ileum, cecum, appendix, and proximal ascending colon. (**C**) The middle colic artery, a branch of the superior mesenteric artery, is the primary blood source for the transverse colon. (**D**) The sigmoid arteries are branches of the inferior mesenteric artery. As their name implies, they distribute primarily to the sigmoid colon. (**E**) The superior rectal artery, which is the continuation of the inferior mesenteric artery into the pelvis, is a major source of blood to the rectum.

Refer to the following image for answer 41:

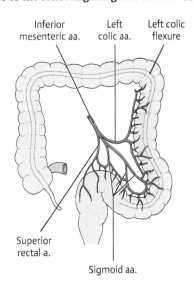

Source: Gilroy AM et al. Atlas of Anatomy. 3rd ed. 2016. Based on: Schuenke M, Schulte E, Schumacher U. THIEME Atlas of Anatomy. Volumes 1-3. Illustrations by Voll M and Wesker K. 2nd ed. New York: Thieme Medical Publishers; 2016

42. Correct: Short gastric (E)

(E) The short gastric arteries, branches of the splenic artery, supply the fundus of the stomach. (A, C) The left and right gastric arteries supply the lesser curvature of the stomach. (B, D) The left and right gastro-epiploic (gastro-omental) arteries supply the greater curvature of the stomach. These vessels also distribute to the greater omentum.

Refer to the following image for answer 42:

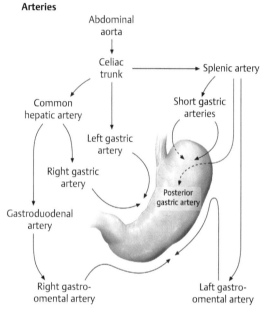

Source: Gilroy AM et al. Atlas of Anatomy. 3rd ed. 2016. Based on: Schuenke M, Schulte E, Schumacher U. THIEME Atlas of Anatomy. Volumes 1-3. Illustrations by Voll M and Wesker K. 2nd ed. New York: Thieme Medical Publishers; 2016

43. Correct: L1–L2 (A)

(A) The renal arteries branch from the abdominal aorta at the L1–L2 vertebral levels. (B) The inferior mesenteric artery branches from the aorta at the L3 vertebral level. (C) The aorta ends at the L4 vertebral level where it divides into the right and left common iliac arteries. (D) The abdominal aorta ends at the L4 vertebral level where it bifurcates into the right and left common iliac arteries. (E) The celiac artery branches from the aorta at the T12 vertebral level.

Refer to the following image for answer 43:

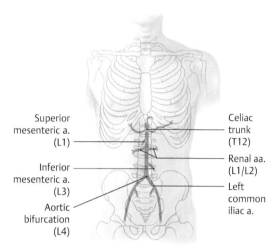

Source: Gilroy AM et al. Atlas of Anatomy. 3rd ed. 2016. Based on: Schuenke M, Schulte E, Schumacher U. THIEME Atlas of Anatomy. Volumes 1-3. Illustrations by Voll M and Wesker K. 2nd ed. New York: Thieme Medical Publishers; 2016

44. Correct: External iliac (B)

(B) The external iliac artery has been crimped and traumatized due to the position of the patient while cycling for long periods of time. This vessel is the parent for most of the blood to the lower limb. (A) The deep femoral artery is a major branch of the femoral artery. Injury to this vessel would not account for the leg and foot symptoms. (C) The internal iliac artery distributes primarily to the pelvis and perineum and injury to it would not account for the lower limb symptoms. (D) The obturator artery is a branch of the internal iliac artery and it distributes to the medial thigh. Injury to this vessel would not account for the leg and foot symptoms. (E) The popliteal artery is the continuation of the femoral artery on the popliteal aspect of the knee. Injury to this vessel would not account for the thigh symptoms.

45. Correct: Renin (E)

(E) Stenosis of a renal artery will stimulate the juxtaglomerular cells of the kidney to release renin. Renin is part of the renin–angiotensin–aldosterone hormone system that regulates plasma sodium levels and blood pressure. (A) Aldosterone is released from the adrenal cortex under stimulation from circulating angiotensin II. (B) Angiotensinogen, produced in the liver, is converted to angiotensin I by renin. (C) Angiotensin II is created from angiotensin I by angiotensin converting enzyme produced by the lungs. (D) Angiotensinogen is produced in the liver. It is converted to angiotensin I by renin.

46. Correct: Internal iliac (C)

Refer to the following image for answer 46:

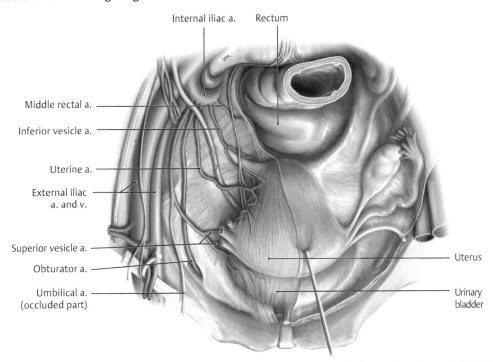

Source: Gilroy AM et al. Atlas of Anatomy. 3rd ed. 2016. Based on: Schuenke M, Schulte E, Schumacher U. THIEME Atlas of Anatomy. Volumes 1-3. Illustrations by Voll M and Wesker K. 2nd ed. New York: Thieme Medical Publishers; 2016

(**C**) The internal iliac artery (anterior division) most often gives rise to the inferior vesical artery, the vessel that was compromised in this patient. (**A**) The common iliac artery does not have any branches other than its terminal branches, the internal and external iliac arteries. (**B**) The inferior gluteal artery does not usually give rise to branches to pelvic viscera. This vessel exits the pelvis through the greater sciatic foramen to distribute to the gluteal region. (**D**) The middle rectal artery is usually a branch of the internal iliac artery. Uncommonly, this vessel may share a common trunk with the inferior vesical artery. (**E**) The obturator artery branches from the anterior division of the internal iliac artery and courses along the lateral pelvic wall to the obturator canal which transmits the vessel into the medial thigh. The obturator artery usually does not give branches to pelvic viscera.

47. Correct: Deep dorsal (A)

(**A**) The deep dorsal vein of the penis drains blood from the erectile tissues. (**B**) The external pudendal vein receives blood from the skin and subcutaneous tissues of the penis, but not the erectile tissues. (**C, D**) The inferior rectal and internal pudendal veins do not directly receive blood from the erectile tissues. Small veins of the deep dorsal vein may communicate with the internal pudendal vein in the pelvis. (**E**) The superficial dorsal vein of the penis drains the skin and subcutaneous tissues of the penis. It joins the external pudendal vein which, in turn, joins the great saphenous vein.

Refer to the following image for answer 47:

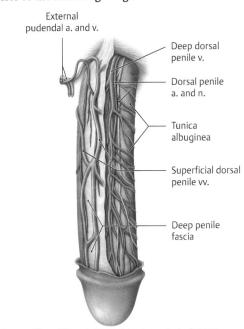

Source: Gilroy AM et al. Atlas of Anatomy. 3rd ed. 2016. Based on: Schuenke M, Schulte E, Schumacher U. THIEME Atlas of Anatomy. Volumes 1-3. Illustrations by Voll M and Wesker K. 2nd ed. New York: Thieme Medical Publishers; 2016

48. Correct: Corpus spongiosum (B)

Refer to the following image for answer 48:

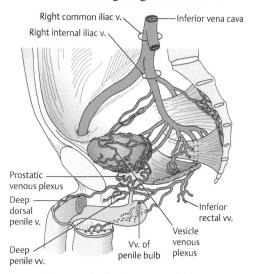

Source: Gilroy AM et al. Atlas of Anatomy. 3rd ed. 2016. Based on: Schuenke M, Schulte E, Schumacher U. THIEME Atlas of Anatomy. Volumes 1-3. Illustrations by Voll M and Wesker K. 2nd ed. New York: Thieme Medical Publishers; 2016

(**B**) The erectile tissues of the penis drain blood into the prostatic and vesical venous plexuses via the deep dorsal vein of the penis. (**A**) The abdominal part of the ureter drains venous blood primarily into the renal vein. (**C**) Venous blood from the rectum will enter the superior, middle, and inferior rectal veins. These veins are tributaries of the inferior mesenteric, internal iliac, and internal pudendal veins, respectively. None of these veins empty into the prostatic venous plexus. (**D**) Venous blood from the sigmoid colon will enter the inferior mesenteric vein via sigmoid veins. (**E**) Venous blood from the upper rectum will drain into the inferior mesenteric vein via the superior rectal vein.

49. Correct: Internal pudendal (D)

(**D**) The tissues of the urogenital triangle of the perineum receive almost all of their blood supply from the internal pudendal artery. This includes the skin, subcutaneous tissues, muscles, and erectile tissues. (**A**) The dorsal artery of the penis is a terminal branch of the internal pudendal artery. It would branch from the internal pudendal artery distal to the area of trauma in this case. (**B**) The external pudendal artery is limited in its distribution to the perineum. It supplies skin at the proximal shaft of the penis and anterior scrotum. (**C, E**) The inferior gluteal and obturator arteries do not supply blood to the perineum.

Refer to the following image for answer 49:

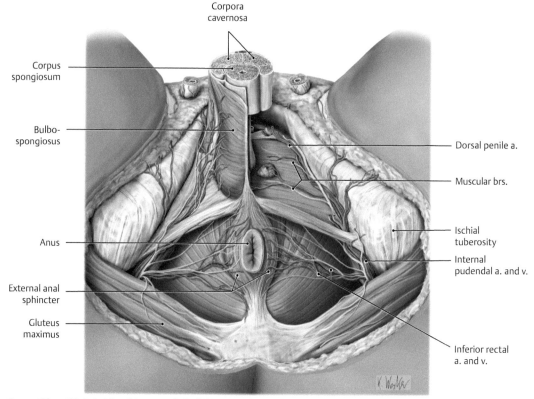

Source: Gilroy AM et al. Atlas of Anatomy. 3rd ed. 2016. Based on: Schuenke M, Schulte E, Schumacher U. THIEME Atlas of Anatomy. Volumes 1-3. Illustrations by Voll M and Wesker K. 2nd ed. New York: Thieme Medical Publishers; 2016

50. Correct: Inferior rectal (B)

Refer to the following images for answer 50:

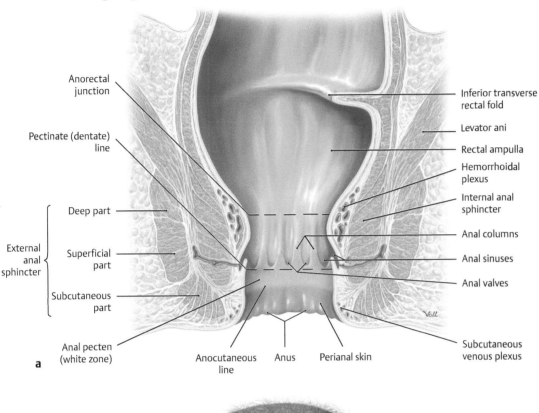

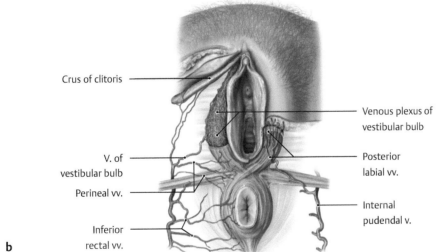

Source: Gilroy AM et al. Atlas of Anatomy. 3rd ed. 2016. Based on: Schuenke M, Schulte E, Schumacher U. THIEME Atlas of Anatomy. Volumes 1-3. Illustrations by Voll M and Wesker K. 2nd ed. New York: Thieme Medical Publishers; 2016

(**B**) This woman's symptoms are related to external hemorrhoids which involve the subcutaneous tributaries (subcutaneous venous plexus; refer to the accompanying images) of the inferior rectal vein. (**A**) The inferior gluteal vein does not receive tributaries from the perineum. (**C**) The femoral vein does not receive tributaries from the anal triangle of the perineum. (**D**) The superficial vein of the clitoris drains the skin and subcutaneous tissue of the clitoris. It empties into the femoral vein and does not receive tributaries from the anal triangle of the perineum. (**E**) The superior rectal veins drain the upper portion of the anal canal. The submucosal veins of the upper anal canal are associated with internal hemorrhoids. They do anastomose with the inferior rectal veins as one of the sites for portal–systemic venous anastomoses.

183

51. Correct: Popliteal (D)

Refer to the following image for answer 51:

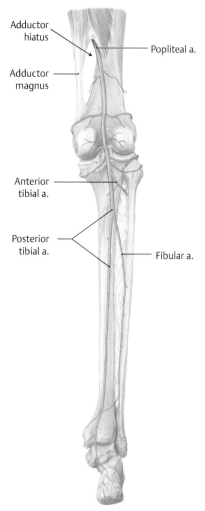

Source: Gilroy AM et al. Atlas of Anatomy. 3rd ed. 2016. Based on: Schuenke M, Schulte E, Schumacher U. THIEME Atlas of Anatomy. Volumes 1-3. Illustrations by Voll M and Wesker K. 2nd ed. New York: Thieme Medical Publishers; 2016

(**D**) The arteriograph indicates that the area of vascular entrapment is in the popliteal fossa. The major artery of this region is the popliteal, a continuation of the femoral artery. (**A, E**) The anterior and posterior tibial arteries are terminal branches of the popliteal artery. This bifurcation occurs at the inferior limit of the popliteal fossa, distal to the point of occlusion in the arteriogram. (**B**) The deep femoral artery is a branch of the femoral artery in the proximal thigh. Only small branches of the deep femoral reach the knee region. (**C**) The femoral artery changes its name to popliteal artery as the vessel passes through the adductor hiatus to enter the popliteal region on the posterior aspect of the knee. The femoral artery, by name, does not enter the popliteal region.

52. Correct: Gastrocnemius (B)

(**B**) The arteriograph indicates that the area of vascular entrapment is in the proximal portion of the popliteal fossa. The medial and lateral heads of gastrocnemius muscle have origin from the condylar (lateral head) and supracondylar (medial head) areas of the popliteal region of the femur. Hypertrophy of gastrocnemius could constrict the popliteal artery, especially during plantar flexion when the muscle contracts. (**A**) Biceps femoris crosses the posterolateral aspect of the knee joint to attach to the fibula. This muscle is not in contact with the popliteal artery. (**C**) Popliteus lies in the floor of the popliteal fossa and its hypertrophy would not entrap the popliteal artery. (**D**) Semi-membranosus crosses the posteromedial aspect of the knee joint to attach to the tibia. This muscle is not in contact with the popliteal artery. (**E**) Soleus has origin from the tibia and fibula at the inferior limit of the popliteal region. The arteriogram indicates that the entrapment is more proximal, on the distal femur.

53. Correct: Posterior tibial (E)

Refer to the following image for answer 53:

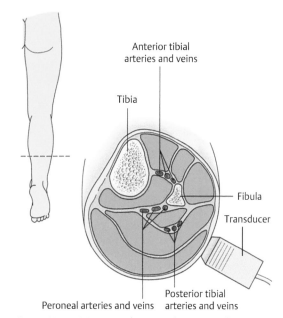

Source: Hennerici M, Neuerburg-Heusler D. Vascular Diagnosis with Ultrasound. 2nd Revised Edition. Stuttgart: Thieme; 2005.

(**E**) The posterior tibial artery in the posterior myofascial compartment of the leg (as it approaches the ankle) will best be appreciated with the transducer in the position shown in the image in the question. (**A**) The anterior tibial artery distributes to the anterior myofascial compartment of the leg and would not be visualized by sonography with the transducer in the position shown. (**B**) The dorsal artery of the foot is the continuation of the anterior tibial artery at the ankle joint. (**C, D**) The lateral and medial plantar arteries are terminal branches of the posterior tibial artery. This occurs on the medial side of the ankle joint.

54. Correct: Lateral circumflex femoral (C)

(**C**) The lateral circumflex femoral artery branches from the deep femoral artery near its origin. The lateral circumflex femoral artery is an important vessel in collateral circulation at the hip joint, being part of the cruciate anastomosis (inferior gluteal, medial circumflex femoral, first perforating, and lateral circumflex femoral). (**A**) The deep circumflex iliac artery is a branch of the external iliac artery. (**B**) The external pudendal artery is a branch of the femoral artery. (**D**) The obturator artery is a branch of the internal iliac artery. (**E**) The perforating arteries (usually four) are branches of the deep femoral artery. They immediately pierce the adductor longus and adductor magnus muscles to reach the muscles of the posterior thigh (hamstrings).

Refer to the following image for answer 54:

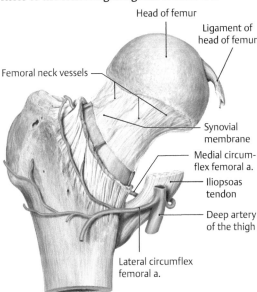

Source: Gilroy AM et al. Atlas of Anatomy. 3rd ed. 2016. Based on: Schuenke M, Schulte E, Schumacher U. THIEME Atlas of Anatomy. Volumes 1-3. Illustrations by Voll M and Wesker K. 2nd ed. New York: Thieme Medical Publishers; 2016

55. Correct: Internal pudendal (B)

Refer to the following image and table for answer 55:

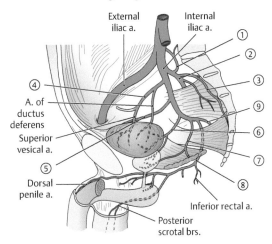

Source: Gilroy AM et al. Atlas of Anatomy. 3rd ed. 2016. Based on: Schuenke M, Schulte E, Schumacher U. THIEME Atlas of Anatomy. Volumes 1-3. Illustrations by Voll M and Wesker K. 2nd ed. New York: Thieme Medical Publishers; 2016

The internal iliac artery gives off five parietal (pelvic wall) and four visceral (pelvic organs) branches. *Parietal branches are shown in italics.		
Branches		
1	*Iliolumbar a.*	
2	*Superior gluteal a.*	
3	*Lateral sacral a.*	
4	Umbilical a.	A. of ductus deferens
		Superior vesical a.
5	*Obturator a.*	
6	Inferior vesical a.	
7	Middle rectal a.	
8	Internal pudendal a.	Inferior rectal a.
		Dorsal penile a.
		Posterior scrotal aa.
9	*Inferior gluteal a.*	

*In the female pelvis, the uterine and vaginal arteries arise directly from the anterior division of the internal iliac artery.

Source: Gilroy AM, Macpherson BR. Atlas of Anatomy. 3rd Edition. New York, NY: Thieme Medical Publishers; 2016.

(**B**) The internal pudendal artery is represented by the number "3" in the arteriogram. It branches from the internal iliac within the pelvis, exiting the pelvis with the superior and inferior gluteal arteries, and then distributing to the perineum. **(A)** The inferior gluteal artery is represented by the number "2" in this arteriogram. It can be seen to exit the pelvis with the superior gluteal and internal pudendal arteries and then distributing to the lower gluteal region. **(C)** The obturator artery is indicated by the *arrow* in this arteriogram. It exits the pelvis via the obturator canal to distribute to the medial thigh. **(D)** The superior gluteal artery is represented by the number "1" in this arteriogram. It can be seen exiting the pelvis with the inferior gluteal and internal pudendal arteries and then distributing to the upper gluteal region. **(E)** The superior vesical artery is a branch of the patent portion of the umbilical artery. It is not clearly appreciated in this arteriogram.

56. Correct: Obturator (C)

(C) The obturator artery is the primary source of blood for this structure, the obturator externus muscle. **(A)** The external iliac artery does not supply any direct branches to obturator externus muscle. **(B)** The internal iliac artery does not supply muscular branches to obturator externus muscle. The obturator artery, which supplies obturator externus muscle, is a branch of the internal iliac artery. **(D)** The lateral circumflex femoral artery does not provide any muscular branches to obturator externus muscle. **(E)** The deep circumflex iliac artery does not supply any muscular branches to the obturator externus muscle.

57. Correct: Anterior tibial (A)

Refer to the following image for answer 57:

(A) Chronic exertional compartment syndrome involves structures of the anterior compartment of the leg. Structures in this compartment are tightly bound by crural fascia and the shaft of the tibia. The anterior tibial vein is the major vein of this compartment. Its deep position renders it vulnerable to compression in cases of edema and swelling of muscles in the compartment. The vein is usually double (concomitant veins). **(B, E)** These are subcutaneous veins (great and small saphenous) and would not be affected directly in compartment syndrome. They do communicate with deep veins and may eventually show some distension. **(C)** The popliteal vein is formed in the knee region with the union of anterior and posterior tibial veins. Its course in the leg is very short. **(D)** The posterior tibial vein is resident to the deep posterior compartment of the leg.

58. Correct: Femoral (A)

(A) The femoral artery is the major artery found in the midportion of the medial thigh. It lies in the adductor canal (subsartorial canal; Hunter's canal) with its companion vein, the saphenous nerve, and the nerve to the vastus medialis muscle. Some authors consider the femoral artery to end at the branch point of the deep artery of the thigh (profunda femoris) and the continuing vessel is termed the superficial (common) femoral artery. **(B, C)** The perforating arteries branch from the deep artery of the thigh (profunda femoris) in the proximal thigh and would not be present in the midthigh. **(D)** The obturator artery branches from the internal iliac and distributes to the medial (adductor) muscles of the thigh. At the midthigh, it is typically present as a series of small muscular branches. **(E)** The popliteal artery represents the continuation

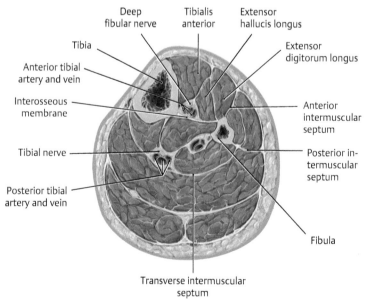

Deep fibular nerve / Tibialis anterior / Extensor hallucis longus / Extensor digitorum longus / Tibia / Anterior tibial artery and vein / Interosseous membrane / Anterior intermuscular septum / Tibial nerve / Posterior intermuscular septum / Posterior tibial artery and vein / Fibula / Transverse intermuscular septum

Source: Gilroy AM et al. Atlas of Anatomy. 3rd ed. 2016. Based on: Schuenke M, Schulte E, Schumacher U. THIEME Atlas of Anatomy. Volumes 1-3. Illustrations by Voll M and Wesker K. 2nd ed. New York: Thieme Medical Publishers; 2016

of the femoral artery in the distal thigh. The femoral artery becomes popliteal as it enters the popliteal region of the posterior knee.

Refer to the following image for answer 58:

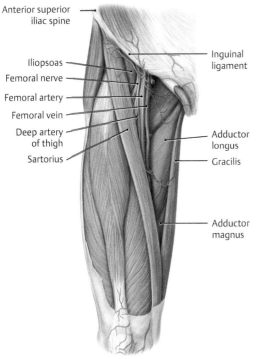

Source: Gilroy AM et al. Atlas of Anatomy. 3rd ed. 2016. Based on: Schuenke M, Schulte E, Schumacher U. THIEME Atlas of Anatomy. Volumes 1-3. Illustrations by Voll M and Wesker K. 2nd ed. New York: Thieme Medical Publishers; 2016

59. Correct: Musculophrenic and pericardiacophrenic (B)

(**B**) The pericardiacophrenic and musculophrenic arteries are both branches of the internal thoracic artery and supply the superior aspect of the diaphragm. Surgeons often refer to the left internal thoracic artery as the left internal mammary artery. (**A**) Neither the anterior nor posterior intercostal arteries supply the diaphragm, although the anterior intercostal is a branch of the internal thoracic. (**C**) The musculophrenic artery is a branch of the internal thoracic artery that supplies the diaphragm, but the superior phrenic is a branch of the thoracic aorta. (**D**) While both the pericardiacophrenic and superior phrenic arteries supply the diaphragm, only the pericardiacophrenic is a branch of the internal thoracic artery (the superior phrenic arises from the thoracic aorta). (**E**) The superior phrenic, which does supply the diaphragm, is not a branch of the internal thoracic artery.

Refer to the following image for answer 59:

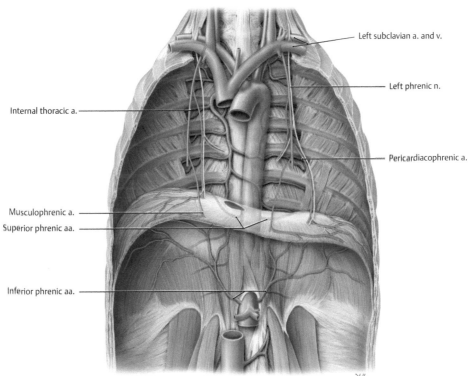

Source: Schuenke M, Schulte E, Schumacher U. THIEME Atlas of Anatomy. General Anatomy and Musculoskeletal System. Illustrations by Voll M and Wesker K. 2nd ed. New York: Thieme Medical Publishers; 2016

187

Chapter 4

Respiratory System

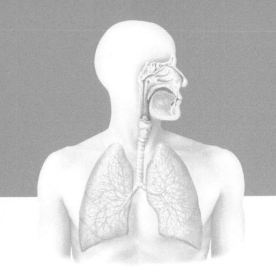

ANATOMICAL LEARNING OBJECTIVES

▶ Describe the anatomy of the thoracic wall, including its skeletal components, muscles, fascial layers, neurovasculature, and its clinically significant anatomical relationships and surface landmarks.

▶ Describe the anatomy of the diaphragm, including its attachments, actions, and neurovasculature.

▶ Describe the anatomy of the superior mediastinum, including its contents and anatomical relationships.

▶ Describe the anatomy of the larynx and tracheobronchial tree, including their characteristic features, neurovasculature, anatomical relationships, and surface landmarks.

▶ Describe the anatomy of the lungs and pleurae, including their innervation, anatomical relationships, and surface landmarks.

▶ Describe the mechanics of breathing, including the role of respiratory muscles and changes in pleural cavity pressure changes.

▶ Describe the anatomy of the nasal cavity and paranasal sinuses, including their characteristic features, neurovasculature, and anatomical relationships.

▶ Describe the anatomy of the oral cavity, including its boundaries, neurovasculature, and anatomical relationships.

▶ Describe the anatomy of the pharynx, its skeletal components, neurovasculature, and anatomical relationships.

▶ Describe the anatomy of the innervation of the respiratory system, including contributions from the phrenic nerve, cranial nerves, and the autonomic nervous system, including their origin, course, and distribution.

▶ Recognize normal and pathological anatomy in standard diagnostic imaging of the upper and lower respiratory tracts.

4.1 Questions

Easy	Medium	Hard

1. A 38-year-old woman presents to the emergency department with chest pain, dyspnea (shortness of breath), and hemoptysis (coughing up blood). The patient, a professional soccer player, recalls taking a hard blow to the back of her right knee. She is diagnosed with a pulmonary embolism secondary to a deep vein thrombosis. In which of the following blood vessels is the thromboembolus most likely to have initially lodged?

A. Arch of aorta

B. Azygos vein

C. Bronchial vein

D. Pulmonary artery

E. Pulmonary vein

2. A 5-year-old girl with an intermittent dry cough of 5-day duration is brought by her parents to the family physician. Although significant respiratory distress is not evident, physical examination reveals reduced ventilation and percussion dullness on the right side of the chest. A chest radiograph reveals increased density consistent with atelectasis (lobar collapse). She is immediately scheduled for bronchoscopy, during which a cherry pit is extracted from her airway. The foreign body was most likely lodged in which of the following airway locations?

A. Carina

B. Left main bronchus

C. Pharyngeal recess

D. Right main bronchus

E. Right superior lobe bronchus

3. A 55-year-old man is admitted to the hospital with a fever, generalized weakness, poor appetite, and a productive cough. Physical examination reveals heart and respiratory rates at the high end of normal, and gingivitis with dental caries. Radiological examination shows consolidation in one of the lung lobes that, combined with infection of the oral cavity, is indicative of aspiration pneumonia. Which lung lobe would most likely be involved in this patient?

A. Left inferior lobe

B. Left superior lobe

C. Right inferior lobe

D. Right middle lobe

E. Right superior lobe

4. A 43-year-old woman with dyspnea (shortness of breath) and right shoulder pain of 6-month duration visits her primary care physician. Physical examination reveals shoulder movement and sensation are normal and no soft-tissue injury. A chest radiograph reveals elevation of the right hemidiaphragm and CT imaging shows an anterior mediastinal mass compressing the anterior aspect of the root of the right lung (refer to the *asterisks* in the accompanying image). A thymic carcinoma is confirmed by CT-guided biopsy. Which of the following structures is most likely affected in this patient to account for the shoulder pain?

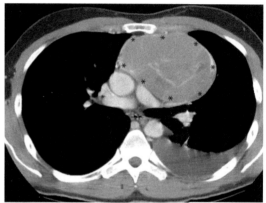

Source: Restrepo C, Zangan S. RadCases. Thoracic Imaging. 1st Edition. Thieme; 2010.

A. Phrenic nerve

B. Suprascapular nerve

C. Sympathetic trunk

D. Thoracic duct

E. Vagus nerve

5. A 43-year-old woman with a chronic cough and chest pain visits her primary care physician. Her history reveals she had a cold 6 weeks earlier and it "had gone to her chest." At the time, she was diagnosed with pneumonia. Physical examination reveals she now has severe, sharp chest pain on the right when breathing deeply or coughing, but that the pain subsides when she holds her breath. Auscultation of her lungs reveals a friction rub (rough, scratching sound) with inspiration and expiration, a classic finding of pleurisy. To reduce the pain, her physician could anesthetize which of the following nerves?

A. Greater splanchnic

B. Intercostal

C. Phrenic

D. Pulmonary plexus

E. Vagus

Consider the following case for questions 6 and 7:

A 32-year-old woman is admitted to the emergency department with a stab wound to the left side of her chest. She is tachycardic (heart rate is elevated), tachypnic (respiratory rate is elevated), hypotensive (arterial pressure is abnormally low), and experiences a sharp pain on the left side of her chest and increasing difficulty in breathing. Lung auscultation reveals absent breath sounds, percussion hyperresonance on the left, and hissing of air through the chest wall with inspiration, but not expiration. Radiographic examination shows widened intercostal spaces on the left (refer to the *arrow* in the accompanying image) and tracheal and mediastinal shift toward the right.

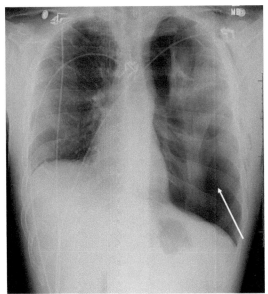

Source: Restrepo C, Zangan S. RadCases. Thoracic Imaging. 1st Edition. Thieme; 2010.

6. Which of the following is the best diagnosis for this patient's condition?

A. Emphysema
B. Hemothorax
C. Open pneumothorax
D. Pleural effusion
E. Tension pneumothorax

7. Emergent needle decompression is used in this patient to allow the air to escape and reduce the intrapleural pressure. Which of the following is the best location to insert the needle?

A. Second intercostal space in the midaxillary line
B. Second intercostal space in the midclavicular line
C. Fifth intercostal space at the left sternal border
D. Seventh intercostal space in the midaxillary line
E. Ninth intercostal space in the midaxillary line

Consider the following case for questions 8 and 9:

A 53-year-old woman is admitted to the hospital with a fever, a productive cough, dyspnea (shortness of breath), and general fatigue. Physical examination reveals decreased breath sounds on the right. Laboratory tests demonstrate an elevated white blood cell count and radiological examination (accompanying images show AP and lateral chest radiographs) indicates consolidation characteristic of pneumonia.

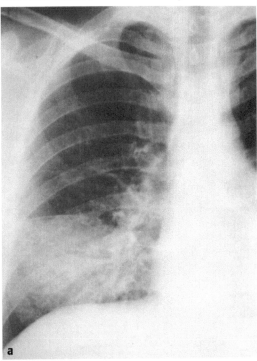

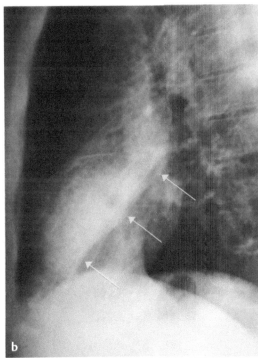

Source: Lange S, Walsh G. Radiology of Chest Diseases. 3rd Edition. Thieme; 2006.

191

8. Which lung lobe is involved in the pneumonia in this patient?

A. Left inferior

B. Left superior

C. Right inferior

D. Right middle

E. Right superior

9. Which fissure is indicated by the *arrows* in image b?

A. Horizontal (minor) fissure of the left lung

B. Horizontal (minor) fissure of the right lung

C. Oblique (major) fissure of the left lung

D. Oblique (major) fissure of the right lung

10. A 78-year-old man with stage IV lung cancer is admitted to the hospital with progressive dyspnea (shortness of breath) over 2 weeks. After completing four cycles of chemotherapy, he develops a right pleural effusion. Thoracentesis is performed to remove the exudate and produce partial relief of the dyspnea. To remove fluid from the pleural cavity while the patient is seated, into which of the following locations would the physician most likely insert the needle?

A. 4th intercostal space at the midaxillary line, along the superior border of the rib 5

B. 6th intercostal space at the midclavicular line, along the inferior border of the rib 6

C. 6th intercostal space at the midclavicular line, along the superior border of the rib 7

D. 8th intercostal space in the midclavicular line, along the superior border of the rib 9

E. 8th intercostal space along the scapular line, at the superior border of the rib 9

11. A 75-year-old woman presents to the emergency department following a head-on motor vehicle accident. Physical examination reveals bruising on her right thorax and severe pain on the right side with breathing. Radiological imaging shows multiple rib fractures along the right midclavicular line. A right intercostal nerve block is administered to relieve the patient's chest pain. At which of the following locations should the needle be inserted?

A. At the angle of the rib, along the inferior border of each rib

B. At the angle of the rib, along the superior border of each rib

C. At the middle of each affected intercostal space

D. In the intercostal space along the sternal border

E. Posteriorly, in the transversospinal muscles of the affected levels

Consider the following case for questions 12 and 13:

A 48-year-old man presents to the clinic with a cough, progressive right shoulder and arm pain and weakness. A history reveals the patient is a long-time, heavy smoker and that the pain started about three months ago. Physical examination shows pain, numbness, and tingling in his right medial forearm and hand, including his ring and little fingers. Radiological imaging shows a large right apical lung tumor (refer to the accompanying image).

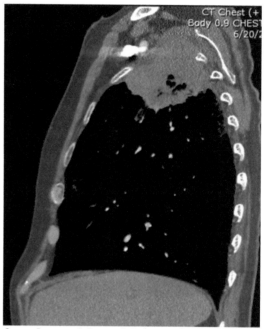

Source: Restrepo C, Zangan S. RadCases. Thoracic Imaging. 1st Edition. Thieme; 2010.

12. Involvement of which of the following structures would likely cause the upper extremity symptoms?

A. Inferior trunk of brachial plexus

B. Medial cutaneous nerve of the forearm

C. Musculocutaneous nerve

D. T1 ventral ramus

E. Ulnar nerve

13. Which of the following additional conditions would most likely be seen in this patient?

A. Erb's palsy

B. Horner's syndrome

C. Pneumonia

D. Retropharyngeal abscess

E. Rotator cuff weakness

14. A 29-year-old man undergoes thoracic surgery and receives a right subclavian venous catheter. Within minutes after removing the catheter, the patient experiences dyspnea (shortness of breath) and sharp, pleuritic pain on right side. A chest tube is introduced and approximately 1.3 L of blood is drained from the right pleural cavity. Which of the following structures is most likely injured by the catheter to cause the hemothorax?

A. Arch of azygos vein

B. Left atrium

C. Right atrium

D. Right brachiocephalic vein

E. Right internal jugular vein

15. A 63-year-old man who is a smoker with a chronic cough presents to a pulmonologist. A chest radiograph reveals a right upper lobe lung mass adjacent and just superior to the hilum of the right lung. CT imaging shows the mass obstructs the right upper lobe bronchus (refer to the *arrow* in the accompanying image). A biopsy is positive for small cell lung carcinoma. Which of the following vessels is most likely compressed by this tumor?

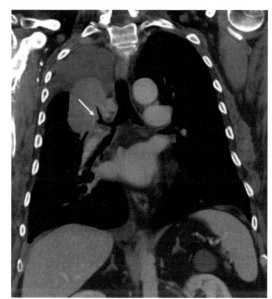

Source: Restrepo C, Zangan S. RadCases. Thoracic Imaging. 1st Edition. Thieme; 2010.

A. Descending aorta

B. Inferior vena cava

C. Right common carotid artery

D. Right subclavian vein

E. Superior vena cava

16. A 58-year-old man with an early diagnosis of lung cancer is brought to surgery for a lingular segmentectomy. Which of the following bronchopulmonary segments would be removed in this patient?

A. Segments I–III

B. Segments I–V

C. Segments IV–V

D. Segments VII–X

17. A 65-year-old woman, who is a long-time heavy smoker and now has shoulder pain, visits her family physician. A patient history reveals she experiences constant, severe left shoulder pain that is exacerbated by walking, sitting, and turning in bed. Physical examination reveals grip weakness and loss of dexterity in her left hand. The patient exhibits a cough, dyspnea (shortness of breath), hoarseness, and a weak voice. CT imaging reveals a mass posterior to the root of the left lung. Which of the following nerves is most likely affected in this patient to account for her respiratory symptoms?

A. Left recurrent laryngeal

B. Phrenic

C. Right recurrent laryngeal

D. T1 ventral ramus

E. Vagus

18. A 44-year-old man involved in a motor vehicle collision is brought to the emergency department with dyspnea (shortness of breath). Physical examination reveals a widening hematoma extending across ribs 4 to 7 from the midclavicular to the midaxillary line on the right. A chest radiograph shows rib fractures at these levels. Bleeding into the pleural cavity is not evident. The trauma team determines that the blood is extravasating immediately superficial to the parietal pleura. In which of the following layers is the blood most likely accumulating?

A. Between external and internal intercostal muscles

B. Between internal intercostal and innermost intercostal muscles

C. Deep to the periosteum of the ribs

D. In the endothoracic fascia layer

E. In the subcutaneous tissue layer

19. A 35-year-old man visits his otolaryngologist following a total thyroidectomy. The patient has developed a hoarse voice. Based on indirect laryngoscopy as shown in the image (viewed from above), which of the following nerves is most likely affected?

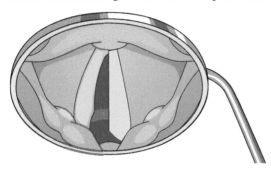

A. Left recurrent laryngeal
B. Right recurrent laryngeal
C. Superior laryngeal, external branch
D. Superior laryngeal, internal branch
E. Vagus

20. A 37-year-old man with hoarseness, sore throat, a dry cough, and a weak voice presents to his primary care physician. A patient history reveals that he works in a dairy factory with a milk-packing machine that emits formaldehyde. Indirect laryngoscopy shows inflammation of the laryngeal vestibule. He is diagnosed with occupational laryngitis. Which of the following nerves provides somatic sensory innervation from the inflamed area?

A. Glossopharyngeal
B. Recurrent laryngeal
C. Superior laryngeal, external branch
D. Superior laryngeal, internal branch
E. Vagus

Consider the following case for questions 21 and 22:

A 65-year-old woman is brought to the emergency department with a swollen tongue after eating shellfish. She exhibits stridor (high pitched breath sounds) and significant dyspnea (shortness of breath) and there is concern that the swelling is progressing into the larynx. The patient is treated for an allergic reaction with epinephrine, methylprednisone, and diphenhydramine, but a lack of improvement necessitates an emergency cricothyrotomy.

21. Which of the following airway spaces does a cannula first enter during a cricothyrotomy?

A. Infraglottic cavity
B. Laryngeal ventricle
C. Laryngeal vestibule
D. Piriform fossa
E. Trachea

22. If a tracheotomy were to be performed in this patient, which of the following structures would be most vulnerable?

A. Inferior thyroid artery
B. Inferior thyroid veins
C. Parathyroid glands
D. Right brachiocephalic vein
E. Superior thyroid artery

23. A 7-year-old girl with a runny nose, nasal congestion, dry cough, and a low grade fever is brought to the pediatrician. During physical examination of the nasal cavity, the physician tilts the patient's head posteriorly and examines the nasal cavity with the aid of an otoscope. Which of the following structures would most likely be seen first through the nostrils (nares)?

A. Choana
B. Inferior nasal concha
C. Middle nasal concha
D. Superior nasal concha
E. Torus tubarius

24. A 43-year-old man presents with nasal obstruction, hyposmia (reduced ability to smell), and rhinorrhea ("runny nose"). CT imaging reveals several nasal opacifications that are consistent with thickened mucosa. Which of the following space(s) is occupied by the mass indicated by the number "4" in the axial CT (refer to the accompanying image)?

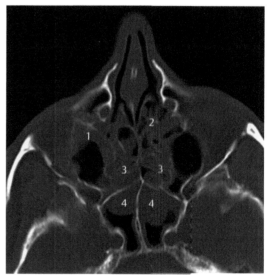

Source: Dunnebier E, Beek E, Pameijer F, Imaging for Otolaryngologists. 1st Edition. Thieme; 2011.

A. Maxillary sinus
B. Nasal cavity
C. Nasopharynx
D. Posterior ethmoidal air cells
E. Sphenoidal sinus

25. A 34-year-old woman visits the primary care clinic with fever (100.4°F/ 38°C), purulent (pus-containing) nasal discharge, and a frontal headache. Her history reveals she has been recovering from an upper respiratory tract infection, but has experienced her current symptoms for about a week. Rhinoscopic examination shows blockage of the frontonasal duct. Which of the following nerves transmits the pain from the affected paranasal sinus?

A. Auriculotemporal

B. Facial

C. Ophthalmic

D. Mandibular

E. Maxillary

26. A 43-year-old man visits his dentist three days after installation of a dental implant to replace his right upper second molar. Physical examination reveals he is in considerable pain in the region of his right zygoma and in the right temporal region. Rhinoscopy shows a purulent (pus-containing) nasal discharge emanating from the lateral wall of the right nasal cavity. Which location in the nasal cavity is most likely the source of the discharge?

A. Choana

B. Inferior nasal meatus

C. Middle nasal meatus

D. Spheno-ethmoidal recess

E. Superior nasal meatus

27. A 34-year-old woman presents to the emergency department after waking up in the middle of the night with blood on her pillow, and a continuous flow of blood from her left nostril. The patient reports a recent sinus infection that she treated with an antihistamine nasal spray. Which arteries contribute to the vascular bed most likely affected in this patient?

A. Ascending pharyngeal, facial, and maxillary

B. Ascending pharyngeal, lingual, and ophthalmic

C. Facial, great auricular, and lingual

D. Facial, maxillary, and ophthalmic

E. Inferior alveolar, maxillary, and ophthalmic

28. A 22-year-old man is admitted to the emergency department following a street fight. Physical and radiological examinations reveal a blowout fracture of the right orbit that involves the orbital plate (lamina papyracea) of the ethmoid bone. Which area on the right side of the nose is most likely to have sensory deficits?

A. External naris (nostril)

B. Inferior meatus

C. Middle meatus

D. Olfactory mucosa

E. Skin over the nasal bones

29. A 42-year-old farm worker presents with dyspnea (shortness of breath), a sore throat, and a cough with purulent (pus-containing) sputum for the last 12 days. He reports he had a cold that got worse. Physical examination reveals pharyngeal inflammation and pain on the right side of his chest when he coughs. Laboratory tests reveal a group A streptococcal infection. Which of the following nerves stimulate the bronchial muscle contractions during this patient's cough?

A. Intercostal

B. Pericardiacophrenic

C. Recurrent laryngeal

D. T3–T5 postganglionic sympathetics

E. Vagus

30. A 55-year-old woman, who is a life-long smoker, presents with a persistent cough, dyspnea (shortness of breath), and right shoulder pain of 3-month duration. Radiological studies show a 3 × 4 cm mass adjacent to the visceral surface of the right superior lung lobe. CT guided-transthoracic needle biopsy confirms a diagnosis of non-small cell lung adenocarcinoma. Which of the following lymph nodes would cells from this tumor most likely enter first if the tumor metastasized through the lymphatics?

A. Bronchopulmonary (hilar)

B. Inferior tracheobronchial (carinal)

C. Intrapulmonary

D. Paratracheal

E. Superior tracheobronchial

Consider the following case for questions 31 and 32

A 28-year-old woman with an acute asthma attack visits the family medicine clinic. She reports she becomes breathless after relatively mild physical activity (e.g., walking). Physical examination shows that the patient has a cough, labored breathing, and a wheezing that is notable at the end of expiration. During the initial physical examination, the surface projection for the tracheal bifurcation is identified.

31. Which of the following anatomical landmarks would be used to localize the position of the feature identified during the physical examination?

A. Manubrium

B. Jugular (suprasternal) notch

C. Sternal angle (of Louis)

D. Superior thoracic aperture

E. Xiphoid process

32. In the accompanying chest radiograph of the patient, which of the following structures is indicated by the *arrows?*

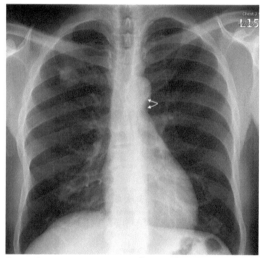

Source: Restrepo C, Zangan S, RadCases. Thoracic Imaging. 1st Edition. Thieme; 2010.

A. Aortopulmonary window

B. Mitral valve

C. Second costal cartilage

D. Superior vena cava

E. Trachea

33. A 43-year-old woman presents with dyspnea (shortness of breath) on exertion. A chest radiograph shows a mass in the aortopulmonary window (refer to the *arrow* in the X-ray below). The mass was surgically removed and a postoperative chest radiograph is shown below. Which of the following structures was most likely compressed by the mass?

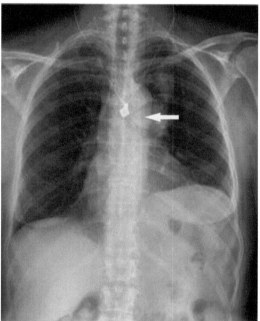

Source: Gunderman R. Essential Radiology. Clinical Presentation, Pathophysiology, Imaging. 2nd Edition. Thieme; 2000.

A. Left phrenic nerve

B. Left pulmonary artery

C. Left recurrent laryngeal nerve

D. Right phrenic nerve

E. Right pulmonary artery

34. A 58-year-old man visits his primary care physician for an annual checkup. During the physical examination, the physician places her stethoscope bell over the seventh intercostal space along the medial (vertebral) border of the right scapula. Which of the following structures is the physician auscultating at this position?

A. Right atrium

B. Right inferior lung lobe

C. Right middle lung lobe

D. Right superior lung lobe

E. Right ventricle

Consider the following case for questions 35 and 36:

A 27-year-old woman with cystic fibrosis presents with persistent dyspnea (difficulty breathing). Her history reveals exertional dyspnea associated with vague chest discomfort, and repeated lung infections. She also reports she has a productive, persistent cough that produces thick mucus (sputum). Physical examination reveals wheezing and inflamed nasal passages. Radiological imaging demonstrates cylindrical bronchiectasis (dilation and destruction of larger bronchi) and airway wall thickening (refer to the accompanying image).

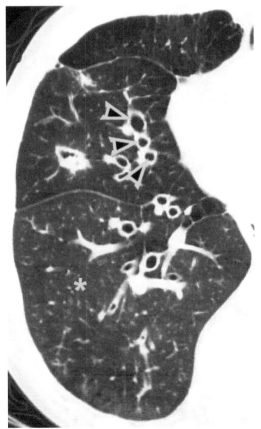

Source: Parker M, Rosado-de-Christenson M, Abbott G. Chest Imaging Case Atlas. 2nd Edition. Thieme; 2012.

35. Which of the following lung lobes is indicated by the *asterisk*?

A. Left inferior lobe

B. Left superior lobe

C. Right inferior lobe

D. Right middle lobe

E. Right superior lobe

36. Which level of the tracheobronchial tree is indicated by the *arrowheads*?

A. Alveolus

B. Lobar bronchus

C. Main bronchus

D. Segmental bronchus

E. Terminal bronchiole

37. A 28-year-old man is admitted to the emergency department with chest trauma on the left and respiratory distress (shallow, rapid breathing) following a motorcycle collision. Physical examination shows the patient is experiencing severe chest pain with inhalation or exhalation, together with paradoxical chest movements. A chest radiograph shows multiple bilateral rib fractures (refer to the accompanying image). The patient is diagnosed with flail chest. Which of the following best describes the paradoxical movements of the thoracic wall in this patient?

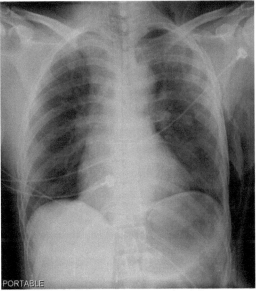

Source: Tisnado J, Ivatury R. Interventional Radiology in Trauma Management. 1st Edition. Thieme; 2015.

A. The "bucket handle" movements are lacking on the affected side

B. The flail segment moves inward with inhalation

C. The flail segment moves outward with inhalation

D. The "pump handle" movements are lacking on the affected side

38. A 15-year-old boy with a history of idiopathic pulmonary hemorrhage presents to the emergency department with acute hemoptysis (blood in sputum from the airway hemorrhage) and dyspnea (shortness of breath). An axial CT demonstrates opacities that appear acinar (refer to the *yellow arrows* in the accompanying image). Which of the following is the most proximal level of the bronchial tree that is directly connected to the acini?

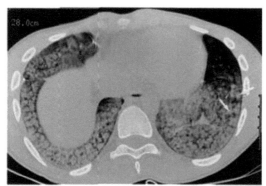

Source: Gunderman R. Essential Radiology. Clinical Presentation, Pathophysiology, Imaging. 2nd Edition. Thieme; 2000.

A. Conducting bronchiole

B. Respiratory bronchiole

C. Small tertiary bronchus

D. Terminal bronchiole

39. A 14-year-old boy with difficulty breathing through his nose is brought to his pediatrician. A patient history indicates he has had progressive dyspnea (shortness of breath). A sagittal CT is obtained to assess his upper air passages (refer to the accompanying image). Which of the following best describes the position of the mass (indicated by the "M" in the image)?

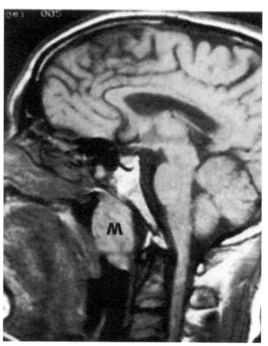

Source: Valvassori G, Mafee M, Becker M. Imaging of the Head and Neck. 2nd edition. Stuttgart: Thieme; 2004.

A. Choanae

B. Nasopharynx

C. Oropharynx

D. Sphenoidal sinus

E. Oral cavity

40. A 38-year-old woman presents with fever of 39 degrees C (102.2 degrees F) and cough. Pleuritic pain is noted upon physical examination. A frontal chest radiograph shows a mass in the lateral aspect of the left lung base and CT imaging (refer to the accompanying image) is used to further localize the mass. In which of the following locations is the portion of the mass indicated by the *asterisk* located?

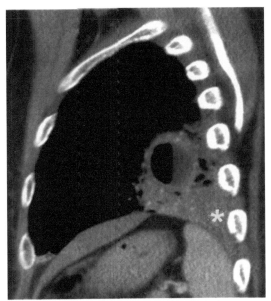

Source: Gunderman R. Essential Radiology. Clinical Presentation, Pathophysiology, Imaging. 3rd Edition. Thieme; 2014.

A. Anterior mediastinum

B. Costodiaphragmatic recess

C. Costomediastinal recess

D. Middle mediastinum

E. Superior mediastinum

41. Shortly after birth a male enters respiratory distress and requires positive pressure ventilation. Physical examination reveals a scaphoid (sunken and hollow) abdomen. A chest radiograph is ordered and the neonate is immediately admitted to the Newborn Intensive Care Unit as the radiograph (refer to the accompanying image) demonstrates a lack of bowel in the abdomen and multiple air-filled loops of bowel in the left hemithorax, consistent with a congenital diaphragmatic hernia (CDH). Which of the following is most consistent with this congenital defect?

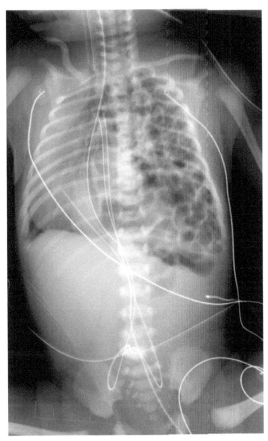

A. Can result in death from lung hypoplasia

B. Is due to failure of neural crest cells to differentiate

C. Is due to failure of the pleuropericardial folds to fuse appropriately

D. Is due to failure of the respiratory diverticulum to branch appropriately

E. More frequently occurs on the right

42. A 45-year-old woman with recurrent pneumonia presents to her primary care physician. Chest radiographs show a dense pulmonary mass in the lower left chest (refer to image a) and an angiogram (refer to image b) shows hypertrophied nonbronchial systemic arteries (*arrows*) supplying the mass. A diagnosis of pulmonary sequestration is indicated. The developmental basis for this diagnosis is abnormal development of which of the following structures?

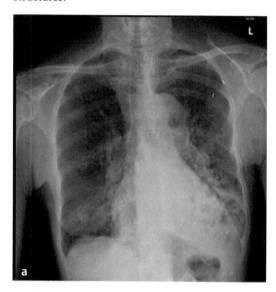

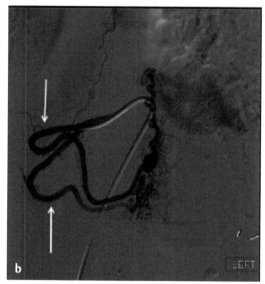

Source: Restrepo C, Zangan S. RadCases Plus Q&A Thoracic Imaging. 2nd Edition. Thieme; 2018

A. Diverticula from the foregut

B. Pleuropericardial membranes

C. Pleuroperitoneal membranes

D. Septum transversum

E. Tracheoesophageal septum

43. A male is delivered at 30 weeks' gestation because of preterm labor. Immediately after delivery, the infant is cyanotic and requires continuous positive airway pressure. He presents with subcostal retractions, grunting, and nasal flaring. Auscultation reveals decreased air entry to the lungs. A chest radiograph reveals a diffuse, ground glass appearance in the lungs, and a diagnosis of respiratory distress syndrome of the newborn (hyaline membrane disease) is made. The diagnosed condition in this infant is most likely due to inadequate development of which of the following structures?

A. Alveolar septa

B. Diaphragm

C. Tracheoesophageal septum

D. Type I pneumocytes

E. Type II pneumocytes

44. At approximately 10 hours postnatally, a cesarean-delivered male infant coughs and chokes on feeding. Physical examination reveals lung crackles on auscultation and increased oral secretions. The obstetrical resident meets resistance when attempting to place a nasogastric tube and an X-ray with contrast reveals a tracheoesophageal fistula. The epithelial lining of the structures that developed abnormally in this infant are derived from which of the following?

A. Endoderm

B. Mesenchyme

C. Neural crest

D. Somatic mesoderm

E. Splanchnic mesoderm

45. A 3-day-old boy is brought to the pediatric clinic with dyspnea (difficulty breathing) and feeding difficulties. He presents with coughing and choking. His mother says he spits up milk immediately after beginning to breastfeed. A chest radiograph reveals he has the most common type of tracheoesophageal fistula. Failure of which of the following accounts for the condition found in this patient?

A. Canalization of the larynx

B. Formation of septum secundum

C. Fusion of the tracheoesophageal ridges

D. Regression of the thyroglossal duct

E. Rupture of the buccopharyngeal membrane

4.2 Answers and Explanations

Easy	Medium	Hard

1. Correct: Pulmonary artery (D)

(**D**) A deep vein thromboembolus, in this case from the lower extremity, travels to the heart most directly via the inferior vena cava and, subsequently, enters the lungs via the pulmonary arteries. (**A**) Since the thromboembolus most likely originated in the popliteal vein, it would have traveled through the venous system. Since it was lodged in the lung, it would not have reached the left heart to enter the arterial system. (**B**) The azygos vein, a tributary of the superior vena cava, would not be a pathway for the thromboembolus since it does not drain the lower extremity. (**C**) Bronchial veins drain into the accessory azygos or superior intercostal veins (left side) or hemiazygos vein (right side). (**E**) Pulmonary veins, which carry oxygen-rich blood from the lungs to the heart, would not be the initial pathway of the thromboembolus from the lower extremity to the lungs.

2. Correct: Right main bronchus (D)

Refer to the following image for answer 2:

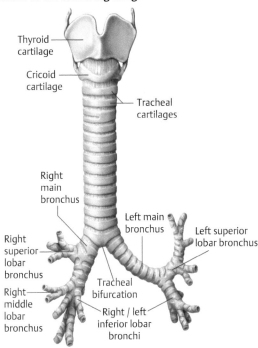

Thyroid cartilage
Cricoid cartilage
Tracheal cartilages
Right main bronchus
Left main bronchus
Left superior lobar bronchus
Right superior lobar bronchus
Right middle lobar bronchus
Tracheal bifurcation
Right / left inferior lobar bronchi

Source: Schuenke M, Schulte E, Schumacher U. THIEME Atlas of Anatomy. Internal Organs. Illustrations by Voll M and Wesker K. 2nd ed. New York: Thieme Medical Publishers; 2016

(**D**) An aspirated foreign body is more likely to lodge in the right main bronchus because is wider and takes a more vertical path than the left as it diverges from the trachea. (**A**) The carina is a ridge on the internal aspect of the airway at the tracheal bifurcation and it is unlikely that an aspirated foreign body will lodge in this location. (**B**) An aspirated foreign body is less likely to lodge in the left main bronchus because it is narrower and takes a more horizontal path than the right. (**C**) The pharyngeal recesses (fossae of Rosenmüller) are bilateral posterolateral extensions of the nasopharynx located between the torus tubarius and salpingopharyngeal fold anteriorly and the pharyngeal wall posteriorly. Their location in the nasopharynx makes it an unlikely location for an aspirated foreign body to lodge. (**E**) Because the right superior lobe bronchus is significantly narrower than the right main bronchus, and is directed superiorly, aspirated foreign bodies are less likely to lodge in this location (assuming the patient aspirated the foreign body while in an upright position).

3. Correct: Right inferior lobe (C)

(**C**) Aspiration pneumonia occurs when food, drink, emesis (vomit), or saliva enters the lungs. The inferior lobe of the right lung is more likely to be involved because the right main bronchus is wider and more vertical than the left, providing a more direct path to the right lung, with gravity favoring passage of the aspirated fluid into the inferior lobe. (**A, B, D, E**) None of these lobes (left inferior, left superior, right middle, right superior) represent the most common location for aspiration pneumonia. The most common site for aspiration pneumonia is the right inferior lobe. In the supine individual, the aspirate may also enter the superior lobes.

4. Correct: Phrenic nerve (A)

(**A**) The thymic tumor shown in the CT image lies anterior to the root of the right lung, where the right phrenic nerve courses inferiorly toward the diaphragm. This resulted in paralysis of the right side of the diaphragm (elevated right hemidiaphragm) and dyspnea. Referred pain from compression of the phrenic nerve (C3–C5) would be sensed from the neck and shoulder dermatomes, which are also supplied by the C3–C5 spinal cord levels. (**B–E**) None of these structures (suprascapular nerve, sympathetic trunk, thoracic duct, and vagus nerve) are located anterior to the root of the lung and, therefore, would not be compressed by the tumor. In addition, involvement of these structures would not result in the dyspnea or pain experienced by the patient.

5. Correct: Intercostal (B)

(**B**) Pleuritic (sharp) chest pain when breathing reflects inflammation of the parietal pleura and the friction rub is caused by the inflamed pleural surfaces as they rub against each other. The parietal pleura is innervated by somatic nerves: intercostal nerves supply costal, peripheral diaphragmatic, and cervical pleurae, whereas the phrenic nerves supply central diaphragmatic and mediastinal pleura.

Because the patient experiences chest pain but not shoulder and neck pain, the intercostal nerves should be targeted. (**C**) While the phrenic nerve does supply sensory innervation to mediastinal and central diaphragmatic pleura, it is not appropriate to perform a nerve block because it would impair the motor function of the diaphragm. (**A, D, E**) The greater splanchnic and vagus nerves, and the pulmonary plexus, do not innervate pleura.

6. Correct: Tension pneumothorax (E)

(**E**) Hissing of air through the chest wall with inspiration, (but not expiration), percussion resonance, and widening of intercostal spaces are all consistent with air entering the pleural cavity on inhalation, but not leaving with exhalation. The minimal lung sounds indicate the lung is not ventilating. Since the volume of air in the affected pleural cavity is building with each breath, the mediastinum is forced to the contralateral side because intrapleural pressure is less than on the affected side (refer to the accompanying image). A consequence of the mediastinal shift is compression of the inferior and superior venae cavae, obstructing venous return. These are all characteristic symptoms of a tension pneumothorax, where a one-way flap of pleura, intercostal muscle, and/or skin prevents air from leaving the pleural cavity with exhalation. (**A**) Emphysema damages the elastic tissue of the lungs and leads to dyspnea. (**C**) An open pneumothorax results from traumatic injury that leaves a wound in the thoracic wall through which air can flow during both inspiration and expiration and, consequently, the intrapleural pressure equals atmospheric pressure. As a result, the mediastinum would shift toward the normal side during inspiration and return to midline (i.e., back toward the pneumothorax) during expiration. (**B, D**) Both a hemothorax and a pleural effusion involve fluid in the pleural space.

Refer to the following image for answer 6:

7. Correct: Second intercostal space in the midclavicular line (B)

(**B**) For an emergency decompression and reduced risk of injury to other structures, the needle is best inserted in the second intercostal space in the midclavicular line. In most patients, this location tends to have less subcutaneous tissue. (**A**) The second intercostal space in the midaxillary line is not easily accessible because it is within the axilla. (**C**) Needle insertion in the fifth intercostal space at the left sternal border may penetrate the pericardial sac. (**D**) Needle insertion in the seventh intercostal space in the midaxillary line may injure the stomach, colon, or diaphragm in the case of an unrecognized diaphragmatic hernia. (**E**) Needle insertion in the ninth intercostal space in the midaxillary line may injure the spleen or stomach.

8. Correct: Right middle (D)

(**D**) The pneumonia is shown in the middle lobe of the right lung

9. Correct: Oblique (major) fissure of the right lung (D)

(**D**) The radiographs show pneumonia in the right lung. The sharp, superior boundary of the horizontal (minor) fissure is visible in image A and a well-defined, posterior boundary of the oblique (major) fissure is visible in image b. (**A, C**) The right lung has both horizontal (minor) and oblique (major) fissures. The left lung, in contrast, has only a single, oblique fissure, that is, it does not have a horizontal fissure. (**B**) The horizontal (minor) fissure in the right lung is shown in image b.

10. Correct: 8th intercostal space along the scapular line, at the superior border of rib 9 (E)

(**E**) The basic anatomical principle underlying selection of a location for inserting a thoracentesis needle is to identify the region of the pleural cavity into which the pleural effusate would collect, and also avoid injury to

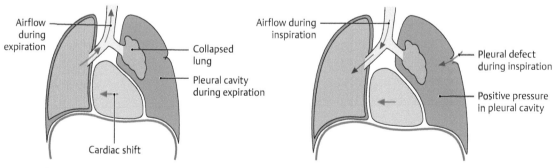

Airflow during expiration — Collapsed lung — Pleural cavity during expiration — Cardiac shift — Airflow during inspiration — Pleural defect during inspiration — Positive pressure in pleural cavity

Source: Schuenke M, Schulte E, Schumacher U. THIEME Atlas of Anatomy. Internal Organs. Illustrations by Voll M and Wesker K. 2nd ed. New York: Thieme Medical Publishers; 2016

the lung and other surrounding organs. Since the costodiaphragmatic recess is most inferior posteriorly, this is usually the most appropriate location to target for this procedure. Therefore, the needle for thoracentesis should be inserted in the eighth intercostal space along the scapular line (i.e., the vertical line through the inferior angle of the scapula) and along the superior edge of the rib that forms the lower border of the space (i.e., the ninth rib). This position is generally inferior to the scapula, which usually overlies ribs 2 to 7, but sufficiently superior to avoid accidental puncture of the liver, spleen, diaphragm, and descending aorta. Insertion of a needle or chest tube along the superior border of a rib avoids injury to the intercostal nerve and vessels, which course along the inferior rib border. (A) Insertion into the fourth intercostal space along the midaxillary line would not be selected because the lung at this position, even in the presence of a pleural effusion, would more likely be adjacent to the parietal pleura. (B, C) The sixth intercostal space at the midclavicular line would not be selected because the costodiaphragmatic recess is more superior anteriorly and is, therefore, not well suited for the procedure. Insertion of a needle or chest tube along the inferior border of a rib would be more likely to injure the intercostal nerve and vessels, which pass along the inferior rib border. (D) The eighth intercostal space is generally not present at the midclavicular line.

Refer to the following image for answer 10:

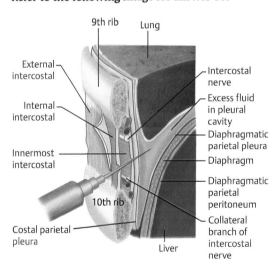

9th rib — Lung

External intercostal

Internal intercostal

Innermost intercostal

10th rib

Costal parietal pleura

Liver

Intercostal nerve

Excess fluid in pleural cavity

Diaphragmatic parietal pleura

Diaphragm

Diaphragmatic parietal peritoneum

Collateral branch of intercostal nerve

---

11. Correct: At the angle of the rib, along the inferior border of each rib (A)

(A) The intercostal nerves, which represent the ventral rami of the T1 to T11 spinal nerves, course within costal grooves along the inferior border of each rib. Smaller, collateral branches also course along the superior border of each rib. An effective intercostal nerve block requires injections to anesthetize both branches. Since the patient had rib fractures along the midclavicular line, it is necessary to provide anesthetic to both the lateral and anterior branches of the intercostal nerves. Application of anesthetic posterior to the midaxillary line will ensure analgesia to both the lateral and anterior cutaneous branches of each intercostal nerve. (B, C) Injection of anesthetic along the superior border of a rib or to the middle of an intercostal space will not direct anesthetic most effectively to the intercostal nerve as it passes through the costal groove. (D) Injection of anesthetic in the intercostal space along the sternal border will affect the anterior cutaneous branch of the intercostal nerve, but not the lateral that branches from the intercostal nerve near the midaxillary line. (E) Injection into the transversospinal muscle group will deliver anesthetic to branches of posterior (dorsal) rami, but not to the intercostal nerve that is formed by a thoracic ventral ramus.

Refer to the following images for answer 11:

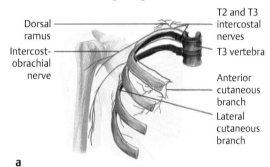

Dorsal ramus

Intercostobrachial nerve

T2 and T3 intercostal nerves

T3 vertebra

Anterior cutaneous branch

Lateral cutaneous branch

a

Source: Schuenke M, Schulte E, Schumacher U. THIEME Atlas of Anatomy. Internal Organs. Illustrations by Voll M and Wesker K. 2nd ed. New York: Thieme Medical Publishers; 2016

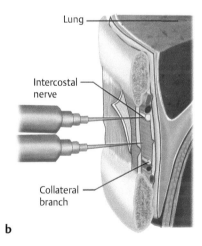

Lung

Intercostal nerve

Collateral branch

b

---

12. Correct: Inferior trunk of brachial plexus (A)

(A) The patient's symptoms of pain, numbness, and tingling in his right medial forearm and hand, including his ring and little fingers, indicate involvement of the C8 and T1 dermatomes. The C8 dermatome, which includes the medial hand and ring and little fingers, is supplied by the ulnar nerve; the distal part of the T1 dermatome includes the medial forearm and is supplied by the medial cutaneous nerve of the forearm. In this patient, the tumor is likely compressing the C8 and T1 brachial plexus roots (ventral rami), thereby affecting the inferior trunk of the brachial plexus, the single structure that contains both C8 and T1 fibers. (**B**) The skin of the medial forearm is supplied by the medial cutaneous nerve of the forearm, which carries T1 fibers. It does not convey C8 fibers. (**C**) The musculocutaneous nerve (C5–C7) supplies muscles of the anterior arm. Fibers from the C6 dorsal root ganglion, which are conveyed to the lateral forearm in the lateral cutaneous nerve of the forearm, are not affected in this patient. (**D**) The medial forearm, the distal part of the T1 dermatome, is supplied by the medial cutaneous nerve of the forearm. Since the symptoms from the medial hand and fingers point to the additional involvement of the C8 ventral ramus, an isolated compression of the T1 dermatome cannot account for the total deficits in this patient. (**E**) The ulnar nerve is involved indirectly in this patient since it conveys C8 sensory fibers from the medial hand and the ring and little fingers (i.e., the C8 dermatome).

13. Correct: Horner's syndrome (B)

(**B**) The sympathetic chain, which passes through the superior thoracic aperture, would also likely be compressed by the apical lung tumor in this patient and lead to the classic signs of a Horner's syndrome due to a reduction or lack of sympathetic innervation on the side of the tumor: anisocoria (i.e., miosis of the affected eye compared to the unaffected eye), ptosis (drooping upper eyelid) and sometimes reverse ptosis (slight elevation of the lower eyelid), and facial erythematosis (flushing) and anhidrosis. (**A**) An Erb's palsy affects the upper part of the brachial plexus,

which is not likely to be compressed by the tumor in this patient. (**C**) Pneumonia is caused by a lung infection is not likely to cause the symptoms in this patient. (**D**) A retropharyngeal abscess is typically caused by a bacterial infection in the potential space between the prevertebral and buccopharyngeal fasciae. It would be unlikely to cause the symptoms in this patient. (**E**) Rotator cuff weakness would result from injury to upper brachial plexus nerves, that is, the C5 and C6 ventral rami, and this is not seen in the symptoms in this patient.

14. Correct: Right brachiocephalic vein (D)

(**D**) Hemothorax, as well as pneumothorax and chylothorax, are possible complications of subclavian venous catheterization. The most likely vessel injured to cause a hemothorax as a result of subclavian catheterization is the right brachiocephalic vein. A catheter advanced along the venous path through the right subclavian vein toward the heart (right atrium) may puncture the right brachiocephalic vein and adjacent cervical pleura, creating a hemothorax. (**A**) The arch of the azygos vein is not along the venous path from the right subclavian vein to the heart (right atrium). (**B**) The left atrium is not along the venous path from the right subclavian vein to the heart (right atrium). (**C**) The right atrium lies within the pericardial sac, this and its thick walls, make it unlikely to be punctured and contribute to the hemothorax. (**E**) The right internal jugular vein is not along the venous path from the right subclavian vein to the heart and, therefore, is unlikely to contribute to the hemothorax.

Refer to the following image for answer 14:

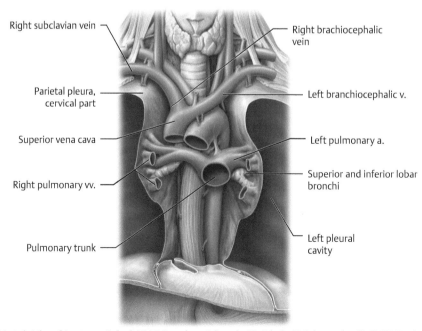

Right subclavian vein

Right brachiocephalic vein

Parietal pleura, cervical part

Left branchiocephalic v.

Superior vena cava

Left pulmonary a.

Right pulmonary vv.

Superior and inferior lobar bronchi

Pulmonary trunk

Left pleural cavity

Source: Gilroy AM et al. Atlas of Anatomy. 3rd ed. 2016. Based on: Schuenke M, Schulte E, Schumacher U. THIEME Atlas of Anatomy. Volumes 1-3. Illustrations by Voll M and Wesker K. 2nd ed. New York: Thieme Medical Publishers; 2016

15.   Superior vena cava (E)

(**E**) At the root of the right lung, the superior vena cava lies anterior to the right main bronchus and pulmonary artery, anterior and slightly to the right of the trachea, and to the right of the ascending aorta. The superior vena cava is a relatively thin-walled, low pressure vessel that can easily be compressed.

(**A–D**) None of these structures (inferior vena cava, right common carotid artery, right subclavian vein, superior vena cava) are adjacent to the hilum of the right lung and would not be compressed by a tumor in this location.

Refer to the following image for answer 15:

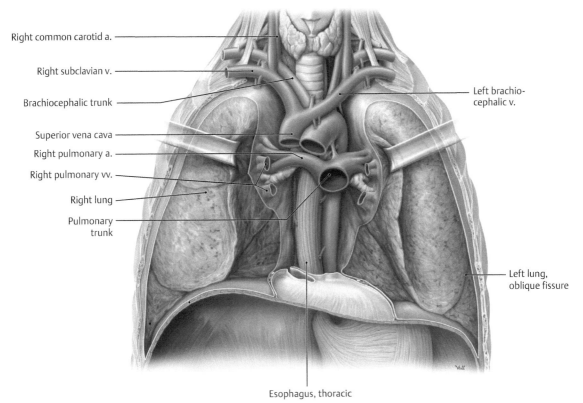

Right common carotid a.
Right subclavian v.
Brachiocephalic trunk
Superior vena cava
Right pulmonary a.
Right pulmonary vv.
Right lung
Pulmonary trunk

Left brachio-cephalic v.

Left lung, oblique fissure

Esophagus, thoracic

Source: Gilroy AM et al. Atlas of Anatomy. 3rd ed. 2016. Based on: Schuenke M, Schulte E, Schumacher U. THIEME Atlas of Anatomy. Volumes 1-3. Illustrations by Voll M and Wesker K. 2nd ed. New York: Thieme Medical Publishers; 2016

16.   Correct: Segments IV–V (C)

Refer to the following image for answer 16:

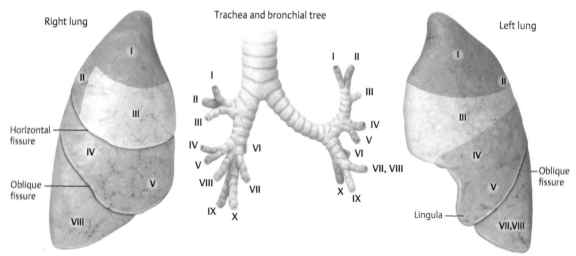

Source: Gilroy AM et al. Atlas of Anatomy. 3rd ed. 2016. Based on: Schuenke M, Schulte E, Schumacher U. THIEME Atlas of Anatomy. Volumes 1-3. Illustrations by Voll M and Wesker K. 2nd ed. New York: Thieme Medical Publishers; 2016

(**C**) Bronchopulmonary segments IV–V are associated with the lingula (see the accompanying image). The lingular portion of the left superior lobe corresponds embryologically to the middle lobe of the right lung, which is also supplied by the same bronchopulmonary segments on the right side. (**A**) Bronchopulmonary segments I–III are associated with portions of the left superior lobe that are superior to the lingula. (**B**) Bronchopulmonary segments I–V are associated with portions of the left superior lobe that are superior to the oblique (major) fissure (i.e., including, but not restricted to, the lingula). (**D**) Bronchopulmonary segments VI–X are associated with the portions of the left inferior lobe that are inferior to the oblique (major) fissure.

17.   Correct: Left recurrent laryngeal (A)

(**A**) The CT indicates a mass posterior to the root of the left lung, which could impact the recurrent laryngeal nerve. Paralysis of the posterior cricoarytenoid muscle, which is innervated by the recurrent laryngeal nerve, causes ipsilateral vocal cord paralysis and results in vocal cord dysfunction, followed by dyspnea (especially on exertion). (**B**) The phrenic nerve passes anterior to the root of the lung and is, therefore, less likely to be compressed by the mass. (**C**) The symptoms and CT indicate the mass is on the left side, making it unlikely the right recurrent laryngeal nerve is involved. (**D**) The patient's upper limb symptoms are consistent with involvement of the T1 and/or C8 ventral rami. Compression of these structures would not account for the respiratory symptoms. (**E**) The left vagus nerve may be compressed; however, its recurrent laryngeal branch is most directly involved in the respiratory symptoms.

18.   Correct: In the endothoracic fascia layer (D)

Refer to the following image for answer 18:

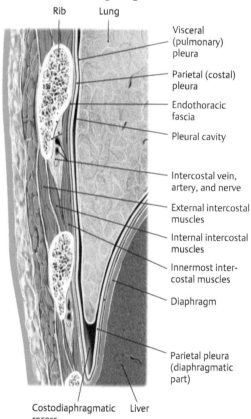

Source: Schuenke M, Schulte E, Schumacher U. THIEME Atlas of Anatomy. Internal Organs. Illustrations by Voll M and Wesker K. 2nd ed. New York: Thieme Medical Publishers; 2016

(**D**) The endothoracic fascia is a thin layer of loose connective tissue located immediately superficial (i.e., external) to the parietal pleura and serves to attach this pleura to the thoracic wall. Because it is a continuous layer, blood extravasating from intercostal vessels can form a widening hematoma. (**A, B**) Although blood from injured intercostal vessels might extravasate between intercostal muscles, these muscular layers are not immediately superficial to the parietal pleura because the endothoracic fascia intervenes. (**C**) Although blood from injured intercostal vessels might extravasate deep to the periosteum of each rib, it is not expected that this would be apparent as a widening hematoma. (**E**) The subcutaneous tissue layer is external to the intercostal muscles and ribs and is not immediately superficial to the parietal pleura.

19. Correct: Left recurrent laryngeal (A)

Refer to the following image for answer 19:

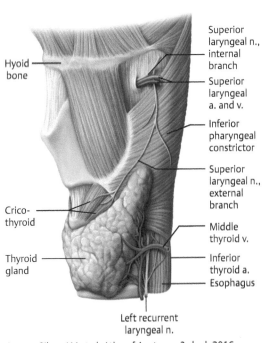

Source: Gilroy AM et al. Atlas of Anatomy. 3rd ed. 2016. Based on: Schuenke M, Schulte E, Schumacher U. THIEME Atlas of Anatomy. Volumes 1-3. Illustrations by Voll M and Wesker K. 2nd ed. New York: Thieme Medical Publishers; 2016

(**A**) During thyroidectomy, a recurrent laryngeal nerve may be injured iatrogenically while ligating the inferior thyroid artery and middle thyroid vein. A recurrent laryngeal nerve palsy affects all intrinsic laryngeal muscles on the side of the lesion except cricothyroid. Paralysis of the posterior cricoarytenoid, the sole abductor of the vocal fold, results in permanent adduction of the affected vocal fold. In this patient, the left vocal fold is adducted, indicating injury of the left recurrent laryngeal nerve. (**B**) If the right recurrent laryngeal nerve was injured, the right vocal fold would be adducted. (**C**) The external branch of the superior laryngeal nerve may be

injured iatrogenically while ligating the superior thyroid artery and vein. This nerve innervates the cricothyroid muscle, which normally tenses the vocal fold. A palsy of this nerve results in a weak voice with decreased pitch. (**D**) The internal branch of the superior laryngeal nerve may be injured iatrogenically while ligating the superior thyroid artery and vein. However, it does not innervate intrinsic laryngeal muscles. (**E**) The vagus nerve (CN X) itself does not have a close relationship to the vasculature of the thyroid gland and is, therefore, not likely to be injured iatrogenically during thyroidectomy.

20. Correct: Superior laryngeal, internal branch (D)

(**D**) Sensory innervation of the laryngeal mucosa superior to the vocal folds is provided by the internal branch of the superior laryngeal nerve, a branch of the vagus (CN X). (**A**) The glossopharyngeal nerve (CN IX) provides somatic sensory innervation from the mucosa of the palatine tonsils, soft palate, posterior one-third of the tongue, and most of the pharynx. (**B**) The sensory innervation for the mucosa on the vocal folds and infraglottic cavity is provided by the inferior laryngeal branch of the recurrent laryngeal nerve, which is a branch of the vagus (CN X). (**C**) The external branch of the superior laryngeal nerve innervates the cricothyroid and inferior pharyngeal constrictor muscles. (**E**) The vagus nerve innervates the larynx through its superior and recurrent laryngeal branches. Other branches of the vagus provide sensory innervation from the external acoustic meatus and skin posterior to the ear, as well as the dura mater of the posterior cranial fossa.

21. Correct: Infraglottic cavity (A)

Refer to the following image for answer 21:

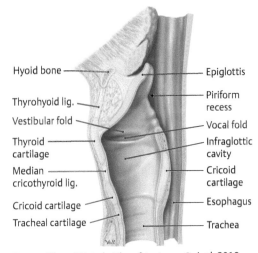

Source: Gilroy AM et al. Atlas of Anatomy. 3rd ed. 2016. Based on: Schuenke M, Schulte E, Schumacher U. THIEME Atlas of Anatomy. Volumes 1-3. Illustrations by Voll M and Wesker K. 2nd ed. New York: Thieme Medical Publishers; 2016

207

(**A**) Cricothyrotomy is a procedure used for emergency tracheal access via the infraglottic cavity. It involves the insertion of a cannula through the median cricothyroid ligament, located between the cricoid and thyroid cartilages. (**B**) The laryngeal ventricle is located between the vestibular and vocal folds, and is superior to the infraglottic cavity. (**C**) The laryngeal vestibule, located between the laryngeal inlet and vestibular fold, forms the supraglottic cavity. (**D**) The piriform fossae (recesses) are located in the laryngopharynx (also known the hypopharynx) on either side of the laryngeal inlet. Since they are not within the larynx, these spaces are not involved in a cricothyrotomy. (**E**) The trachea extends inferior to the cricoid cartilage. As such, it is not part of the larynx. While the cannula will ultimately enter the trachea, the first space it enters is the infraglottic cavity.

22. Correct: Inferior thyroid veins (B)

Refer to the following image for answer 22:

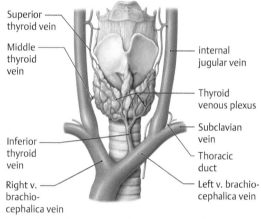

Superior thyroid vein

Middle thyroid vein

internal jugular vein

Thyroid venous plexus

Subclavian vein

Inferior thyroid vein

Thoracic duct

Right v. brachiocephalica vein

Left v. brachiocephalica vein

Source: Schuenke M, Schulte E, Schumacher U. THIEME Atlas of Anatomy. Head, Neck, and Neuroanatomy. Illustrations by Voll M and Wesker K. 2nd ed. New York: Thieme Medical Publishers; 2016

(**B**) The inferior thyroid veins drain inferiorly along the anterior aspect of the trachea from the thyroid gland to the left brachiocephalic vein. Since they arise from the thyroid venous plexus as midline structures, they may be injured when the thyroid isthmus is divided to insert the cannula through the tracheal rings. (**A**) The inferior thyroid arteries arise from the thyrocervical trunks and enter the inferior aspect of the thyroid gland on either side of the midline. Since they are not midline structures, they are not likely to be injured during the tracheotomy. (**C**) The parathyroid glands lie on the posterior aspect of the thyroid gland lobes. Since they are not midline structures, they are not likely to be injured during the tracheotomy. (**D**) The right brachiocephalic vein lies posterior to the manubrium of the sternum and to the right side of the midline. It is not likely to be injured during the tracheotomy. (**E**) The superior thyroid artery (and

vein) extends from the superior pole of each thyroid lobe. Since they are not midline structures, they are not likely to be injured during the tracheotomy.

23. Correct: Inferior nasal concha (B)

(**B**) The inferior nasal concha (nasal conchae are commonly referred to clinically as the turbinates) is the most anterior and inferior concha and would be visible first, especially in a patient whose nasal mucosa is inflamed. (**A**) The choana, also known as the posterior nasal aperture, is located in the posterior aspect of the nasal cavity, is not visible with this type of inspection. (**C**) The middle nasal concha may be visible, but its anterior aspect would most likely be superior and posterior to the inferior concha. (**D**) The superior nasal concha is more superior and posterior than the inferior and middle conchae and would not be visible. (**E**) The torus tubarius (tubal elevation), an elevation of cartilage and mucous membrane that covers the base of the pharyngotympanic (Eustachian or auditory) tube, is located in the nasopharynx. It would not be visible by an external inspection of the nasal cavity.

24. Correct: Sphenoidal sinus (E)

(**E**) The sphenoidal sinuses (a septum is evident) are indicated by the number "4" in the axial CT. (**A**) The number "1" indicates the thickened wall of the right maxillary sinus. (**B**) The nasal cavity is not indicated. (**C**) The nasopharynx is not indicated. (**D**) The "3s" indicates the thickened walls of ethmoidal air cells.

25. Correct: Ophthalmic (C)

(**C**) The frontonasal duct connects the frontal paranasal sinus with the nasal cavity, where it opens into the middle meatus. The mucous membranes of the paranasal sinuses (frontal, ethmoidal, sphenoidal, maxillary) receive sensory innervation from branches of the ophthalmic (CN V1) and maxillary (CN V2) nerves. The frontal sinus is innervated by the supraorbital and anterior ethmoidal nerves, both branches of the ophthalmic nerve. (**A, B, D, E**) None of these nerves (auriculotemporal, facial, mandibular, maxillary) innervate the frontal sinus.

26. Correct: Middle nasal meatus (C)

(**C**) The dental implant in this patient most likely protruded into the right maxillary sinus and caused a sinus infection and drainage through its ostium into the middle nasal meatus. (**A, B, D, E**) The opening of the maxillary sinus is not located in these anatomical spaces (choana or nasal meatus).

27. Correct: Facial, maxillary, and ophthalmic (D)

(**D**) Three arteries anastomose to form a vascular plexus (Little's or Kiesslebach's area) on the nasal septum: the ophthalmic (via its anterior ethmoidal branch), the maxillary (via its sphenopalatine and greater palatine branches), and the facial (via the septal branch of the superior labial). (**A**) The ascending pharyngeal artery does not contribute to the arterial plexus on the nasal septum. (**B**) The ascending pharyngeal and lingual arteries do not contribute to the arterial plexus on the nasal septum. (**C**) The great auricular and lingual arteries do not contribute to the arterial plexus on the nasal septum. (**E**) The inferior alveolar artery does not contribute to the arterial plexus on the nasal septum.

28. Correct: External naris (nostril) (A)

(**A**) An orbital blowout fracture that involves the orbital plate (lamina papryceae) of the ethmoid bone will likely damage the anterior ethmoidal nerve (a branch of the ophthalmic nerve, CN V1). This nerve supplies sensory innervation from the anterosuperior nasal cavity; the external nasal branch of the anterior ethmoidal branch supplies the skin of the dorsum of the nose inferior to the nasal bones—excluding the external nares (which are supplied by CN V2). (**B, C**) The mucosa of the inferior and middle meatus is innervated by branches of the greater palatine nerve (a branch of CN V2) that would not be injured by the orbital fracture. (**D**) The olfactory mucosa is innervated by the olfactory nerve (CN I). (**E**) The skin over the nasal bones (bridge of the nose) is innervated by branches of the ophthalmic nerve (infra- and supratrochlear nerves).

29. Correct: Vagus (E)

(**E**) The vagus nerve supplies the smooth muscle of the bronchial tree and stimulates bronchoconstriction. (**A–D**) The intercostal, pericardiacophrenic, recurrent laryngeal, and T3–T5 postganglionic sympathetic nerves do not supply the smooth muscle of the bronchial tree.

30. Correct: Intrapulmonary (C)

(**C**) Lymphatics from the deep lymphatic plexus of the lungs, which start along the bronchioles, drain first to intrapulmonary nodes and then to the bronchopulmonary (hilar) nodes. (**A**) Bronchopulmonary (hilar) nodes receive lymph from intrapulmonary nodes. (**B, E**) Tracheobronchial nodes, which collect lymph from the lung as a whole, drain to paratracheal nodes. (**D**) Paratracheal nodes receive lymph from tracheobronchial nodes and drain to the bronchomediastinal lymph trunks.

Refer to the following image for answer 30:

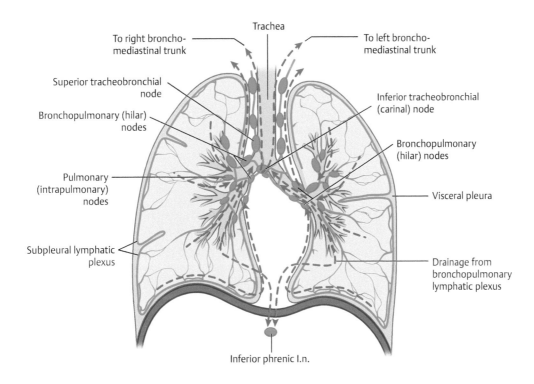

209

31. Correct: Sternal angle (of Louis) (C)

Refer to the following image for answer 31:

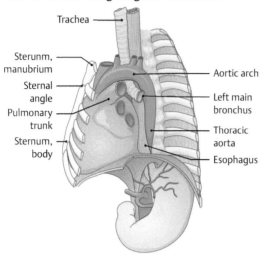

Trachea

Sterunm, manubrium

Sternal angle

Pulmonary trunk

Sternum, body

Aortic arch

Left main bronchus

Thoracic aorta

Esophagus

Source: Gilroy AM et al. Atlas of Anatomy. 3rd ed. 2016. Based on: Schuenke M, Schulte E, Schumacher U. THIEME Atlas of Anatomy. Volumes 1-3. Illustrations by Voll M and Wesker K. 2nd ed. New York: Thieme Medical Publishers; 2016

(**C**) The trachea bifurcates posterior to the sternal angle, which is formed at the junction of the manubrium and sternal body. This anatomical landmark lies at the level of the T4 and T5 intervertebral disc. (**A, B, D, E**) The manubrium (T3–T4), jugular (suprasternal) notch (T2), superior thoracic aperture (T1–T3), and xiphoid process (T9) do not lie at the level of the tracheal bifurcation.

32. Correct: Aortopulmonary window (A)

(**A**) The aortopulmonary window is a mediastinal space visible in a frontal chest radiograph. It is bounded by the aortic arch (superiorly), the left pulmonary artery (inferiorly), the ascending aorta (anteriorly), the descending aorta (posteriorly), the trachea, left main bronchus and esophagus (medially), and the hilum of the left lung (laterally). (**B–E**) The mitral valve, second costal cartilage, superior vena cava, and trachea are not indicated by the circle.

33. Correct: Left phrenic nerve (A)

(**A**) The contents of the aortopulmonary window include the left phrenic, vagus and recurrent laryngeal nerves, ligamentum arteriosum, left bronchial arteries, and lymph nodes. The postoperative radiograph shows significant left hemidiaphragm elevation compared to the right, consistent with a left phrenic nerve palsy. (**B**) The left pulmonary artery comprises the inferior boundary of the aortopulmonary window. While it can be compressed by a mass in the aortopulmonary window, this would not account for the left hemidiaphragm elevation. (**C**) The left recurrent laryngeal nerve,

as well as the left vagus nerve, can be compressed by a mass in the aortopulmonary window, but this would not account for the left hemidiaphragm elevation. (**D, E**) The aortopulmonary window is a mediastinal space that can be seen in frontal chest radiographs. Structures on the right are, therefore, not involved.

34. Correct: Right inferior lung lobe (B)

(**B**) Breath sounds from the inferior lung lobes can be auscultated on the posteroinferior surface of the back. The oblique fissure, which divides the right superior and inferior lobes, extends laterally on the back from the level of the T4 or T5 spinous process. (**A, E**) The right atrium and ventricle would not be auscultated on the back. (**C**) The right middle lobe would be auscultated in the fourth intercostal space in the midclavicular line. (**D**) The right superior lung would be auscultated either anteriorly in the second intercostal space in the midclavicular line, or posteriorly between the C7 and T3 vertebrae.

35. Correct: Right inferior lobe (C)

(**C**) The right inferior lobe is indicated by the *asterisk* in the CT: two fissures are evident and the inferior lobe is more posterior. (**A, B, D, E**) The left inferior and superior lobes, and the right middle and superior lobes are not indicated by the *asterisk*.

36. Correct: Segmental bronchus (D)

(**D**) Since there is a single, lobar (secondary) bronchus for each lung lobe, the multiple bronchial profiles in the lung parenchyma represent segmental (tertiary) bronchi, that is, the next level of branching of the bronchial tree. Segmental bronchi serve individual bronchopulmonary segments, which are pyramidal. In this patient, the bronchi are dilated and destruction of larger bronchi is caused by chronic infection and inflammation. (**A, E**) Alveoli and terminal bronchioles are located in the periphery of each lung lobe and not close to the hilum as seen in this CT image. (**B**) The multiple bronchial profiles are not consistent with a lobar bronchus, of which there is one for each lung lobe. (**C**) The main (primary) bronchi arise from the trachea in the middle mediastinum and extend laterally into the root of the lung. Each main bronchus gives rise to lobar bronchi (three on the right and two on the left) as it enters the hilum of the lung.

37. Correct: The flail segment moves inward with inhalation (B)

(**B**) With multiple rib fractures, a segment of the chest wall becomes disconnected from the remainder of the chest wall. Upon inhalation and the production of negative pressure in the pleural cavity, the detached segment moves inward with the parietal pleura rather than outward with the rib cage.

Conversely, the detached segment moves outward with exhalation. (**A**) The "bucket handle" movements of the chest wall involve the *lower* ribs: when they are elevated they also move laterally. While these movements may be impaired on the affected side, they do not describe the paradoxical movements associated with flail chest. (**C**) The normal chest wall moves outward with inhalation. (**D**) The "pump handle" movements of the chest wall involve the *upper* ribs: when they are elevated they also move anteriorly. While these movements may be impaired on the affected side, they do not describe the paradoxical movements associated with flail chest.

38. Correct: Respiratory bronchiole (B)

Refer to the following image for answer 38:

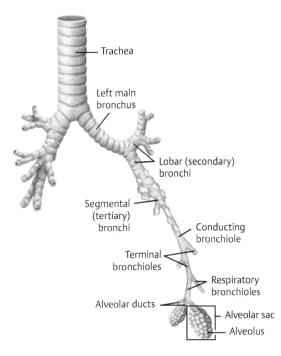

(**B**) Respiratory bronchioles, the continuations of terminal bronchioles, give rise to the respiratory units of the lung known as acini. Each acinus consists of an alveolar duct that opens into clusters of alveoli (as many as 3,000 alveoli may open into a single alveolar duct). Each respiratory bronchiole may also open directly into a relatively small number of alveoli. They are considered the first portion of the airway where gas exchange can occur. (**A**) Conducting bronchioles are continuations of tertiary bronchioles, before terminal bronchioles are formed. They are not connected directly to alveoli. (**C**) Tertiary (segmental) bronchi are continuations of secondary (lobar) bronchi. They are not connected directly to alveoli. (**D**) Terminal bronchioles are continuations of conducting bronchioles. They

are the most distal part of the *conducting* portion of the respiratory system and are not connected directly to alveoli.

39. Correct: Nasopharynx (B)

(**B**) The mass, a rhinoscleroma (a chronic granulomatous disease of the respiratory tract caused by the bacterium Klebsiella rhinoscleromatis) is located in the nasopharynx.

40. Correct: Costomediastinal recess (B)

(**B**) This patient has bacterial pneumonia, which is visualized in the costodiaphragmatic recess.

41. Correct: Can result in death from lung hypoplasia (A)

(**A**) Pulmonary hypoplasia is a common consequence of congenital diaphragmatic hernia as the mass effect of abdominal contents in the thorax can impede the development of the lungs. (**B**) Neural crest cells do not contribute to the development of the diaphragm. (**C**) Congenital diaphragmatic hernia generally results from the incomplete closure of the pericardioperitoneal (pleural) canals, and this involves the fusion of the pleuroperitoneal membranes with other components of the diaphragm. The pleuropericardial folds divide the pleural and the pericardial spaces and are not components of the diaphragm. (**D**) Branching of the respiratory diverticulum does not normally affect the development of the diaphragm. However, because abdominal organs can move into the thoracic cavity when the diaphragm is not fully developed, the abdominal contents can exert a mass effect that can prevent the lung on that side from developing fully. (**E**) Usually, the defect in congenital diaphragmatic hernia occurs on the left posterolateral side. This is thought to be related to the fact that the right pericardioperitoneal canal normally closes earlier than the left.

42. Correct: Diverticula from the foregut (A)

(**A**) Pulmonary sequestration is a congenital abnormality characterized by a mass of lung tissue thought to develop as an anomalous out-pocketing from the foregut endoderm. The normal respiratory diverticulum (lung bud) develops from the foregut endoderm; however, the anomalous mass in a sequestration does not connect with the tracheobronchial tree and is supplied by systemic arteries. An intralobar sequestration shares the visceral pleura of the adjacent lung, while the extralobar type is contained within its own visceral pleura, separate from the involved lung. (**B**) The pleuropericardial membranes form the separation between the pleural and pericardial cavities and do not form lung tissue. (**C, D**) The pleuroperitoneal membranes, together with the septum transversum, contribute to the diaphragm and do not form lung tissue. (**E**) The tracheoesophageal septum develops from the tracheoesophageal ridges and partitions the esophagus from the trachea, thus dividing the respiratory from the gastrointestinal system.

43. Correct: Type II pneumocytes (E)

(**E**) Type II pneumocytes, also called type II alveolar epithelial cells, differentiate between 24 and 34 weeks of gestation, and produce and secrete surfactant. Surfactant is necessary to reduce the surface tension at the air/liquid interface in the lung. When there is insufficient surfactant, alveoli collapse and a "glassy" hyaline membrane composed of proteins and dead cells lines the alveoli, making breathing difficult. (**A**) The alveolar period (alveolar phase) in lung development begins in utero after about 32 to 36 weeks, and lasts until about 8 years of age. Alveoli increase in number and are divided by septa during this period. (**B**) Although abnormal development of the diaphragm could present with respiratory distress, it would not present with the other symptoms in this infant. (**C**) The tracheoesophageal septum forms the partition that separates the trachea from the esophagus. Abnormal development of the tracheoesophageal septum will more likely result in tracheoesophageal fistula, with or without esophageal atresia. (**D**) Type I pneumocytes form the majority of the epithelial lining of the lungs, they are the cells responsible for gas exchange that takes place in the alveoli. They do not directly contribute to respiratory distress syndrome/hyaline membrane disease, which is a consequence of insufficient production of surfactant by the type II pneumocytes.

44. Correct: Endoderm (A)

Refer to the following image for answer 44:

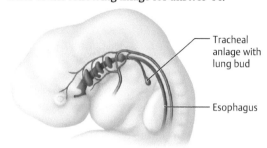

Source: Gilroy AM et al. Atlas of Anatomy. 3rd ed. 2016. Based on: Schuenke M, Schulte E, Schumacher U. THIEME Atlas of Anatomy. Volumes 1-3. Illustrations by Voll M and Wesker K. 2nd ed. New York: Thieme Medical Publishers; 2016

(**A**) The lower respiratory tract develops as a single respiratory diverticulum or lung bud from the anterior wall of the foregut and is therefore derived from endoderm. (**B, D, E**) The mesenchyme associated with the lower respiratory tract is from the splanchnic mesoderm, not somatic mesoderm—it forms the connective tissue, smooth muscle, and associated vessels. (**C**) Neural crest cells do not contribute to the epithelial lining of the lower respiratory tract.

Refer to the following image for answer 43:

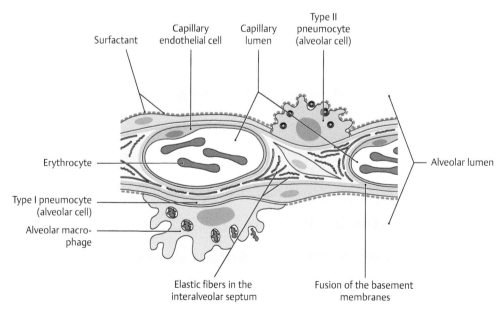

Source: Gilroy AM et al. Atlas of Anatomy. 3rd ed. 2016. Based on: Schuenke M, Schulte E, Schumacher U. THIEME Atlas of Anatomy. Volumes 1-3. Illustrations by Voll M and Wesker K. 2nd ed. New York: Thieme Medical Publishers; 2016

45. Correct: Fusion of the tracheoesophageal ridges (C)

(**C**) The tracheoesophageal ridges are longitudinal ridges that fuse to separate the respiratory diverticulum from the foregut. Incomplete separation leads to the most common form of tracheoesophageal fistula with esophageal atresia. (**A**) Incomplete canalization of the larynx results in a laryngeal web which may partially obstruct the larynx, but should not influence feeding and swallowing. (**B**) The septum secundum forms in the developing heart to separate the right and left atria. It becomes part of the interatrial septum. (**D**) The thyroglossal duct is a diverticulum from the floor of the primitive oral cavity. The duct extends into the neck and its distal part gives rise to the thyroid gland. The proximal portion of the duct regresses and its only remnant is a small, short, blind pouch (foramen cecum) on the dorsum of the tongue at the junction of the tongue's oral and pharyngeal parts. The thyroglossal duct is not related to tracheoesophageal fistula. (**E**) The buccopharyngeal (oropharyngeal) membrane lies at the junction of the primitive mouth and pharynx. It represents the point where ectoderm and endoderm meet. It usually ruptures at the fourth week of development and is not related to tracheoesophageal fistula.

Refer to the following images for answer 45:

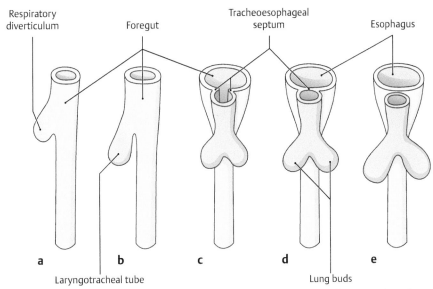

Source: Schuenke M, Schulte E, Schumacher U. THIEME Atlas of Anatomy. Internal Organs. Illustrations by Voll M and Wesker K. 2nd ed. New York: Thieme Medical Publishers; 2016

Chapter 5
Urinary System

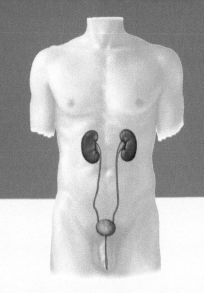

ANATOMICAL LEARNING OBJECTIVES

▶ Describe the anatomy of the abdominal components of the urinary system, the kidneys and ureters, including their neurovasculature, anatomical relationships, and relevant surface anatomy.

▶ Describe the anatomy of the abdominal components of the urinary system, distal ureters and urinary bladder, including their neurovasculature, anatomical relationships, and relevant surface anatomy.

▶ Describe the anatomy of the urethra, including its neurovasculature and anatomical relationships.

▶ Describe the anatomical basis for the control of micturition.

▶ Describe the development of the genitourinary system.

▶ Describe the anatomy of the pelvic reproductive and digestive organs as they relate to the urinary system.

▶ Describe the anatomy of the bony pelvis.

▶ Recognize normal and pathological anatomy in standard diagnostic imaging of the urinary system.

5.1 Questions

Easy	Medium	Hard

1. A 24-year-old woman with burning micturition and pain in the right lumbar region presents to a primary care physician. As the physician performs a bimanual palpation in the area of pain, the patient is asked to take a deep breath. A firm rounded mass is palpated on the right side that descends during inspiration. Which part of the kidney is palpated?

A. Inferior pole

B. Lateral margin

C. Renal hilum

D. Renal pelvis

E. Superior pole

2. A 32-year-old woman presents with intermittent pain in the right lower abdominal quadrant. She reports that the pain started several weeks ago and subsides when she lies down. Ultrasonography performed with the patient upright shows that the hilum of the right kidney is lower than normal and, although the right ureter is normal in length, it has a kink. Which of the following is the most likely cause for this patient's condition?

A. Ectopic kidney

B. Horseshoe kidney

C. Nephrolith

D. Nephroptosis

E. Renal cysts

3. A 43-year-old man presents with intermittent, sudden-onset, excruciating right lower back pain. The pain has progressed over the past 12 hours and sometimes radiates to his genitalia and adjacent thigh. He describes urination as difficult and says his urine is "pink." Ultrasonography indicates a 10 mm dense mass in the right ureter at the L5 to S1 vertebral level. Considering this individual's symptoms, at which of the following locations along the ureter is the calculus most likely lodged?

A. At the pelvic brim

B. Where it crosses the ductus deferens

C. Where it crosses rib 12

D. Where it is continuous with the renal pelvis

E. Where it passes through the wall of the urinary bladder

4. A 58-year-old, multiparous, postmenopausal woman is concerned with occasional "leakage" of urine. She is in good physical condition and participates in competitive cycling on a regular basis. She reports that the leakage occurs even during mild exertion, such as laughing, sneezing, or coughing. Weakness of which of the following structures most likely caused this condition?

A. Broad ligaments

B. Detrusor muscle

C. Pelvic floor muscles

D. Pubovesical ligaments

E. Transverse cervical (cardinal) ligaments

5. A 53-year-old man presents with acute renal failure secondary to recurrent urolithiasis (obstructive stone disease). After his most recent obstruction was corrected by lithotripsy, his renal function only modestly improved and he was placed on hemodialysis. The dialysis was complicated by several episodes of sepsis and, consequently, he was scheduled for a renal transplant with his twin brother as donor of his left kidney. Which of the following accounts for why the left kidney is harvested for the transplant?

A. It is more accessible due to its lower position

B. It is more likely to have multiple renal arteries

C. The left renal vein is nearly three times as long as the right

D. There are fewer branches to the suprarenal gland from the left renal artery

E. The suprarenal gland is located entirely on the upper pole of the left kidney

6. A 63-year-old woman with a history of autosomal dominant polycystic kidney disease presents with severe chronic abdominal pain. Patient history indicates she has recently lost a considerable amount of weight. Renal ultrasonography reveals multiple cysts are compressing her stomach, and she is scheduled for a nephrectomy. During surgery, which of the following relationships should be remembered?

A. The left kidney lies lower than the right

B. The left renal vein lies anterior to the aorta and the left renal artery

C. The perirenal fat lies external to the renal fascia

D. The renal fascia does not surround the suprarenal gland

E. The right renal artery is shorter than the left

7. A 38-year-old woman who undergoes contrast-enhanced CT for vague abdominal pain is incidentally found to have a horseshoe kidney (refer to the accompanying image). During development, the lower poles of the kidneys fuse across the midline at the L3 to L5 vertebral levels and the kidneys fail to ascend to the normal adult position (usually above the L3 vertebra). Which vessel most likely prevents the ascent of the structure indicated by the *asterisks* in the CT?

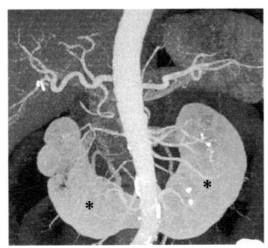

Source: Hamm B, Asbach P, Beyersdorff D et al. Direct Diagnosis in Radiology. Urogenital Imaging. 1st Edition. Thieme; 2008.

A. Abdominal aorta

B. Celiac trunk

C. Inferior mesenteric artery

D. Inferior vena cava

E. Superior mesenteric artery

8. A 38-year-old man presents with dull right upper abdominal quadrant pain and a history of right percutaneous nephrolithotomy. He exhibits costovertebral angle tenderness (CVAT; Goldflam's sign) on physical examination. Ultrasonography indicates hydronephrosis with hydroureter caused by an obstructing calculus. Which of the following is indicated by the *arrow* in this sonogram of the affected organ (refer to the accompanying image)?

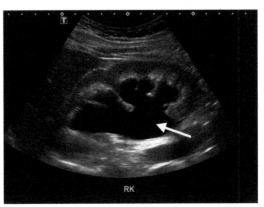

Source: Yu E, Jaffer N, Chung T et al. RadCases. Emergency Radiology. 1st Edition. Thieme; 2015.

A. Major calyx

B. Minor calyx

C. Renal papilla

D. Renal pelvis

E. Renal pyramid

9. A 3-year-old girl who still uses diapers is brought to the pediatrician by her mother. On physical examination, urine is detected coming from the girl's vagina. Ultrasonography of the kidneys reveals two renal pelves on the right side. On consultation, a pediatric urologist determines that there is an abnormal opening in the child's vagina. Duplication of which of the following structures is likely responsible for the child's incontinence?

A. Kidney

B. Ureter

C. Urethra

D. Urinary bladder

E. Vagina

10. A newborn male presents with hydronephrosis detected in utero. A cystourethrogram (refer to the accompanying image) performed after birth demonstrates reflux into a dilated ureter (*arrowhead*) and a dilation in the region indicated by the *arrow*. A diagnosis of posterior urethral valves is made. The dilated region distal to the urinary bladder (*arrow*) is derived from which of the following?

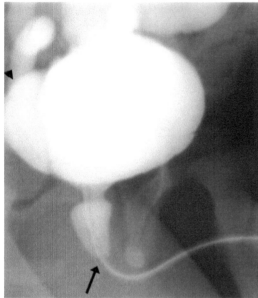

Source: Gunderman R, Delaney L. RadCases. Pediatric Imaging. 1st Edition. Thieme; 2010.

A. Mesonephric duct
B. Metanephric blastema
C. Paramesonephric duct
D. Ureteric bud
E. Urogenital sinus

11. A 68-year-old man with deteriorating renal function reports to his nephrologist for evaluation. The nephrologist orders an ultrasound, which reveals hydronephrosis. A noncontrast CT image of the urinary bladder (refer to the accompanying image) obtained for additional evaluation shows bladder hypertrophy (*asterisk*) and multiple bladder diverticulae (*arrowheads*). Blood supply to the superior portion of the structure identified by the *asterisk* is a direct branch of which of the following arteries?

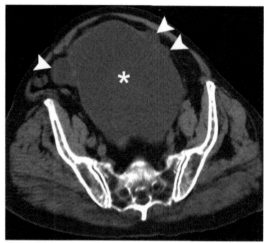

Source: Chopra S. RadCases. Genitourinary Imaging. 1st Edition. Thieme; 2011.

A. External iliac
B. Internal iliac
C. Internal pudendal
D. Obturator
E. Umbilical

12. An 8-year-old boy is brought to the pediatrician by his mother who reports that, although he never wets his pants during the day, he frequently wets the bed at night. The pediatrician counsels the mother that most bedwetting is due to a developmental delay and not to physical illness or emotional problems. He suggests that inadequate voluntary control of the external urethral sphincter might be responsible. The sphincter discussed for this patient is primarily associated with which of the following structures?

A. Bladder neck
B. Glans penis
C. Membranous urethra
D. Prostatic urethra
E. Spongy urethra

13. A 5-year-old girl with a recent history of urinary tract infection is brought to her pediatrician for a follow-up examination. The physician orders a voiding cystourethrogram (refer to the accompanying image), which indicates a defect in the valve-like mechanism that normally prevents reflux of urine (*arrows* indicate hydronephrosis as a result of the reflux). This sphincter-like mechanism involves which two structures?

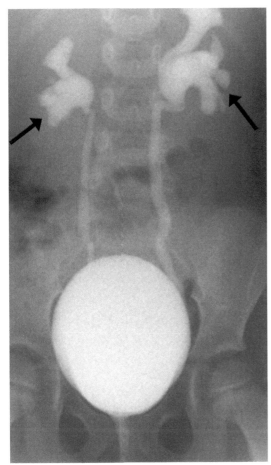

Source: Gunderman R, Delaney L. RadCases. Pediatric Imaging. 1st Edition. Thieme; 2010.

A. Renal pelvis and calyces
B. Renal pelvis and ureters
C. Ureters and bladder wall
D. Urethra and external urethral orifice
E. Urethra and internal urethral orifice

Consider the following case for questions 14 and 15:

A 68-year-old woman with concerns of urinary frequency, urgency, nocturia, and urge incontinence presents to her gynecologist. She has had these symptoms for several years, but thought they were a normal consequence of aging. Recently, however, she finds that she urinates more frequently and sometimes cannot make it to the bathroom in time. The physician suspects that the muscles that override involuntary emptying of the urinary bladder are weakened.

14. The weakened muscles are supplied by which of the following nerves?

A. Deep branch of the perineal
B. Inferior rectal
C. Pelvic splanchnic
D. Sacral splanchnic
E. Superficial branch of the perineal

15. Which of the following nerves regulate involuntary control of micturition?

A. Deep branch of the perineal
B. Inferior rectal
C. Pelvic splanchnics
D. Sacral splanchnics
E. Superficial branch of the perineal

16. A 38-year-old woman is readmitted to the hospital with urinary incontinence and abdominal pain 8 days after a laparoscopic hysterectomy. Surgical exploration reveals partial ligation of her ureters. At which of the following locations are the ligated structures most susceptible to iatrogenic injury during a hysterectomy?

A. Adjacent to the suspensory ligament of the ovary
B. As they cross the pelvic brim
C. As they cross under the uterine artery
D. As they enter the urinary bladder

17. A 48-year-old woman with a history of urinary calculi presents to the emergency department after 2 days of fever and left flank pain. Physical examination confirms severe left flank tenderness. Ultrasonography reveals calyceal stones and swelling of the left kidney and CT reveals an abscess in the lower pole with focal perirenal fat blurring, indicative of fluid infiltration. Where is the fluid located?

A. Deep to the kidney capsule

B. Deep to perirenal (Gerota's) fascia

C. Superficial to the pararenal fat

D. Superficial to perirenal (Gerota's) fascia

E. Within pararenal fat

18. A 56-year-old man with bilateral swellings in his groin presents to his primary care physician. Axial noncontrast CT imaging (refer to the accompanying image) shows herniation of the urinary bladder (*asterisk*) into the right inguinal canal. The left inguinal canal contains a herniated loop of bowel (*arrow*). What specific abnormality is seen in the right inguinal canal?

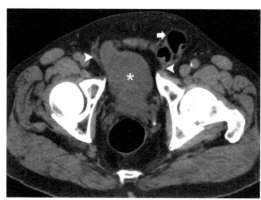

Source: Chopra S. RadCases. Genitourinary Imaging. 1st Edition. Thieme; 2011.

A. Cystocele

B. Hydrocele

C. Patent urachus

D. Rectocele

E. Undescended testis

19. A 23-year-old woman gives birth to a full-term male. Two days after being discharged from the hospital, the mother brings her newborn child to the pediatrician because she has observed leakage from his umbilical stump. Imaging shows an extension of contrast from the urinary bladder into the umbilical stump (refer to the *arrow* in the accompanying image). Which of the following congenital anomalies is present in this neonate?

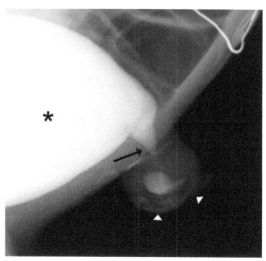

Source: Gunderman R, Delaney L. RadCases. Pediatric Imaging. 1st Edition. Thieme; 2010.

A. Gastroschisis

B. Meckel's diverticulum

C. Meckel's fistula

D. Omphalocele

E. Patent urachus

20. A 25-year-old woman with a 6-month history of urinary hesitancy and weak urine stream presents to her primary care physician. A history reveals that she sustained a lower spinal cord injury from a motor vehicle accident 2 years previously. Cystoscopy reveals a normal urethra with no obstruction, and a trabeculated urinary bladder. Urodynamic studies indicate a diagnosis of detrusor sphincter dyssynergia, a condition that results from dyscoordination between the detrusor muscle of the bladder and the external urethral sphincter muscle. Somatic innervation to the latter muscle arises from which of the following spinal cord segments?

A. L5–S1

B. S1–S3

C. S1–S4

D. S2–S4

E. S3–Co1

21. A 38-year-old male construction worker is taken to the emergency department after suffering direct trauma to his perineum by falling astride scaffolding. Physical examination reveals blood at the external urethral meatus, a perineal hematoma, and acute urinary retention. A retrograde cystourethrogram confirms urethral rupture. A suprapubic approach is used to place a catheter in the urinary bladder to divert urine and allow the damaged urethra to heal. This procedure is used to avoid piercing which of the following structures?

A. Detrusor muscle

B. Membranous layer (Scarpa's) of superficial fascia

C. Peritoneum

D. Rectus sheath

E. Superficial layer (Camper's) of superficial fascia

22. A 26-year-old man presents in the emergency department with minor head and right flank injury after a motorcycle accident. Physical examination reveals hematomas of the right chest and flank. Contrast-enhanced CT (refer to the accompanying image) shows absence of perfusion in the lower third of the right kidney (*arrow*) indicating an infarct with perinephric hemorrhage (*asterisk*). Which of the following renal vessels was probably infarcted in this patient?

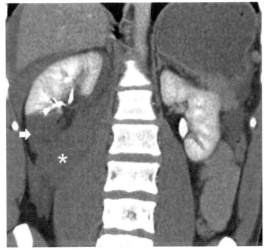

Source: Chopra S. RadCases. Genitourinary Imaging. 1st Edition. Thieme; 2011.

A. Arcuate

B. Interlobar

C. Interlobular

D. Right renal

E. Segmental

23. A 27-year-old man was brought to the emergency department after being hit by a bus. He presents with hematuria and a suspected pelvic fracture. A cystogram (refer to the accompanying image) shows a full urinary bladder (*asterisk*) that is abnormally elongated, and streaks of extravasated contrast are visible in the surrounding tissues (*arrows*). The imaging also reveals bilateral fractures of the superior pubic rami (*arrowheads*). Which of the following best describes the location of the extravasated contrast in the image?

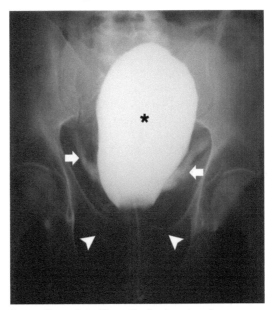

Source: Chopra S. RadCases. Genitourinary Imaging. 1st Edition. Thieme; 2011.

A. Extraperitoneal

B. Intraperitoneal

C. Perineal

D. Retroperitoneal

E. Subcutaneous

24. A 32-year-old man with chronic left flank pain, hematuria, and occasional renal hypertension presents to his primary care physician. Ultrasonography of the abdomen (refer to the accompanying image) demonstrates a focal narrowing of his left renal vein. Evaluation using contrast-enhanced MRI of the kidneys confirms compression of the left renal vein and a significant increase in flow velocity along this vein is noted on pulse Doppler. Which of the following structures is compressing the vein (*red arrow*)?

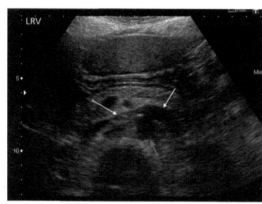

Source: Azar N, Donaldson C. RadCases: Ultrasound Imaging. 1st Edition. Thieme; 2015.

A. Duodenum
B. Inferior mesenteric artery
C. Inferior vena cava
D. Pancreas
E. Superior mesenteric artery

25. A 28-year-old woman is admitted to the emergency department after sustaining injury in a motor vehicle accident. The attending physician orders imaging to rule out intra-abdominal injury. A CT scan reveals a fracture of the right 12th rib. Which of the following viscera is most susceptible to injury in this patient?

A. Duodenum
B. Gallbladder
C. Kidney
D. Pancreas
E. Spleen

26. A 55-year-old man with dull abdominal pain that has increased over time presents to his primary care physician. CT imaging reveals hydronephrosis of the right kidney and a retroperitoneal mass. Ureteroscopy reveals compression of the right ureter near its junction with the renal pelvis and retroperitoneal fibrosis is suspected. The patient is scheduled for surgery to remove the mass and decompress the ureter. Which of the following best describes the arterial supply to the compressed area of this structure?

A. Common iliac
B. Internal iliac
C. Renal
D. Superior mesenteric
E. Superior vesicle

Consider the following case for questions 27 and 28:

A 16-year-old boy with end-stage renal disease is scheduled for bilateral nephrectomy and a living donor renal transplant from his older sister. A posterior lumbotomy (thoracolumbar/retroperitoneal) approach via a vertical incision from the 12th rib to the iliac crest is used. The incision passes through subcutaneous fat, latissimus dorsi muscle, and thoracolumbar fascia, just lateral to the erector spinae and quadratus lumborum muscles.

27. Which of the following nerves traverse this operating field?

A. Genitofemoral, ilioinguinal, and iliohypogastric
B. Genitofemoral, femoral, and obturator
C. Ilioinguinal, iliohypogastric, and obturator
D. Ilioinguinal, iliohypogastric, and subcostal
E. Ilioinguinal, obturator, and femoral

28. Which of the following structures is most anterior in the hilum of the diseased organs?

A. Renal artery
B. Renal vein
C. Renal pelvis
D. Suprarenal gland
E. Ureter

29. A 37-year-old man with spasmodic and excruciating right groin pain of approximately 3-hour duration presents to the emergency department. On physical examination, a retracted right testis is noted and the patient is referred to the urology department. Urinalysis reveals hematuria and an intravenous urogram shows two small calculi in his right distal ureter. The pain in this patient will most likely be referred to cutaneous areas innervated by which of the following spinal cord levels?

A. L3–L4

B. L4–L5

C. S2–S4

D. T9–T10

E. T11–L2

30. A 45-year-old man presents with left flank pain. MRI with contrast and enhancement reveals an obstructing ureteric calculus and masses on both kidneys. Renal cell carcinoma is suspected and anterior transabdominal laparoscopic partial nephrectomies are performed. On the right side, which of the following are most susceptible to iatrogenic injury during this anterior approach?

A. Duodenum

B. Liver

C. Pancreas

D. Spleen

E. Stomach

31. A 34-year-old man with an umbilical discharge associated with lower abdominal pain presents to his primary care physician. Examination shows purulent discharge originating from a tender, red, swelling inferior to the umbilicus. MRI shows a communication between the urinary bladder and the swelling. The swollen tissue is a derivative of which of the following embryonic structures?

A. Allantois

B. Ductus arteriosus

C. Ductus venosus

D. Urogenital sinus

E. Urorectal septum

5.2 Answers and Explanations

Easy	Medium	Hard

1. Correct: Inferior pole (A)

(**A**) The right kidney is often palpable in a thin person during a bimanual examination when the abdominal muscles are relaxed. A bimanual examination is performed by pressing simultaneously on the flank anteriorly at the costal margin and posteriorly between the 12th rib and iliac crest. During inspiration, the kidneys descend due to contraction of the diaphragm and consequently the inferior pole of the right kidney can be palpated. The left kidney is not typically palpable as it lies at a higher vertebral level and its inferior pole does not descend inferior to the posterior costal margin. (**B**) The lateral margin of the kidney is not accessible for palpation by bimanual examination except at its inferior pole. (**C**) The renal hilum is not accessible for palpation by bimanual examination as it is located medially and does not lie near the posterior costal margin. (**D**) The renal pelvis is not accessible for palpation by bimanual examination as it is located medially and does not lie near the posterior costal margin. (**E**) The superior pole of the kidney is not accessible for palpation by bimanual examination as it is located close to the diaphragm and does not descend inferior to the posterior costal margin during inspiration.

2. Correct: Nephroptosis (D)

(**D**) Nephroptosis, a dropped or sagging kidney, can be differentiated from an ectopic kidney by ureter length. Since the two layers of renal (Gerota's) fascia are not fused inferiorly, the kidney may descend as much as 3 cm when the patient is upright, causing a ureter of normal length to develop a kink. Intermittent pain in the right lower quadrant that subsides when the patient is supine is believed to be caused by tension on the renal vasculature and intermittent or partial obstruction of the kinked ureter. Nephroptosis is usually treated by nephropexy (kidney fixation). (**A**) The ureter of an ectopic kidney, a congenital defect in which the kidney develops in an abnormal position, is usually short and not kinked. Symptoms of an ectopic kidney are not affected by the patient's position. (**B**) A horseshoe kidney is a congenital anomaly in which the ureters are shorter than normal because during development the inferior poles of the kidneys fuse and the fused kidneys are prevented from ascending to a normal position by the inferior mesenteric artery. (**C**) The severe abdominal pain from an obstructing calculus (nephrolith or renal stone) is the result of the hydronephrosis. Non-obstructing nephroliths usually do not cause pain. The patient may also have additional symptoms such as vomiting and urinary frequency. (**E**) Renal cysts are typically seen as fluid-filled sacs within the kidney.

3. Correct: At the pelvic brim (A)

(**A**) The location of pain depends on the site of obstruction and usually occurs at one of the three points of narrowing along the course of the ureter: (1) where the renal pelvis narrows to form the ureter; (2) where the ureter crosses the pelvic brim; and (3) where the ureter passes through the wall of the urinary bladder. The sonogram places the calculus at the L5–S1 vertebral level, which corresponds to the pelvic brim. Lower ureteric obstruction causes radiating pain to the external genitalia, whereas upper ureteric obstruction (renal pelvis) causes flank pain. Afferent inpulses from the ureters follow sympathetic fibers primarily to the T11–L2 segments of the spinal cord, and pain is referred to dermatomes supplied by these spinal cord segments. As the calculus moves along a ureter, the pain is described to progress from "loin (lumbar region) to groin (external genitalia)." (**B**) The ureter and ductus deferens cross on the posterolateral aspect of the urinary bladder at the midsacral vertebral level. Since the ureter and ductus deferens are not in contact with one another, there would not be a constriction in the ureter at this location. (**C**) The ureter does not cross rib 12. The ureter begins at the midlumbar vertebral level, inferior to rib 12. (**D**) The renal pelvis is continuous with the ureter at the midlumbar vertebral level and the calculus in this case is at the lower lumbar level. (**E**) The ureter passes through the bladder wall at the midsacral level. The calculus has been localized at the lower lumbar/upper sacral level.

Refer to the following image for answer 3:

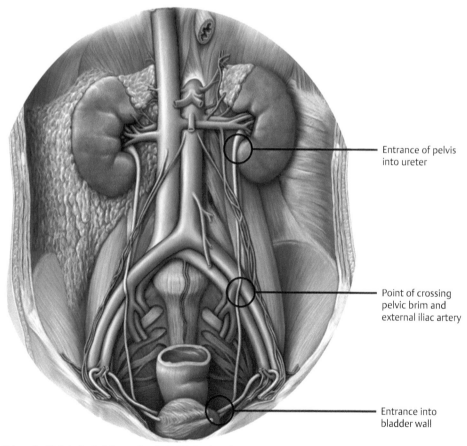

Entrance of pelvis into ureter

Point of crossing pelvic brim and external iliac artery

Entrance into bladder wall

Source: Schuenke M, Schulte E, Schumacher U. THIEME Atlas of Anatomy. Internal Organs. Illustrations by Voll M and Wesker K. 2nd ed. New York: Thieme Medical Publishers; 2016

4. Correct: Pelvic floor muscles (C)

(**C**) The normal function of the female pelvic organs (i.e., urinary bladder, vagina, uterus, rectum) is dependent primarily on the tone of levator ani muscles. Reduced tone in these pelvic floor muscles allows pelvic organs to assume altered positions, which commonly impacts their functioning. Vaginal deliveries and surgeries of the perineum and pelvis are the most common causes of compromise to the pelvic floor muscles. (**A**) The broad ligament, a double layer of peritoneum that forms a mesentery for the uterus, uterine tubes, and ovary, provide only minimal support for these structures; it is not associated with the urinary bladder or urethra. (**B**) Weakness of the detrusor muscle of the bladder wall is unlikely to cause urinary incontinence. Its weakness would lead to an inability to completely empty the bladder. (**D**) Although the paired pubovesical ligaments help maintain the urinary bladder in its midpelvic position on the transverse plane, they offer little resistance to the bladder "sinking" inferiorly in the pelvic cavity. (**E**) The transverse cervical ligament lies at the base of the broad ligament and conveys vessels and nerves to and from the uterus. It plays a minor role in support of the bladder.

Refer to the following image for answer 4:

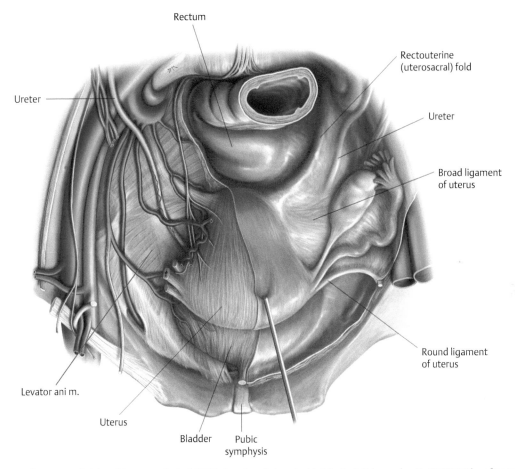

Source: Gilroy AM et al. Atlas of Anatomy. 3rd ed. 2016. Based on: Schuenke M, Schulte E, Schumacher U. THIEME Atlas of Anatomy. Volumes 1-3. Illustrations by Voll M and Wesker K. 2nd ed. New York: Thieme Medical Publishers; 2016

5. Correct: The left renal vein is nearly three times as long as the right (C)

Refer to the following image for answer 5:

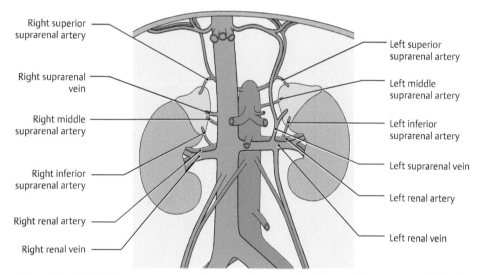

Right superior suprarenal artery

Right suprarenal vein

Right middle suprarenal artery

Right inferior suprarenal artery

Right renal artery

Right renal vein

Left superior suprarenal artery

Left middle suprarenal artery

Left inferior suprarenal artery

Left suprarenal vein

Left renal artery

Left renal vein

Source: Schuenke M, Schulte E, Schumacher U. THIEME Atlas of Anatomy. Internal Organs. Illustrations by Voll M and Wesker K. 2nd ed. New York: Thieme Medical Publishers; 2016

(**C**) Since the inferior vena cava is located to the right of the midline, the left renal vein must cross the lumbar vertebral bodies to enter the inferior vena cava. Thus, the left renal vein is nearly three times longer than the right renal vein, which facilitates the vascular grafting in the recipient. (**A**) The right kidney is at a more inferior level than the left on the posterior abdominal wall. This is due to the larger right lobe of the liver, which occupies more of the subdiaphragmatic area on the right side. (**B**) Studies show that the right kidney is more likely to have multiple renal arteries. The left kidney, with one renal artery, would offer fewer challenges in the harvest procedure. (**D**) Typically, each renal artery provides only one branch (middle suprarenal artery) to the suprarenal gland. (**E**) The left suprarenal gland is usually located on the superior pole and superomedial aspect of the left kidney. In general, the position of the suprarenal gland is not a factor in kidney harvest since a septum of renal fascia separates the suprarenal gland from the kidney.

6. Correct: The left renal vein lies anterior to the aorta and the left renal artery (B)

(**B**) The left renal vein courses anterior to the aorta and left renal artery. (**A**) The left kidney is approximately one vertebral level higher, not lower, than the right kidney. (**C**) The perirenal fat is internal, not external, to the renal fascia. (**D**) The renal fascia does surround the suprarenal gland. (**E**) The right renal artery is longer, not shorter, than the left renal artery.

Refer to the following image for answer 6:

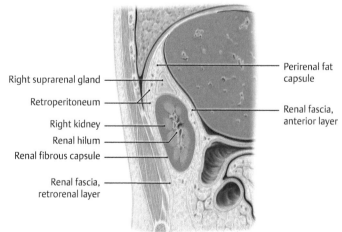

Right suprarenal gland

Retroperitoneum

Right kidney

Renal hilum

Renal fibrous capsule

Renal fascia, retrorenal layer

Perirenal fat capsule

Renal fascia, anterior layer

Source: Gilroy AM et al. Atlas of Anatomy. 3rd ed. 2016. Based on: Schuenke M, Schulte E, Schumacher U. THIEME Atlas of Anatomy. Volumes 1-3. Illustrations by Voll M and Wesker K. 2nd ed. New York:Thieme Medical Publishers; 2016

7. Correct: Inferior mesenteric artery (C)

Refer to the following image for answer 7:

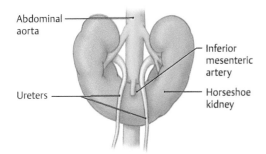

Source: Schuenke M, Schulte E, Schumacher U. THIEME Atlas of Anatomy. Internal Organs. Illustrations by Voll M and Wesker K. 2nd ed. New York: Thieme Medical Publishers: 2016

(**C**) A horseshoe kidney develops when the lower poles of the kidneys fuse across the midline at the L3–L5 vertebral levels and the kidneys fail to ascend to the normal adult position (usually above the L3 vertebra) because the inferior mesenteric artery impedes its upward progression. (**A**) The abdominal aorta itself would not impede the ascent of the horseshoe kidney. (**B**) The celiac trunk would not impede ascent because it is located superior (i.e., at the T12 vertebral level) to the final position of the horseshoe kidney. (**D**) The inferior vena cava itself would not impede the ascent of the horseshoe kidney. (**E**) The superior mesenteric artery would not impede ascent because it is located superior to the final position of the horseshoe kidney.

8. Correct: Renal pelvis (D)

Refer to the following image for answer 8:

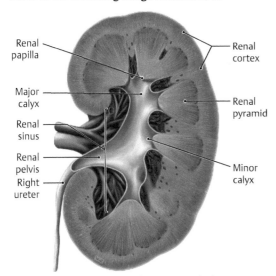

Source: Gilroy AM et al. Atlas of Anatomy. 3rd ed. 2016. Based on: Schuenke M, Schulte E, Schumacher U. THIEME Atlas of Anatomy. Volumes 1-3. Illustrations by Voll M and Wesker K. 2nd ed. New York: Thieme Medical Publishers; 2016

(**D**) The renal pelvis, the portion of the collecting system between the major calyces and the ureter, is dilated in this patient as a result of a ureteric obstruction. Enlargement of the collecting system of the kidney may include the major and minor calyces (as shown in the ultrasound with the question). (**A, B**) Both the minor and major calyces are also enlarged in this patient (*asterisks*). The minor renal calyces are funnel-shaped tubes whose proximal ends encircle the renal papillæ and unite to form two or three short major calyces. (**C, E**) The renal papilla and pyramids, which are parts of the renal medulla, become compressed by the enlarged collecting system in hydronephrosis. The renal pyramids are regions in the medulla, each of which has a nipple-like projection (renal papilla) into a minor calyx.

9. Correct: Ureter (B)

(**B**) An ectopic ureter usually opens into the urogenital tract below the bladder because it gets pulled down with the developing mesonephric duct and opens with it into the caudal part of the urogenital sinus (Weigert–Meyer rule). Because this part of the urogenital sinus gives rise to the urethra and part of the vagina, the ectopic ureteric orifice may be located in either of these structures. This accounts for the continuous dribbling of urine since there is no urinary bladder or urinary sphincter between the ectopic ureter and the vaginal vestibule. Normally, the oblique passage of the ureter through the posterior wall of the bladder, together with the bladder musculature, act as a sphincter for the ureter. (**A**) The duplicated renal pelvis and incontinence are indicative of a duplicated ureter. There is no evidence of a duplicated kidney, and a duplicated kidney would not lead to incontinence. (**C**) The duplicated renal pelvis and incontinence are indicative of a duplicated ureter, not a duplicated urethra. (**D**) The duplicated renal pelvis and incontinence are indicative of a duplicated ureter, not a duplicated urinary bladder. (**E**) A duplicated vagina would not lead to incontinence.

10. Correct: Urogenital sinus (E)

(**E**) The structure indicated by the *arrow* is the urethra, which is derived from the urogenital sinus (an endodermal derivative). Posterior urethral valves are extra flaps of tissue that develop within the male urethra. This extra tissue blocks the normal flow of urine, which may lead to bladder hypertrophy and hydronephrosis. (**A**) The mesonephric (Wolffian) ducts form the male reproductive ducts including the epididymis, ductus deferens, seminal gland, and ejaculatory ducts. While they open into the urogenital sinus and will eventually descend into the prostate as they form the ejaculatory ducts, they do not contribute to the urethra. (**B**) The metanephric blastema forms the excretory units of the definitive kidney, the metanephros. It does not contribute to the urethra. (**C**) The paramesonephric (Müllerian) ducts form the female reproductive ducts including the uterine tubes, uterus, cervix and upper portion of the vagina. While they open into the urogenital sinus and will induce the sinovaginal bulbs that will eventually form the lower vagina, they do not contribute to the urethra. (**D**) The ureteric buds, which form the ureters and collecting ducts of the definitive kidney, develop as outgrowths of the mesonephric ducts that grow into the metanephric blastema and induce the formation of the excretory units that will become the nephrons of the definitive kidney.

11. Correct: Umbilical (E)

(**E**) The superior vesical artery, which supplies the superior aspect of the urinary bladder, is a direct branch of the umbilical artery (which is a branch of the internal iliac artery). (**A–D**) The external iliac, internal iliac, internal pudendal, and obturator do not normally supply a direct branch to the superior aspect of the urinary bladder.

12. Correct: Membranous urethra (C)

(**C**) The external urethral sphincter is voluntary skeletal muscle that surrounds the male urethra just superior to the perineal membrane, the portion of the urethra in males known as the membranous urethra. Fibers from this muscle typically extend superiorly along the prostatic urethra. (**A**) The urinary bladder neck is adjacent to the prostate gland. It is surrounded by circular smooth muscle that forms the involuntary internal urethral sphincter. (**B**) The distal urethra contains the dilated navicular fossa, which is located in the glans penis. There is no sphincteric mechanism in this part of the urethra. (**D**) The prostatic urethra is surrounded by the prostate gland and has no sphincteric mechanism. (**E**) The spongy urethra is located in the penis and courses within the corpus spongiosum on the ventral aspect of the penis and has no sphincteric mechanism.

13. Correct: Ureters and bladder wall (C)

(**C**) The antireflux mechanism of the urinary system is located where the ureters traverse the urinary bladder wall, at the vesicoureteric junction (VUJ). The VUJ is thought to function as a passive sphincter whereby the ureters, as they obliquely traverse the posterior bladder wall, become compressed as the bladder fills, thereby preventing reflux of urine into the ureters. (**A, B, D, E**) There is no sphincteric mechanism within the kidney, between the kidney and ureter, or at either the internal or external urethral orifices that prevents urine reflux.

14. Correct: Deep branch of the perineal (A)

(**A**) The deep perineal nerves are branches of the pudendal nerves. They supply the muscles of the anterior perineum, including the external urethral sphincter that functions in voluntary control of urination. (**B**) The inferior rectal nerves, also branches of the pudendal nerve, innervate the external anal sphincter muscle, which does not have a role in urinary continence. (**C**) Involuntary urinary bladder emptying results from the detrusor reflex. The detrusor muscle remains relaxed to allow the bladder to store urine. Distension of the bladder as it fills leads to contraction of the detrusor muscle. The efferent limb of the reflex is mediated through parasympathetic preganglionic neurons that are conveyed to the urinary bladder via pelvic splanchnic nerves (S2–S4). In the male, these nerves also stimulate relaxation of the internal urethral sphincter during bladder emptying. (**D**) The sacral splanchnic nerves convey sympathetic fibers to the pelvic viscera. These nerves have a role in the tonic contraction of the internal urethral sphincter in males, the involuntary sphincter of the urinary bladder. (**E**) The superficial branches of the perineal nerve become the posterior labial nerves in females and posterior scrotal nerves in males and provide sensory innervation from the skin of those respective areas.

15. Correct: Pelvic splanchnics (C)

(**C**) Pelvic splanchnic nerves (S2–S4) convey preganglionic parasympathetic fibers for the involuntary detrusor reflex. The detrusor muscle remains relaxed to allow the bladder to store urine. Distension of the bladder as it fills leads to contraction of the detrusor muscle. In the male, these nerves also stimulate relaxation of the internal urethral sphincter during bladder emptying. (**A**) The deep perineal nerves are also branches of the pudendal nerve and supply the muscles of the anterior perineum. Among these muscles is the external urethral sphincter muscle that functions in voluntary control of urination. (**B**) The inferior rectal nerves, also branches of the pudendal nerve, innervate the external anal sphincter muscle, which does not have a role in urinary continence. (**D**) The sacral splanchnic nerves convey sympathetic fibers to the pelvic viscera. These nerves have a role in the tonic contraction of the internal urethral sphincter in the male, the involuntary sphincter of the urinary bladder. (**E**) The superficial branches of the perineal nerve become the posterior labial nerves in females and posterior scrotal nerves in males, and provide sensory innervation from the skin of those respective areas.

16. Correct: As they cross the uterine artery (C)

(**C**) The female ureters are most susceptible to iatrogenic injury during a hysterectomy as they cross inferior to the uterine artery and vein (recall the commonly used mnemonic for this relationship is "water under the bridge"). These structures lie in the transverse cervical (cardinal or Mackenrodt's) ligament, which is located in the base of the mesometrium portion of the broad ligament. (**A, B**) The ureters are susceptible to iatrogenic injury during an oophorectomy as they cross the pelvic brim and course adjacent to the suspensory ligament of the ovary (infundibulopelvic ligament). (**D**) The ureters

are susceptible to iatrogenic injury during colorectal surgery as they enter the urinary bladder.

Refer to the following image for answer 16:

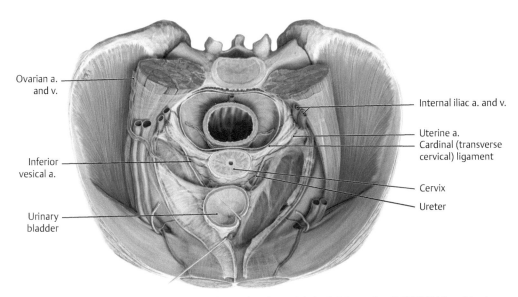

Source: Gilroy AM et al. Atlas of Anatomy. 3rd ed. 2016. Based on: Schuenke M, Schulte E, Schumacher U. THIEME Atlas of Anatomy. Volumes 1-3. Illustrations by Voll M and Wesker K. 2nd ed. New York: Thieme Medical Publishers; 2016

---

17. Correct: Deep to perirenal (Gerota's) fascia (B)

(**B**) The fluid observed in the image is within the perirenal fat, which lies between the perirenal (Gerota's) fascia and the kidney capsule. Typically, this layer of fatty tissue is approximately 2 to 3 cm thick and blurring of this layer on CT or MRI indicates edema and inflammation. (**A**) The kidney capsule separates kidney parenchyma from perirenal fat. (**C–E**) The pararenal (paranephric) fat is superficial to the perirenal fascia and represents the external-most layer of fat associated with the kidney.

18. Correct: Cystocele (A)

(**A**) Herniation of the urinary bladder is a cystocele. (**B–E**) Hydrocele, patent urachus, rectocele, or undescended testis are not involved in herniation of the urinary bladder.

19. Correct: Patent urachus (E)

(**E**) Leakage of urine at the umbilicus suggests the presence of a patent urachus. The patent urachus, confirmed by the cystourethrogram, is a cranial extension of the urinary bladder. During development, the bladder extends into the umbilical cord via a channel called the urachus, which normally regresses to a fibrous cord before birth. Failure of the urachus to regress can lead to a variety of anomalies, including patent urachus, urachal sinus, urachal

diverticulum, or urachal cyst. (**A, D**) Gastroschisis and omphalocele are congenital anomalies that affect the digestive, not the urinary system. In gastroschisis, there is a defect in the anterior abdominal wall that allows a portion of the abdominal gastrointestinal tract to herniate secondarily into the defect. In omphalocele, the developing gastrointestinal tract that normally herniates into the umbilical cord fails to leave the umbilical cord and return to the abdominal cavity. (**B, C**) Meckel's diverticulum and a Meckel's fistula each represent remnants of the yolk stalk that fail to fully regress.

20. Correct: S2–S4 (D)

(**D**) The external urethral sphincter muscle is a voluntary muscle innervated by deep perineal branches of the pudendal nerve that arises from sacral spinal segments S2–S4. (**A–C, E**) The pudendal nerve does not arise from spinal segments L5–S1, or Co1.

21. Correct: Peritoneum (C)

(**C**) During a suprapubic cystostomy the urinary bladder is approached through the anterior abdominal wall, a catheter is inserted directly through the bladder wall through a midline incision 2-3 cm superior to the pubic symphysis. This approach allows access to the urinary bladder without entering the peritoneal cavity. (**A**) The detrusor muscle forms the smooth muscle of the urinary bladder wall and

229

would be penetrated by the catheter. (**B, D, E**) To gain access to the urinary bladder through the anterior abdominal wall the subcutaneous fascia, both the superficial fatty (Camper's) and membranous

(Scarpa's) layers, as well as the rectus sheath, would be pierced by the catheter.

Refer to the following image for answer 21:

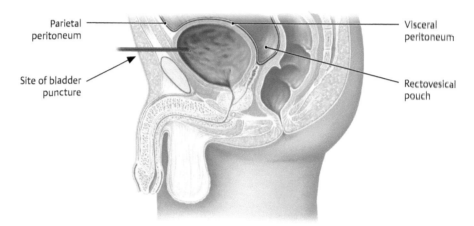

Source: Schuenke M, Schulte E, Schumacher U. THIEME Atlas of Anatomy. Internal Organs. Illustrations by Voll M and Wesker K. 2nd ed. New York: Thieme Medical Publishers; 2016

---

22.   Correct: Segmental (E)

(**E**) Typically, each renal artery forms anterior and posterior branches that, in turn, form segmental arteries that supply the five lobes of the kidney. The segmental arteries are end arteries; each segmental artery forms a succession of branches—interlobar (**B**), arcuate (**A**), and interlobular (**C**) The complete loss of renal perfusion to a lower lobe indicates that segmental arteries were infarcted, resulting in

loss of blood supply from its branches. (**A–C**) Since these arteries (arcuate, interlobar, and interlobular) are branches of the segmental arteries, infarction of these vessels alone would not result in the complete loss of blood supply in the lower lobe. (**D**) Infarction in the renal artery would result in complete loss of blood supply to the right kidney.

Refer to the following image for answer 22:

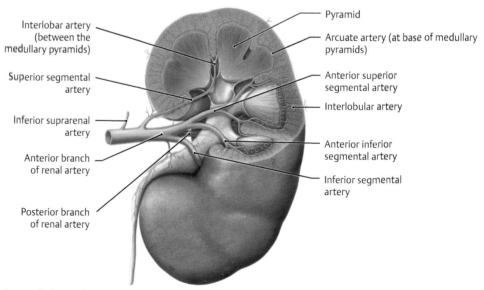

Source: Schuenke M, Schulte E, Schumacher U. THIEME Atlas of Anatomy. Internal Organs. Illustrations by Voll M and Wesker K. 2nd ed. New York: Thieme Medical Publishers; 2016

23. Correct: Extraperitoneal (A)

(**A**) The extravasated contrast is extraperitoneal since it has infiltrated the tissues around the urinary bladder, which is itself extraperitoneal. A bladder rupture into the extraperitoneal space often results from pieces of fractured pelvic bones that pierce the inferolateral surface of the urinary bladder. In the pelvic cavity, the extraperitoneal space is often termed "subperitoneal." (**B**) If the extravasated contrast was intraperitoneal, the CT cystogram would more likely show contrast material outlining loops of bowel, between folds of mesentery, or in the paracolic gutters. (**C**) If the extravasated contrast was in the perineum, the rupture would have more likely occurred in the urethra and would be inferior to the pelvic diaphragm and not in the pelvic cavity. (**D**) If the extravasated contrast was retroperitoneal it would be along the posterior abdominal wall. (**E**) Subcutaneous extravasation of contrast material would likely present as a relatively diffuse pattern, neither outlining bowel nor any organs.

24. Correct: Superior mesenteric artery (E)

(**E**) As the left renal vein crosses the midline to reach the inferior vena cava it passes through the angle formed by the superior mesenteric artery (anteriorly) and the abdominal aorta (posteriorly). Left renal vein compression at this point results in increased left renal vein pressure and may lead to hematuria, proteinuria, left flank pain, nausea, and vomiting. This compression of the left renal vein is known as "nutcracker syndrome." (**A–D**) None of these structures (duodenum, inferior mesenteric artery, inferior vena cava, and pancreas) is in a position to compress the left renal vein. It should be noted that the third (horizontal) part of the duodenum may also be compressed because it is also located in the angle between the superior mesenteric artery and the abdominal aorta, just inferior to the left renal vein.

Refer to the following image for **answer 24**:

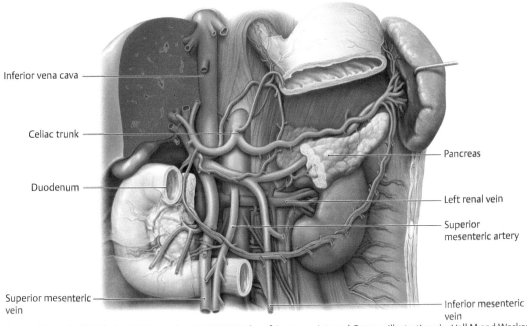

Source: Schuenke M, Schulte E, Schumacher U. THIEME Atlas of Anatomy. Internal Organs. Illustrations by Voll M and Wesker K. 2nd ed. New York: Thieme Medical Publishers; 2016

25.   Correct: Kidney (C)

Refer to the following image for answer 25:

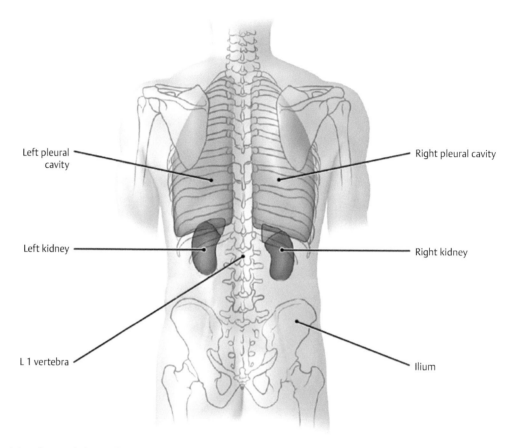

Left pleural cavity

Right pleural cavity

Left kidney

Right kidney

L 1 vertebra

Ilium

Source Schuenke M, Schulte E, Schumacher U. THIEME Atlas of Anatomy. Internal Organs. Illustrations by Voll M and Wesker K. 2nd ed. New York: Thieme Medical Publishers; 2016

(**C**) The kidneys and spleen are the only structures listed that are in contact with the ribs. In this patient, the spleen is likely not injured because it is located on the left side. Due to the larger size of the right lobe of the liver, the right kidney extends superiorly only to the level of rib 12. In contrast, the left kidney extends superiorly to rib 11 as the kidney is not typically present at this location. (**A**) The duodenum begins at the pylorus on the transpyloric plane (L1) and ends at the duodenojejunal junction at the L3 vertebral level. (**B**) The gallbladder rests against the inferior surface of the liver in the right upper quadrant. It is not normally in contact with rib 12. (**D**) The pancreas is located retroperitoneally on the transpyloric plane, anterior to the bodies of the L1 and L2 vertebrae. (**E**) The spleen is located in the left upper abdominal quadrant, posterolateral to the stomach and superior to the left kidney. It is related to ribs 9 to 11 on the left.

26. Correct: Renal (C)

Refer to the following image for answer 26:

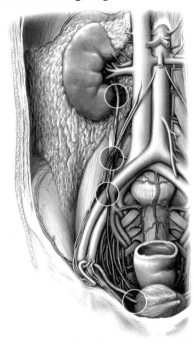

Source: Gilroy AM et al. Atlas of Anatomy. 3rd ed. 2016. Based on: Schuenke M, Schulte E, Schumacher U. THIEME Atlas of Anatomy. Volumes 1-3. Illustrations by Voll M and Wesker K. 2nd ed. New York: Thieme Medical Publishers; 2016

(**C**) The proximal ureter is supplied by branches of the renal and gonadal arteries, as well as direct branches from the abdominal aorta. (**A–C**) The common and internal iliac arteries, and some of their branches (e.g., superior vesicle), distribute to the distal (pelvic) ureter. (**D, E**) The superior mesenteric and superior vesicle arteries do not supply blood to the proximal ureter.

27. Correct: Ilioinguinal, iliohypogastric, and subcostal (D)

(**D**) The ilioinguinal (L1), iliohypogastric (L1), and subcostal (T12) nerves lie between the quadratus lumborum and the kidney and traverse the operating field. (**A**) The genitofemoral nerve (L1–L2) lies medial to the operating field. It usually emerges from the anterior aspect of psoas major muscle and descends on that muscle toward the inguinal ligament. (**B, C, E**) The femoral (L2–L4) and obturator (L2–L4) nerves lie medial to the operating field. Both nerves parallel the psoas major muscle with the femoral appearing at the muscle's lateral side and the obturator along the medial side.

Refer to the following image for answer 27:

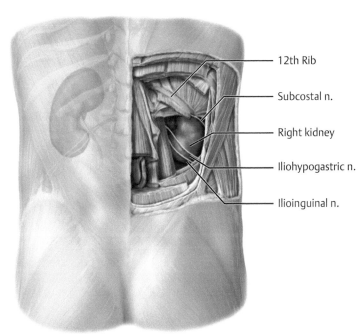

- 12th Rib
- Subcostal n.
- Right kidney
- Iliohypogastric n.
- Ilioinguinal n.

Source: Gilroy AM et al. Atlas of Anatomy. 3rd ed. 2016. Based on: Schuenke M, Schulte E, Schumacher U. THIEME Atlas of Anatomy. Volumes 1-3. Illustrations by Voll M and Wesker K. 2nd ed. New York: Thieme Medical Publishers; 2016

28. Correct: Renal vein (B)

Refer to the following image for answer 28:

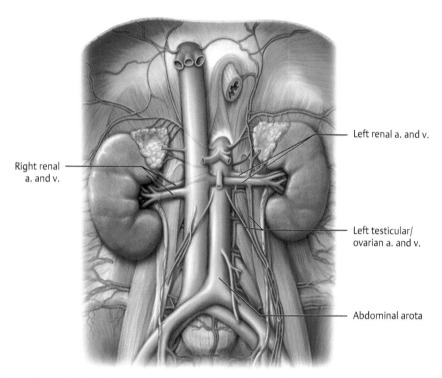

Right renal a. and v.

Left renal a. and v.

Left testicular/ ovarian a. and v.

Abdominal arota

Source: Gilroy AM et al. Atlas of Anatomy. 3rd ed. 2016. Based on: Schuenke M, Schulte E, Schumacher U. THIEME Atlas of Anatomy. Volumes 1-3. Illustrations by Voll M and Wesker K. 2nd ed. New York: Thieme Medical Publishers; 2016

(**B**) In the renal hilum, the renal veins course anterior to the renal arteries and the renal pelvis. Multiple renal veins converge to form the right and left renal veins, which then join the inferior vena cava. (**A, C**) The renal artery and renal pelvis are not the most anterior structures in the renal hilum. (**D, E**) The suprarenal gland and ureter are not located in the renal hilum.

29. Correct: T11–L2 (E)

(**E**) Ureteric pain is referred to cutaneous areas that are innervated by spinal cord levels that supply the ureter, mainly T11–L2. Excessive ureteric distension by a calculus as it progresses along the ureter typically results in severe pain (ureteric colic) that radiates from the flank (or loin) to the inguinal region (or groin), and external genitalia (primarily the scrotum or labium majus). The pain may also extend into the anterior proximal thigh because this region is supplied by the genitofemoral nerve (L1–L2), which also innervates the cremaster muscle. The stimulation of the pain fibers in the genitofemoral nerve due to the calculi in the lower ureter will result in contraction of the cremaster muscle and testicular elevation. (**A–D**) Pain from the ureter does not refer to the cutaneous areas supplied by nerves originating from the T9–T10, L3–L5, or S2–S4 spinal segments.

30. Correct: Duodenum (A)

Refer to the following image for answer 30:

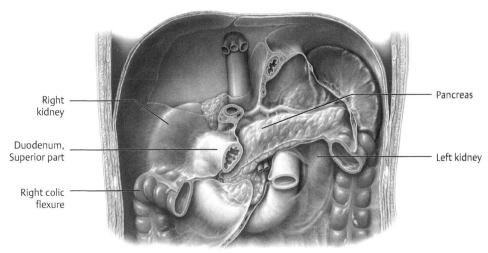

Right kidney

Pancreas

Duodenum, Superior part

Left kidney

Right colic flexure

Source: Gilroy AM et al. Atlas of Anatomy. 3rd ed. 2016. Based on: Schuenke M, Schulte E, Schumacher U. THIEME Atlas of Anatomy. Volumes 1-3. Illustrations by Voll M and Wesker K. 2nd ed. New York: Thieme Medical Publishers; 2016

(**A**) The descending or second part of the duodenum is immediately adjacent to the hilum of the right kidney and would need to be considered for potential iatrogenic injury in an anterior approach to the right kidney. (**B**) The right lobe of the liver is associated with the upper pole of the right kidney, but the duodenum is of greater vulnerability due to its relationship to the medial border of the kidney. (**C**) The right kidney is separated from the head of the pancreas by the descending portion of the duodenum. (**D, E**) The spleen and stomach are not associated with the right kidney.

31. Correct: Allantois (A)

(**C**) This individual has a patent urachus, which is a derivative of the allantois. The developing bladder is continuous with the allantois superiorly and, during the weeks 5 to 7, the allantois forms the urachus. In the adult, the lumen of the urachus is normally obliterated and forms the median umbilical ligament that extends from the umbilicus to the apex of the bladder. (**A**) The ductus arteriosus connects the left pulmonary artery to the arch of the aorta as an extracardiac shunt for fetal blood. After birth, it becomes the ligamentum arteriosum. (**B**) The ductus venosus connects the left umbilical vein to the inferior vena cava and, after birth, it becomes the ligamentum venosum. (**D**) The urogenital sinus is the ventral part of the cloaca, formed after the cloaca is partitioned by the urorectal septum. (**E**) The urorectal septum divides the cloaca into dorsal and ventral parts.

Chapter 6

Digestive System

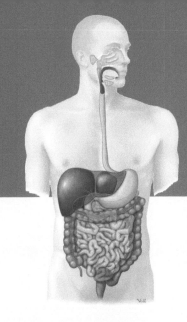

ANATOMICAL LEARNING OBJECTIVES

- ▶ Describe the anatomy of the digestive organs in the head and neck, including their neurovasculature, role in deglutition, and their anatomical relationships.
- ▶ Describe the anatomy of the anterior and lateral abdominal walls, including their layers, muscles (attachments, actions), and innervation.
- ▶ Describe the anatomy of the peritoneum and peritoneal cavity, including its innervation and anatomical relationships.
- ▶ Describe the anatomy of the digestive organs in the abdominal and pelvic cavities, including their neurovasculature and anatomical relationships.
- ▶ Describe the surface anatomy of the abdominal organs and list the abdominal viscera that lie within each abdominal quadrant.
- ▶ Describe the anatomy of the digestive organs in the pelvic cavity, including their neurovasculature and anatomical relationships.
- ▶ Describe the anatomy of the unpaired branches of the abdominal aorta, including their branches, distribution, and anatomical relationships.
- ▶ Describe the anatomy of the hepatic portal system, including its anastomoses with systemic blood vessels.
- ▶ Describe the anatomy of the diaphragm, including its divisions, attachments, neurovasculature, and anatomical relationships.

- ▶ Describe the anatomy of the facial muscles, including their attachments, action(s) and innervation.
- ▶ Differentiate regions of the gastrointestinal tract based on variations in the mucosa, submucosa, muscularis, and serosa/adventitia.
- ▶ Describe the characteristics of hernias in the groin region and how inguinal hernias develop, including the anatomy and clinical presentation of such hernias.
- ▶ Describe the developmental anatomy of the digestive system.
- ▶ Describe the features of the anal canal that help maintain continence.
- ▶ Describe the origin, course, and distribution of the facial nerve (CN VII).
- ▶ Explain the anatomical basis for referred pain.
- ▶ Recognize normal and pathological anatomy in standard diagnostic imaging of the digestive system.

6.1 Questions

Easy	Medium	Hard

1. A 45-year-old woman is admitted to the emergency department with severe abdominal pain that radiates to her back. Physical examination demonstrates abdominal tenderness upon palpation and CT imaging reveals a pancreatic cyst (refer to the *arrow* in the accompanying image). Into which of the following spaces would fluid first enter if the cyst were to rupture through the peritoneum on the anterior surface of the involved organ?

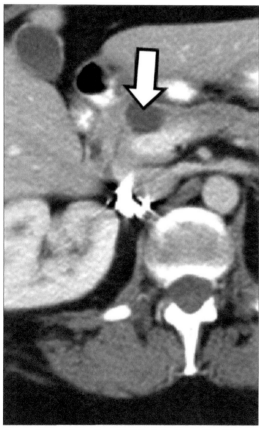

Source: Riascos R, Bonfante E, Calle S. RadCases Plus Q&A: Neuro Imaging. 2nd Edition. Thieme; 2018.

A. Greater sac
B. Hepatorenal recess
C. Left subphrenic recess
D. Lesser sac
E. Rectouterine pouch

2. A 63-year-old man is admitted to the emergency department after having been found in the street vomiting blood (hematemesis). A review of his medical history shows that he has a cirrhotic liver due to alcoholism. Endoscopy reveals lower esophageal varices (refer to the accompanying image). Increased pressure in which of the following vessels results in the observed varices?

Esophageal varices

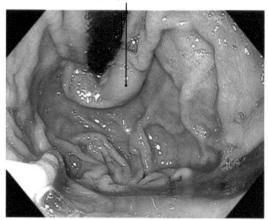

Source: Al-Osaimi A, Caldwell S. Medical and Endoscopic Management of Gastric Varices. Seminars in Interventional Radiology 2011; 28(03): 273–282.

A. Aorta
B. Left gastric artery
C. Left renal vein
D. Portal vein
E. Superior vena cava

3. A 45-year-old man with signs of liver failure presents to the physician. Liver function tests confirm advanced liver disease and he is placed on a transplant list. During donor hepatectomy, a Pringle maneuver (compression of the hepatoduodenal ligament) is performed. Which of the following vessels is compressed during the performed maneuver?

A. Common hepatic artery
B. Gastroduodenal artery
C. Hepatic artery proper
D. Inferior vena cava
E. Left gastric artery

4. A 48-year-old man presents to the emergency department with colicky pain, abdominal distension, vomiting, fever, and dehydration. The patient history shows that he was previously admitted to the hospital for atrial fibrillation. Paralytic ileus is suspected and a mesenteric arteriogram is performed to locate the suspected embolus and area of ischemia. The arteriogram will most likely show an embolus obstructing the blood flow in which of the following?

A. Arterial arcades

B. Inferior mesenteric artery

C. Marginal artery (of Drummond)

D. Right colic artery

E. Vasa rectae

5. A 45-year-old woman with fever, chills, and abdominal pain in the right upper abdominal quadrant visits her primary care physician. Physical examination reveals abdominal tenderness and guarding, and the patient exhibits a positive Murphy's sign (examiner's fingers placed at right costal border on the midclavicular line; pain is elicited when patient inhales). Further evaluation confirms gallbladder disease and she is referred for cholecystectomy (gallbladder removal). The artery to be ligated during the removal of the diseased organ is typically located in the angle between the liver, the common hepatic duct, and which of the following structures?

A. Celiac trunk

B. Common hepatic artery

C. Cystic duct

D. Hepatic artery proper

E. Portal vein

6. A 72-year-old woman with known systemic sclerosis presents with melena (black feces) to her primary care physician. Gastroscopy reveals esophageal varices and an ultrasound scan of her abdomen shows a small liver with coarse texture, splenomegaly, and a distended splenic vein. The splenic and superior mesenteric veins unite to form the portal vein posterior to which of the following parts of the pancreas?

A. Body

B. Head

C. Neck

D. Tail

Consider the following case for questions 7 and 8:

A 74-year-old woman with heartburn, loss of appetite, and general fatigue visits her primary care physician. Imaging with a barium swallow shows well-defined gastric folds that extend through the esophageal hiatus.

7. Which of the following conditions is most likely in this patient?

A. Coronary artery disease

B. Esophageal motility disorder

C. Esophagitis

D. Paraesophageal hernia

E. Sliding hiatal hernia

8. Which of the following components of the diaphragm is directly related to this pathology?

A. Central tendon

B. Costal fibers

C. Left crus

D. Right crus

E. Sternal fibers

9. A 58-year-old man presents to the emergency department with a distended abdomen. Physical examination and ultrasound confirm ascites (fluid in the peritoneal cavity). Paracentesis is performed via the anterior abdominal wall, lateral to the semilunar line. Which of the following will the needle immediately encounter after passing through all muscle layers?

A. Extraperitoneal fat

B. Fatty layer of subcutaneous fascia (Camper's fascia)

C. Membranous layer of subcutaneous fascia (Scarpa's fascia)

D. Parietal peritoneum

E. Transversalis fascia

Consider the following case for questions 10 and 11:

A 22-year-old man presents to a rural clinic with a three-day history of diffuse, periumbilical pain associated with vomiting. The pain has now become sharp, constant, and localized to the right lower quadrant. During physical examination, the right lower quadrant pain is aggravated by movement, the abdomen is soft with rebound tenderness, and there is abdominal wall guarding. The patient has low-grade pyrexia (elevated temperature). Acute appendicitis is suspected and he is treated with intravenous antibiotics and referred for further evaluation.

10. The original diffuse pain in this patient was most likely transmitted via which of the following nerves?

A. Greater splanchnic

B. Inferior hypogastric

C. Least splanchnic

D. Lesser splanchnic

E. Superior hypogastric

11. Which of the following transmits the pain impulses elicited during the physical examination?

A. Greater splanchnic nerve

B. Least splanchnic nerve

C. Lumbosacral trunk (L4–L5)

D. Thoracoabdominal nerves T7–T9

E. Thoracoabdominal nerves T10–T11

12. Following surgery to repair an intertrochanteric femoral fracture, a 65-year-old woman presents with abdominal distension and pain. Physical examination reveals marked abdominal dilation and a lack of bowel sounds. A CT scan shows a massively dilated colon. Medications to increase intestinal motility are administered to prevent ischemic bowel necrosis due to the increased pressure from the dilation (refer to the accompanying image). Which of the following regions of the large intestine in this patient is most susceptible to ischemic necrosis from increased luminal pressure?

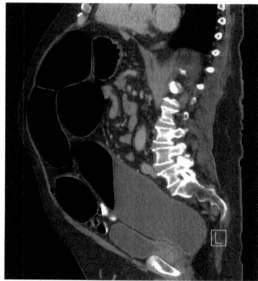

Source: Image provided courtesy of David Bloom, MD, Beaumont Health System

A. Ascending colon

B. Descending colon

C. Left colic (splenic) flexure

D. Right colic (hepatic) flexure

E. Sigmoid colon

13. A 25-year-old man who has returned recently from a 2-month visit to Asia presents with abdominal pain, vomiting, and a gradually increasing fever. Physical examination shows a distended and tender abdomen. Further evaluation leads to a diagnosis of typhoid fever with inflammation of Peyer's patches. Which of the following is the most likely location of the inflammation in this patient?

A. Duodenum

B. Esophagus

C. Ileum

D. Jejunum

E. Stomach

14. A 54-year-old woman with constipation and abdominal distension presents to a primary care physician. Physical examination of the abdomen detects a hard mass in the left lower quadrant. Which distended structure is most likely palpated in this patient?

A. Cecum

B. Ileum

C. Left colic (splenic) flexure

D. Rectum

E. Sigmoid colon

15. A 78-year-old man with jaundice presents to his primary care physician. Testing and imaging lead to a diagnosis of carcinoma in an upper abdominal organ. During surgical removal of the affected organ, the gastroduodenal and inferior pancreaticoduodenal arteries are ligated. What is the most likely site of the cancer?

A. Body of pancreas

B. Fundus of gallbladder

C. Fundus of stomach

D. Head of pancreas

E. Pylorus of stomach

16. A deceased 64-year-old woman is brought to the coroner's office for autopsy after a suspected poisoning. The assistant coroner notes that a portion of the intestine lacks luminal circular folds and its mesentery near the intestinal wall contains abundant fat and numerous short, anastomosing vessels. Based on these features, which of the following is being observed?

A. Distal ileum

B. Distal jejunum

C. First part of duodenum

D. Fourth part of duodenum

E. Proximal jejunum

Consider the following case for questions 17 and 18:

A group of researchers are studying parotid secretion flow rates in 35 healthy volunteers (28 ± 5 years of age). Stimulation of saliva production is achieved by application of a 3% citric acid solution, four times per minute, to the rim of the posterior one-third of the tongue. Saliva samples are collected for 2 minutes at 07:30 am (before breakfast) and at 10:00 am (2 hours after a standard breakfast) for 3 consecutive days.

17. Which of the following is an ideal site for placing a saliva collection cup?

A. In the oral vestibule adjacent to a first maxillary molar

B. In the oral vestibule adjacent to a second mandibular molar

C. In the oral vestibule adjacent to a second maxillary molar

D. In the oral vestibule adjacent to a third mandibular molar

E. In the oral vestibule adjacent to a third maxillary molar

18. Afferent impulses resulting from the citric acid stimulation are conducted from the involved area of the tongue by which of the following nerves?

A. Chorda tympani

B. Glossopharyngeal

C. Greater palatine

D. Internal laryngeal

E. Lingual

Consider the following case for questions 19 and 20:

An 11-year-old boy is brought to the emergency department following a roll-over accident of an all-terrain vehicle. The boy indicates that one end of the handlebar impacted on his upper abdomen. He is complaining of upper abdominal pain and physical examination reveals tenderness on deep palpation along the left costal margin. A CT scan reveals a laceration with hemorrhage to an upper abdominal organ (refer to the accompanying image).

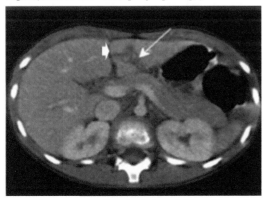

Source: Staatz G, Honnef D, Piroth W et al. Direct Diagnosis in Radiology. Pediatric Imaging. 1st Edition. Thieme; 2007.

19. Which of the following organs has the laceration revealed in the accompanying CT (indicated by *long arrow*)?

A. Head of pancreas

B. Left lobe of liver

C. Right lobe of liver

D. Spleen

E. Transverse colon

20. Which of the following structures occupies the area at the tip of the *short arrow* in the accompanying CT?

A. Common hepatic artery

B. Cystic duct

C. Falciform ligament

D. Portal vein

E. Proper hepatic artery

21. A 76-year-old man visits his primary care physician for an annual examination. Physical examination, with the patient standing, reveals a swelling at the right superficial inguinal ring. Ultrasonography indicates a direct inguinal hernia. Which of the following is the most likely location for the neck of the hernia sac?

A. Inferior to the inguinal ligament

B. Medial to the inferior epigastric vessels

C. Medial to pubic tubercle

D. Medial to the semilunar line

E. Superior to the arcuate line

22. A 50-year-old man is admitted to the emergency department after a motor vehicle collision. The patient is hemodynamically unstable and a FAST examination (focused assessment with sonography in trauma) is positive for peritoneal hemorrhage (hemoperitoneum). Subsequent CT imaging reveals a three centimeter tear along the anterior border of the spleen and he is scheduled for an emergency splenectomy. At which of the following locations should the blood supply to the organ being removed be ligated without compromising the vasculature of other organs?

A. Immediately distal to the origin of the greater pancreatic artery

B. Immediately distal to the origin of the short gastric arteries

C. Immediately distal to the origin of the splenic artery from the celiac trunk

D. Immediately proximal to the branching of the left gastro-omental artery

E. Immediately proximal to the origin of the greater pancreatic artery

241

23. A 16-year-old girl with sickle cell disease presents to her primary care physician for a regularly scheduled check-up. During the physical examination, an organ is palpated that extends 2 cm inferior to the left costal margin, posterior to the midaxillary line. Which of the following organs is most likely increased in size and palpable in this patient?

A. Abdominal aorta

B. Duodenum

C. Left kidney

D. Spleen

E. Stomach

24. A 50-year-old man is admitted to the emergency department after an automobile accident. Ultrasound confirms a ruptured spleen and a splenectomy was performed. During a follow-up visit 2 weeks after the surgery, the patient indicates he is experiencing left shoulder pain. This pain is most likely due to fluid collecting in which of the following regions?

A. Costodiaphragmatic recess

B. Left paracolic gutter

C. Right paracolic gutter

D. Subhepatic space

E. Subphrenic recess

25. A 17-year-old girl with severe abdominal pain, fever, and vomiting is brought by her parents to the emergency department. Physical examination localizes the pain to the right iliac fossa and ultrasound confirms appendicitis. An open appendectomy is performed. Which of the following most closely represents the surface projection for the base/root of the infected organ?

A. One-half of the distance between the anterior superior iliac spine and the umbilicus

B. One-half the distance between the umbilicus and the pubic tubercle

C. One-third of the distance from the anterior superior iliac spine to the umbilicus

D. Two centimeters inferior to the umbilicus on the midline

E. Two-thirds of the distance from the anterior superior iliac spine to the umbilicus

26. A 17-year-old girl is brought to the clinic for chronic amenorrhea. A history reveals that she has not had a menstrual period for 3 months, and that she had been dieting for the past 7 months. The patient also indicates that she has had "stomach" (epigastric) pain, belching (eructation), and yellowish (bilious) vomiting. Physical examination shows a body weight of 35.9 kg (79 lb), height 1.6 m (5 feet 2 inches), and a body mass index of 15.5. A CT scan shows the angle between the abdominal aorta and superior mesenteric artery to be less than 20 degrees and a diagnosis of superior mesenteric artery (Wilkie's) syndrome is made. Which of the following parts of the digestive tract is most likely compressed by the narrow angle between the two vessels?

A. Duodenal–jejunal junction

B. Horizontal (third) part of duodenum

C. Ileocecal junction

D. Pyloris of stomach

E. Transverse colon

27. A 38-year-old woman is brought to the emergency department after she sustained a stab injury. On examination, a 2-cm-long entry wound is seen in the umbilical region and ultrasound shows a pneumoperitoneum (air within the peritoneal cavity) caused by a perforation of the proximal jejunum. A posterior-anterior radiograph with the patient standing will most likely show the air is located in which of the following?

A. Hepatorenal recess

B. Rectouterine pouch

C. Retropubic space

D. Subphrenic recess

E. Vesicouterine pouch

28. A 42-year-old woman presents with fever, right upper abdominal quadrant pain, and muscle guarding on inspiration. During ultrasonography the patient experiences focal pain when pressure is applied by the transducer probe over the location of the gallbladder fundus. At which of the following locations is the ultrasound probe most likely located when the focal pain is produced?

A. Rib 7 along the midaxillary line

B. Rib 7 along the midclavicular line

C. Rib 9 along the midaxillary line

D. Rib 9 along the midclavicular line

E. Rib 11 along the midaxillary line

F. Rib 11 along the midclavicular line

29. A 52-year-old man presents to the emergency department with sudden onset of severe, sharp abdominal pain. Physical examination discloses generalized abdominal tenderness, guarding, and rigidity. Ultrasound shows fluid posterior to the stomach and a perforation of the posterior wall of the stomach. Which of the following peritoneal ligaments forms the inferior boundary of the space in which the fluid has collected?

A. Gastrocolic

B. Gastrophrenic

C. Gastrosplenic

D. Hepatoduodenal

E. Triangular

30. A 9-year-old boy with a history of skeletal and cardiac birth defects is brought to his pediatrician for a semiannual checkup. A radiograph reveals air in an organ just inferior to the diaphragm (refer to the accompanying image). Which of the following structures most likely contains the air shown in the radiograph (*arrow*)?

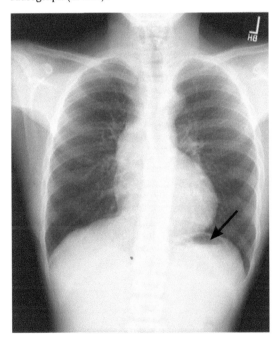

Source: Gunderman R, Delaney L. RadCases. Pediatric Imaging. 1st Edition. Thieme; 2010.

A. Cardia of the stomach

B. Descending (second) part of the duodenum

C. Fundus of stomach

D. Inferior (third) part of the duodenum

E. Pylorus of stomach

31. A 35-year-old man with chronic abdominal pain, nausea, and vomiting presents to his primary care physician. Physical examination reveals the pain to be localized to the epigastric region. The initial workup is inconclusive and a subsequent CT scan of the abdomen reveals an annular pancreas (refer to the *arrow* in the accompanying image) surrounding the duodenum (*asterisk*). Which part of the intestinal tract is encircled by the pancreas in this patient?

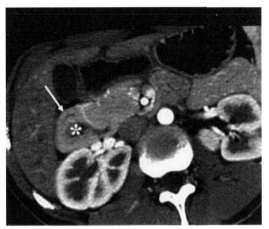

Source: Brambs H. Direct Diagnosis in Radiology. Gastrointestinal Imaging. 1st Edition. Thieme; 2007.

A. Ascending (fourth)

B. Descending (second)

C. Inferior (horizontal; third)

D. Superior (first)

32. A 22-year-old woman presents to the emergency department with severe abdominal pain and vaginal bleeding. A history indicates that she cannot recall when she had her last period and she acknowledges she could be pregnant. Physical examination shows abdominal rigidity and tenderness and a pelvic examination discloses a cervical motion tenderness. Ultrasound indicates fluid in the rectouterine pouch (of Douglas) and a ruptured ectopic pregnancy is suspected. The first attempt to sample the fluid by culdocentesis through the posterior vaginal fornix yields a fecal aspirate. Which of the following organs was most likely inadvertently punctured during the procedure?

A. Cecum

B. Descending colon

C. Proximal portion of jejunum

D. Rectum

E. Sigmoid colon

Consider the following case for questions 33 and 34:

An 81-year-old man presents to the emergency department with severe abdominal pain and hypotension. A patient history reveals that he had experienced heartburn and upper abdominal discomfort for the past 2 days, but he reports no nausea or vomiting, and his other bowel habits are normal. CT imaging reveals gas in the retroperitoneum.

33. From which of the following portions of the gastrointestinal tract is the gas most likely escaping to enter the retroperitoneum?

A. Ampulla of duodenum (duodenal cap)
B. Descending part of duodenum
C. Jejunum
D. Pyloric antrum of stomach
E. Transverse colon

34. The gastroduodenal artery is ligated during the surgical repair of the lesion. Which of the following arteries will continue to supply blood to the pancreas in this patient?

A. Hepatic artery proper
B. Inferior mesenteric
C. Left gastric
D. Superior mesenteric
E. Right gastric

Consider the following case for questions 35 and 36:

A 60-year-old man with a 4-week history of intermittent chest pain that radiates to his back presents to his primary care physician. Evaluation for a cardiac source for the chest pain is not conclusive, but subsequent epigastric pain, indigestion, feeling bloated after eating, and heartburn raises a concern of a stomach lesion (refer to the *arrow* in the accompanying image).

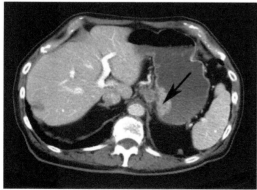

Source: Gunderman R. Essential Radiology. Clinical Presentation, Pathophysiology, Imaging. 3rd Edition. Thieme; 2014.

35. The mass (*arrow*) is most likely located in which of the following areas of the effected organ?

A. Cardia
B. Fundus
C. Greater curvature
D. Lesser curvature
E. Pylorus

36. During a gastrectomy in this patient, an additional tumor is detected in the fundus of the stomach. Which of the following arteries would need to be ligated that most directly supplies the area of the tumor?

A. Gastroduodenal
B. Left gastric
C. Left gastro-omental
D. Short gastric
E. Splenic

37. A 54-year-old man is admitted to the emergency department after indicating that for the previous 5 days he has been producing blood-tinged vomit (hematemesis) and has black stools (hematochezia). A history reveals active alcoholism and chronic hepatitis C. Physical examination shows a rounded abdomen, an enlarged, palpable liver, and moderate epigastric tenderness. A superior mesenteric venogram is ordered. Which of the following veins (*arrow*) exhibits the filling defect in the accompanying image?

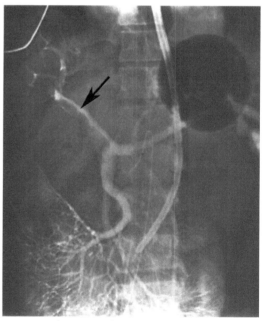

Source: Savader S, Trerotola S. Venous Interventional Radiology with Clinical Perspectives. 2nd Edition. Thieme; 2000.

A. Inferior mesenteric
B. Inferior vena cava
C. Portal
D. Splenic
E. Superior mesenteric

38. A 70-year-old woman with a history of alcoholism presents with hemoptysis (coughing up blood). A coronal, post-intravenous contrast CT of the abdomen and pelvis shows features consistent with portal hypertension (refer to the accompanying image). Which of the following organs is indicated by the *asterisk* in the CT?

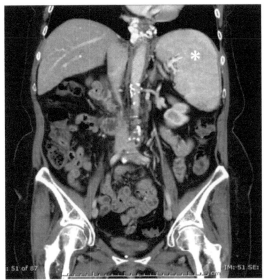

Source: Gunderman R. Essential Radiology. Clinical Presentation, Pathophysiology, Imaging. 3rd Edition. Thieme; 2014.

A. Fundus of stomach

B. Kidney

C. Liver

D. Pancreas

E. Spleen

39. A 34-year-old woman is referred to the gastroenterology clinic because she has had frequent, small volume, loose, bloody stools for the last 5 weeks. A patient history reveals that she has urgency to move her bowels and sometimes has left lower abdominal pain that diminishes after a bowel movement. Occasionally, she has low grade fevers. A contrast enema shows a dilated colon with numerous pseudopolyps and she is diagnosed with ulcerative colitis. Which characteristic feature of the effected bowel is most obviously lacking in the accompanying image?

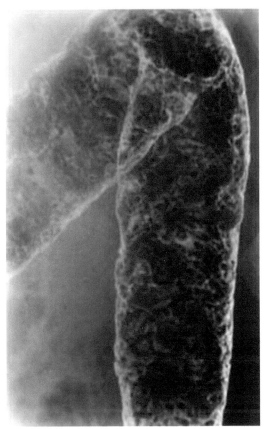

Source: Brambs H. Direct Diagnosis in Radiology. Gastrointestinal Imaging. 1st Edition. Thieme; 2007.

A. Circular folds

B. Haustra

C. Omental appendices

D. Pectinate line

E. Taeniae coli

40. A 54-year-old woman is admitted to the hospital after a motor vehicle accident. The patient is awake and alert, with stable vital signs. She is experiencing abdominal pain. A CT scan shows disruption of the pancreatic parenchyma with a small amount of peripancreatic fluid at the pancreatic head. Endoscopic retrograde cholangiopancreatography (ERCP) is ordered to evaluate the biliary and pancreatic ducts (refer to the accompanying image). In order to fill the biliary and pancreatic ducts as shown in the ERCP, into which of the following would the catheter need to be introduced?

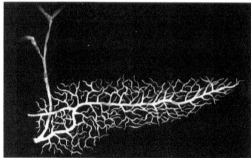

Source: Gunderman R. Essential Radiology. Clinical Presentation Pathophysiology, Imaging. 3rd Edition. Thieme; 2014.

A. Bile duct
B. Common hepatic duct
C. Cystic duct
D. Main pancreatic duct
E. Major duodenal papilla

41. A 59-year-old woman is referred to the gastroenterology clinic because she has noticed streaks of bright red blood on the toilet paper, and blood and mucus is visible on the surface of the stool. A history reveals that she sometimes experiences perianal itching and slight oozing from the anus that is not associated with defecation. Physical examination shows painless, hyperplastic vascular cushions that prolapse from the anus with a Valsalva maneuver (refer to the accompanying image). Anoscopy is used to diagnose grade III internal hemorrhoids. Tributaries of which of the following veins will be found in the prolapsed tissue?

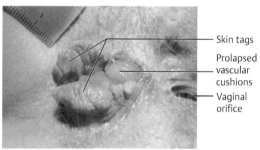

Skin tags

Prolapsed vascular cushions

Vaginal orifice

Source: Rohde, H. Lehratlas der Proktologie. Thieme, Stuttgart; 2006

A. Inferior rectal
B. Inferior vesical
C. Internal pudendal
D. Left colic
E. Superior rectal

42. The parents of a 3-month-old boy bring him to the pediatrician with concerns that the infant is experiencing recurring, intermittent bouts of loud crying during which he brings his knees to his chest. They relate that recently they have noticed small amounts of blood and mucus in his diapers. Imaging reveals that the child has a Meckel's diverticulum and, just proximal to that, there is intussusception ("telescoping" of a segment of bowel). Which portion of the intestinal tract is involved in this child's condition?

A. Duodenum
B. Ileum
C. Jejunum
D. Sigmoid colon
E. Transverse colon

43. A 63-year-old man is brought to the emergency department with constant abdominal pain and a feeling of nausea over the past 12 hours. The pain is localized to the left lower quadrant. A history indicates that he is overweight, leads a sedentary life, and suffers frequent bouts of constipation. Physical examination reveals increased abdominal pain when the left lower quadrant is compressed. His body temperature is 37.5°C (99.6°F). Coronal CT imaging results in a diagnosis of diverticulitis (refer to the *arrows* in the accompanying image) that involves which of the following portions of the intestinal tract?

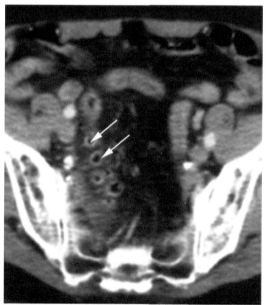

Source: Prokop M, Galanski M, van der Molen A et al. Spiral and Multislice. Computed Tomography of the Body. 1st Edition. Thieme; 2002.

A. Ascending colon
B. Descending colon
C. Rectum
D. Sigmoid colon
E. Transverse colon

Consider the following case for questions 44 and 45:

A 53-year-old woman with concerns about changes in her bowel habits visits her primary care physician. She indicates experiencing recurring episodes of lower bowel pain, bloating, abdominal discomfort, and a low energy level. She frequently uses laxatives to combat constipation and sometimes notices red blood streaks on her stools. She indicates she has lost approximately 55 kg (25 lb) over the past 6 months "without really trying." The initial evaluation is inconclusive and she is referred for further testing that leads to a diagnosis of rectal carcinoma.

44. Which of the following represents the average length of the section of bowel with pathology in this patient?

A. Fifty centimeters (~ 20 inches)
B. Seven centimeters (~ 3 inches)
C. Thirty centimeters (~ 12 inches)
D. Twelve centimeters (~ 5 inches)
E. Two hundred centimeters (~ 79 inches)

45. Which of the following represents the skeletal landmark for the junction of the diseased region of bowel with the region just proximal?

A. Body of S3 vertebra
B. Iliac crest
C. Ischial spine
D. Pelvic brim
E. Sacral promontory

46. A 28-year-old woman comes to the emergency department with sudden onset of severe abdominal cramping. Her history indicates she has vomited several times over the past several days and she is uncertain of when she last had a bowel movement. Physical examination reveals moderate abdominal distension. Imaging discloses a greatly distended region of colon with a point of constriction in the false pelvis (refer to the accompanying image). Sections of the colon proximal to the constriction also show distension while the area of the colon distal to the narrowing is collapsed. She is diagnosed with colonic volvulus (twisting of a section of colon). Which of the following mesenteries would be involved in the volvulus in this patient?

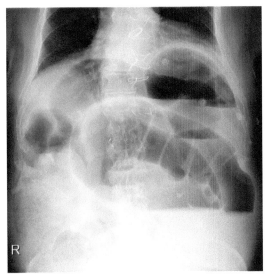

Source: Baxter A. Emergency Imaging. A Practical Guide. 1st Edition. Thieme; 2015.

A. Greater omentum
B. Lesser omentum
C. Mesentery of the small intestine
D. Sigmoid mesocolon
E. Transverse mesocolon

47. A 39-year-old woman is brought to the emergency department because she has "something stuck in my throat" that is causing discomfort and pain when she swallows. She indicates that 2 hours ago she inadvertently swallowed a fish bone which lodged in her throat. Drinking copious amounts of fluids and swallowing soft solids has failed to dislodge the bone. Fiber optic nasopharyngoscopy reveals a fish bone lodged in the right piriform recess. In which of the following regions is the bone lodged?

A. Esophagus

B. Laryngopharynx (hypopharynx)

C. Nasopharynx

D. Oral cavity proper

E. Oropharynx

48. A 46-year-old man visits his primary care physician because of intermittent episodes of pain along his jaw and floor of the mouth on the left side. He says the pain becomes worse at mealtime and then subsides over the next few hours. Physical examination reveals an enlarged, tender gland just inferior to the body of the mandible on the left side. Examination of the oral cavity exposes a calculus, visible through the mucosa, on the left side of the oral cavity floor. The calculus is located in which of the following?

A. Parotid duct

B. Sublingual duct

C. Submandibular duct

D. Thyroglossal duct

49. A 42-year-old woman is brought to the emergency department with upper abdominal pain that has become progressively worse over the past 2 days. She rates the pain as severe and indicates it frequently radiates to her back. During the initial evaluation she vomited. History indicates that she was incidentally diagnosed with cholelithiasis (gallstones) 2 years ago, but has remained asymptomatic and without treatment. A blood test indicates her serum amylase level is 580 U/L and lipase is 460 U/L (normal: 40–140 U/L and 0–160 U/L, respectively). A diagnosis of acute pancreatitis associated with gallstones is made. In which of the following would a gallstone be lodged to account for the patient's symptoms?

A. Bile duct

B. Common hepatic duct

C. Cystic duct

D. Gallbladder

E. Hepatopancreatic ampulla

50. A 38-year-old man presents to the emergency department concerned that he is having a stroke because, over the previous 4 hours, he is having increasing problems with leakage of food and liquids from the right side of his mouth. Following physical examination, he is diagnosed with facial nerve (Bell's) palsy. Paralysis of which of the following muscles is responsible for the patient's presenting symptom?

A. Buccinator

B. Genioglossus

C. Hyoglossus

D. Superior pharyngeal constrictor

E. Temporalis

Consider the following case for questions 51 and 52:

A 45-year-old man with previously diagnosed Huntington's disease (Huntington's chorea) presents to the otolaryngology clinic with dysarthria (difficulty with speech articulation) and dysphagia (difficulty swallowing). A history reveals that 4 years ago the appearance of involuntary movements of his limbs and face led to a Huntington's disease diagnosis. The dysphagia is a recent concern, with occasional aspiration of liquids and progressive difficulty eating solid food. During the physical examination the patient is not able to elevate the lateral margins of the tongue to form a central trough. Videofluorography of a barium swallow shows that fluid is retained in the valleculae and piriform recesses (fossa), indicative of incomplete pharyngeal elevation.

51. Impairment of which of the following muscles accounts for the tongue deficit?

A. Hyoglossus

B. Musculus uvulae

C. Mylohyoid

D. Palatoglossus

E. Styloglossus

52. Which of the following muscles is most likely impaired during swallowing?

A. Superior pharyngeal constrictor

B. Inferior pharyngeal constrictor

C. Palatoglossus

D. Styloglossus

E. Stylopharyngeus

53. A 49-year-old woman with a history of rectal carcinoma and recent resection presents with left lower quadrant pain one day after surveillance colonoscopy. An abdominal CT is ordered. Which of the following regions of the gastrointestinal tract is indicated by the *arrow* in the CT (refer to the accompanying image)?

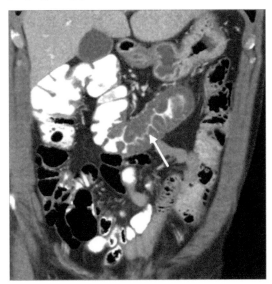

Source: Yu E, Jaffer N, Chung T et al. RadCases. Emergency Radiology. 1st Edition. Thieme; 2015.

A. Ascending colon

B. Cecum

C. Descending colon

D. Rectum

E. Transverse colon

54. A 60-year-old man with long-standing cirrhosis and portal vein thrombosis presents for a repeat splenic artery embolization to improve his portal hypertension by decreasing portal blood flow. Digital subtraction angiography of the celiac axis demonstrates complete occlusion of the splenic artery. Which of following organs is supplied directly by the artery indicated by the *arrow* in the accompanying image?

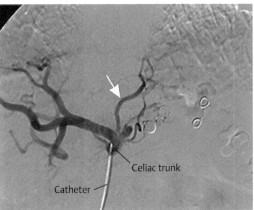

Source: Lubarsky M, Ray C, Funaki B. Embolization Agents— Which One Should Be Used When? Part 2: Small-Vessel Embolization. Semin Intervent Radiol. 2010 Mar; 27(1): 99–104.

A. Duodenum

B. Left lobe of liver

C. Pancreas

D. Right lobe of liver

E. Stomach

55. A 43-year-old man with sharp, shooting pain and pruritus (itching) in the anal region presents to his primary care physician. A history reveals that the symptoms are chronic, and that the pain intensity increases when defecating and while sitting. He reports that he has frequent episodes of constipation with hard stools and blood-streaked toilet tissue. Physical examination reveals an anal fissure in the posterior midline, inferior to the pectinate line. Which of the following nerves carries sensory information from the affected area in this patient?

A. Hypogastric

B. Inferior rectal

C. Pelvic splanchnic

D. Perineal

E. Sacral splanchnic

56. A 61-year-old man is in recovery following his first colonoscopy. The physician shows him images taken during the procedure and informs the patient that there are no signs of disease. The patient inquires about the part of bowel in the images that shows the lumen to have prominent transverse folds. Which area of the digestive tract has the characteristic observed by the patient?

A. Ascending colon
B. Descending colon
C. Rectum
D. Sigmoid colon
E. Transverse colon

57. A 31-year-old woman with a 10-year history of Crohn's disease visits her gastroenterologist because of severe abdominal cramping. Follow-up testing and imaging reveals that scar tissue has created an obstruction of a section of small intestine (refer to the *arrows* in the accompanying image). Which part of the small intestine is most likely obstructed in this patient?

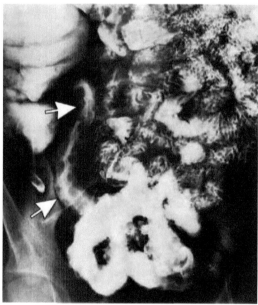

Source: Burgener F, Kormano M, Pudas T. Differential Diagnosis in Conventional Radiology. 3rd edition. Stuttgart: Thieme; 2007.

A. Distal ileum
B. Distal jejunum
C. Duodenum
D. Proximal ileum
E. Proximal jejunum

58. A 26-year-old woman, who had no prenatal care, delivers vaginally and without complications a male at 39 weeks. The baby shows no distress at birth, but presents with a large umbilical swelling that appears to contain loops of intestine (refer to the *arrows* in the accompanying image). He is transferred to the Newborn Intensive Care Unit, where a pediatric gastroenterologist is consulted. A radiograph of the abdomen reveals that the infant has an omphalocele. Which of the following is associated with this type of defect?

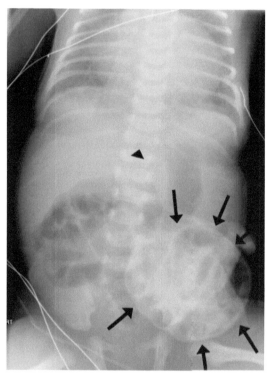

Source: Gunderman R, Delaney L. RadCases. Pediatric Imaging. 1st Edition. Thieme; 2010

A. A membrane covering the herniation
B. Accompanying ectopia cordis
C. Accompanying situs inversus
D. Bladder exstrophy
E. Lack of membrane covering

59. A 10-year-old girl is brought by her parents to the emergency department with abdominal pain and nausea that began 9 hours earlier. Prior to the onset of the pain, the patient was totally normal. Abdominal examination reveals rebound tenderness in the right lower quadrant. Ultrasound of the abdomen shows no signs of acute appendicitis, but fluid is detected in the pelvic cavity. Subsequent laparoscopic examination reveals perforation of the ileum approximately 2 feet from the ileocecal valve. An ileal segmental resection is performed and histological examination of the resected ileum reveals pancreatic tissue. Which of the following embryological structures failed to obliterate/regress in this patient?

A. Allantois

B. Cloaca

C. Umbilical vein

D. Urachus

E. Vitelline duct

60. A female infant is born prematurely to a woman whose pregnancy was complicated by polyhydramnios. The baby presents with abdominal distension and absent bowel sounds. Within a few hours after birth, the baby begins to produce bilious vomit. Gas is observed in the stomach and the superior part of the duodenum ("double bubble" sign) on radiographs (refer to the accompanying image). The congenital abnormality exhibited by this infant is most likely due to failure of which of the following?

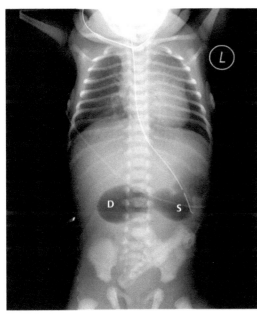

Source: Yu E, Jaffer N, Chung T et al. RadCases. Emergency Radiology. 1st Edition. Thieme; 2015

A. Endodermal tube to canalize

B. Esophagus to separate completely from the trachea

C. Midgut rotation

D. Physiological herniation

E. Smooth muscle development

61. A male infant is delivered at 38 weeks of gestation via cesarean delivery. At 15 weeks of gestation, elevated alpha-fetoprotein levels were detected and, consequently, a level II ultrasound (to identify fetal anomalies) was scheduled. The ultrasound revealed free intestine protruding from the anterior abdominal wall and floating in the amniotic cavity. At birth, intestinal loops are visible herniating through a defect in the anterior abdominal wall to the right of the umbilical stump. Which of the following is most correct regarding this congenital anomaly?

A. It frequently leads to lung hypoplasia

B. It generally occurs within the umbilical stump

C. It occurs due to weakness in developing abdominal wall muscles

D. It results from failure of the intestinal loops to return to the abdomen

E. It is usually covered by amnion

62. An 8-year-old girl with a 7-year history of feeling full after only a few bites, and recurrent vomiting after eating, is brought to the pediatric gastroenterologist. She has been treated for chronic gastroenteritis, but the problems persisted. The gastroenterologist orders an abdominal CT, which reveals an annular pancreas (pancreatic tissue encircling a portion of her intestines). A laparoscopic surgical bypass of the annular pancreas is performed and the girl makes a full recovery. Which portion of the gastrointestinal tract is most likely stenotic as a result of the congenital anomaly seen in this patient?

A. Duodenal–jejunal junction

B. First part of duodenum

C. Fourth part of duodenum

D. Second part of the duodenum

E. Third part of duodenum

251

6.2 Answers and Explanations

Easy	Medium	Hard

1. Correct: Lesser sac (D)

Refer to the following image for answer 1:

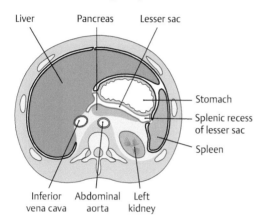

Source: Gilroy AM et al. Atlas of Anatomy. 3rd ed. 2016. Based on: Schuenke M, Schulte E, Schumacher U. THIEME Atlas of Anatomy. Volumes 1-3. Illustrations by Voll M and Wesker K. 2nd ed. New York: Thieme Medical Publishers; 2016

(**D**) The lesser sac (omental bursa) is the portion of the peritoneal cavity that lies between the pancreas (posteriorly) and stomach and lesser omentum (anteriorly). The pancreas is a retroperitoneal organ covered by peritoneum only on its anterior aspect. If a pancreatic cyst were to rupture through the peritoneum on the anterior surface of the pancreas, the fluid would initially collect in the lesser sac. (**A**) If fluid in the lesser sac passes through the epiploic foramen, the passage between the greater and lesser sac, it would enter the greater sac. (**B**) The hepatorenal recess (Morison's pouch) is a portion of the greater sac located between the liver and the right kidney and suprarenal gland. It would not be the first place fluid from a ruptured pancreatic cyst would collect. (**C**) The left subphrenic recess is a space between the diaphragm and the liver, to the left of the falciform ligament. Since it is within the greater sac, it would not be the first place fluid would collect. (**E**) The rectouterine pouch (of Douglas) is the inferior-most extension of the greater sac in women that is located between the rectum and uterus. Because fluid from the cyst is within the lesser sac, it is not likely that the fluid would reach the rectouterine pouch.

2. Correct: Portal vein (D)

(**D**) In cirrhosis of the liver, blood flow through the portal vein is compromised, which results in portal hypertension (increased pressure within the portal vein). In the lower third of the esophagus, there is a portosystemic anastomosis between the esophageal tributaries of the left gastric vein (part of the hepatic portal system) and esophageal tributaries of the azygos vein (part of the systemic or caval system of veins). In liver disease, increased blood flow and pressure in submucosal esophageal veins results their distension and leads to varices. The esophageal varices may rupture and result in vomiting of blood (hematemesis). (**A, B**) The aorta and left gastric artery are systemic arteries and are not affected by portal hypertension caused by the cirrhotic liver. (**C, E**) The left renal vein and superior vena cava are systemic veins and are not involved in portosystemic anastomoses.

Refer to the following image for answer 2:

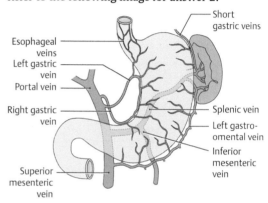

Source: Schuenke M, Schulte E, Schumacher U. THIEME Atlas of Anatomy. Internal Organs. Illustrations by Voll M and Wesker K. 2nd ed. New York: Thieme Medical Publishers; 2016

3. Correct: Hepatic artery proper (C)

(**C**) The hepatoduodenal ligament, the free margin of the lesser omentum, contains the portal triad: hepatic artery proper, bile duct, and portal vein. During donor hepatectomy, a Pringle maneuver uses a Satinski clamp to compress the hepatic artery proper and the portal vein to prevent excessive bleeding. (**A**) The common hepatic artery, a branch of the celiac trunk, does not pass through the hepatoduodenal ligament and would not be compressed during this procedure. (**B**) The gastroduodenal artery typically arises from the common hepatic artery. It does not pass through the hepatoduodenal ligament and would not be compressed during this procedure. (**D**) The inferior vena cava is not contained within the hepatoduodenal ligament. It forms the posterior boundary of the epiploic foramen and can be iatrogenically damaged by an improperly placed clamp on hepatoduodenal ligament. (**E**) The left gastric artery, a branch of the celiac trunk does not pass through the hepatoduodenal ligament and would not be compressed during this procedure.

Refer to the following image for answer 3:

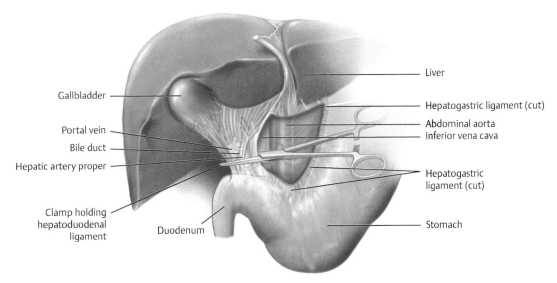

4. Correct: Vasa rectae (E)

Refer to the following image for answer 4:

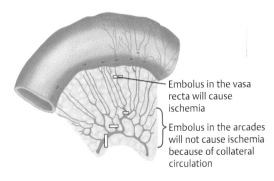

(E) The vasa rectae of the small intestine are end arteries (there is no collateral circulation to the intestinal wall they supply). Therefore, obstruction of these arteries by emboli will most likely result in ischemia of the bowel. (A) An embolus in an arterial arcade will not cause ischemia to a section of bowel since they have a collateral circulation. (B) An embolus in the inferior mesenteric artery will not cause ischemia to the bowel since there is collateral circulation via the marginal artery (of Drummond). (C) An embolus in the marginal artery (of Drummond) will not cause ischemia as there is collateral circulation. (D) An embolus in the right colic artery will not cause ischemia as there is collateral circulation through the marginal artery (of Drummond).

5. Correct: Cystic duct (C)

(C) During cholecystectomy (gallbladder removal), the cystic artery that supplies the gallbladder has to be ligated to minimize bleeding. This artery is typically found in the cystohepatic triangle (of Calot), whose boundaries are: the visceral surface of the right lobe of the liver (superiorly), the common hepatic duct (medially), and the cystic duct (laterally). (A) The celiac trunk is a direct branch of the abdominal aorta and is not located in the cystohepatic triangle. (B) The common hepatic artery is a direct branch of the celiac trunk and is not located in the cystohepatic triangle. (D) The hepatic artery proper, located lateral to the common hepatic duct, is part of the portal triad and is not located in the cystohepatic triangle. (E) The portal vein, located posterior to the common hepatic duct, is part of the portal triad and is not located in the cystohepatic triangle.

Refer to the following image for answer 5:

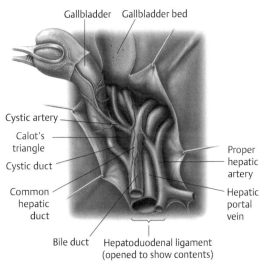

Source: Schuenke M, Schulte E, Schumacher U. THIEME Atlas of Anatomy. Internal Organs. Illustrations by Voll M and Wesker K. 2nd ed. New York: Thieme Medical Publishers; 2016

6. Correct: Neck (C)

(**C**) The splenic and superior mesenteric veins unite posterior to the neck of the pancreas, and anterior to the inferior vena cava, to form the portal vein at the L1 vertebral level. (**A**) The body of the pancreas is located anterior to the aorta and to the left of the superior mesenteric vessels at the L2 vertebral level.

(**B**) The head of the pancreas is located to the right of the superior mesenteric vessels, close to the second part of the duodenum. (**D**) The tail of the pancreas is related to the hilum of the spleen and the left kidney.

Refer to the following image for answer 6:

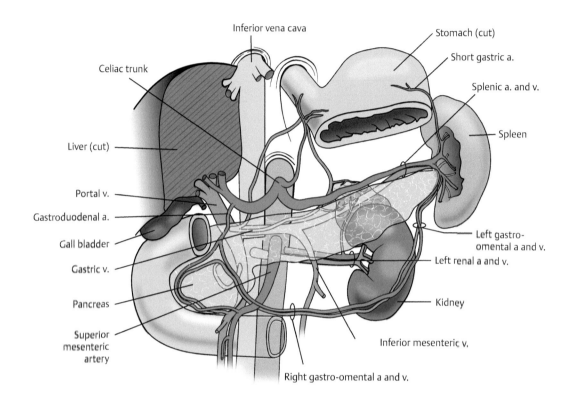

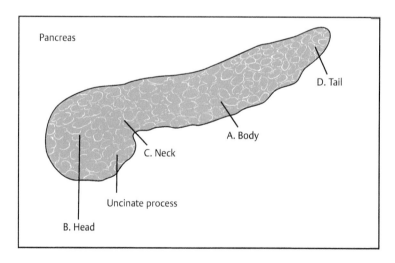

7. Correct: Sliding hiatal hernia (E)

Refer to the following image for answer 7:

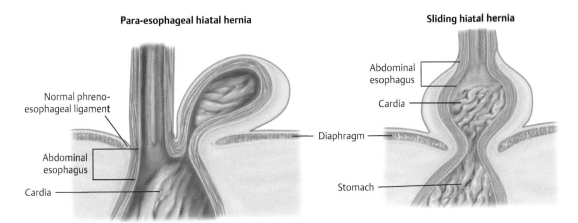

Para-esophageal hiatal hernia

Normal phreno-esophageal ligament

Abdominal esophagus

Cardia

Diaphragm

Sliding hiatal hernia

Abdominal esophagus

Cardia

Stomach

(**E**) A sliding hiatal (hiatus) hernia is characterized by the displacement of the gastroesophageal junction superior to the diaphragm. The abdominal portion of the esophagus and the cardia and parts of the fundus of the stomach slide superiorly through the esophageal hiatus (refer to the accompanying image b). This hernia is suspected in patients with symptoms of gastroesophageal reflux disease (GERD), including pyrosis (heartburn), regurgitation, and dysphagia (difficulty swallowing). (**A–C**) Patients with coronary artery disease, esophageal motility disorder, or esophagitis might present with symptoms similar to GERD. However, in these patients the gastroesophageal junction is not displaced. (**D**) A paraesophageal hernia is characterized by superior displacement of the fundus of stomach through the esophageal hiatus. The gastroesophageal junction and cardia of the stomach remain in their abdominal location.

8. Correct: Right crus (D)

(**D**) The right crus of the diaphragm arises from the L1 to L3 vertebral bodies and splits to form the esophageal hiatus. In a hiatal hernia, the portion of the stomach that protrudes through the esophageal hiatus into the thorax is in contact with muscle fibers from the right crus. (**A–C, E**) The central tendon of the diaphragm, muscle fibers from the costal and sternal attachments, and the left crus are not associated with the esophageal hiatus.

9. Correct: Transversalis fascia (E)

Refer to the following image for answer 9:

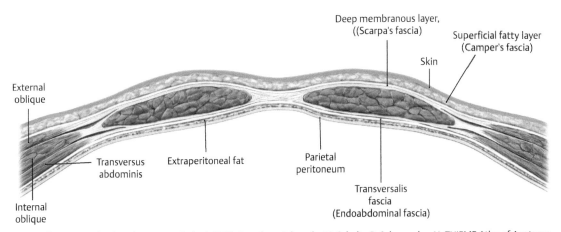

Deep membranous layer, ((Scarpa's fascia)

Superficial fatty layer (Camper's fascia)

Skin

External oblique

Transversus abdominis

Extraperitoneal fat

Parietal peritoneum

Transversalis fascia (Endoabdominal fascia)

Internal oblique

Source: Gilroy AM et al. Atlas of Anatomy. 3rd ed. 2016. Based on: Schuenke M, Schulte E, Schumacher U. THIEME Atlas of Anatomy. Volumes 1-3. Illustrations by Voll M and Wesker K. 2nd ed. New York: Thieme Medical Publishers; 2016

(E) During paracentesis, a large-bore needle is used to drain ascites for diagnostic or therapeutic purposes. The semilunar line marks the lateral edge of the rectus abdominis muscle. The abdominal oblique and transversus abdominis muscles lie lateral to this line. The needle will enter the peritoneal cavity after it passes, in order, through the following layers of the anterior abdominal wall: skin → superficial fascia (fatty layer/Camper's fascia) → superficial fascia (membranous layer/Scarpa's fascia) → external abdominal oblique muscle → internal abdominal oblique muscle → transversus abdominis muscle → transversalis fascia (endoabdominal fascia) → extraperitoneal fat → parietal peritoneum. (**A, D**) Extraperitoneal fat and parietal peritoneum are deep to the transversalis fascia and, therefore, would not be pierced immediately after the needle passes through transversus abdominis. (**B, C**) Both the fatty (Camper's) and membranous (Scarpa's) layers of superficial fascia are superficial to transversus abdominis. Therefore, they would not be pierced immediately after the needle passes through this muscle.

10. Correct: Lesser splanchnic (D)

(**D**) Generalized periumbilical pain that gradually localizes in the right lower quadrant is a classic sign of appendicitis. In the early stages of acute appendicitis, distension of the appendix and inflammation of its visceral peritoneum causes diffuse pain and discomfort in the periumbilical region (i.e., the T10 dermatome near the midline). Visceral sensory fibers from the appendix travel via the superior mesenteric plexus and lesser splanchnic nerve (sympathetic) to reach the neuronal cell bodies in the T10–T11 dorsal root ganglia. As the disease progresses, the parietal peritoneum near the appendix can become irritated and inflamed, which results in acute pain that is localized to the right lower abdominal quadrant. Somatic afferent fibers from the parietal peritoneum of the right lower quadrant are carried in the T10–T11 thoracoabdominal, subcostal

(T12) and iliohypogastric (L1) nerves. (**A–C, E**) the greater and least splanchnic nerves, and the superior and inferior hypogastric plexuses do not transmit visceral sensory fibers from the appendix.

11. Correct: Thoracoabdominal nerves T10–T11 (E)

(**E**) Generalized periumbilical pain that gradually localizes in the right lower quadrant is a classic sign of appendicitis. As the disease progresses, the parietal peritoneum around the appendix can become irritated and inflamed, which results in acute pain that is localized to the right lower abdominal quadrant. Somatic afferent fibers from the parietal peritoneum of the right lower quadrant are carried in the T10–T11 thoracoabdominal, subcostal (T12), and iliohypogastric (L1) nerves. In the early stages of acute appendicitis, distension of the appendix, and inflammation of its visceral peritoneum causes a diffuse periumbilical pain and discomfort. Visceral afferent fibers from the appendix travel via the superior mesenteric plexus and lesser splanchnic nerve (sympathetic nerves) to reach the neuronal cell bodies in the T10–T11 dorsal root ganglia. As the disease progresses, the parietal peritoneum around the appendix can become irritated and inflamed which results in acute pain that is localized to the right lower abdominal quadrant. Somatic afferent fibers from the parietal peritoneum of the right lower quadrant are carried in the T10–T11 thoracoabdominal, subcostal (T12) and iliohypogastric (L1) nerves. (**A–D**) The greater and least splanchnic nerves, the lumbosacral trunk, and the T7–T9 thoracoabdominal nerves do not transmit pain from the right lower quadrant.

12. Correct: Left colic (splenic) flexure (C)

Refer to the following images for answer 12:

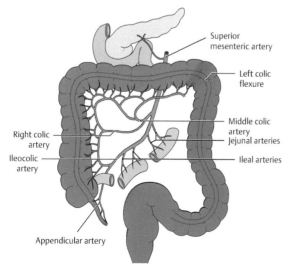

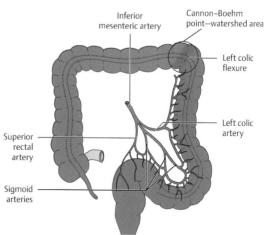

Source: Schuenke M, Schulte E, Schumacher U. THIEME Atlas of Anatomy. Internal Organs. Illustrations by Voll M and Wesker K. 2nd ed. New York: Thieme Medical Publishers; 2016

(**C**) The superior and inferior mesenteric arteries, which supply the intestines, anastomose via the marginal artery (of Drummond; juxtacolic artery) at the left colic (splenic) flexure. This region (known as the Cannon–Böhm point) is considered a "watershed" area in that it is most vulnerable to ischemia. Factors that contribute to increased susceptibility to ischemia are fewer arterial branches to the bowel at this point, and the splenic flexure is usually more superior and less mobile than the hepatic flexure. This patient has acute colonic pseudo-obstruction (ACPO, or Ogilvie's syndrome), which is characterized by acute dilation of the colon in the absence of a mechanical obstruction. The dilated intestinal segment has a greater wall tension that obstructs blood flow and causes ischemia and, eventually, necrosis. (**A, B, D, E**) The blood supply to the ascending colon, descending colon, right colic flexure, and sigmoid colon typically are not affected by bowel distension since the marginal artery (of Drummond) provides numerous branches to the intestinal wall in these regions.

13. Correct: Ileum (C)

(**C**) In advanced stages of typhoid fever, there may be inflammation of the lymphoid tissues in the intestinal wall, especially the Peyer's patches (part of the gut-associated lymphoid tissue, or GALT) of the ileum. Peyer's patches are oval to round thickenings of lymphoid follicles along the antimesenteric border. They are found in the lamina propria layer and may extend into the submucosa. Typhoid fever, which is caused by the bacterium Salmonella typhi, is spread by eating or drinking food or water contaminated with the feces of an infected person. People that travel to the developing world are at increased risk. Potential complications of typhoid fever involving GALT include luminal obstruction, bleeding, and perforation of the intestine. (**A, B, D, E**) Peyer's patches are not found in the duodenum, esophagus, jejunum, or stomach. Therefore, the inflamation is not located in any of these regions.

14. Correct: Sigmoid colon (E)

(**E**) The sigmoid colon is located in the left lower quadrant of the abdomen. With chronic constipation, fecal material will collect in the sigmoid colon, possibly causing distension to the point of being palpable. (**A**) The cecum is located in the right lower quadrant and would not be the structure palpated in this patient. (**B**) Loops of ileum may be located in the lower left abdominal quadrant but would most likely not be distended with fecal material to the point of being palpable. (**C**) The junction of the transverse and descending colon forms the left colic (splenic) flexure. It is located in the left upper quadrant and is fixed by the phrenicocolic (Hensing's) ligament. (**D**) The rectum collects feces and will distend, especially with constipation. The rectum begins opposite the S3 vertebral body, placing it in the true pelvis and, therefore, not palpable via the anterior abdominal wall.

15. Correct: Head of pancreas (D)

Refer to the following image for answer 15:

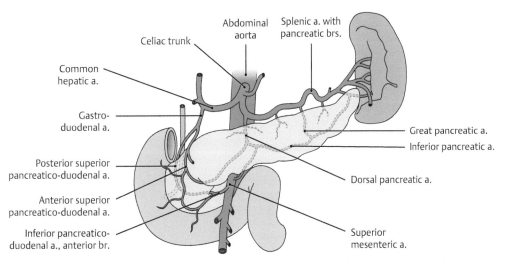

Source: Gilroy AM et al. Atlas of Anatomy. 3rd ed. 2016. Based on: Schuenke M, Schulte E, Schumacher U. THIEME Atlas of Anatomy. Volumes 1-3. Illustrations by Voll M and Wesker K. 2nd ed. New York: Thieme Medical Publishers; 2016

(**D**) The head of the pancreas, which is partly surrounded by the C-shaped duodenum, is supplied primarily by the gastroduodenal (derived from the celiac trunk) and inferior pancreaticoduodenal (derived from the superior mesenteric artery) arteries. These arteries must be ligated before the pancreatic head is removed. One cause of jaundice is obstruction of the bile duct posterior to the head of the pancreas as it passes to the second (descending) part of the duodenum. Carcinoma of the head of the pancreas could compress or obstruct the bile duct. (**A**) The body of the pancreas is supplied by branches from the splenic artery, which is a branch of celiac trunk. (**B**) The cystic artery, a branch of right hepatic artery, supplies the gallbladder fundus. (**C**) The fundus of the stomach is supplied by short gastric arteries, which are branches of the splenic artery. (**E**) The pylorus of the stomach is supplied by pyloric arteries, which are branches of the right gastric and right gastro-omental arteries.

16. Correct: Distal ileum (A)

(**A**) The distal ileum, which is typically located in the right lower abdominal quadrant, lacks luminal circular folds (plicae circulares), the fat in its mesentery encroaches onto the ileal wall, and the mesentery contains several generations of branching and anastomosing arteries (arterial arcades). The arteries that reach the intestinal wall (vasa recta) are shorter that those found in other regions of the small intestine. (**B, E**) The jejunum has luminal circular folds (plicae circulares) and typically has a thicker wall than the distal ileum. The jejunum also has fewer arterial arcades in the mesentery and fat distribution in the mesentery tends to not reach the intestinal wall, creating "windows" in the mesentery. (**C**) The first (superior) part of the duodenum (ampulla or duodenal cap) has luminal circular folds. It does have a mesentery, the hepatoduodenal ligament, but the mesentery does not contain arterial arcades. (**D**) The fourth (ascending) part of duodenum contains luminal circular folds and lacks a mesentery (is retroperitoneal) except at the duodenal–jejunal junction where it is attached to the diaphragm by the suspensory ligament of the duodenum (of Treitz).

17. Correct: In the oral vestibule adjacent to a second maxillary molar (C)

(**C**) The parotid (Stensen's) duct opens into the oral vestibule adjacent to the second maxillary molar.

The duct lies on the lateral surface of the masseter muscle and pierces the buccinator muscle to open into the vestibule (**A, B, D, E**) The parotid duct does not open into the oral cavity opposite any other molar teeth.

Refer to the following image for answer 17:

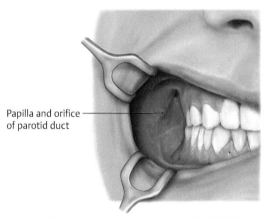

Papilla and orifice of parotid duct

Source: Schuenke M, Schulte E, Schumacher U. THIEME Atlas of Anatomy. Head, Neck, and Neuroanatomy. Illustrations by Voll M and Wesker K. 2nd ed. New York: Thieme Medical Publishers; 2016

18. Correct: Glossopharyngeal (B)

(**B**) The lingual branch of glossopharyngeal nerve (CN IX) innervates the posterior one-third of the tongue. It carries both general and special (taste) sensation. (**A**) The chorda tympani nerve (a branch of CN VII) contains afferent fibers for taste from the anterior two-thirds of the tongue and efferent preganglionic parasympathetic fibers for the submandibular and sublingual salivary glands. (**C**) The greater palatine nerve is sensory for the mucosa of the hard palate and the medial maxillary gingivae. (**D**) The internal laryngeal nerve, a branch of the superior laryngeal nerve from CN X, innervates a small area of tongue anterior to the epiglottis. It carries both general and taste sensations. (**E**) The lingual nerve, a branch of CN V3, innervates the anterior two-thirds of the tongue. It carries fibers for general sensation (temperature, touch) and its distal portion contains fibers from chorda tympani (via CN VII) that carry taste sensation from this part of the tongue.

19. Correct: Left lobe of liver (B)

Refer to the following image for answer 19:

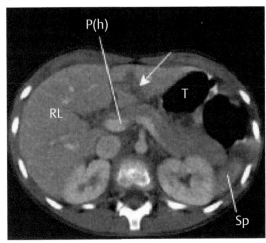

Source: Staatz G, Honnef D, Piroth W et al. Direct Diagnosis in Radiology. Pediatric Imaging. 1st Edition. Thieme; 2007.

(**B**) The structure with the laceration is the left lobe of the liver. (**A, C–E**) All of these structures (P[h], head of pancreas; RL, right lobe of liver; Sp, spleen; T, transverse colon) are visible in the CT, but none of them has the laceration.

20. Correct: Falciform ligament (C)

(**C**) The falciform ligament, a remnant of the fetal ventral mesentery, is a fold of peritoneum that separates the right and left lobes of the liver and attaches it to the anterior abdominal wall. The falciform ligament contains the round ligament of the liver (ligamentum teres hepatis, a fibrous remnant of the fetal umbilical vein) and the paraumbilical veins that contribute to a portosystemic venous anastomosis. (**A, B, D, E**) None of these structures (common hepatic artery, cystic duct, portal vein, proper hepatic artery) occupy the space between the right and left lobes of the liver.

Refer to the following image for answer 20:

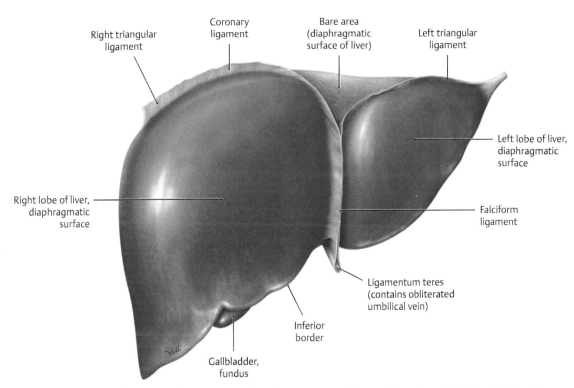

Source: Schuenke M, Schulte E, Schumacher U. THIEME Atlas of Anatomy. Internal Organs. Illustrations by Voll M and Wesker K. 2nd ed. New York: Thieme Medical Publishers; 2016

21. Correct: Medial to the inferior epigastric vessels (B)

Refer to the following image for answer 21:

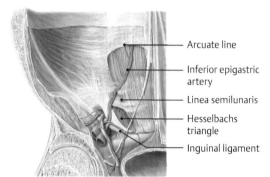

Arcuate line

Inferior epigastric artery

Linea semilunaris

Hesselbachs triangle

Inguinal ligament

Source: Gilroy AM et al. Atlas of Anatomy. 3rd ed. 2016. Based on: Schuenke M, Schulte E, Schumacher U. THIEME Atlas of Anatomy. Volumes 1-3. Illustrations by Voll M and Wesker K. 2nd ed. New York: Thieme Medical Publishers; 2016

(**B**) A swelling in the inguinal region of a 76-year-old man that emerges through the superficial ring is most likely a direct inguinal hernia. A direct inguinal hernia passes through the medial inguinal fossa (Hesselbach's triangle) which is bounded laterally by the inferior epigastric vessels (i.e., the neck of the hernial sac is medial to these vessels), medially by the semilunar line (the lateral margin of the rectus sheath), and inferiorly by the inguinal ligament. (**A, C–E**) None of these relationships (inferior to the inguinal ligament, medial to the pubic tubercle, medial to the semilunar line, superior to the arcuate line) describe the position of the neck of a hernial sac in a direct inguinal hernia as it passes through the medial inguinal fossa (Hesselbach's triangle).

22. Correct: Immediately distal to the origin of the short gastric arteries (B)

Refer to the following image for answer 22:

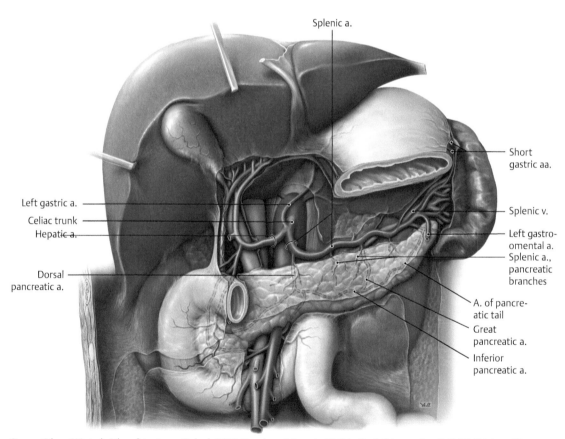

Splenic a.

Short gastric aa.

Splenic v.

Left gastric a.

Celiac trunk

Hepatic a.

Left gastro-omental a.

Splenic a., pancreatic branches

Dorsal pancreatic a.

A. of pancreatic tail

Great pancreatic a.

Inferior pancreatic a.

Source: Gilroy AM et al. Atlas of Anatomy. 3rd ed. 2016. Based on: Schuenke M, Schulte E, Schumacher U. THIEME Atlas of Anatomy. Volumes 1-3. Illustrations by Voll M and Wesker K. 2nd ed. New York: Thieme Medical Publishers; 2016

(**B**) To effectively remove the spleen and not compromise the blood supply to the pancreas and stomach, the splenic artery must be ligated immediately distal to the origin of the short gastric arteries that distribute to the fundus of the stomach. These vessels are the last branches of the splenic artery before it distributes to the spleen. (**A**) Ligation of the splenic artery immediately distal to the origin of the greater pancreatic artery would compromise the blood supply to the fundus (short gastric arteries) and the greater curvature of the stomach (left gastro-omental artery). (**C**) Ligation of the splenic artery immediately distal to the origin of the splenic artery from the celiac trunk would disrupt the blood supply to the pancreas (pancreatic branches and the dorsal pancreatic artery) and stomach (short gastric and left gastro-omental arteries). (**D**) Ligation of the splenic artery immediately proximal to the branching of the left gastro-omental artery would compromise the blood supply to greater curvature and fundus of the stomach. (**E**) Ligation of the splenic artery immediately proximal to the origin of the greater pancreatic artery would compromise the blood supply to part of the pancreas, as well as the fundus and greater curvature of the stomach.

23. Correct: Spleen (D)

(**D**) The spleen is an intraperitoneal organ located close to the 9th to 11th ribs in the left upper abdominal quadrant posterior to the midaxillary line. The healthy spleen is not palpable. In sickle cell disease, it may enlarge due to sequestration of damaged red blood cells and become palpable if it extends inferior to the costal margin. (**A**) The abdominal aorta is located to the left side of the midline and is not palpable near the costal margin. (**B**) The duodenum is located in the right upper quadrant. (**C**) The left kidney is located in the left upper quadrant, superior to the costal margin. The healthy kidney is not palpable and would not be expected to be enlarged in sickle cell disease. (**E**) The stomach is located primarily in the left upper quadrant and does not extend posterior to the midaxillary line.

24. Correct: Subphrenic recess (E)

(**E**) Following splenectomy, the patient has a postoperative infection with fluid collection in the left upper quadrant. The fluid most likely extends superiorly to the left subphrenic recess, especially when the patient is supine. Here, the fluid causes irritation of the diaphragmatic (parietal) peritoneum, which is innervated by the phrenic nerve (C3–C5). Consequently, the pain associated with irritation of the peritoneum is referred to the C3 to C5 dermatomes in the left shoulder region. (**A**) The costodiaphragmatic recesses are the pleural spaces into which the lungs expand during inspiration. The fluid within the abdominal cavity cannot spread into the thoracic cavity. (**B, C**) The left and right paracolic gutters are the lateral grooves between the descending and ascending colon and their respective posterolateral abdominal walls. Fluid in the abdominopelvic cavity can spread in the paracolic gutters to the supracolic or infracolic compartments. It is unlikely, however, that this fluid can directly cause the irritation of the diaphragmatic peritoneum. (**D**) The subhepatic space is a portion of the supracolic compartment inferior to the liver and would not directly contact parietal peritoneum on the diaphragm. However, fluid that collects here may extend superiorly to the right subphrenic recess when the person is supine and cause irritation of the diaphragmatic peritoneum and the resultant referral of pain to the right shoulder.

25. Correct: One-third of the distance from the anterior superior iliac spine to the umbilicus (C)

(**C**) The surface projection for the base of the vermiform appendix (i.e., the position at which it is attached to the cecum) is commonly located approximately one-third of the distance from the anterior superior iliac spine to the umbilicus. This position, known as McBurney's point, represents the location used to assess rebound tenderness associated with acute appendicitis. (**A, B, D, E**) None of these surface points overlie the root of the vermiform appendix.

Refer to the following image for answer 25:

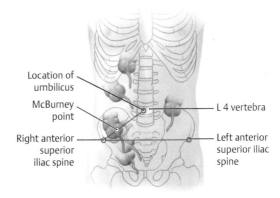

Location of umbilicus
McBurney point
Right anterior superior iliac spine
L 4 vertebra
Left anterior superior iliac spine

Source: Schuenke M, Schulte E, Schumacher U. THIEME Atlas of Anatomy. Internal Organs. Illustrations by Voll M and Wesker K. 2nd ed. New York: Thieme Medical Publishers; 2016

26. Correct: Horizontal (third) part of duodenum (B)

(**B**) The horizontal (third) part of the duodenum is located between the abdominal aorta (anteriorly) and the superior mesenteric artery and vein (posteriorly) at the L3 vertebral level. (**A, C–E**) The duodenal–jejunal and ileocecal junction, the pylorus of stomach, and transverse colon do not lie in the angle between the abdominal aorta and the superior mesenteric artery.

27. Correct: Subphrenic recess (D)

Refer to the following image for answer 27:

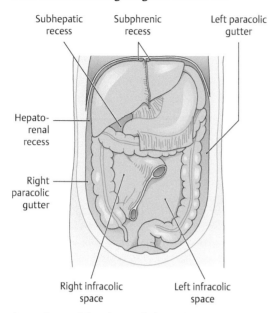

Source: Source: Schuenke M, Schulte E, Schumacher U. THIEME Atlas of Anatomy. Internal Organs. Illustrations by Voll M and Wesker K. 2nd ed. New York: Thieme Medical Publishers; 2016

(**D**) The subphrenic recess is located between the anterior and superior parts of the liver and the diaphragm. The coronary ligament forms the posterosuperior boundary of the space and the falciform ligament divides it into left and right portions. Air that collects in the peritoneal cavity, commonly from a perforated abdominal viscus, will most likely collect in this space and appear as an air bubble below the diaphragm in a chest radiograph of the upright patient. (**A**) The hepatorenal recess (Morison's pouch) is the space located between the liver and the right kidney. (**B**) The rectouterine pouch (of Douglas; cul-de-sac) is in the pelvic cavity and represents the most inferior portion of the greater sac of the peritoneal cavity in women. (**C**) The retropubic space (of Retzius) is located between the pubic symphysis and urinary bladder. (**E**) The vesicouterine pouch is a pelvic portion of the peritoneal cavity located between the uterus and bladder in women.

28. Correct: Rib 9 along the midclavicular line (D)

(**D**) The surface projection of the gallbladder is at the ninth rib along the midclavicular line. The sonographer places the probe at this location and applies pressure while directly visualizing the gallbladder. If the patient expresses pain during inhalation, it is considered a positive Murphy's sign (which is indicative of an inflamed gallbladder associated with cholecystitis). (**A–C, E, F**) The surface projection of the gallbladder is not associated with rib 7, rib 11, or the midaxillary line.

29. Correct: Gastrocolic (A)

Refer to the following image for answer 29:

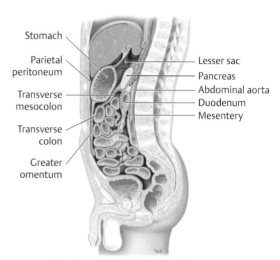

Source: Schuenke M, Schulte E, Schumacher U. THIEME Atlas of Anatomy. Internal Organs. Illustrations by Voll M and Wesker K. 2nd ed. New York: Thieme Medical Publishers; 2016

(**A**) With a gastric ulcer that has perforated the posterior wall of the stomach, gastric fluid will initially collect in the lesser sac (omental bursa), a portion of the peritoneal cavity. The inferior recess of the lesser sac extends into the gastrocolic ligament (part of the greater omentum) that connects the greater curvature of the stomach to the transverse colon. The extent of the inferior recess varies depending on the degree of fusion of adjacent layers of the gastrocolic ligament. (**B**) The gastrophrenic ligament is a part of the greater omentum that connects the greater curvature of stomach with the diaphragm. (**C**) The gastrosplenic ligament is a part of the greater omentum that connects the greater curvature of stomach with the hilum of the spleen. (**D**) The hepatoduodenal ligament is a part of the lesser omentum that connects the porta hepatis of the liver to the superior part of the duodenum. (**E**) The triangular ligament connects the superior surface of the liver to the diaphragm. It continues as the falciform ligament anteriorly.

30. Correct: Fundus of stomach (C)

(**C**) Air or gas is commonly seen on a radiograph of the gastrointestinal tract. Typically, air accumulates in the fundus of the stomach when the patient is standing. It appears as a radiolucent area directly under the left hemidiaphragm. (**A, B, D, E**) Under nonpathological conditions, reliable and predictable collections of air are not seen in the cardia or pylorus of the stomach, or in the second or third parts of the duodenum.

31. Correct: Descending (second) (B)

(**B**) In a case of an annular pancreas, the descending (second) part of the duodenum is surrounded by a ring of pancreatic tissue that is continuous with the head of the pancreas. This portion of the duodenum may be partially or completely occluded and result in signs of intestinal obstruction: chronic abdominal pain, nausea, and vomiting. (**A, C, D**) An annular pancreas typically does not surround the ascending, inferior, or superior parts of the duodenum.

32. Correct: Rectum (D)

(**D**) The rectouterine pouch (of Douglas) is the inferior-most extension of the peritoneal cavity (greater sac). It is located in the female pelvic cavity between the rectum and uterus (in men, this space is represented by the rectovesical pouch). Fluid (e.g., blood, ascites, pus) can collect in this recess when the woman is standing. During culdocentesis, a needle is inserted through the posterior fornix of the vagina to access the rectouterine pouch. Since the rectum forms the posterior border of the rectouterine pouch, it is not unusual for the rectum to be punctured during culdocentesis, resulting in fecal material in the aspirate. This is seldom a serious clinical situation. (**A–C, E**) The proximal jejunum, cecum, descending, and sigmoid colon do not typically occupy, nor form the posterior boundary of, the rectouterine pouch.

33. Correct: Descending part of duodenum (B)

(**B**) Retroperitoneal gas can result from rupture of a hollow viscus that is retroperitoneal. The portions of the gastrointestinal tract where this is possible include most of the duodenum (except the ampulla/duodenal cap), as well as the ascending and descending colon. (**A, C–E**) The ampulla of the duodenum (duodenal cap), jejunum, pyloric antrum of stomach, and transverse colon, each have a mesentery and, therefore, are intraperitoneal. A lesion/rupture of one of these organs may release air or fluid (depending on the organ) into the greater or lesser peritoneal sacs.

Refer to the following image for answer 33:

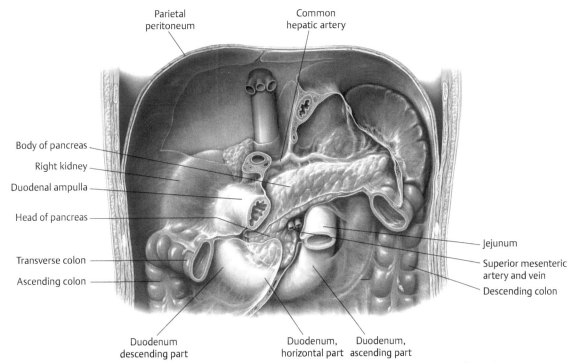

Source: Schuenke M, Schulte E, Schumacher U. THIEME Atlas of Anatomy. Internal Organs. Illustrations by Voll M and Wesker K. 2nd ed. New York: Thieme Medical Publishers; 2016

34. Correct: Superior mesenteric (D)

Refer to the following images for answer 34:

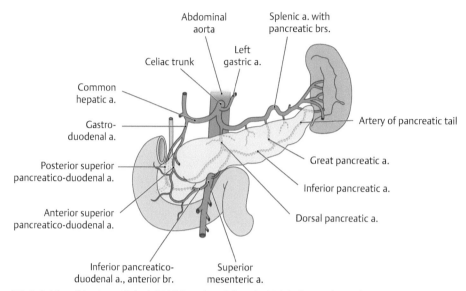

Source: Gilroy AM et al. Atlas of Anatomy. 3rd ed. 2016. Based on: Schuenke M, Schulte E, Schumacher U. THIEME Atlas of Anatomy. Volumes 1-3. Illustrations by Voll M and Wesker K. 2nd ed. New York: Thieme Medical Publishers; 2016

(**D**) The pancreas is supplied by arteries derived from the celiac trunk and superior mesenteric (SMA) artery. The superior pancreaticoduodenal arteries are derived from the gastroduodenal (which was ligated in this patient). The dorsal, inferior, and great pancreatic arteries arise from the splenic, and the inferior pancreaticoduodenal arteries arise from the SMA. (**A–C, E**) The hepatic artery proper, and inferior mesenteric and right and left gastric arteries do not supply the pancreas.

35. Correct: Lesser curvature (D)

(**D**) The mass, a gastric adenocarcinoma, (*arrow* in the accompanying CT in A) is located along the lesser curvature ("L" in accompanying CT in A; yellow area in the accompanying image B) of the stomach. (**C, E**) The greater curvature ("G" in the accompanying CT in A) and pyloric region ("P" in the accompanying CT in A) are also labeled in accompanying image B. The cardia and fundus of the stomach are located superior to this CT section (A) and are not visible.

Refer to the following images for answer 35:

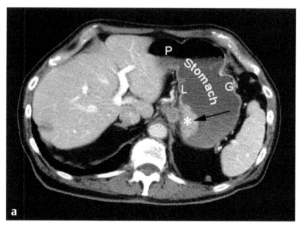

Source: Gunderman R. Essential Radiology. Clinical Presentation, Pathophysiology, Imaging. 3rd Edition. Thieme; 2014.

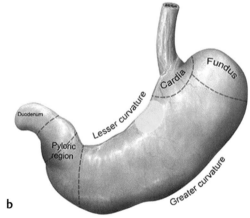

Source: Gilroy AM et al. Atlas of Anatomy. 3rd ed. 2016. Based on: Schuenke M, Schulte E, Schumacher U. THIEME Atlas of Anatomy. Volumes 1-3. Illustrations by Voll M and Wesker K. 2nd ed. New York: Thieme Medical Publishers; 2016

36. Correct: Short gastric (D)

Refer to the following image for answer 36:

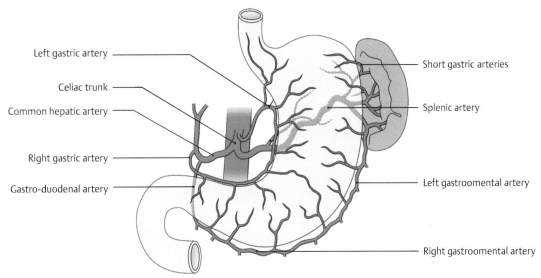

Left gastric artery

Celiac trunk

Common hepatic artery

Right gastric artery

Gastro-duodenal artery

Short gastric arteries

Splenic artery

Left gastroomental artery

Right gastroomental artery

Source: Schuenke M, Schulte E, Schumacher U. THIEME Atlas of Anatomy. Internal Organs. Illustrations by Voll M and Wesker K. 2nd ed. New York: Thieme Medical Publishers; 2016

(**D**) The short gastric arteries arise from the splenic artery and provide the primary blood supply to the fundus of the stomach. (**A**) The gastroduodenal artery is a terminal branch of the common hepatic artery and gives rise to branches that distribute to the duodenum, head of the pancreas, and greater curvature of the stomach. (**B**) The left gastric artery, which is typically the smallest branch of the celiac trunk, supplies the superior portion of the lesser curvature of the stomach. (**C**) The left gastro-omental artery is a branch of the splenic and supplies the left side of the greater curvature. (**E**) The splenic artery, typically the largest branch of the celiac trunk, gives rise to the short gastric arteries that distribute to the fundus of the stomach.

37. Correct: Portal (C)

(**C**) The portal vein ("P" in the accompanying venogram in A) exhibits an extensive filling defect that is consistent with a thrombus (*arrows* in the accompanying image a). (**A, B, D**) The inferior mesenteric, splenic, and superior mesenteric veins do not exhibit filling defects. (**E**) The inferior vena cava is not seen in either of the accompanying images. The typical arrangement of veins that form the portal is shown in accompanying image b.

Refer to the following images for answer 37:

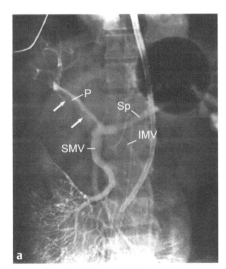

a

Source: Savader S, Trerotola S. Venous Interventional Radiology with Clinical Perspectives. 2nd Edition. Thieme; 2000.

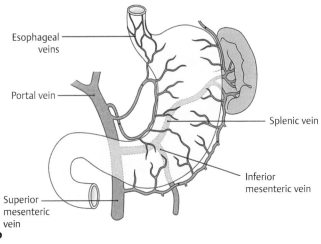

Esophageal veins

Portal vein

Splenic vein

Inferior mesenteric vein

Superior mesenteric vein

b

Source: Schuenke M, Schulte E, Schumacher U. THIEME Atlas of Anatomy. Internal Organs. Illustrations by Voll M and Wesker K. 2nd ed. New York: Thieme Medical Publishers; 2016

38. Correct: Spleen (E)

Refer to the following image for answer 38:

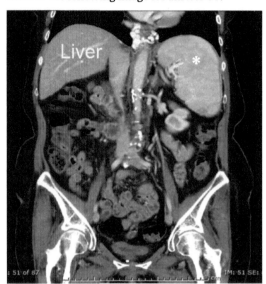

Source: Gunderman R. Essential Radiology. Clinical Presentation, Pathophysiology, Imaging. 3rd Edition. Thieme; 2014.

(**E**) The organ indicated is the enlarged spleen, secondary to portal hypertension caused by the patient's alcoholism. The spleen (*asterisk* in the accompanying image) is normally located in the left upper quadrant, along the posterior abdominal wall and just below the diaphragm. (**A, B, D**) The stomach, kidneys, and pancreas are not readily visible in this image. (**C**) The right lobe of the liver is apparent in the right upper quadrant.

39. Correct: Haustra (B)

(**B**) Ulcerative colitis is a chronic, inflammatory condition that affects the mucosa of the colon resulting in a thickening of the bowel wall in the distended state and an absence of haustra, which is a characteristic feature of the normal colon). This creates the abnormal, smooth, tube-like appearance that is evident in the image of the large intestine at the splenic (right colic) flexure. (**A**) Circular folds (plicae circulares) are characteristic of the small intestine, especially the jejunum and proximal ileum. (**C**) Omental appendices (appendices epiploicae) are small, fat-filled pouches attached along the external surface of the colon. While they are characteristic of the colon, they are not visualized in the image. (**D**) The pectinate (dentate) line, which represents the junction of the hindgut and proctodeum during development, is a feature of the anal canal in which a scalloped border is formed by the anal valves and sinuses. (**E**) Taeniae coli are longitudinal bands of muscle on the external surface of the colon. While they are characteristic of the colon, they are not visualized in the image.

40. Correct: Major duodenal papilla (E)

(**E**) The major duodenal papilla is a small elevation in the descending (second) part of the duodenum that contains the opening of the hepatopancreatic ampulla (of Vater), a short duct formed by the convergence of the bile duct (common bile duct) and the main pancreatic duct (of Wirsung). Introduction of contrast via the hepatopancreatic ampulla will permit filling of the biliary tree and the pancreatic ducts (as seen in the accompanying images). (**A–D**) Injection of contrast into any one component of the biliary tree or into the main pancreatic duct would not fill all biliary and pancreatic ducts. The bile duct and the main pancreatic duct converge to form the hepatopancreatic ampulla and only injection at this site would assure filling of all bile and pancreatic ducts.

Refer to the following images for answer 40:

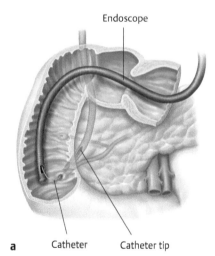

Source: Schuenke M, Schulte E, Schumacher U. THIEME Atlas of Anatomy. Internal Organs. Illustrations by Voll M and Wesker K. 2nd ed. New York: Thieme Medical Publishers; 2016

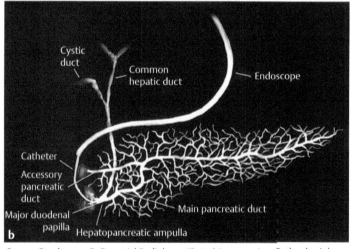

Source: Gunderman R. Essential Radiology. Clinical Presentation, Pathophysiology, Imaging. 3rd Edition. Thieme; 2014.

41. Correct: Superior rectal (E)

Refer to the following image for answer 41:

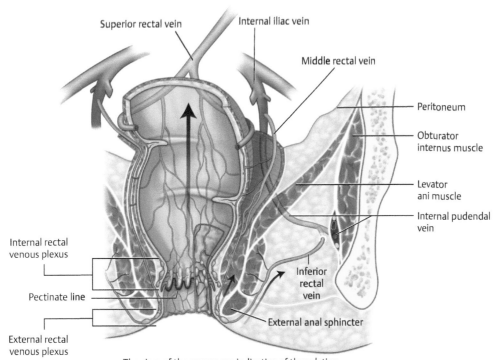

The sizes of the arrows are indicative of the relative volume of blood flowing through the superior, middle and inferior rectal veins

(**E**) Blood in the submucosal internal rectal (hemorrhoidal) venous plexus above the pectinate line of the anal canal drains primarily to the superior rectal vein, a tributary of the inferior mesenteric vein. This venous plexus is characterized by engorged anastomotic vessels that are organized into "anal cushions." With degeneration of the connective tissue in the mucous membrane overlying the anal cushions, they can descend along the anal canal as internal hemorrhoids and, with severity, prolapse through the anus. In addition, the engorged anal mucosa is easily traumatized, especially with the passage of stool, and is prone to bleeding. This blood is a brighter red than typical venous blood due to its relatively high oxygen content brought about by arteriovenous anastomoses. The lack of pruritis (itching) and perianal pain is consistent with the fact that the epithelium lining the prolapsed anal cushion is supplied by visceral afferent fibers. This is in contrast to external hemorrhoids that are associated with sharp, somatic pain because the skin over the thrombosed external rectal venous plexus has somatic innervation (via the inferior rectal nerve). (**A, C**) Blood in the external rectal (hemorrhoidal) venous plexus drains preferentially to the inferior rectal vein, which is a tributary of the internal pudendal vein. (**B**) The inferior vesical vein drains portions of the urinary bladder and does not receive blood from the anal canal. (**D**) The left colic vein, a tributary of the inferior mesenteric vein, does not receive blood from the anal canal.

42. Correct: Ileum (B)

(**B**) Meckel's diverticulum is a short, blind pouch extending from the wall of the ileum. It represents the developmental failure of complete degeneration of the vitelline (omphalomesenteric) duct. Meckel's diverticulum is said to follow a rule of "2s": it is approximately 2 inches long, is approximately 2 feet from the ileocecal junction, and is present in 2% of the general population. Since the intussusception is near the Meckel's diverticulum, the pathology involves the ileum. Intussusception is the leading cause of bowel obstruction in infants and it is suggested there is increased risk for telescoping of a section of the ileum in infants with a Meckel's diverticulum as the diverticulum serves as an "anchor" point for a section of bowel to slide inside an adjacent portion. (**A, C–D**) The intussusception is located just proximal to a Meckel's diverticulum, a feature always associated with the ileum.

43. Correct: Sigmoid colon (D)

(**D**) Small pouches (diverticula) most often form in the colon. The portion of the large bowel indicated in the CT image (at the level of the false pelvis) is the sigmoid colon. The presence of intestinal diverticula is

267

known as diverticulosis. When these small pouches become inflamed and/or infected, the diagnosis is diverticulitis. (**A, B, E**) While diverticula may form in any region of the colon, the ascending, transverse, and descending portions of the colon are not shown in the CT. (**C**) The rectum, part of the large intestine but not part of the colon, is not seen in the CT.

44. Correct: Twelve centimeters (~ 5 inches) (D)

(**D**) The human rectum averages 12 cm (4.5 inches) in length. (**A–C, E**) None of these other measurements accurately reflect the average length of the rectum.

45. Correct: Body of S3 vertebra (A)

Refer to the following image for answer 45:

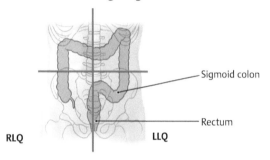

RLQ   LLQ

Source: Gilroy AM et al. Atlas of Anatomy. 3rd ed. 2016. Based on: Schuenke M, Schulte E, Schumacher U. THIEME Atlas of Anatomy. Volumes 1-3. Illustrations by Voll M and Wesker K. 2nd ed. New York: Thieme Medical Publishers; 2016

(**A**) The body of the S3 vertebra is generally considered to mark the junction of the sigmoid colon and rectum. (**B–E**) The iliac crest, ischial spine, pelvic brim and sacral promontory are not accurate landmarks for delineating the rectosigmoid junction.

46. Correct: Sigmoid mesocolon (D)

Refer to the following image for answer 46:

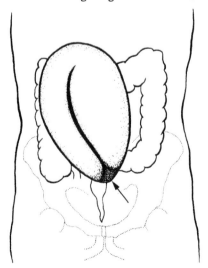

Source: Burgener F, Kormano M, Pudas T. Differential Diagnosis in Conventional Radiology. 3rd edition. Stuttgart: Thieme; 2007.

(**D**) This patient has volvulus of the sigmoid colon. As the sigmoid colon twists (volvulus), the sigmoid mesocolon (mesentery) will also undergo twisting. At the point of rotation, a narrowing or complete occlusion of the intestinal lumen will develop. The colon proximal to the stricture will show distension while segments of the colon distal to the narrowing will often be collapsed. The appearance in imaging is described as resembling a coffee bean. (**A**) The greater omentum extends between the greater curvature of the stomach and the transverse colon. (**B**) The lesser omentum extends between the lesser curvature of the stomach and the liver and first part of the duodenum. (**C**) The mesentery of the small intestine suspends most of the small intestine from the posterior abdominal wall. (**E**) The transverse mesocolon suspends the transverse colon from the posterior abdominal wall.

47. Correct: Laryngopharynx (hypopharynx) (B)

Refer to the following image for answer 47:

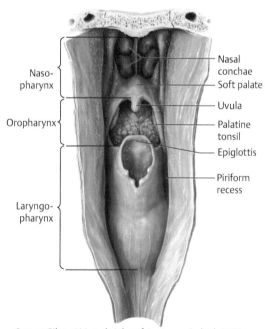

Source: Gilroy AM et al. Atlas of Anatomy. 3rd ed. 2016. Based on: Schuenke M, Schulte E, Schumacher U. THIEME Atlas of Anatomy. Volumes 1-3. Illustrations by Voll M and Wesker K. 2nd ed. New York: Thieme Medical Publishers; 2016

(**B**) The piriform recesses (fossae, sinuses) are paired, shallow depressions in the lateral walls of the laryngopharynx (hypopharynx). When swallowing, the epiglottis closes over the laryngeal inlet, diverting the food bolus laterally toward the piriform recesses. Hard particles such as pointed bones, seeds, and kernels in the bolus may become lodged in a piriform recess. (**A, C–E**) The piriform recess is not located in the esophagus, nasopharynx, oropharynx, or oral cavity proper.

48. Correct: Submandibular duct (C)

Refer to the following image for answer 48:

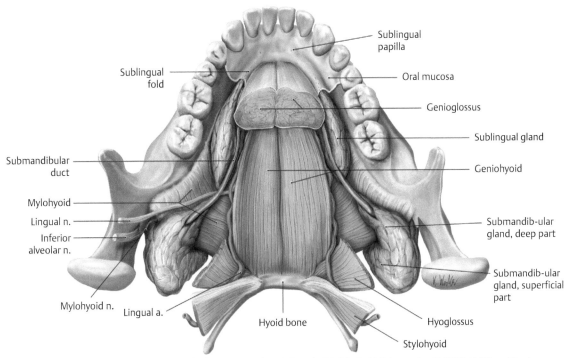

Source: Gilroy AM et al. Atlas of Anatomy. 3rd ed. 2016. Based on: Schuenke M, Schulte E, Schumacher U. THIEME Atlas of Anatomy. Volumes 1-3. Illustrations by Voll M and Wesker K. 2nd ed. New York: Thieme Medical Publishers; 2016

(**C**) The calculus (sialolith) is located in the submandibular duct, which courses in the submucosa of the floor of the oral cavity. The duct extends from the deep part of the submandibular gland and opens into the oral cavity at the sublingual papilla on the side of the frenulum of the tongue. Submandibular calculi usually form in the gland and enter the duct, where they may become lodged. If the calculus completely occludes the duct, pain and swelling occurs in the gland as secretions accumulate. Mealtime, and thinking about eating, stimulates the gland to increase secretions which explains why symptoms increase at these times. (**A**) Calculi may become lodged in the parotid (Stensen's) duct, causing pain and swelling of the parotid gland. However, the parotid gland is located posterior to the ramus of the mandible and its duct opens into the oral vestibule opposite the maxillary second molar tooth. (**B**) The sublingual gland rarely develops calculi and this gland drains directly into the floor of the oral cavity via 8 to 20 small, short ducts. The ducts open onto a narrow ridge of mucosa (sublingual fold) that overlies the gland itself. (**D**) The thyroglossal duct is an embryonic structure that buds from the floor of the developing oral cavity/pharynx. The distal part of the duct gives rise to the thyroid gland. Normally, the only remnant of the duct is a small blind diverticulum on the dorsum of the adult tongue (foramen cecum). In some individuals, a remnant of the distal portion of the duct forms the pyramidal lobe of the thyroid gland.

49. Correct: Hepatopancreatic ampulla (E)

Refer to the following image for answer 49:

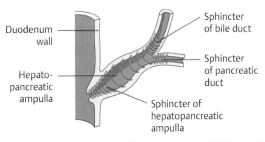

Source: Gilroy AM et al. Atlas of Anatomy. 3rd ed. 2016. Based on: Schuenke M, Schulte E, Schumacher U. THIEME Atlas of Anatomy. Volumes 1-3. Illustrations by Voll M and Wesker K. 2nd ed. New York: Thieme Medical Publishers; 2016

(**E**) The gallstone would be lodged in the hepatopancreatic ampulla to account for the development of acute pancreatitis. The bile duct (common bile duct) from the liver and gallbladder unites with the main pancreatic duct to form the hepatopancreatic ampulla. Blockage of the ampulla prevents pancreatic and liver secretions from entering the duodenum. The combination of bile entering the pancreas by retrograde flow and accumulation of pancreatic enzymes will lead to inflammation of the pancreas. (**A–D**) A gallstone located in the bile duct (common bile duct), common hepatic duct, cystic duct or gall bladder would not cause pancreatitis.

269

50. Correct: Buccinator (A)

(A) The buccinator and orbicularis oris muscles, with the tongue, work together to keep a bolus of food between the occlusal surfaces of the molar teeth during chewing. The buccinator muscle is innervated by the facial nerve (CN VII) and is, therefore, affected in Bell's palsy. (B–E) The genioglossus, hyoglossus, superior pharyngeal constrictor, and temporalis muscles are not innervated by the facial nerve and would not be affected in Bell's palsy.

51. Correct: Styloglossus (E)

(E) The styloglossus muscle retrudes and elevates the sides of the tongue to form a trough on the dorsum of the tongue to facilitate movement of a bolus into the pharynx. (A) The hyoglossus muscle depresses the sides of the tongue, an action opposite that of styloglossus. (B) Musculus uvulae shorten and pull the uvula of the soft palate superiorly. (C) The mylohyoid muscle elevates the floor of the mouth and, in turn, the tongue during swallowing. (D) Palatoglossus muscle acts to elevate the posterior portion of the tongue and, acting together, the paired muscles can close off the oral cavity from the oropharynx.

52. Correct: Stylopharyngeus (E)

(E) The stylopharyngeus muscle, with the other longitudinal pharyngeal muscles (palatopharyngeus and salpingopharyngeus) assist in elevation of the pharynx during swallowing. Muscles that elevate the larynx will also have a role in elevation of the pharynx since the pharynx is attached to the larynx via the inferior pharyngeal constrictor muscle. (A, B) The pharyngeal constrictors do not elevate the pharynx. (C) The palatoglossus muscle acts to elevate the posterior portion of the tongue and, acting together, the paired muscles can close off the oral cavity from the oropharynx. (D) The styloglossus retrudes and elevates the sides of the tongue.

53. Correct: Transverse colon (E)

(E) The portion of the bowel indicated by the *arrow* is the transverse colon. (A, C) Portions of the ascending (A) and descending (C) colon are visible. (B, D) The cecum and rectum are not readily apparent in this image.

54. Correct: Stomach (E)

(E) The left gastric artery (LGA in the accompanying arteriogram in image a) supplies the lesser curvature of the stomach and lower esophagus. Other branches of the celiac trunk are shown in accompanying image b. (A–D) The left gastric artery does not distribute to the duodenum, liver or pancreas.

Refer to the following images for answer 54:

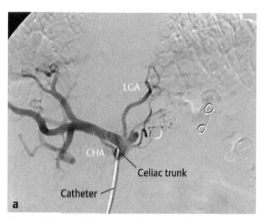

Source: Lubarsky M, Ray C, Funaki B. Embolization Agents—Which One Should Be Used When? Part 2: Small-Vessel Embolization. Semin Intervent Radiol. 2010 Mar; 27(1): 99–104.

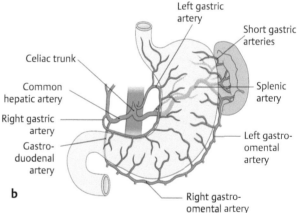

Source: Schuenke M, Schulte E, Schumacher U. THIEME Atlas of Anatomy. Internal Organs. Illustrations by Voll M and Wesker K. 2nd ed. New York: Thieme Medical Publishers; 2016

55. Correct: Inferior rectal (B)

(**B**) Most anal fissures occur in the posterior midline, in the region known as the anoderm that is between the pectinate (dentate) line and the anal margin. Anal fissures are commonly caused by hard stools as they pass through the lower anal canal. This region is innervated by the somatic inferior rectal nerve, a branch of the pudendal, which accounts for the sharp pain (especially during defecation), pruritus, and burning sensation. (**A, C, E**) The hypogastric, pelvic splanchnic, and sacral splanchnic nerves are visceral (autonomic) nerves and, therefore, do not transmit somatic pain from the lower anal canal. (**D**) The perineal nerve, also a branch of the pudendal, generally supplies structures in the urogenital triangle, including the labia majora and scrotum.

56. Correct: Rectum (C)

(**C**) The interior of the rectum is marked consistently by three large transverse rectal folds (two on the right and one on the left) that overlie thickened parts of the external muscle layer of the rectal wall. These folds correspond to the three lateral flexures of the rectum (superior and inferior on the left side and middle on the right) when the rectum is viewed from the anterior. (**A, B, D, E**) While the ascending, transverse, descending, and sigmoid colon possess semilunar luminal folds, they are not as prominent as in the rectum.

Refer to the following image for answer 56:

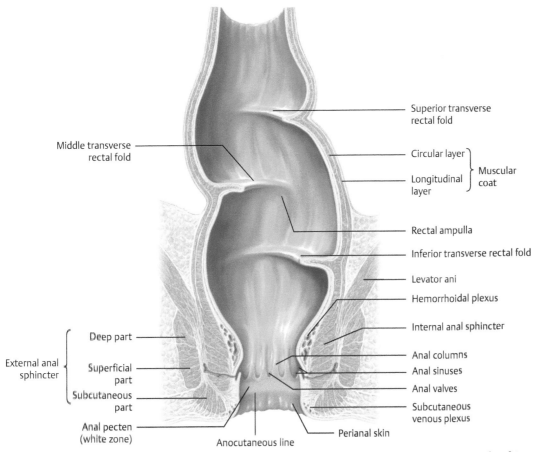

Source: Gilroy AM et al. Atlas of Anatomy. 3rd ed. 2016. Based on: Schuenke M, Schulte E, Schumacher U. THIEME Atlas of Anatomy. Volumes 1-3. Illustrations by Voll M and Wesker K. 2nd ed. New York: Thieme Medical Publishers; 2016

57. Distal ileum (A)

(**A**) Crohn's disease is a chronic inflammatory bowel disease that most often involves the terminal small intestine (ileum) and/or the colon. The bowel wall becomes thickened and scarred, potentially resulting in obstruction. (**B–E**) The duodenum, jejunum and proximal ileum are less often involved in Crohn's disease.

58. Correct: A membrane covering the herniation (A)

Refer to the following image for answer 58:

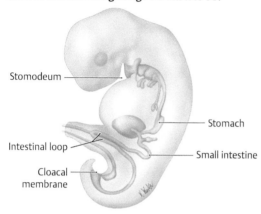

Source: Schuenke M, Schulte E, Schumacher U. THIEME Atlas of Anatomy. Internal Organs. Illustrations by Voll M and Wesker K. 2nd ed. New York: Thieme Medical Publishers; 2016

(A) An omphalocele is defined as a midline abdominal wall defect with herniated viscera covered by a membrane consisting of amnion on the outer surface and visceral peritoneum on the inner surface. During normal development, the midgut lengthens faster than the abdominal cavity can accommodate and protrudes into the umbilical cord. This normal process of "physiological herniation" begins at 6 weeks, with the herniated midgut normally returning to the abdomen by week 10. If the midgut loop fails to return, the intestines protrude into the umbilical cord, and grow along with the embryo. At birth, they will retain the coverings of the umbilical cord, which appears as a membrane covering the herniated viscera. (**B**) Ectopia cordis is a rare congenital defect due to a failure of fusion of the anterior chest wall that results in complete or partial displacement of the heart outside the thoracic cavity. (**C**) Situs inversus is not related to anterior abdominal wall defects, it occurs when all or part of the viscera are reversed from their normal position inside the abdominal or thoracic cavity. (**D**) Bladder exstrophy is an abdominal wall defect where the urinary bladder is open to the surface. It results from defective formation of abdominal muscles that normally develop in association with the cloacal membrane. (**E**) Another congenital defect that presents with herniated intestines at birth is gastroschisis. Here, the intestines herniate secondarily to their return to the abdomen during physiological herniation due to inadequate development of anterior abdominal wall muscles. The herniated intestines in gastroschisis are not covered with amnion and usually herniate to the right of the umbilicus.

59. Correct: Vitelline duct (E)

(**E**) Failure of regression of the vitelline (or omphalomesenteric) duct can lead to a Meckel's diverticulum, as seen in this patient. The vitelline duct, an embryonic structure that connects the yolk sac to the midgut, normally regresses or obliterates by week 12 of development. Several anomalies can result from this failure: Meckel's diverticulum, a patent vitelline duct, a vitelline ligament, or a vitelline sinus or cyst. Meckel's diverticulum occurs in approximately 2% of the population, is usually approximately 2 feet from the ileocecal valve, and is 2 inches long. Meckel's diverticulum often presents by the age of 2 if there is ectopic gastric or pancreatic tissue, since these cause ulceration and intestinal bleeding, but can be asymptomatic or appear later in life. A Meckel's diverticulum may remain silent throughout life, or may present incidentally. (**A, B, D**) The allantois is a diverticulum from the cloaca that projects into the umbilical cord. It normally regresses and its remnant is found in the median umbilical ligament in adults. If it fails to regress and retains its lumen it is called a patent urachus, which can result in discharge of urine from the umbilical stump in a newborn. (**C**) Remnants of the umbilical vein will form the ligamentum teres hepatis. It originates at the umbilicus and passes superiorly in the free margin of the falciform ligament and has no relationship to the midgut loop.

Refer to the following images for answer 59:

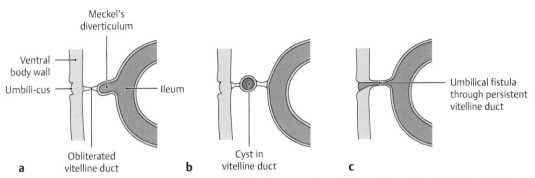

Source: Schuenke M, Schulte E, Schumacher U. THIEME Atlas of Anatomy. Internal Organs. Illustrations by Voll M and Wesker K. 2nd ed. New York: Thieme Medical Publishers; 2016

60. Correct: Endodermal tube to canalize (A)

(**A**) The symptoms and findings are characteristic of duodenal atresia in which there is a congenital absence of a duodenal lumen and intestinal obstruction due to failure of the endodermal tube to canalize. In duodenal atresia, increased levels of amniotic fluid occur during pregnancy (polyhydramnios) and symptoms of intestinal obstruction present in the newborn. The increased amniotic fluid results from the inability of the fetus to swallow and absorb the amniotic fluid. The "double bubble" sign is due to a dilated, fluid-filled stomach and proximal duodenum, and bilious vomiting is a consequence of atresia distal to the bile duct. These findings are a consequence of the failure of canalization, the process where the endoderm proliferates and fills the developing gut tube, followed by canal formation and creation of a lumen. (**B**) When the esophagus fails to be completely separated from the trachea, a tracheoesophageal fistula with or without esophageal atresia generally results. In this congenital anomaly, the infant often presents with coughing or choking, frothy oral secretions, and difficulty in breathing and feeding, and a nasogastric tube cannot be passed beyond the fistula or atresia. (**C**) Failure of midgut rotation (malrotation) can be complete or incomplete and will generally present as cramping, crying, and vomiting. It often results in intestinal blockage or volvulus, and can prevent the proper passage of food. (**D**) Physiological herniation is the normal process whereby the midgut loop herniates into the umbilical cord during weeks 6 to 10, and then returns to the abdominal cavity once it enlarges sufficiently. Failure of the midgut loop to return to the abdominal cavity will lead to omphalocele. (**E**) Abnormal smooth muscle development is generally associated with pyloric stenosis. In pyloric stenosis, the pylorus muscles thicken and block food from entering the duodenum. Pyloric stenosis generally presents with projectile vomiting. The enlarged pylorus can sometimes be palpated in the right upper quadrant or epigastrium, and is described as feeling like an olive.

61. Correct: It occurs due to weakness in developing abdominal wall muscles (C)

Refer to the following image for answer 61:

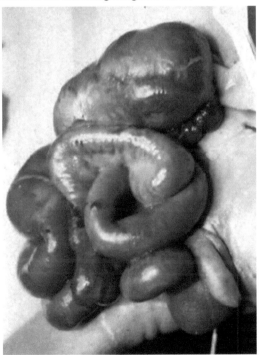

Source: Riccabona M. Pediatric Imaging Essentials. Radiography, Ultrasound, CT, and MRI in Neonates and Children. 1st Edition. Thieme; 2013

(C) Gastroschisis develops when the intestines herniate though the abdominal wall secondarily to physiological herniation, generally as a result of the failure of the anterior abdominal muscles to develop appropriately. The opening is often on the right side of the umbilical stump. In the most severe cases, the stomach and/or liver can also herniate. Since the intestines develop outside the body in the amniotic fluid, they are unprotected and can become irritated, swollen, and damaged. (A) Lung hypoplasia is more commonly associated with a congenital diaphragmatic hernia. (B, D, E) In omphalocele, the midgut herniates into the umbilical cord, fails to return to the abdominal cavity and, thus, continues to develop in the umbilical cord. Because the intestines develop in the umbilical stump in omphalocele, they are covered by amnion.

62. Correct: Second part of the duodenum (D)

(D) The pancreas develops from two endodermal outgrowths of the primitive gut, the dorsal and ventral pancreatic buds at the foregut/midgut junction, approximately at the level of the second part of the duodenum. The dorsal bud generates most of the pancreas whereas the ventral bud arises beside the bile duct and forms part of the head and uncinate process of the pancreas. (A–C, E) The pancreas develops in association with the second part of the duodenum and this portion of the duodenum is the portion most likely to be obstructed by an annular pancreas and not these other segments.

Refer to the following images for answer 62:

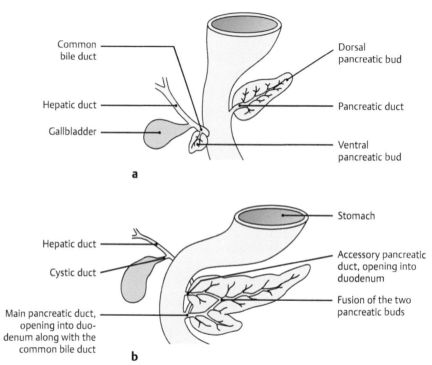

Source: Schuenke M, Schulte E, Schumacher U. THIEME Atlas of Anatomy. Internal Organs. Illustrations by Voll M and Wesker K. 2nd ed. New York: Thieme Medical Publishers; 2016

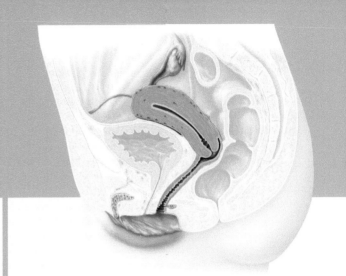

Chapter 7

Female Reproductive System

ANATOMICAL LEARNING OBJECTIVES

▶ Describe the anatomy of the female breast, including its neurovasculature and anatomical relationships.

▶ Describe the anatomy of the female pelvic organs, including their neurovasculature, peritoneal coverings, and anatomical relationships.

▶ Describe the anatomy of the pelvic floor, including its anatomical relationships and functional significance.

▶ Describe the anatomy of the female perineum, including its neurovasculature and anatomical relationships.

▶ Describe the anatomy relevant to a pelvic examination.

▶ Explain the stages of the female reproductive cycle.

▶ Recognize normal and pathological anatomy in standard diagnostic imaging of the female reproductive system.

7.1 Questions

Easy	Medium	Hard

1. During a scheduled annual examination of a 27-year-old woman, the gynecologist notes that the patient's external uterine os is stellate (star-shaped). Based on this observation, which of the following can be said of this patient?

A. She has had at least one cesarean delivery

B. She has had at least one vaginal delivery

C. She has never had a vaginal delivery

D. She is a virgin

E. She is pregnant

2. During a scheduled annual examination of a 45-year-old woman, the gynecologist cannot distinguish the fundus of the uterus by bimanual examination. Ultrasound reveals that the fundus is pressing against the rectum. Which of the following most likely describes the position of the patient's uterus?

A. Anteflexed

B. Anteverted

C. Normal

D. Retroflexed

E. Retroverted

Consider the following case for questions 3 and 4:

A second-year medical student is instructed by a physician, with the aid of a standardized patient, in the proper method of a pelvic examination. The student is instructed to palpate a pelvic ligament via the lateral vaginal fornix and to appreciate an arterial pulse in this ligament.

3. What ligament is the student palpating in this patient?

A. Pubocervical

B. Pubovesical

C. Sacrotuberous

D. Transverse cervical

E. Uterosacral

4. From which of the following arteries will the student distinguish a pulse during this procedure?

A. Inferior vesical

B. Internal iliac

C. Middle rectal

D. Uterine

E. Vaginal

5. A 41-year-old nulliparous woman presents with concerns about a recently self-detected dimple in the skin of her left breast. Physical examination shows a conspicuous skin depression in the upper lateral quadrant of that breast, and a mammogram reveals a spiculated mass within the same quadrant (refer to the *arrows* in accompanying image). Which of the following is the most likely cause of the skin dimple?

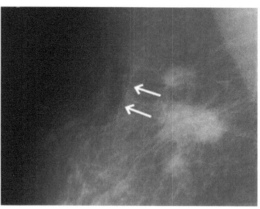

Source: Heywang-Köbrunner S, Schreer I, Barter S. Diagnostic Breast Imaging. Mammography, Sonography, Magnetic Resonance Imaging, and Interventional Procedures. 1st Edition. Thieme; 2014.

A. The mass has eroded the dermis in the area of the dimple

B. The mass has occluded some lobar ducts

C. The mass is compromising the blood and lymphatic supply for part of the breast

D. The mass is placing traction on the fibrous septa within the breast

E. There is a decreased amount of fat to maintain the breast contour

6. During laparoscopic surgery to treat an ovarian cyst in a 14-year-old girl, the surgeon notes a portion of the broad ligament that extends from the sides of the body of the uterus to the lateral wall of the pelvis. Which of the following structures lies between the layers of peritoneum in this part of the broad ligament?

A. Fimbria of the uterine tube

B. Internal iliac artery

C. Ovarian artery

D. Round ligament of the uterus

E. Vesicular appendage (mesonephric duct remnant)

7. A 34-year-old woman with a tender swelling at her vaginal opening presents to the physician. Physical examination reveals a reddened, cyst-like nodule on the right side of the introitus. Which of the following is the most likely cause for this condition?

A. Cystocele

B. Greater vestibular (Bartholin's) gland cyst

C. Sexually transmitted disease

D. Urinary tract infection

E. Vaginal wall cyst (Gartner's duct cyst)

8. A couple has not practiced birth control for 2 years, hoping for a pregnancy. Recently, they have been counseled to time intercourse to coincide with the woman's ovulation. Assuming that all goes as planned, in which of the following is an ovum most likely to be fertilized?

A. Ampulla of uterine tube

B. Infundibulum of uterine tube

C. Intramural portion of uterine tube

D. Isthmus of uterine tube

E. Uterine cavity

9. A 44-year-old multiparous, premenopausal woman explains to the physician that she has experienced many years of debilitating menstrual pain and heavy menstrual flow. She elects to undergo a vaginal hysterectomy. Which of the following is most vulnerable for iatrogenic injury when the major artery to the organ being removed is ligated?

A. Internal iliac artery

B. Internal pudendal artery

C. Suspensory ligament of the ovary

D. Sympathetic trunk

E. Ureter

10. A 38-year-old woman with a history of alcoholism visits the emergency department with abdominal pain and distension. Ultrasound (refer to the accompanying image) reveals fluid in the pelvic cavity. Which of the following peritoneal recesses most likely contains the fluid?

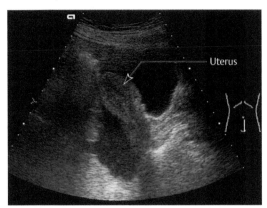

Source: Schmidt G, Greiner L, Nürnberg D. Differential Diagnosis in Ultrasound Imaging. 2nd Edition. Thieme; 2014.

A. Inferior recess of omental bursa

B. Lesser sac

C. Rectouterine pouch

D. Right paracolic gutter

E. Vesicouterine pouch

11. A 25-year-old primigravida (pregnant for the first time) woman is in active labor. The fetal heart sounds are of concern and the delivery room team decides an episiotomy would help the delivery. A mediolateral incision is performed. A midline incision is not performed because of concern for damage to which of the following muscles?

A. External anal sphincter

B. External urethral sphincter

C. Ischiocavernosus

D. Puborectalis

E. Superficial transverse perineal

12. A 31-year-old woman is scheduled for her annual physical examination. During her pelvic examination she finds the cold vaginal speculum uncomfortable. Which of the following spinal cord segments will receive the afferent impulses from the area of discomfort?

A. L2–L4

B. L3–L5

C. L4–S1

D. L5–S2

E. S2–S4

13. A 23-year-old woman with mild lower abdominal pain and dyspareunia (pain during intercourse) of approximately 6-weeks duration comes to the physician. She is relatively certain she is not pregnant. A pelvic examination indicates a mass on her right ovary. Transvaginal ultrasound reveals an anechoic ovarian cyst (refer to the accompanying image). Which of the following nerves will conduct pain from this cystic organ?

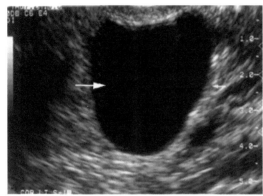

Source: Benson C, Bluth E, Ralls P et al. Ultrasound: A Practical Approach to Clinical Problems. 2nd Edition. New York: 2007.

A. Iliohypogastric

B. Obturator

C. Parasympathetic

D. Sympathetic

E. Vagus

14. A 19-year-old woman with mild vaginal bleeding, abdominal discomfort, nausea, and breast tenderness presents to the obstetrics and gynecology clinic. A history indicates she is sexually active with multiple partners, consumes 2 or 3 alcoholic beverages and smokes 15 to 20 cigarettes each day. She has missed her last two menstrual cycles and acknowledges that she could be pregnant. A blood test for human chorionic gonadotropin confirms pregnancy but transvaginal ultrasound reveals a small, empty uterus. Which of the following is the most likely site of implantation?

A. Loop of ileum

B. Mesometrium

C. Serosal surface of uterus

D. Surface of ovary

E. Uterine tube

15. A 12-year-old girl with abdominal cramping and progressive difficulty urinating is brought to the pediatrician. Although the symptoms suggest menstrual discomfort, she indicates she has had no menstrual flow. Physical examination reveals a dark red mass between the labia minora. She is diagnosed with an imperforate hymen. Which of the following is the normal expected age for perforation?

A. Eighteen months

B. Nine years

C. Perinatal period

D. Seven years

E. Three years

16. A 44-year-old woman comes to her primary care physician with chronic back and neck pain associated with breast size disproportionate to her height and weight. Subsequently, she elects to undergo breast reduction surgery that requires removal and repositioning of the nipples and areola. At her 6-month postoperative examination, sensation has not returned to the nipples and areola. Which of the following nerves normally conveys sensations from the area of skin removed and repositioned in this patient?

A. Anterior ramus of T4

B. Long thoracic nerve

C. Medial pectoral nerve

D. Medial supraclavicular nerve

E. Thoracodorsal nerve

17. A 38-year-old woman with concerns over the past four months about irregular menstrual bleeding and bleeding between menstrual periods, presents to her gynecologist. She is hypertensive and has a body mass index (BMI) of 32 (healthy weight for middle-age adult = BMI of 18.5–24.9). Hysterosonography (ultrasonography following injection of saline) is performed and the result is shown. The polyp (P) in the presented image is located in which of the following areas?

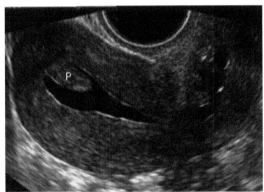

Source: Dogra V, Saad W. Ultrasound. Guided Procedures. 1st Edition. Thieme; 2009.

A. Body of uterus
B. Cervix of uterus
C. Fundus of uterus
D. Posterior vaginal fornix

18. A 44-year-old gravida 6, para 5 (six pregnancies, five deliveries) woman visits her gynecologist because she recently discovered a lump in her vagina that causes pain during intercourse. She indicates she is experiencing urgency to urinate and urination is often painful. She works for a local freight company and does considerable lifting as part of her job requirements. Physical examination reveals a soft bulge in the anterior vaginal wall near the vestibule. Which of the following is the most likely structure causing the bulge in this patient?

A. Cervix
B. Loop of ileum
C. Rectum
D. Sigmoid colon
E. Urinary bladder

19. A 58-year-old woman presents to her gynecologist with concerns that she experiences a "heaviness and pulling sensation" in her pelvis that tends to be more pronounced later in the day, especially if she has been on her feet for extended periods. She also frequently takes a stool softener as her bowel movements can be difficult otherwise. Her history indicates she has had three vaginal deliveries. Physical examination reveals the cervix is 2 cm from the vestibule. Which of the following structures is most likely compromised in this patient?

A. Broad ligament
B. External urethral sphincter
C. Ischiococcygeus (coccygeus) muscle
D. Obturator internus muscle
E. Pubococcygeus muscle

20. A 34-year-old woman visits her gynecologist because of urinary incontinence and a purulent vaginal discharge. Three weeks ago she experienced an obstructed labor during the vaginal delivery of a 4.5 kg (9.14 lb) baby. Physical examination reveals an abnormal tract between the urinary bladder and the adjacent vagina (vesicovaginal fistula). This diagnosis is confirmed by cystography (refer to the accompanying image), which shows contrast leaking from the bladder (B) into the vagina (arrows). Which of the following arteries provides blood to the area of the urinary bladder that has become necrotic and resulted in the fistula?

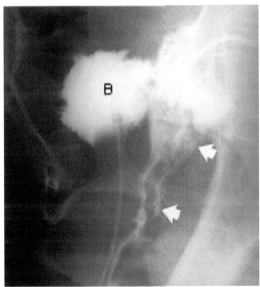

Source: Kadir S. Teaching Atlas of Interventional Radiology. Non-Vascular Interventional Procedures. 1st Edition. Thieme; 2006.

A. Inferior epigastric
B. Inferior rectal
C. Inferior vesical
D. Internal pudendal
E. Superior vesical

Consider the following case for questions 21 and 22:

A 32-year-old woman with suspected urinary bladder pathology is referred for MR imaging of her pelvis (refer to the accompanying image).

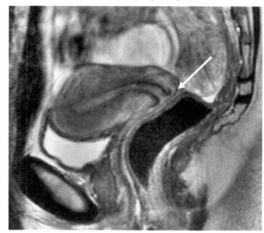

Source: Hamm B et al. MRT von Abdomen und Becken, 2 Aufl. Thieme, Stuttgart; 2006

21. Which of the following is indicated by the *arrow* on the MRI?

A. Anal canal
B. Cervical canal
C. Posterior fornix
D. Ureter
E. Urethra

22. Which of the following best describes the position of the uterus in the MRI?

A. Anteverted and anteflexed
B. Anteverted and retroflexed
C. Retroverted and anteflexed
D. Retroverted and retroflexed

23. A 28-year-old woman visits her gynecologist 10 days after the vaginal delivery of her first child, a 4.3kg (9.5lb) boy. She is experiencing perineal pain and a foul-smelling vaginal discharge. Physical examination reveals a midline anovaginal fistula. Which of the following muscles attaches to tissues involved in the fistula?

A. Bulbospongiosus
B. External urethral sphincter
C. Ischiocavernosus
D. Ischiococcygeus (coccygeus)
E. Obturator internus

24. A 28-year-old woman in labor requests analgesia and is administered a local anesthetic by bilateral pudendal nerve block. Which of the following structures would retain sensory innervation following this procedure?

A. External anal sphincter
B. External urethral sphincter
C. Glans clitoris
D. Iliococcygeus muscle
E. Ischiocavernosus muscle

25. A woman of indeterminate age is brought to the emergency department by ambulance after being found semiconscious in an alleyway. Physical evaluation reveals contusions on her face and both thighs, as well as hematomas in the labia majora. Evidence suggests she has been physically and sexually assaulted. Branches of which of the following arteries have been traumatized to account for the contusions of her external genitalia?

A. Deep artery of the clitoris
B. Dorsal artery of the clitoris
C. Inferior rectal
D. Internal pudendal
E. Superficial circumflex iliac

26. Transvaginal ultrasound on a 31-year-old woman with symptoms of endometriosis reveals fluid in her rectouterine pouch. The fluid is sampled by culdocentesis. Which of the following will be pierced by the needle used to sample the fluid?

A. Endometrium
B. Myometrium
C. Peritoneum
D. Simple columnar epithelium
E. Skeletal muscle

27. A newlywed couple, both 23 years old, visits their primary care physician because the woman is experiencing progressive, increasing pain during sexual intercourse (dyspareunia). During the past 2 weeks, her vaginal orifice constricted to the degree that penetration was not possible. She relates having no symptoms at other times and she uses tampons during her periods without discomfort. Physical examination reveals no pathology of her genitourinary system. She is diagnosed with vaginismus. Spasms in which of the following muscles is most likely involved in this condition?

A. Bulbospongiosus
B. Deep transverse perineal
C. Iliococcygeus
D. Ischiocavernosus
E. Obturator internus

28. Three days after falling astraddle a tree branch, a 30-year-old arborist visits her gynecologist because of pain, swelling, and bruising to her perineum. She also indicates there is pain during urination. Physical examination confirms hematomas in the labia majora and tissues of the vaginal vestibule. Pain is experienced when she provides a urine sample. Urinalysis is negative for urinary tract infection and she is referred for further evaluation. Urethroscopy reveals a longitudinal tear in the urethra superior to the perineal membrane. Which of the following also pierces this membrane?

A. Anorectal junction

B. Corpus cavernosum

C. Duct of the greater vestibular (Bartholin's) gland

D. Pudendal nerve

E. Vagina

29. A 48-year-old woman with a history of human papillomavirus (HPV) presents with progressively increasing itching and burning. She indicates redness has developed on her labia majora and she notices blood on her underclothing. Physical examination reveals three small ulcers in the skin of the labia majora. She is referred for further evaluation which leads to a diagnosis of vulvar carcinoma. In preparation for resection of the cancer, an anesthesiologist administers a bilateral pudendal nerve block and a second series of injections into the mons pubis. The second area of anesthetic administration will block impulse transmission in which of the following?

A. Dorsal nerve of the clitoris

B. Ilioinguinal nerve

C. Inferior rectal nerve

D. L5 ventral ramus

E. Posterior labial nerve

30. A 39-year-old woman with genital pruritus (itching) of several-months duration visits her gynecologist. A sexual history indicates fewer than five partners over the past two decades. Physical examination reveals several small, raised, pink lesions on the mucous membrane of the vaginal vestibule. She is diagnosed with genital warts (HPV). Which of the following nerves will conduct impulses generated by the itching?

A. Genitofemoral

B. Ilioinguinal

C. Inferior rectal

D. Posterior labial

E. Sacral parasympathetic

31. A 12-year-old girl is brought to her pediatrician with abrupt onset of excruciating pelvic pain accompanied by nausea and vomiting. Doppler ultrasound demonstrates a soft-tissue mass with minimal peripheral flow and no evidence of central flow on the right lateral pelvic wall. The main vessels that supply the organ with compromised blood flow pass through which of the following pelvic ligaments?

A. Ligament of the ovary

B. Round

C. Suspensory ligament of the ovary

D. Transverse cervical

E. Uterosacral ligament

32. A 26-year-old woman presents to the emergency department with acute onset of lower left quadrant pain and nausea. Her history reveals she is undergoing assisted reproduction treatment. A pregnancy test is negative and there is no obvious vaginal discharge or odor. Ultrasound reveals numerous cystic structures and Doppler ultrasound shows reduced blood flow to her left ovary. The resident suspects ovarian torsion and consults with surgery. An emergency laparoscopic surgery is performed to detorse the left ovary and neighboring uterine tube. The latter structure develops from which of the following?

A. Mesonephric duct

B. Mesonephric tubules

C. Paramesonephric duct

D. Primordial germ cells

E. Urogenital sinus

33. A newborn with an XX karyotype is diagnosed with ambiguous genitalia. Routine neonatal screening for 21-hydroxylase deficiency, detects 17-hydroxyprogesterone indicative of congenital adrenal hyperplasia. Ultrasound confirms the presence of ovaries, uterine tubes and a uterus. These results confirm a diagnosis of congenital adrenal hyperplasia and suggest that the small phallus observed in this patient is in fact an enlarged clitoris. Which of the following embryological structure(s) responded to the androgens in utero to produce the enlarged structure?

A. Genital tubercle

B. Labioscrotal folds

C. Urethral folds

D. Urogenital folds

E. Vestibule

34. A 36-year-old woman experiencing vague bilateral inguinal pain in her fifth month of pregnancy is referred to surgery as her obstetrician suspected inguinal hernias. On physical examination, visible masses are observed in the region of her superficial inguinal rings when she is erect, but they recede completely when she is supine. Ultrasound shows dilated spaces and Doppler ultrasound reveals that these spaces contain blood. The surgeon decides that the masses are varicosities associated with the remnants of an embryonic structure that normally courses from the inferior pole of the gonad and through the inguinal canal to the labioscrotal swellings. In females, this structure gives rise to which of the following structures?

A. Broad ligament and transverse cervical ligament

B. Mesosalpinx, mesovarium, and mesometrium

C. Round ligament of the uterus and proper ligament of the ovary

D. Scrotal ligament

E. Suspensory ligament of the ovary

35. A 21-year-old female presents with amenorrhea to the obstetrics and gynecology department. She reports that she is married but has been unable to conceive. On physical examination, the patient has normal breasts and external genitalia; however, a speculum examination reveals a hypoplastic vagina and no cervix is visible. Karyotyping reveals she is 46 XY and she is diagnosed with complete androgen insensitivity syndrome. Derivatives of which of the following would not be detected by ultrasound in this patient?

A. Gonadal ridge

B. Medullary sex cords

C. Metanephric blastema

D. Paramesonephric ducts

E. Ureteric bud

36. A 14-year-old girl is referred to the endocrinology clinic by her pediatrician due to her unusually short stature, underdeveloped breasts and amenorrhea. A hormonal study reveals elevated luteinizing hormone and follicle-stimulating hormone and reduced estradiol levels suggesting ovarian failure. An ultrasound shows that the patient has streak ovaries, and karyotyping revealed an XO genotype. She is diagnosed with Turner syndrome and is placed on estrogen replacement therapy. Which of the following statements is most correct concerning the gonads in this individual?

A. Cortical sex cords do not develop during establishment of the ovary

B. Primordial germ cells enter the ovary, but most primordial follicles regress before puberty

C. Primordial germ cells never enter the ovary to form primary oocytes and primordial follicles

D. Medullary sex cords do not develop during establishment of the ovary

E. Neither cortical nor medullary sex cords develop during establishment of the ovary

37. A 4-month-old female infant is brought to the pediatrician by her mother with the concern that the baby has a bulge in her right groin. On physical examination, a firm, oval, cystic swelling is found in the baby's inguinal region. The swelling is translucent and cannot be reduced. Ultrasound identifies a cystic mass of 3.2 cm that is subsequently excised. Pathological examination reveals that the excised tissue is peritoneum, which confirms a diagnosis of hydrocele of the canal of Nuck. The excised structure was derived from which of the following embryonic structures?

A. Cloacal membrane

B. Labioscrotal folds

C. Processus vaginalis

D. Urogenital folds

E. Urogenital sinus

38. A 53-year-old postmenopausal woman with concerns of vaginal bleeding for the last 20 days presents to her gynecologist. On pelvic examination, her uterus is enlarged and mobile, shows a possible myoma of the uterus and an adnexal mass. She undergoes a hysterectomy, bilateral salpingo-oophorectomy, and pelvic lymphadenectomy. Pathology reports the adnexal mass is a rare mesonephric carcinoma derived from remnants of mesonephric tubules. During normal development these structures will form which homologous structure(s) in the male and female, respectively?

A. Bulbourethral gland: bulbs of the vestibule

B. Efferent ductules: vestigial structures

C. Epididymis: uterine tubes

D. Prostate: paraurethral glands

E. Uterus masculinus: uterus

7.2 Answers and Explanations

Easy	Medium	Hard

1. Correct: She has had at least one vaginal delivery (B)

Refer to the following image for answer 1:

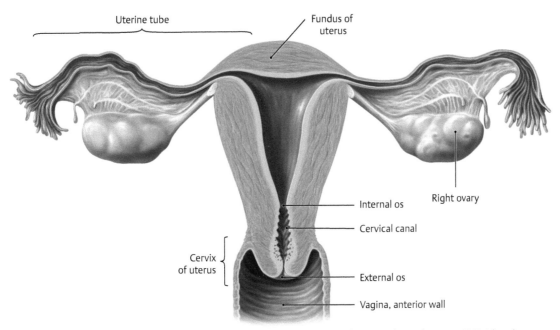

Uterine tube

Fundus of uterus

Internal os

Right ovary

Cervical canal

Cervix of uterus

External os

Vagina, anterior wall

Source: Gilroy AM et al. Atlas of Anatomy. 3rd ed. 2016. Based on: Schuenke M, Schulte E, Schumacher U. THIEME Atlas of Anatomy. Volumes 1-3. Illustrations by Voll M and Wesker K. 2nd ed. New York: Thieme Medical Publishers; 2016

(**B**) The external os of the cervix has a round-to-slightly-oval appearance in women who have never had a vaginal delivery. With the first vaginal delivery, the shape of the external os is permanently changed to a stellate appearance. (**A, C–E**) None of these conditions or situations alters the shape of the external os.

2. Correct: Retroverted (E)

(**E**) The uterus in this patient is retroverted. Version refers to the angle, which is formed at the external cervical os by the longitudinal axes of the cervical canal and the vagina (refer to accompanying image a, angle 2). Flexion refers to the angle formed at the internal os by the longitudinal axes of the uterine cavity and the cervical canal (refer to accompanying image a, angle 1). The normal uterine position is anteverted and anteflexed (**A–C**): anteflexion (**A**) occurs when there is a near 170-degree angle at the internal os (refer to accompanying image a, angle 1), whereas anteversion (**B**) occurs when there is a near 90-degree angle at the external os (refer to accompanying image a, angle 2). These angles place in the body of the uterus on the superior surface of the non-distended urinary bladder and, as a result, the fundus should be palpable by a bimanual examination (refer to accompanying image b). In this patient, however, the uterine fundus is in contact with the rectum. This occurs when the uterus is retroverted, implying that the angle at the external os is significantly greater than the 90 degrees associated with the anteverted uterus (refer to accompanying image b). (**D**) Retroflexion occurs when angle at the internal os is significantly greater than the 170 degrees associated with the normal anteflexed position.

Refer to the following image for answer 2:

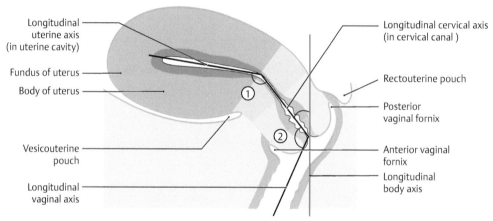

a

Source: Gilroy AM et al. Atlas of Anatomy. 3rd ed. 2016. Based on: Schuenke M, Schulte E, Schumacher U. THIEME Atlas of Anatomy. Volumes 1-3. Illustrations by Voll M and Wesker K. 2nd ed. New York: Thieme Medical Publishers; 2016

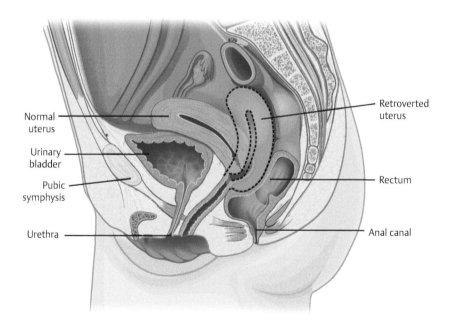

b

3. Correct: Transverse cervical (D)

Refer to the following image for answer 3:

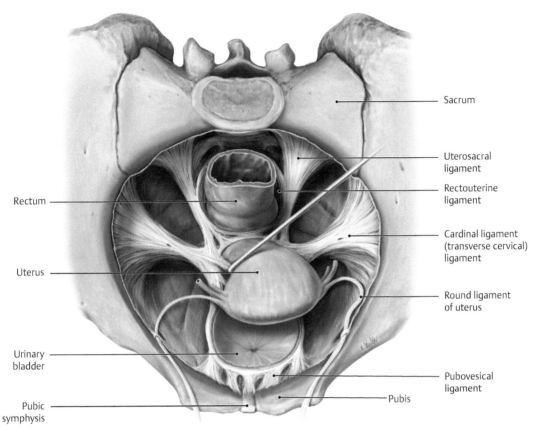

Source: Gilroy AM et al. Atlas of Anatomy. 3rd ed. 2016. Based on: Schuenke M, Schulte E, Schumacher U. THIEME Atlas of Anatomy. Volumes 1-3. Illustrations by Voll M and Wesker K. 2nd ed. New York: Thieme Medical Publishers; 2016

(**D**) Thickenings of endopelvic fascia form the transverse cervical (cardinal or Mackenrodt's) ligaments that radiate from the lateral pelvic walls to the supravaginal cervix. This ligament can be palpated via the lateral vaginal fornix and, together with the musculature of the pelvic floor, provides most of the support for the uterus. (**A, E**) The pubocervical and uterosacral ligaments are also endopelvic fascial thickenings that extend from the pubis and sacrum, respectively, to attach to the supravaginal cervix. They cannot be palpated readily via the lateral vaginal fornix. (**B, C**) The pubovesical and sacrotuberous ligaments cannot be palpated transvaginally.

4. Correct: Uterine (D)

Refer to the following image for answer 4:

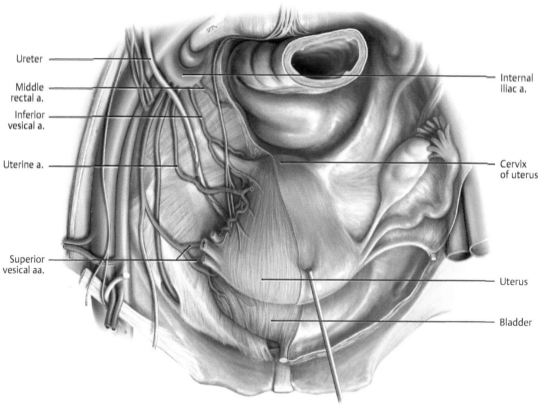

Ureter

Middle rectal a.

Inferior vesical a.

Uterine a.

Superior vesical aa.

Internal iliac a.

Cervix of uterus

Uterus

Bladder

Source: Gilroy AM et al. Atlas of Anatomy. 3rd ed. 2016. Based on: Schuenke M, Schulte E, Schumacher U. THIEME Atlas of Anatomy. Volumes 1-3. Illustrations by Voll M and Wesker K. 2nd ed. New York: Thieme Medical Publishers; 2016

(**D**) The uterine artery, a branch of the internal iliac artery, courses within the transverse cervical ligament to reach the uterus near the junction of the supravaginal cervix and the body of the uterus. The pulse of the uterine artery can normally be palpated through the wall of the lateral vaginal fornix. (**A–C, E**) A pulse within the inferior vesical, internal iliac, middle rectal, or vaginal arteries usually cannot be palpated or distinguished by transvaginal palpation.

5. Correct: The mass is placing traction on the fibrous septa within the breast (D)

Refer to the following image for answer 5:

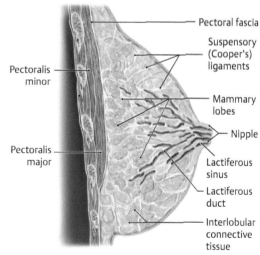

Pectoralis minor

Pectoralis major

Pectoral fascia

Suspensory (Cooper's) ligaments

Mammary lobes

Nipple

Lactiferous sinus

Lactiferous duct

Interlobular connective tissue

Source: Gilroy AM et al. Atlas of Anatomy. 3rd ed. 2016. Based on: Schuenke M, Schulte E, Schumacher U. THIEME Atlas of Anatomy. Volumes 1-3. Illustrations by Voll M and Wesker K. 2nd ed. New York: Thieme Medical Publishers; 2016

(**D**) Skin dimpling of the breast is due to traction on the connective tissue septa that divide the breast into 12 to 20 lobes. The most common cause of traction on the septa is malignant carcinoma of the breast. These adenocarcinomas are invasive and will create traction on the septa. These septa, best developed in the upper quadrants of the breast as suspensory (Cooper's) ligaments, are connected to the dermis and any traction on them will manifest as skin dimples of varying size. (**A, B, E**) While these may occur with breast carcinomas, they will not lead to skin dimpling. (**C**) The blood supply may actually be increased due to the vascular demands of tumors.

6. Correct: Round ligament of the uterus (D)

(**D**) The portion of the broad ligament that extends laterally from the sides of the body of the uterus is the mesometrium. The round ligament of the uterus, a vestigial remnant of the gubernaculum, lies between the double layer of peritoneum that forms the mesometrium. (**A–C, E**) The fimbriae of the uterine tube, internal iliac artery, ovarian artery and vesicular appendix are not located in this part of the broad ligament.

Refer to the following image for answer 6:

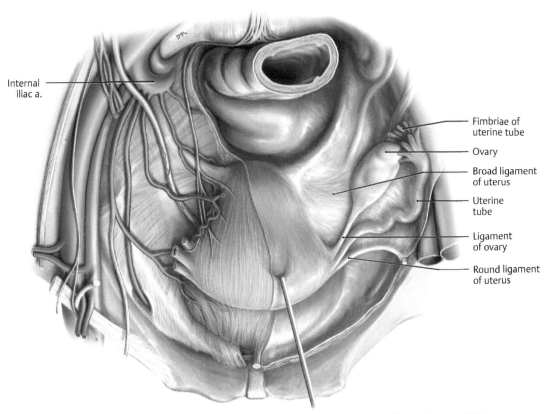

Internal iliac a.

Fimbriae of uterine tube

Ovary

Broad ligament of uterus

Uterine tube

Ligament of ovary

Round ligament of uterus

Source: Gilroy AM et al. Atlas of Anatomy. 3rd ed. 2016. Based on: Schuenke M, Schulte E, Schumacher U. THIEME Atlas of Anatomy. Volumes 1-3. Illustrations by Voll M and Wesker K. 2nd ed. New York: Thieme Medical Publishers; 2016

7.   Correct: Greater vestibular (Bartholin's) gland cyst (B)

(**B**) The paired greater vestibular (Bartholin's) glands lie at the posterior edge of the bulbs of the vestibule, deep to the bulbospongiosus muscles. The duct of each gland opens into the vestibule in the groove between the hymen or its remnants (hymenal caruncles) and the labium minus on each side. A duct may become occluded and secretions accumulate and form a cyst (Bartholin's cyst). The cysts are almost always unilateral. (**A**) A cystocele is a bulge in the anterior wall of the vagina caused by a displaced urinary bladder. (**C, D**) These conditions (sexually transmitted disease, urinary tract infection) are not likely since the lesion is focal and unilateral. (**E**) Remnants of Gartner's duct, if present, may become cystic later in life. These form in the vaginal wall, not the introitus.

Refer to the following image for answer 7:

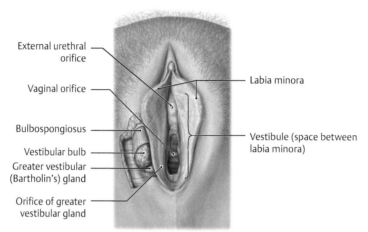

External urethral orifice
Vaginal orifice
Bulbospongiosus
Vestibular bulb
Greater vestibular (Bartholin's) gland
Orifice of greater vestibular gland
Labia minora
Vestibule (space between labia minora)

Source: Gilroy AM et al. Atlas of Anatomy. 3rd ed. 2016. Based on: Schuenke M, Schulte E, Schumacher U. THIEME Atlas of Anatomy. Volumes 1-3. Illustrations by Voll M and Wesker K. 2nd ed. New York: Thieme Medical Publishers; 2016

8.   Correct: Ampulla of uterine tube (A)

(**A**) Fertilization of an ovum occurs most often in the ampulla of the uterine (Fallopian) tube. (**B–E**) Fertilization is infrequent in these regions of the female reproductive tract (infundibulum of uterine tube, intramural portion of uterine tube, isthmus of uterine tube, uterine cavity).

Refer to the following image for answer 8:

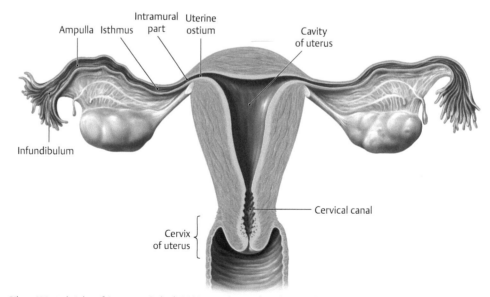

Ampulla   Isthmus   Intramural part   Uterine ostium   Cavity of uterus
Infundibulum
Cervical canal
Cervix of uterus

Source: Gilroy AM et al. Atlas of Anatomy. 3rd ed. 2016. Based on: Schuenke M, Schulte E, Schumacher U. THIEME Atlas of Anatomy. Volumes 1-3. Illustrations by Voll M and Wesker K. 2nd ed. New York: Thieme Medical Publishers; 2016

9. Correct: Ureter (E)

Refer to the following image for answer 9:

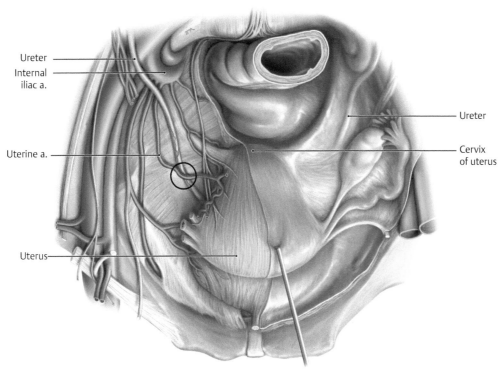

Source: Gilroy AM et al. Atlas of Anatomy. 3rd ed. 2016. Based on: Schuenke M, Schulte E, Schumacher U. THIEME Atlas of Anatomy. Volumes 1-3. Illustrations by Voll M and Wesker K. 2nd ed. New York: Thieme Medical Publishers; 2016

(**E**) The ureter and uterine artery cross each other approximately 2 cm lateral to the uterine cervix, with the ureter passing inferior to the artery. This anatomical relationship gives rise to the mnemonic "water under the bridge," with the water represented by the ureter/urine and the bridge by the uterine artery (*circle* in accompanying image). Ligation of the uterine artery during hysterectomy requires special attention to avoid damage to the ureter. (**A–D**) The internal iliac artery, internal pudendal artery, suspensory ligament of the ovary and sympathetic trunk are located far enough away from the uterus that they should not be injured during a hysterectomy.

10. Correct: Rectouterine pouch (C)

Refer to the following image for answer 10:

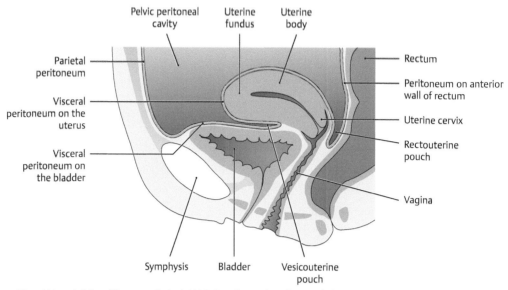

Source: Gilroy AM et al. Atlas of Anatomy. 3rd ed. 2016. Based on: Schuenke M, Schulte E, Schumacher U. THIEME Atlas of Anatomy. Volumes 1-3. Illustrations by Voll M and Wesker K. 2nd ed. New York: Thieme Medical Publishers; 2016

(**C**) The rectouterine pouch (cul-de-sac or pouch of Douglas) is the most inferior part of the greater sac of the peritoneal cavity in the female. Gravity will cause fluid that accumulates in the peritoneal cavity to collect in this recess. Liver disease is a common cause of peritoneal ascites. (**A, B, D**) These peritoneal recesses are not located in the pelvis. (**E**) The vesicouterine pouch is the other peritoneal recess located in the female pelvis. Fluid is less likely to collect here because its size and capacity are variable, due primarily to the constant changes in the relationship between the urinary bladder and uterus as the urinary bladder fills and empties.

11. Correct: External anal sphincter (A)

(**A**) A midline episiotomy involves an incision from the posterior wall of the vagina into the perineal body. The most vulnerable muscle in this procedure is the external anal sphincter. Many of the fibers of this muscle insert on the perineal body and an incision into the perineal body has the potential to damage the muscle, which may lead to fecal incontinence. For this reason, a midline episiotomy is widely avoided. (**B**) The external urethral sphincter lies anterior to the vagina and would not be impacted by a midline episiotomy. (**C**) The ischiocavernosus muscle lies lateral to the vagina and perineal body and would not be impacted by a midline episiotomy. (**D**) The puborectalis muscle lies deep to the external anal sphincter and a properly placed midline episiotomy would not involve the puborectalis. The puborectalis is susceptible to trauma by the passage of the baby through the lower birth canal. (**E**) While

the superficial transverse perineal muscle is attached to the perineal body and would, therefore, be vulnerable to damage in a mediolateral episiotomy. Loss of function of this muscle is likely to have minimal effect on the support mechanism of the pelvic floor.

Refer to the following images for answer 11:

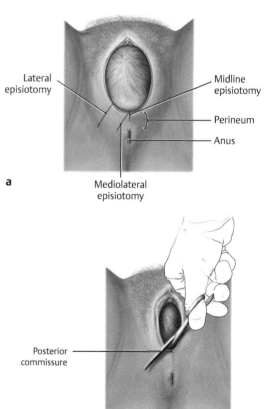

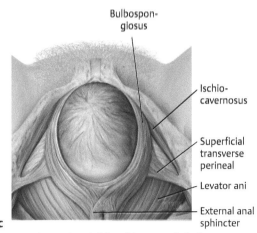

Bulbospon-
glosus

Ischio-
cavernosus

Superficial
transverse
perineal

Levator ani

External anal
sphincter

c

Source: Gilroy AM et al. Atlas of Anatomy. 3rd ed.
2016. Based on: Schuenke M, Schulte E, Schumacher U.
THIEME Atlas of Anatomy. Volumes 1-3. Illustrations by
Voll M and Wesker K. 2nd ed. New York: Thieme Medical
Publishers; 2016

12. Correct: S2–S4 (E)

Refer to the following image for answer 12:

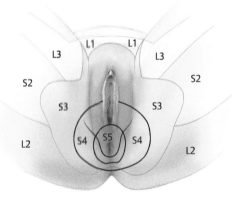

(**E**) Only the lower one-fifth of the vagina has somatic innervation and is sensitive to pain and temperature. The pudendal nerve (S2–S4) conveys somatic sensory innervation from this part of the vagina. (**A–D**) Lumbar spinal cord segments do not distribute to the perineum.

13. Correct: Sympathetic (D)

(**D**) Sensory fibers from the ovary accompany the sympathetic nerves that originate in the T10 and T11 segments of the spinal cord. Pain from the ovary also may be referred to the paraumbilical region (dermatomes T10–T11). In severe cases, if the ovary is inflamed, there may be pain in the medial thigh due to irritation of the obturator nerve in its course along the pelvic wall. (**A–C, E**). The iliohypogastric, obturator and vagus nerves, as well as visceral afferents traveling with parasympathetic nerves, do not conduct sensory afferents from the ovary.

14. Correct: Uterine tube (E)

(**E**) By far, the most common site for ectopic implantation is the luminal wall of the uterine tube (tubal pregnancy). Ectopic implantation is often a consequence of uterine tube inflammation and scarring. The ciliated epithelial cells lining the uterine tube are essential for moving a fertilized ovum toward the uterine cavity and their disruption may cause the blastocyst to implant ectopically. Tobacco use increases the risk for ectopic pregnancy. (**A–D**) A fertilized ovum rarely implants ectopically on the ileum, mesometrium, surface of the ovary, or serosal surface of the uterus.

15. Correct: Perinatal period (C)

(**C**) The hymen normally perforates just before, or soon after birth. With an imperforate hymen, during the first menstrual cycle, menses is prevented from draining from the vagina. The accumulated menses distends the hymen to produce a red mass in the vestibule. Vaginal distension may also compress the urethra, compromising the flow of urine. (**A–B, D–E**) The hymen normally becomes perforate during the perinatal period.

16. Correct: Anterior ramus of T4 (A)

(**A**) The nipple and areola lie in the T4 dermatome. Sensory impulses from this area are conveyed by branches of the anterior ramus of the T4 spinal nerve. (**B, C, E**) These nerves (long thoracic, medial pectoral, thoracodorsal) are motor branches of the brachial plexus. (**D**) The suprascapular nerves (medial, intermediate, lateral) are sensory branches of the cervical plexus and distribute to the lower neck.

17. Correct: Fundus of uterus (C)

Refer to the following image for answer 17:

Fundus   Uterine
of uterus   cavity

Body of
uterus

P

Uterine
cervix

Body of
uterus

Source: Dogra V, Saad W. Ultrasound. Guided Procedures.
1st Edition. Thieme; 2009.

(**C**) The saline injected into the uterus in this patient outlines the uterine cavity and the polyp (P) is in the uterine fundus. Hypertension and obesity are contributing factors for development of uterine polyps. (**A, B, D**) The polyp in this patient is not located in the uterine cervix or body, or in the posterior vaginal fornix.

18. Correct: Urinary bladder (E)

(**E**) A bulge in the anterior wall of the vagina is often caused by prolapse of either the urinary bladder (cystocele) or urethra (urethrocele). These two structures are dependent on the pelvic floor musculature to support and maintain their normal position in the pelvic cavity. Loss of pelvic floor muscle (levator ani) tone will cause pelvic organs to sag toward the pelvic floor, compromising their normal function and that of surrounding organs. Chronic increases in abdominal pressure (heavy lifting, constipation) will contribute to downward displacement of pelvic organs. (**A**) The cervix opens into the lumen of the upper vagina. This vaginal part of the cervix would be observed within the vagina, not as a bulge in the wall. (**B, D**) Other organs (uterus, urinary bladder, rectum) separate loops of ileum and the sigmoid colon from the vagina. Pressure against the anterior vaginal wall by a loop

of ileum or the sigmoid colon would be rare. (**C**) The rectum lies posterior to the vagina. A rectocele would manifest in the posterior wall of the vagina.

19. Correct: Pubococcygeus muscle (E)

(**E**) A primary support for the female genitourinary organs is the levator ani muscle. The pubococcygeus and puborectalis portions of levator ani are most important in providing organ support. Injury or loss of tone to the pubococcygeus allows pelvic organs (especially the urinary bladder and uterus) to "sag" and is most common in multiparous women. With the loss of support, the uterus may prolapse into the vagina and the cervix may project into or past the vestibule. Also, multiple vaginal deliveries may cause the uterus to become aligned with the vagina (retroverted and/or retroflexed uterus). In extreme cases, the uterus may be in contact with the rectum, compressing the rectum and affecting bowel movements. (**A, B, D**) None of these structures (broad ligament, external urethral sphincter, obturator internus muscle) provide significant support for genitourinary structures. (**C**) The ischiococcygeus (coccygeus) muscle is a component of the pelvic diaphragm (but not part of levator ani) and does not play a major role in support of genitourinary organs.

Refer to the following image for answer 19:

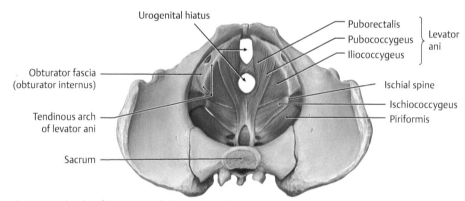

Source: Gilroy AM et al. Atlas of Anatomy. 3rd ed. 2016. Based on: Schuenke M, Schulte E, Schumacher U. THIEME Atlas of Anatomy. Volumes 1-3. Illustrations by Voll M and Wesker K. 2nd ed. New York: Thieme Medical Publishers; 2016

20. Correct: Inferior vesical (C)

(**C**) The posterior aspect of the female urinary bladder is in contact with the anterior wall of the vagina. This area of the urinary bladder receives its arterial supply from the inferior vesical artery, a branch of the vaginal artery. The vaginal artery arises from the uterine artery or directly from the internal iliac. Prolonged distension of the vagina (i.e., difficult childbirth) may compress the walls of the posterior bladder and vagina, compromising the blood supply. This may result in necrosis and formation of a vesicovaginal fistula. The patient may not realize that the urine is leaking from the vagina when a fistula exists because of the close relationship of the urethra to the anterior vaginal wall. (**A, B, D**) The inferior epigastric, inferior rectal, and internal pudendal arteries do not distribute to the urinary bladder. (**E**) The superior vesical artery distributes to the anterosuperior parts of the urinary bladder.

Refer to the following images for answer 20:

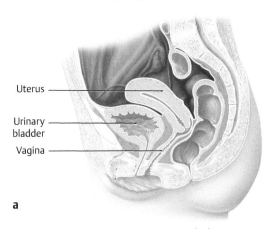

a

Source: Gilroy AM et al. Atlas of Anatomy. 3rd ed. 2016. Based on: Schuenke M, Schulte E, Schumacher U. THIEME Atlas of Anatomy. Volumes 1-3. Illustrations by Voll M and Wesker K. 2nd ed. New York: Thieme Medical Publishers; 2016

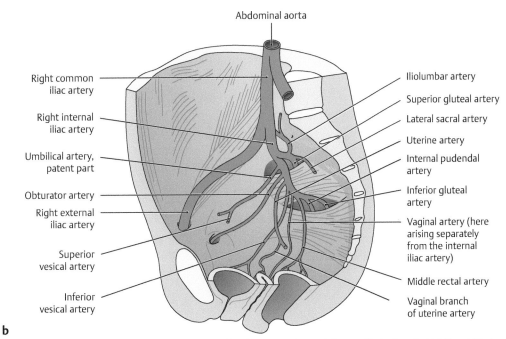

b

Source: Schuenke M, Schulte E, Schumacher U. THIEME Atlas of Anatomy. Internal Organs. Illustrations by Voll M and Wesker K. 2nd ed. New York: Thieme Medical Publishers; 2016

21. Correct: Posterior fornix (C)

(**C**) The cervix projects into the lumen of the vagina, creating a circular recess in the upper vaginal canal. This recess, the vaginal fornix, has anterior, posterior, and lateral parts. The posterior fornix is the largest and is closely related to the peritoneal cavity (rectouterine pouch). (**A**) The anal canal is located more inferiorly, at the pelvic floor. (**B**) The cervical canal lies at a near-right angle to the vaginal canal and lies anterior to the area indicated by the *arrow*. (**D**) The ureter is not visible in this sagittal section. (**E**) The urethra lies anterior to the vagina and passes through the pelvic floor.

22. Correct: Anteverted and anteflexed (A)

(**A**) The position of the uterus in this woman is within the normal range. The most common position of the uterus when the urinary bladder is empty is anteverted and anteflexed. These terms refer to the angulations that occur at the external and internal os, respectively. Anteversion refers to the angle at the junction of the vagina and cervical canal and should be approximately 90 degrees. Anteflexion occurs at the junction of the cervical canal and uterine cavity and should be approximately 170 degrees. (**B–D**) Retroversion and retroflexion describe variations in the position of the uterus. Retroversion describes an increased angulation (> 90 degrees) at the external os. Retroflexion describes an increased angulation (> 170 degrees) at the internal os. Since the position of the uterus is normal in this woman, the other positional descriptions are incorrect.

Refer to the following image for answer 22:

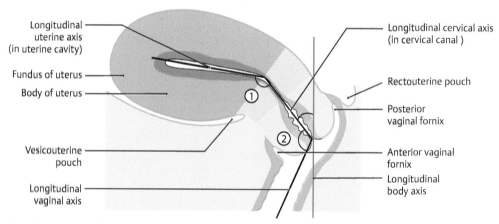

Source: Gilroy AM et al. Atlas of Anatomy. 3rd ed. 2016. Based on: Schuenke M, Schulte E, Schumacher U. THIEME Atlas of Anatomy. Volumes 1-3. Illustrations by Voll M and Wesker K. 2nd ed. New York: Thieme Medical Publishers; 2016

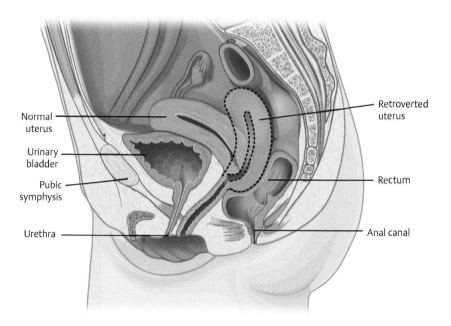

23. Correct: Bulbospongiosus (A)

(**A**) The perineal body is a subcutaneous, fibromuscular perineal mass that lies on the median plane between the posterior vaginal wall and the anal canal. The bulbospongiosus, superficial and deep transverse perineal, and external anal sphincter muscles all have attachment to the perineal body. Difficult vaginal deliveries may cause tearing of the posterior vaginal wall that may extend into the perineal body and anal canal, creating an anovaginal fistula. An episiotomy may be performed to reduce the chance of trauma to the vagina. (**B–E**) The external urethral sphincter, ischiocavernosus, ichicoccygeus, and obturator obternus muscles do not attach to the perineal body.

24. Correct: Iliococcygeus muscle (D)

Refer to the following image for answer 24:

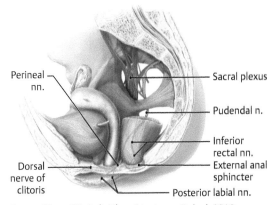

Perineal nn.
Sacral plexus
Pudendal n.
Inferior rectal nn.
Dorsal nerve of clitoris
External anal sphincter
Posterior labial nn.

Source: Gilroy AM et al. Atlas of Anatomy. 3rd ed. 2016. Based on: Schuenke M, Schulte E, Schumacher U. THIEME Atlas of Anatomy. Volumes 1-3. Illustrations by Voll M and Wesker K. 2nd ed. New York: Thieme Medical Publishers; 2016

(**D**) A pudendal nerve block will anesthetize structures innervated by the pudendal nerve. The iliococcygeus muscle is a part of the levator ani muscle and is not supplied by the pudendal nerve. The iliococcygeus muscle receives innervation from the S4 spinal nerve directly from the sacral plexus and from branches of the inferior rectal nerve. (**A, B, E**) The external anal and urethral sphincter and ischiocavernosus muscles receive innervation from branches of the pudendal nerve. (**C**) Sensory impulses from the clitoris are conveyed by the dorsal nerve of the clitoris, a branch of the pudendal nerve.

25. Correct: Internal pudendal (D)

(**D**) Hematomas in the labia majora are most often associated with trauma to the highly vascularized bulbs of the vestibule. These erectile tissues receive their blood supply from branches of the internal pudendal artery and injuries to them are usually associated with athletic and iatrogenic injuries or sexual assault. (**A–C**) These arteries (deep artery and dorsal arteries of the clitoris, and inferior rectal) are branches of the internal pudendal artery, but none of them distribute to the labia majora or bulbs of the vestibule. (**E**) The superficial circumflex iliac artery, a branch of the femoral, does not distribute to the genitalia.

26. Correct: Peritoneum (C)

(**C**) Culdocentesis involves introducing the tip of a needle into the rectouterine pouch of the peritoneal cavity by piercing the wall of the posterior vaginal fornix. The needle will pass through the structures of the vaginal wall and the peritoneum closely associated with the posterior vaginal fornix. (**A, B**) The endometrium and myometrium are layers of the uterus. No part of the uterus is pierced during a culdocentesis. (**D**) The vagina is lined by stratified squamous epithelium in postpubertal women and the peritoneum is lined by simple squamous epithelium. (**E**) The musculature of the vaginal wall is smooth and nonstriated.

Refer to the following image for answer 26:

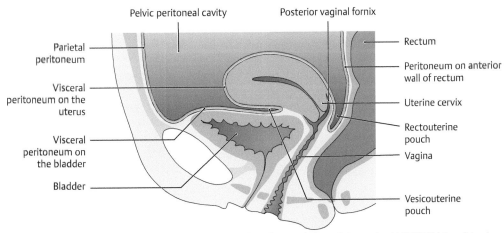

Pelvic peritoneal cavity
Posterior vaginal fornix
Parietal peritoneum
Rectum
Peritoneum on anterior wall of rectum
Visceral peritoneum on the uterus
Uterine cervix
Visceral peritoneum on the bladder
Rectouterine pouch
Vagina
Bladder
Vesicouterine pouch

Source: Gilroy AM et al. Atlas of Anatomy. 3rd ed. 2016. Based on: Schuenke M, Schulte E, Schumacher U. THIEME Atlas of Anatomy. Volumes 1-3. Illustrations by Voll M and Wesker K. 2nd ed. New York: Thieme Medical Publishers; 2016

27. Correct: Bulbospongiosus (A)

Refer to the following image for answer 27:

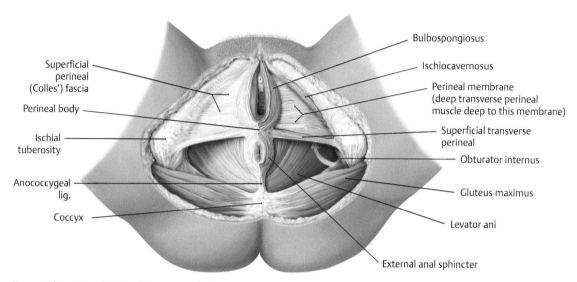

Superficial perineal (Colles') fascia

Perineal body

Ischial tuberosity

Anococcygeal lig.

Coccyx

Bulbospongiosus

Ischiocavernosus

Perineal membrane (deep transverse perineal muscle deep to this membrane)

Superficial transverse perineal

Obturator internus

Gluteus maximus

Levator ani

External anal sphincter

Source: Gilroy AM et al. Atlas of Anatomy. 3rd ed. 2016. Based on: Schuenke M, Schulte E, Schumacher U. THIEME Atlas of Anatomy. Volumes 1-3. Illustrations by Voll M and Wesker K. 2nd ed. New York: Thieme Medical Publishers; 2016

(**A**) Vaginismus is a condition in which the vaginal walls are compressed by spasms in the skeletal muscles surrounding the introitus. The primary muscles involved are the paired bulbospongiosus muscles, which flank the vaginal orifice, and the pubovaginalis part of levator ani muscle. The two muscles have a sphincteric action on the vagina. The causes of vaginismus are not well understood, but anxiety related to sexual intercourse is thought to be a major factor. Pelvic pain related to vaginismus is a universal complaint, but researchers are uncertain which occurs first: pain causing vaginismus or vaginismus leading to painful intercourse. Kegel exercises are of proven benefit in treatment. (**B–E**) The deep transverse perineal, iliococcygeus, ischiocavernosus, and obturator internus muscles do not have a direct action on the vaginal walls.

28. Correct: Vagina (E)

(**E**) In the female, the urethra and vagina pierce the perineal membrane as they pass between the pelvic cavity and the perineum. (**A–D**) None of these structures (anorectal junction, corpus cavernosum, duct of greater vestibular (Bartholin's) gland, pudendal nerve) pierce the perineal membrane.

29. Correct: Ilioinguinal nerve (B)

(**B**) Ilioinguinal and iliohypogastric nerves (L1) conduct sensory impulses from the skin of the inguinal and suprapubic regions, including the mons pubis (L1 dermatome). These nerves also provide motor innervation to the anterior abdominal wall muscles. A history of human papillomavirus increases the risk for developing vulvar cancer. (**A, C–E**) None of these nerves (dorsal nerve of the clitoris, ilioinguinal, inferior rectal, posterior labial) carry sensory information from the mons pubis.

30. Correct: Posterior labial (D)

(**D**) The posterior labial branches of the pudendal nerve carry sensory impulses from the vaginal vestibule. The genital type of HPV is the most common sexually transmitted disease in the United States. It is estimated that 50% of sexually active people will contract genital HPV. In most cases, the body's immune system destroys the virus before symptoms develop. (**A–C**) None of these nerves (genitofemoral, ilioinguinal, inferior rectal) distribute to the vaginal vestibule. (**E**) Somatic sensation from the vaginal vestibule does not travel in parasympathetic nerves.

31. Correct: Suspensory ligament of the ovary (C)

Refer to the following images for answer 31:

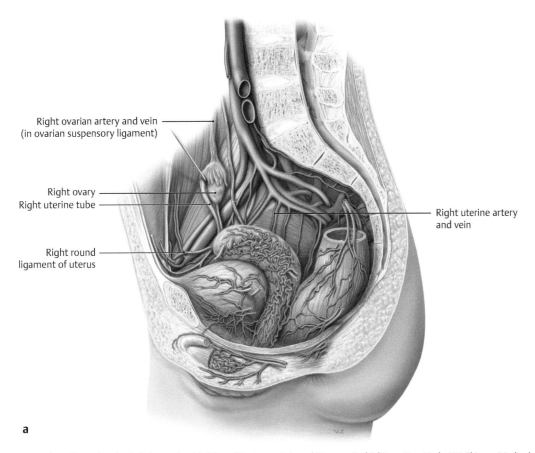

Right ovarian artery and vein
(in ovarian suspensory ligament)

Right ovary

Right uterine tube

Right round
ligament of uterus

Right uterine artery
and vein

a

Source: Schuenke M, Schulte E, Schumacher U. Atlas of Anatomy. Internal Organs. 2nd Edition. New York, NY: Thieme Medical Publishers; 2016. Illustration by Voll M and Wesker K.

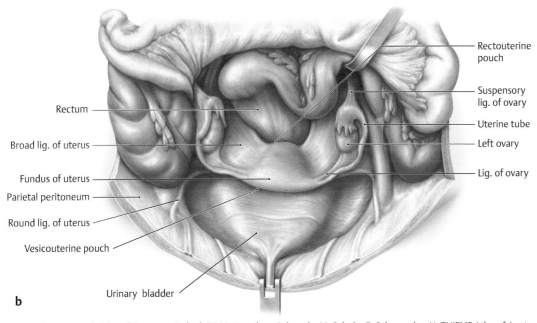

Rectouterine
pouch

Suspensory
lig. of ovary

Uterine tube

Left ovary

Lig. of ovary

Rectum

Broad lig. of uterus

Fundus of uterus

Parietal peritoneum

Round lig. of uterus

Vesicouterine pouch

Urinary bladder

b

Source: Gilroy AM et al. Atlas of Anatomy. 3rd ed. 2016. Based on: Schuenke M, Schulte E, Schumacher U. THIEME Atlas of Anatomy. Volumes 1-3. Illustrations by Voll M and Wesker K. 2nd ed. New York: Thieme Medical Publishers; 2016

(**C**) The ovaries are supplied by arteries that originate from the abdominal aorta and lengthen to accompany the ovaries as they descend into the pelvis during development. The suspensory ligament of the ovary, also known as the infundibulopelvic or IP ligament, is a fold of peritoneum that extends from the lateral pelvic wall to the ovary (refer to the accompanying images). The ligament contains the ovarian vessels as they pass over the pelvic brim to enter the mesosalpinx portion of the broad ligament to reach the ovaries. A few authors consider the IP ligament a portion of the broad ligament. Torsion of the ovary (adnexal torsion) causes twisting of its pedicle, i.e., the IP ligament. This results in a compromised venous return, leading to stromal edema and internal hemorrhage of the ovary. In prepubescent patients, there may be congenital malformations of the reproductive organs or elongated uterine tubes. (**A**) The ligament of the ovary (also called the proper ovarian ligament) is a fibromuscular band that extends from the medial aspect of the ovary to the lateral aspect of the uterus, just inferior to the junction of the uterine tube and uterus (refer to image b). It supports the ovary on the posterior aspect of the broad ligament and is the proximal remnant of the gubernaculum ovary. It does not convey the ovarian vessels to the ovary. (**B**) The round ligament of the uterus, the distal remnant of the gubernaculum ovary, courses anterolaterally in the broad ligament and passes through the inguinal canal to the labium majus, where it blends into the tissue of the mons pubis. It does not convey the ovarian vessels to the ovary. (**D**) The transverse cervical ligament (not shown), also known as Mackenrodt's or the cardinal ligament, is a thickened band of endopelvic fascia that is located at the base of the broad ligament. It extends from the lateral wall of the pelvis to the cervix and conveys the uterine vessels. It lies superior to the ureters on each side of the cervix. (**E**) The uterosacral ligament (not shown) is a condensation of endopelvic fascia that extends from the cervix to the anterior aspect of the sacrum on each side. It creates the rectouterine peritoneal fold on each side of the rectum. It does not convey the ovarian vessels, but is associated with the pelvic splanchnic nerves.

32. **Correct: Paramesonephric duct (C)**

Refer to the following images for answer 32:

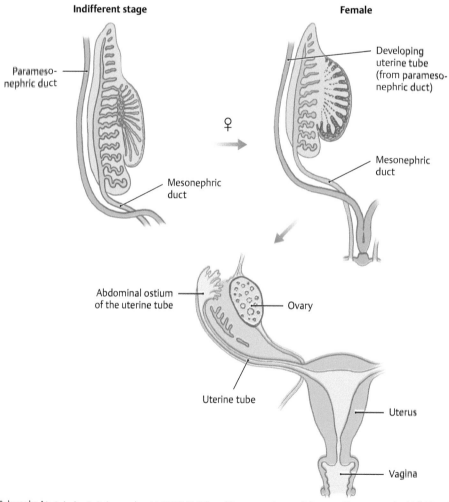

Source: Schuenke M, Schulte E, Schumacher U. THIEME Atlas of Anatomy. Internal Organs. Illustrations by Voll M and Wesker K. 2nd ed. New York: Thieme Medical Publishers; 2016

(C) The uterine tubes, together with the uterus and upper one-third of the vagina, are derived from the paramesonephric (Müllerian) ducts. Assisted reproductive technologies can increase the risk for ovarian torsion because the hormones that induce ovulation may cause the ovaries to enlarge and/or develop multiple cysts, and these may increase the risk of ovarian torsion. (A) The mesonephric (Wolffian) ducts will develop into the male genital ducts, which include the vas (ductus) deferens and epididymis, and also the seminal gland. (B) The mesonephric tubules are remnants of the excretory ducts that form in the mesonephros, and will form the efferent ductules that connect the testis to the epididymis. (D) Primordial germ cells do not contribute to the female reproductive ducts. (E) The urogenital sinus is the anterior portion of the cloaca after it is partitioned by the urorectal septum. It will form the lower portion of the vagina, the urinary bladder and urethra in the female and does not contribute to either the ovaries or the uterine tube.

33. Correct: Genital tubercle (A)

(A) The clitoris forms from the genital tubercle. Congenital adrenal hyperplasia is caused by abnormalities in the enzymes required for the production of the steroid hormones cortisol and/or aldosterone. 17-hydroxyprogesterone is produced in the process of making the hormone cortisol. In congenital adrenal hyperplasia there is decreased adrenal cortisol and aldosterone and increased male sex hormone is produced. The genital tubercle responds to the androgens and will form the phallus in males; in females, excess androgens cause the clitoris to become enlarged. (B) The labioscrotal folds will form the labia majora in females and scrotum in males, and do not contribute to the developing clitoris. (C, D) The urethral folds or urogenital folds are derived from the cloacal folds. In males they fuse to form the spongy urethra and ventral aspect of the penis, in females they form the labia minora. (E) The vestibule forms in females in the absence of fusion of the urethral folds as occurs in males.

Refer to the following images for answer 33:

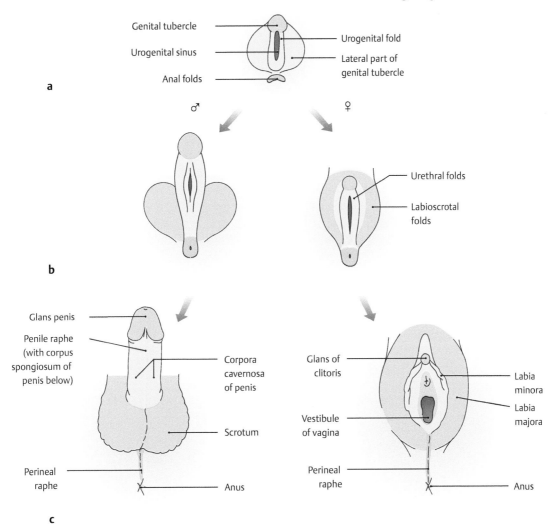

Source: Schuenke M, Schulte E, Schumacher U. THIEME Atlas of Anatomy. General Anatomy and Musculoskeletal System. Illustrations by Voll M and Wesker K. 2nd ed. New York: Thieme Medical Publishers; 2016

34. Correct: Round ligament of the uterus and proper ligament of the ovary (C)

Refer to the following image for answer 34:

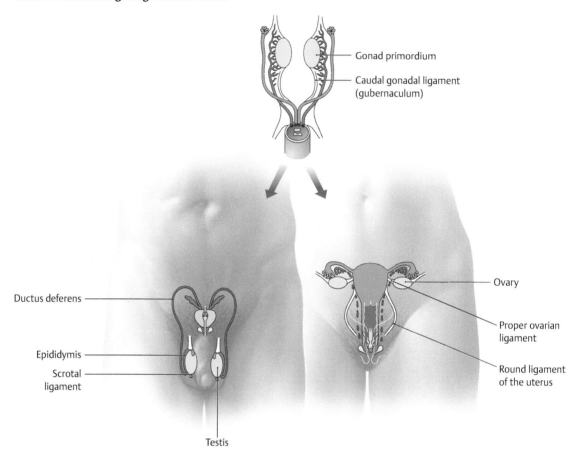

Source: Schuenke M, Schulte E, Schumacher U. THIEME Atlas of Anatomy. Internal Organs. Illustrations by Voll M and Wesker K. 2nd ed. New York: Thieme Medical Publishers; 2016

(**C**) This patient has varicosities of the veins associated with the round ligament, which is derived from the gubernaculum. The gubernaculum in females develops into two vestigial structures: the round ligament of the uterus and the ligament of the ovary. (**A**) The broad ligament and transverse cervical ligaments are not derived from the gubernaculum. (**B**) The mesosalpinx, mesovarium, and mesometrium are all parts of the broad ligament and are not derived from the gubernaculum. (**D**) The scrotal ligament is the derivative of the gubernaculum in the male. (**E**) The suspensory ligament of the ovary (infundibulopelvic or ligament) is a peritoneal fold that partially encloses the ovarian vessels and extends from the ovary to the lateral wall of the pelvis.

35. Correct: Paramesonephric ducts (D)

(**D**) Female internal genital structures are derived from the paramesonephric (Müllerian) ducts and these would not develop in this individual because 46 XY karyotypes have testes and Sertoli cells in the testes produce Müllerian-inhibiting substance, also called anti-Müllerian hormone. Müllerian-inhibiting substance produced by the testes prevents development of derivatives of the paramesonephric (Müllerian) ducts (uterine tubes, uterus, and upper vagina) in genetic males. (**A**) This individual has testes derived from the gonadal ridge because testicular development is dependent on the presence of testes determining factor, the product of the SRY gene located on the Y chromosome. Although her testes produce testosterone, the lack of functional androgen receptors result in the lack of differentiation of male genital duct structures and external genitalia that would normally be dependent on testosterone. (**B**) The medullary sex cords will develop into the seminiferous tubules as this individual has testes. (**C, E**) The metanephric blastema and ureteric bud will develop into the adult kidney and ureter and are not necessarily dependent on androgens for their development.

36. Correct: Primordial germ cells enter the ovary, but most primordial follicles regress before puberty (B)

(**B**) In Turner syndrome, primordial germ cells enter the ovary early in its development to become oogonia and primary oocytes by the fifth month. Follicle cells will develop from the cortical cords and surround the primary oocytes, but these primordial follicles are lost much more rapidly than in unaffected individuals and ovarian tissue is replaced with fibrous tissue forming streak ovaries. (**A, C–E**) In classic Turner syndrome, the ovaries initially develop normally, primordial follicles will form from primary oocytes and cortical cord cells. During formation of the ovary medullary cords form but regress, whereas they are retained in the developing testes.

37. Correct: Processus vaginalis (C)

(**C**) The female homologue of a hydrocele is a cyst of the canal of Nuck. It results from a patent processus vaginalis in the female inguinal canal. The processus vaginalis is an outpocketing of the peritoneum that traverses the abdominal wall during development to enter the scrotum in males and the labium majus in females. The processus usually loses its connection with the peritoneum to form the tunica vaginalis in males and canal of Nuck in females. A patent canal of Nuck can predispose to an inguinal hernia or a hydrocele. (**A**) The cloacal membrane is not related to hydroceles; it breaks down once the cloaca is divided by the urorectal septum to form the urogenital openings anteriorly and anus posteriorly. (**B**) The labioscrotal folds will form the labia majora in females and the scrotum in males and are not outgrowths of the peritoneum. (**D**) The urogenital folds are derived

from the cloacal folds and will form the labia minora in females and the spongy urethra in males and are not outgrowths of the peritoneum. (**E**) The urogenital sinus is the ventral compartment formed once the cloaca is divided by the urorectal septum and is not an outgrowth of the peritoneum.

Refer to the following image for answer 37:

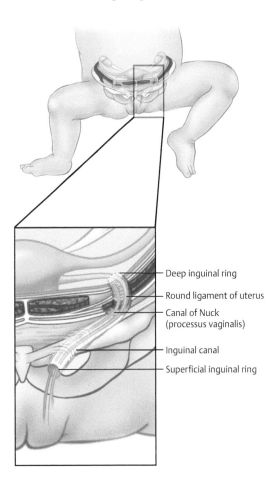

Deep inguinal ring

Round ligament of uterus

Canal of Nuck (processus vaginalis)

Inguinal canal

Superficial inguinal ring

38. Correct: Efferent ductules: vestigial structures (B)

(**B**) Efferent ductules arise from the remnants of the mesonephric tubules in males, but are retained only as vestigial structures in females. Mesonephric tubules are primitive excretory ducts. Most disappear and the nephrons of the definitive kidney assume their role, except for those that form the efferent ductules in males. In females, the mesonephric tubules form the epo-ophoron and paro-ophoron in the mesovarium. These vestigial structures are usually of little concern unless they become cystic. Mesonephric carcinoma is extremely rare. (**A**) The bulbourethral gland and bulbs of the vestibule are not homologous structures and are not formed from remnants of the mesonephric tubules. The bulbourethral glands develop from the urogenital sinus and the bulbs of the vestibule develop from the urethral folds. (**C**) The epididymis is derived from the mesonephric duct, whereas the uterine tubes develop from the paramesonephric duct; neither are derivatives of the mesonephric tubules. (**D**) The prostate in males and the paraurethral glands in females are homologous structures derived from the urogenital sinus and are not derivatives of the mesonephric tubules. (**E**) The uterus masculinus is a remnant of the paramesonephric ducts in the male, whereas the uterus is formed from fusion of the paramesonephric ducts distally. While homologous, neither is derived from mesonephric tubules.

Refer to the following image for answer 38:

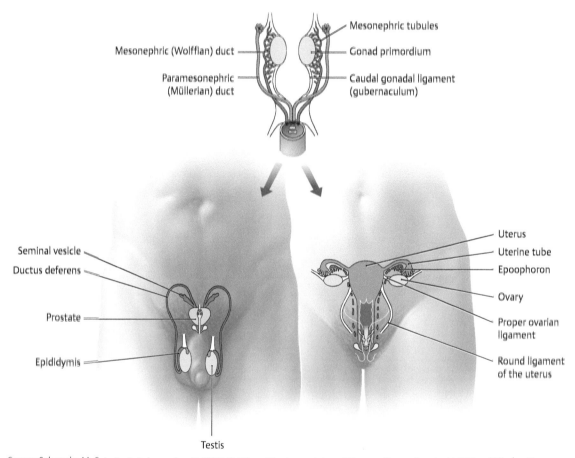

Source: Schuenke M, Schulte E, Schumacher U. THIEME Atlas of Anatomy. Internal Organs. Illustrations by Voll M and Wesker K. 2nd ed. New York: Thieme Medical Publishers; 2016

Chapter 8

Male Reproductive System

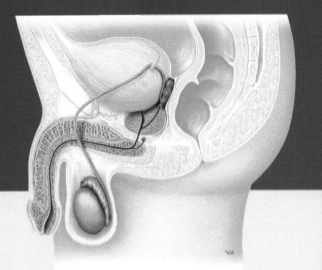

ANATOMICAL LEARNING OBJECTIVES

▶ Describe the anatomy of the bony pelvis, including features that distinguish male from female.

▶ Describe the anatomy of the inguinal region in the male, including the development and characteristics of inguinal hernias.

▶ Describe the anatomy of the spermatic cord, including its fascial coverings, neurovasculature, and contents.

▶ Describe the anatomy of the testis, including its layers, neurovasculature, and development.

▶ Describe the anatomy of the male perineum, including its subdivisions, fasciae and compartments, muscles, erectile tissues, neurovasculature, and anatomical relationships.

▶ Describe the anatomy of the scrotum, including its layers, neurovasculature, and contents.

▶ Describe the anatomy of the penis.

▶ Describe the anatomy of the male pelvic reproductive organs, including their neurovasculature and anatomical relationships.

▶ Describe the anatomy of the urinary organs in the male pelvis, including their neurovasculature and anatomical relationships.

▶ Describe the anatomy of the male urethra, including its neurovasculature and anatomical relationships.

▶ Describe the anatomy of the digestive organs in the male pelvis, including their neurovasculature and anatomical relationships.

▶ Describe the development of male genito-urinary system.

▶ Describe the anatomical basis for pain sensation from pelvic organs.

▶ Describe the origin, course, and distribution of the branches of the genitofemoral nerve.

▶ Describe the stages and anatomical basis of the male sexual response, including its neural regulation.

8.1 Questions

Easy	Medium	Hard

Consider the following case for questions 1 to 3:

A 60-year-old man presents to the urology clinic with nocturia, difficulty urinating, and a decreased urine stream. A digital rectal examination identifies nodules on his prostate, and his prostate-specific antigen (PSA) level, determined by fluorimetric assay, is elevated. A radical prostatectomy is scheduled after a biopsy indicates cancerous cells. During the surgery, there is iatrogenic damage to the prostatic nerve plexus.

1. What of the following is the most likely complication of this injury?

A. Erectile dysfunction
B. External anal sphincter dysfunction
C. Loss of sensation from the penis
D. Loss of sensation from the posterior scrotum
E. Loss of voluntary control of the bladder

2. Which of the following spinal cord segments contain the preganglionic parasympathetic neurons that were injured?

A. T11–T12
B. T12–L2
C. L1–L4
D. S2–S4
E. S5–Co1

3. If other pelvic parasympathetic fibers were injured, which of the following additional complications might be anticipated?

A. Inability to empty the bladder
B. Loss of inhibition of bladder contraction
C. Loss of internal urethral sphincter contraction
D. Loss of external urethral sphincter function

4. A 24-year-old-man with a painful, swollen glans penis presents to the emergency department. The patient reports he is on his honeymoon and was sexually active for an extended period. The physician notes that the patient has a retracted foreskin (paraphimosis). Before the procedure to release the paraphimosis is performed, a nerve block is administered. Which of the following branches of the pudendal nerve should be targeted for local anesthesia?

A. Anterior scrotal
B. Deep perineal
C. Dorsal nerve of the penis
D. Posterior scrotal
E. Superficial perineal

5. A 41-year-old ironman athlete with a symptom of constant penile pain, 12 to 24 hours after long-distance cycling, reports to his urologist. His history reveals frequent penile pain after sexual intercourse. A nerve block test is performed to determine if the symptoms are the result of nerve injury (bicycle seat neuropathy). Anesthesia is injected along the course of the nerve to determine if this alleviates the pain. Which of the following nerves is targeted in this test?

A. Inferior rectal
B. Inferior gluteal
C. Obturator
D. Posterior femoral cutaneous
E. Pudendal

Consider the following case for questions 6 and 7:

A 75-year-old man with a history of smoking, diabetes, obesity, and elevated cholesterol presents to his urologist. The patient reports an inability to sustain an erection despite the use of erectile dysfunction medications. The physician suspects the erectile dysfunction is a result of vascular disease.

6. Which of the following arteries is most likely affected?

A. Deferential
B. External iliac
C. Inferior epigastric
D. Internal pudendal
E. Lateral sacral

7. The urologist decides that an appropriate treatment to improve the erectile dysfunction is a direct injection of prostaglandin E1 into the penis. Injection is generally performed directly into the corpus cavernosum. During the procedure, the needle would pass through which of the following layers in order?

A. Skin, deep perineal (Buck's) fascia, superficial penile fascia, dartos fascia, tunica albuginea
B. Skin, perineal membrane, superficial penile fascia, deep perineal fascia
C. Skin, superficial penile fascia, deep penile (Buck's) fascia, tunica albuginea
D. Skin, superficial penile fascia, tunica albuginea, deep perineal (Buck's) fascia
E. Skin, superficial penile fascia, tunica albuginea, perineal membrane

8. A 42-year-old man reports to his urologist for bilateral, laparoscopic hernia repair and requests a simultaneous vasectomy. In order to avoid a separate scrotal incision, a bilateral vasectomy is done by a laparoscopic approach at the time of extraperitoneal hernia repair. Which of the following would be found in the patient's ejaculate if analyzed at 3-month post-procedure?

A. Prostatic fluid only

B. Seminal fluid and prostatic fluid

C. Sperm and seminal fluid

D. Sperm only

E. Sperm, seminal fluid, and prostatic fluid

9. An 18-year-old man is brought to the emergency department after receiving a traumatic injury to his pelvis in a motorcycle accident. During the physical examination, blood is observed at the external urethral orifice and a pelvic fracture is suspected. A retrograde urethrogram reveals a tear of the membranous urethra. Blood and urine from this injury would most likely collect in which of the following spaces?

A. Beneath the deep (Buck's) fascia of the penis

B. Deep to the dartos fascia of the scrotum and penis

C. Lower abdominal wall deep to the membranous (Scarpa's) superficial fascia

D. Subperitoneal (infraperitoneal)

E. Superficial to the perineal (Colles') fascia

10. A recently married 28-year-old-man with concerns about his sexual performance presents to his primary care provider. He reports production of very little, if any, ejaculate on orgasm and his urine is often cloudy after intercourse. Which of the following nerves is most likely involved in generating this patient's symptoms?

A. Least splanchnic

B. Lumbosacral trunk

C. Pelvic splanchnic

D. Pudendal

E. Sacral splanchnic

11. A 32-year-old man with a history of a left-side scrotal swelling and heaviness for the last 6 months presents to his primary care provider. He relates that the swelling is painless and has progressively increased in size. Ultrasound of the scrotum reveals a large cyst and calcifications. Post-orchiectomy gross pathological examination reveals a solitary, nonencapsulated tumor. Metastasis from the tumor would most likely enter which of the following veins?

A. Inferior vena cava

B. Left inferior epigastric

C. Left internal iliac

D. Left internal pudendal

E. Left renal

12. A 40-year-old man who had a vasectomy 3 years previously presents to his urologist. He has recently remarried and wishes to father a child with his wife. A surgical attempt to reverse the vasectomy fails and the urologist decides to harvest sperm directly from the patient's reproductive tract for artificial insemination. In which of the following locations would he most likely be able to harvest viable sperm from this patient?

A. Ampulla of the ductus deferens

B. Duct of the seminal gland

C. Ejaculatory duct

D. Epididymis

E. Prostatic urethra

13. A body is discovered in an automobile that caught fire when it was driven off a cliff and landed in a ravine. The remains are taken to the coroner's office for examination and identification. As part of the examination, the pelvic bones are evaluated to determine the gender of the victim. By comparing the normal dimensions for the male and female bony pelvis, which of the following features would indicate that the victim is male?

A. Larger pelvic inlet

B. Larger pelvic outlet

C. Rounder pelvic inlet

D. Smaller subpubic angle

E. Straighter sacral curvature

14. A 70-year-old man with dysuria (difficulty or pain during urination) and urgency presents to his urologist. The physician performs a digital rectal examination and orders a prostate specific antigen (PSA) blood test. Further testing suggests that benign prostatic hyperplasia (BPH) is causing the patient's symptoms. Which of the following structures is most likely displaced in this patient?

A. External urethral sphincter (sphincter urethrae)

B. Interureteric crest

C. Prostatic utricle

D. Seminal colliculus

E. Uvula of the bladder

15. A 65-year-old man reports to his urologist for a transurethral resection of the prostate (TURP) procedure to alleviate symptoms of benign prostatic hyperplasia (BPH). During the TURP procedure, a portion of the posterior wall of the prostatic urethra is removed. Which of the following structures is likely to be disrupted during this procedure?

A. Ampulla of ductus deferens

B. Bulbo-urethral gland

C. Ejaculatory duct

D. Navicular fossa

E. Seminiferous tubule

16. A 43-year-old-man reports to his urologist because he and his wife feel that a vasectomy is their preferred method of birth control. During the procedure, a bilateral incision is made in the upper scrotum in order to ligate the ductus (vas) deferens. Which of the following order of layers, after the skin, must be breached in order to perform the ligation?

A. External spermatic fascia, cremaster muscle and fascia, internal spermatic fascia, superficial (dartos) fascia

B. Internal spermatic fascia, cremaster muscle and fascia, external spermatic fascia, superficial (dartos) fascia

C. Internal spermatic fascia, cremaster muscle and fascia, external spermatic fascia, tunica vaginalis

D. Subcutaneous (dartos) fascia, external spermatic fascia, cremaster muscle and fascia, internal spermatic fascia

E. Subcutaneous (dartos) fascia, external spermatic fascia, internal spermatic fascia, tunica vaginalis

17. A 66-year-old man is hospitalized for inguinal hernia repair. While he is in preoperative care, a fourth-year medical student is asked to insert a Foley catheter. During the procedure, the student injures the urethra just inferior to the perineal membrane. Although blood is noted in the external urethral orifice, it is assumed the injury is confined to the urethra. In which of the following spaces might there be extravasation of urine from this type of injury?

A. Between the deep (Buck's) and the superficial penile fascia

B. Between the superficial (Camper's) and membranous (Scarpa's) layer of fascia of the anterior abdominal wall

C. Between the superficial perineal (Colles') fascia and the superficial penile fascia

D. Deep to the deep penile (Buck's) fascia

18. A 55-year-old man with a scrotal swelling presents to his urologist. He has a past history of scrotal trauma from a sports injury. Transverse sonographic imaging of the left side of the scrotum shows a normal-appearing testicle (refer to the *arrow* in the accompanying image) surrounded by an anechoic (fluid-filled) area (*asterisk*). The man is told that he has a hydrocele. In which of the following potential spaces is the fluid most likely located?

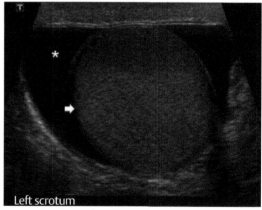

Left scrotum

Source: Chopra S. RadCases. Genitourinary Imaging. 1st Edition. Thieme; 2011.

A. Between the dartos layer and the external spermatic fascia

B. Between the external spermatic fascia and cremasteric fascia

C. Between the parietal and visceral layers of the tunica vaginalis

D. Between the scrotal skin and the dartos fascia

E. Deep to the tunica albuginea

19. A 31-year old man presents to the emergency department with abdominal pain and urine retention. He had been binge drinking, "passed out," and awoke several hours later with severe abdominal pain and an inability to void. The patient's recollection of events is sketchy and there are no obvious physical signs of trauma. CT imaging and a cystogram (refer to the accompanying image) reveal a pelvic fracture and rupture of the bladder at its neck. The *arrows* indicate extravasated urine and blood in tissue planes surrounding the bladder (because the amount of extravasated fluid is small, it appears streaky). Blood and urine from this injury would most likely collect in which of the following potential spaces?

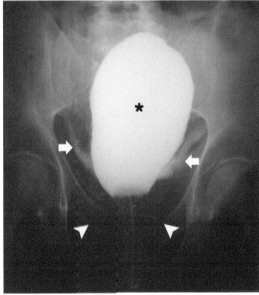

Source: Chopra S. RadCases. Genitourinary Imaging. 1st Edition. Thieme; 2011.

A. Anterior lower abdominal wall deep to Scarpa's (membranous layer of superficial) fascia

B. Beneath the deep (Buck's) fascia of the penis

C. Beneath the superficial perineal (Colles') fascia

D. Deep to the dartos fascia of the scrotum and penis

E. Subperitoneal (infra- or retroperitoneal)

20. A 21-year-old gymnast suffers a pelvic fracture after a serious fall from the parallel bars. At 3 months after the accident, the patient is experiencing difficulty urinating. His physician suspects that the fracture led to traction of nerve roots resulting in transient bladder paralysis that will resolve with time. Which of the following nerve(s) is most likely affected to account for the current symptoms?

A. Ilioinguinal

B. Lumbar splanchnic

C. Pelvic splanchnic

D. Pudendal

E. Superior hypogastric

Consider the following case for questions 21 and 22:

A 16-year-old boy presents to the emergency department following an automobile accident. Radiographs of the pelvis (refer to the accompanying image) show a vertically oriented fracture (*white arrows*) and diastasis (separation) of a joint (*black arrows*) typical of an "open book" fracture of the pelvis.

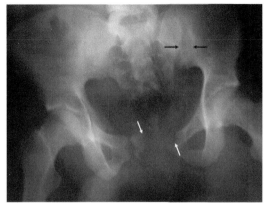

Source: Garcia G. RadCases: Musculoskeletal Radiology. 1st Edition. Thieme; 2010.

21. Which of the following is fractured in this patient (*white arrows*)?

A. Acetabulum

B. Body of ilium

C. Iliac fossa

D. Ischium

E. Pubis

22. Where is the diastasis in this patient (*black arrows*)?

A. Ala of sacrum and auricular surface of ilium

B. Apex of sacrum and coccyx

C. Inferior pubic ramus and ramus of ischium

D. Right and left pubic bodies

E. Superior pubic ramus and ilium

23. A 28-year-old carpenter was forcibly struck in his suprapubic region by a loose piece of scaffolding. Cystography (refer to the accompanying image) shows the urinary bladder (*white arrow*) to be nearly empty. Contrast is seen outlining bowel loops (*arrowheads*). No obvious pelvic fracture is present. In which of the following spaces is the contrast medium (*asterisk*) located?

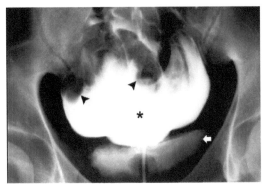

Source: Chopra S. RadCases. Genitourinary Imaging. 1st Edition. Thieme; 2011.

A. Extraperitoneal
B. Intraperitoneal
C. Perineal
D. Retropubic
E. Subpubic

Consider the following case for questions 24 and 25:

A 24-year-old man presents with long-standing bilateral inguinal swellings to his primary care provider. A CT image at the level of the inguinal canals (refer to the accompanying image) reveals a mass in the right inguinal canal (*arrow*) and a hernia (*arrowhead*) in the left inguinal canal. The mass in the right inguinal canal is likely an undescended testis. An image at a more superior level on the left shows the location of the neck of the hernia to be consistent with an indirect inguinal hernia.

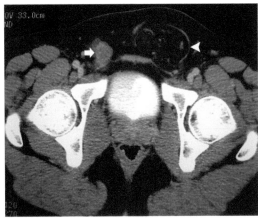

Source: Chopra S. RadCases. Genitourinary Imaging. 1st Edition. Thieme; 2011.

24. Which of the following statements is true regarding this type of hernia?

A. It does not pass through the deep inguinal ring
B. It lies medial to the median umbilical fold
C. It may pass through the superficial inguinal ring
D. Its neck lies medial to the inferior epigastric vessels
E. It will always pass through the superficial inguinal ring

25. With the right testicle located in the inguinal canal, which of the following structures will pass through the superficial inguinal ring on this side?

A. Epididymis
B. Gubernaculum testis
C. Pampiniform venous plexus
D. Testicular artery
E. Vas (ductus) deferens

26. A 35-year old man with a bulge in his right groin presents to his primary care provider. During the physical examination, the physician reduces the bulge into the abdomen when the patient is supine. A diagnosis of direct inguinal hernia is made and a herniorrhaphy (open hernia repair surgery) is performed. During a follow-up evaluation, the physician discovers that the cremasteric reflex is absent on the treated side. Iatrogenic injury to which of the following nerves is responsible for the motor (efferent) deficit in this reflex?

A. Femoral branch of genitofemoral
B. Genital branch of genitofemoral
C. Iliohypogastric
D. Ilioinguinal
E. Posterior scrotal

Consider the following case for questions 27 and 28:

A 32-year-old man with chronic testicular pain and a significant psychiatric history presents to the emergency department with a self-inflicted scrotal laceration. He reports that the chronic testicular pain had become unbearable so he self-amputated both of his testicles. Significant arterial bleeding is evident, and the major vessels responsible were clamped with hemostats.

27. The clamped vessels are direct branches of which of the following arteries?

A. Abdominal aorta
B. External iliac
C. Inferior epigastric
D. Internal iliac
E. Internal pudendal

28. Visceral pain from the amputation would be referred to which of the following dermatomes?

A. L1

B. L4–L5

C. S2–S4

D. T5–T9

E. T10–T11

29. A 33-year-old man presents with lower back pain to his primary care provider. On neurological examination, he is found to have weak dorsiflexion and radiography reveals degenerative changes at the L3–L4 and L4–L5 vertebral levels and spondylolisthesis at L4–L5. During retroperitoneal interbody fusion, the genitofemoral nerve is inadvertently severed when the psoas major muscle is retracted. Loss of which of the following would most likely result from injury to this nerve?

A. Cremasteric reflex

B. Hip flexion

C. Innervation to the pyramidalis muscle

D. Sensation over the most lateral aspect of the thigh

E. Sensory innervation from the dorsum of penis

30. A 28-year-old man is admitted with a 2-day history of progressive pain and swelling in the perianal region. On examination, he has local tenderness, erythema (redness) and swelling, and a mild fever. He is diagnosed with a perianal abscess and is administered antibiotics prior to drainage of the abscess under general anesthesia. Which of the following structures would be most susceptible to injury during the drainage procedure?

A. Bulbourethral glands

B. Inferior gluteal nerve

C. Inferior rectal nerve

D. Membranous urethra

E. Obturator nerve

31. A 37-year-old man had arthroscopic right knee surgery. An ultrasound-guided transgluteal approach was used to administer a sciatic nerve block on the right side. On routine postoperative surgical review 6 weeks later, among other symptoms, the patient indicates that he is experiencing erectile dysfunction and partial loss of sensation over the right aspect of his penis. Iatrogenic injury to the pudendal nerve is suspected. Which of the following is least likely to be affected by the injury to this nerve?

A. External anal sphincter

B. External urethral sphincter

C. Ischiocavernosus muscle

D. Skin of the medial thigh

E. Skin of the scrotum

32. At the routine 6-month evaluation of a male infant, it is discovered he has bilateral cryptorchidism with otherwise normal male external genitalia. His karyotype is 46 XY. Imaging at 1 year of age in preparation for correcting the cryptorchidism reveals a uterus and uterine tubes. His anti-Müllerian hormone level is undetectable and a diagnosis of persistent Müllerian duct syndrome is made. Which of the following structures does not normally arise from the homologous ducts in individuals of this child's gender?

A. Ampulla of ductus deferens

B. Ductus deferens

C. Epididymis

D. Prostate

E. Seminal gland (vesicle)

33. A 12-year-old boy is seen by his pediatrician after suffering a straddle injury to his perineal region while attempting BMX-style stunts with his bicycle. A cysto-urethrogram indicates that the injury resulted in rupture of the spongy urethra, corpus spongiosum, and Buck's (deep perineal) fascia, with the extravasation of blood and urine. Extravasated fluids are least likely to drain into which of the following?

A. Anal triangle

B. Abdominal wall

C. Penis

D. Scrotum

E. Superficial perineal space (pouch)

34. A 3-week-old male, born at 38-weeks of gestation, presents for his first visit to the pediatric clinic. His parents are concerned about a bulge in his scrotum that has been present since birth. The mass has not changed in size and there is no reduction with compression when the mass is palpated. Transillumination of the scrotum readily defines the surface of a testicle with a translucent zone surrounding it. Which of the following diagnoses is most likely?

A. Hydrocele

B. Testicular cancer

C. Testicular torsion

D. Undescended testis

E. Varicocele

35. A 64-year-old man who has had type 2 diabetes for 14 years and erectile dysfunction (ED) for 8 years elects to use a vacuum device for his ED. Vacuum devices mechanically create penile blood engorgement and consist of a vacuum chamber or cylinder, a pump to produce negative pressure, and a band that fits around the base of the penis once it is erect (constriction ring). Which of the following nerves would normally be directly responsible for eliciting the vascular engorgement that is being created artificially with the vacuum device?

A. Parasympathetic efferent

B. Somatic afferent

C. Somatic efferent

D. Sympathetic efferent

E. Visceral afferent

36. A 63-year-old man with a known history of benign prostatic hyperplasia (BPH) reports to his urologist for a follow-up. He complains of continued frequency of urination and slow initiation of a urine stream. The urologist performs a digital rectal examination to determine the size and consistency of the patient's prostate. Which of the following is least likely to be palpable?

A. Evidence of urinary retention in the bladder

B. Inflamed and swollen seminal glands (vesicles)

C. Lateral lobes of the prostate

D. Median lobe of the prostate

E. Posterior lobe of the prostate

37. A 25-year-old man, whose wife recently discovered a painless, firm lump on his right testicle, presents to his primary care provider. Physical examination, ultrasound and radiographic testing confirm the presence of a right testicular mass. Serum evaluation for tumor markers indicates a testicular malignancy. Advanced imaging shows the cancer has spread to lymph nodes. Which of the following lymph nodes are likely to be involved?

A. Deep inguinal

B. External iliac

C. Internal iliac

D. Lumbar (lateral aortic)

E. Superficial inguinal

38. A 23-year-old male mixed martial arts competitor presents to the emergency department after a kick to the groin has caused numbness in his scrotum. Physical examination reveals that the numbness is confined to his anterior scrotum. Which of the following nerves is most likely injured?

A. Femoral

B. Genitofemoral

C. Iliohypogastric

D. Ilioinguinal

E. Posterior scrotal

39. A 12-year-old boy is brought to the emergency department with the chief complaint of acute onset of left-side scrotal pain of several hours' duration. His left hemiscrotum is edematous (swollen) and erythematous (red), and the cremasteric reflex is absent on that side. Color Doppler ultrasound reveals absence of blood flow to the left testicle and epididymis. The diagnosis is testicular torsion with "bell clapper deformity." Which of the following abnormalities most significantly contributes to this deformity?

A. Abnormal attachment of tunica vaginalis

B. Communicating hydrocele

C. Direct inguinal hernia

D. Indirect inguinal hernia

E. Patent processus vaginalis

40. A 35-year-old man with left scrotal pain and swelling for the last week presents to his primary care provider. He also reports feeling feverish. Elevation of the affected hemiscrotum relieves the pain (Prehn's sign). Transverse ultrasound imaging through the left hemiscrotum demonstrates enlargement of the body of the epididymis. Which of the following is the embryological origin of the inflamed structure?

A. Mesonephric duct

B. Mesonephric tubules

C. Paramesonephric duct

D. Seminiferous (testis) cords

E. Urogenital sinus

41. A 45-year-old man with fever, chills, and mild pain in his perineum and lower abdomen presents to his primary care provider. He also experiences painful urination and urinary difficulty. Physical examination reveals suprapubic tenderness, a distended bladder, and an enlarged and tender prostate. A urine sample indicates infection and a diagnosis of prostatitis is made. Which of the following nerves would convey the referred pain experienced by this individual?

A. Pelvic splanchnic

B. Perineal

C. Posterior scrotal

D. Pudendal

E. Sacral splanchnic

42. Following an uncomplicated pregnancy, a 25-year-old woman gives birth to a full-term male. On physical examination, the newborn has a midshaft opening on the ventral aspect of his penis. Which of the following conditions describes this anomaly?

A. Epispadias

B. Exstrophy of the bladder

C. Hypospadias

D. Paraphimosis

E. Priapism

43. A 25-year-old man and his wife report to the fertility clinic as they have been unsuccessful in their efforts to conceive. After a fertility workup, it is determined that the wife's reproductive function is normal, but the man has oligospermia (low sperm count). On physical examination, both his testes are normal in size, with no palpable masses. The spermatic cord on the left, however, has the feel of a "bag of worms." Which of the following conditions most likely exist in this patient?

A. Hematocele

B. Hydrocele

C. Spermatocele

D. Testicular torsion

E. Varicocele

44. A 40-year-old man with penile discomfort presents to his urologist. On physical examination, the urologist notes that the prepuce cannot be fully retracted from the glans. The patient was recently treated for balanitis (inflammation of the glans penis). Which of the following conditions most likely exist in this patient?

A. Epispadias

B. Exstrophy of the bladder

C. Hypospadias

D. Phimosis

E. Priapism

45. A 30-year-old man with infertility presents to his urologist. He reports that he experiences the sensation of orgasm but only produces a few drops of semen from the external urethral orifice. He further indicates that he "dribbles" fluid for some time after experiencing orgasm. This occurs even when his penis has returned to the flaccid state. Electro-ejaculation is used to obtain semen with viable sperm. Which of the following nerves would normally regulate the process that is absent in this patient?

A. Genitofemoral and ilioinguinal

B. Great splanchnic and pelvic splanchnic

C. Ilioinguinal and iliohypogastric

D. Lesser splanchnic and pelvic splanchnic

E. Sacral splanchnic and perineal

Consider the following case for questions 46 and 47:

A 70-year-old man is scheduled for a prostate biopsy following inconclusive results of a rectal digital examination and an elevated serum prostate specific antigen (PSA) level. The urologist uses a transrectal ultrasound-guided approach. After administering periprostatic anesthesia, a biopsy needle is advanced through the anterior rectal wall adjacent to the ultrasound probe, and then guided into the prostate to obtain the biopsy samples.

46. Which of the following structures is also likely to be immediately affected by the anesthesia?

A. Deep transverse perineal muscle

B. Hemorrhoidal plexus

C. Seminal gland (vesicle)

D. Spongy urethra

E. Ureter

47. After biopsy confirms a diagnosis of prostate cancer, the man consults with several physicians and decides to undergo a traditional "open" radical prostatectomy. Which of the following approaches would be most appropriate to employ for this type of surgery for the diseased organ?

A. Intraperitoneal

B. Retropubic

C. Supravesical

D. Transurethral

48. A 2-month-old infant is brought to the pediatrician by his parents because they are concerned that he still "has no testicles." On physical examination, no testes are palpable in either the scrotum or the inguinal canals. Further examination reveals that the infant has a micropenis and that there is a vaginal introitus with a urethral orifice. Laboratory studies indicate the patient has congenital adrenal hyperplasia (CAH) and that this female infant has virilized external genitalia. Which of the following accurately describes homologous structures that were likely misidentified in this individual?

A. Bulbs of the vestibule and bulbourethral (Cowper's) glands

B. Greater vestibular glands and bulb of the penis

C. Labia majora and bulb of the penis

D. Labia majora and penile urethra

E. Vestibule and penile urethra

49. A 59-year-old man with a 6-month history of difficulty voiding and the sensation that he cannot completely empty his bladder reports to his urologist. He has had two episodes of urinary tract infections but denies dysuria (burning with urination) or urethral discharge. The urologist places the cystoscope through the external urethral orifice into the navicular fossa. Which of the following tissues surrounds this portion of the male urethra?

A. Corpus spongiosum

B. External urethral sphincter muscle

C. Pelvic diaphragm

D. Prostate

E. Seminal colliculus

Consider the following case for questions 50 and 51:

A full-term male is delivered vaginally to a 36-year-old mother. At delivery, it is noted that the baby has a large scrotum. In the delivery room the midwife palpates the enlarged scrotum and detects both testicles, however when she presses gently on the newborn's abdomen, the scrotum swells.

50. Which of the following congenital conditions is most likely present in this baby?

A. Communicating hydrocele

B. Femoral hernia

C. Maldescended testis

D. Umbilical hernia

E. Varicocele

51. The mother brings the child to the pediatric surgeon after his second birthday for a surgical repair. At the level of the testicle, between which of the following layers will the surgeon find accumulated fluid?

A. Cremasteric fascia and internal spermatic fascia

B. Dartos and external spermatic fascia

C. Ductus deferens and the internal spermatic fascia

D. Internal and external spermatic fascia

E. Visceral and parietal layers of tunica vaginalis

8.2 Answers and Explanations

Easy	Medium	Hard

Refer to the following image for answers 1 and 2:

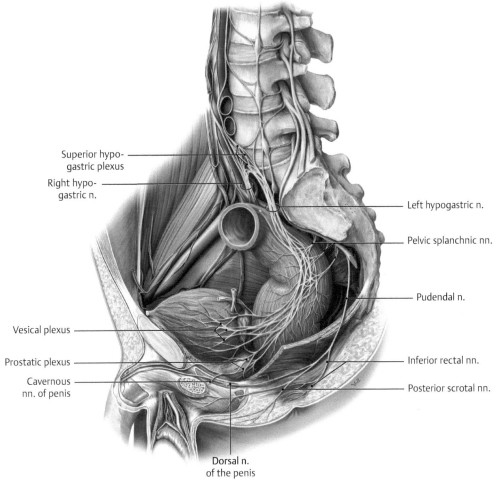

Superior hypo-gastric plexus

Right hypo-gastric n.

Left hypogastric n.

Pelvic splanchnic nn.

Pudendal n.

Vesical plexus

Prostatic plexus

Cavernous nn. of penis

Inferior rectal nn.

Posterior scrotal nn.

Dorsal n. of the penis

Source: Gilroy AM et al. Atlas of Anatomy. 3rd ed. 2016. Based on: Schuenke M, Schulte E, Schumacher U. THIEME Atlas of Anatomy. Volumes 1-3. Illustrations by Voll M and Wesker K. 2nd ed. New York: Thieme Medical Publishers; 2016

1. Correct: Erectile dysfunction (A)

(**A**) The cavernous nerves travel in the prostatic nerve plexus and leave the pelvis with the urethra before distributing to the corpus spongiosum and corpora cavernosa. They convey parasympathetic fibers to the erectile tissue of the penis, facilitating erection. The cavernous nerves, as they travel through the prostatic plexus, are susceptible to injury during a prostatectomy and damage would most likely result in erectile dysfunction (refer to the accompanying image). (**B**) Injury to the inferior rectal nerve would result in dysfunction of the external anal sphincter and likely result in fecal incontinence. The inferior rectal nerve, a branch of the pudendal nerve, courses through the ischioanal fossa and does not contribute to the prostatic nerve plexus. (**C**) Loss of sensation from the penis would result from injury to the

dorsal nerve of the penis, a branch of the pudendal nerve. The latter exits the pelvis via the greater sciatic foramen and then enters the perineum through the lesser sciatic foramen. It does not travel through the prostatic nerve plexus. (**D**) Loss of sensation from the posterior scrotum would result from injury to the posterior scrotal nerves, branches of the pudendal nerve. (**E**) Loss of voluntary control of the bladder would result from injury to the deep branch of the perineal nerve, a branch of the pudendal that innervates the external urethral sphincter. The pudendal nerve is located in the perineum and does not contribute to the prostatic nerve plexus. Voluntary control of urinary continence is dependent on contraction of the external urethral sphincter, whereas involuntary control is mediated by the detrusor reflex, whose efferent limb is mediated by parasympathetic innervation.

2. Correct: S2–S4 (D)

(**D**) The cell bodies of preganglionic parasympathetic fibers that travel in the cavernous nerves are found at spinal cord levels S2–S4. Their axons travel to the prostatic plexus via the pelvic splanchnic nerves (nervi erigentes) that branch from the ventral rami of S2–S4 (refer to the accompanying image). (**A–C, E**) Spinal cord levels L1-L4, S5-Co1, T11-T12, and T12-L2 do not contain any parasympathetic neurons. Preganglionic parasympathetic cell bodies are located only in brainstem nuclei and S2-S4 spinal cord segments.

3. Correct: Inability to empty the bladder (A)

(**A**) The detrusor reflex, the involuntary reflex involved in urinary bladder empting, is stimulated by receptors in the bladder wall that respond to stretch. In response to stretching of the bladder wall, parasympathetic stimulation leads to contraction of the detrusor muscle and urinary bladder emptying. Injury to these parasympathetic fibers would likely result in the inability to empty the urinary bladder. (**B, C**) Postganglionic sympathetic fibers inhibit detrusor muscle contraction and stimulate contraction of the internal urethral sphincter. If these fibers were injured there would be loss of internal sphincter function and urinary incontinence would result. (**D**) Contraction of the external anal sphincter is under control of the inferior rectal branches of the pudendal nerve. Although the pudendal nerve also originates from spinal segments S2–S4, these somatic efferent fibers do not travel with the pelvic splanchnic nerves.

4. Correct: Dorsal nerve of the penis (C)

(**C**) The dorsal nerve of the penis is a terminal branch of the pudendal nerve on each side (the other terminal branch being the perineal nerve). It passes inferior to the pubic symphysis, just deep to the deep fascia of the penis (Buck's fascia), and conveys sensory innervation from the penis. (**A**) The anterior scrotal nerve, an anterior cutaneous branch of the ilioinguinal nerve, conveys sensory innervation from the skin of the anterior scrotum. (**B**) The deep branch of the perineal nerve is distributed to the muscles of the urogenital triangle. It does not convey sensory innervation from the penis. (**D**) The posterior scrotal nerve, derived from the superficial branch of the perineal nerve, conveys sensory innervation from the posterior scrotum. (**E**) The superficial perineal nerve, a branch of the perineal branch of the pudendal nerve, gives rise to posterior scrotal nerves.

Refer to the following image for answer 4:

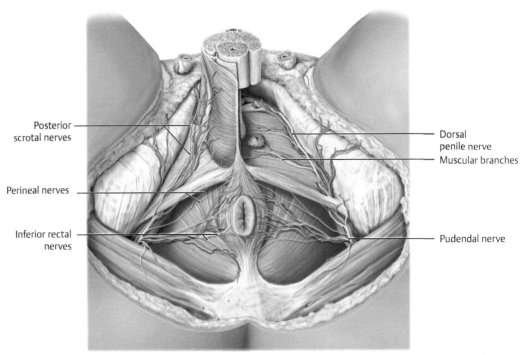

Source: Schuenke M, Schulte E, Schumacher U. THIEME Atlas of Anatomy. General Anatomy and Musculoskeletal System. Illustrations by Voll M and Wesker K. 2nd ed. New York: Thieme Medical Publishers; 2016

5. Correct: Pudendal (E)

(**E**) Irritation of the pudendal nerve (pudendal neuralgia) is often a source of perineal pain for avid cyclists (bicycle seat neuropathy). The nerve can be irritated anywhere along its course. In this case, branches of the pudendal that supply structures in the urogenital triangle, notably the perineal branches and dorsal nerve of the penis, were affected. Testing for pudendal neuralgia involves CT-guided injection of anesthetic, either in the region of the ischial spine or pudendal (Alcock's) canal. (**A**) The inferior rectal nerve may be irritated by similar activities, but symptoms would present differently and involve structures in the anal region. (**B**) The inferior gluteal nerve supplies the gluteus maximus muscle and irritation of this nerve would not produce the symptoms seen in this patient. (**C**) The obturator nerve supplies muscles of the medial thigh and irritation of this nerve would not produce the symptoms seen in this patient. (**D**) The posterior cutaneous nerve of the thigh arises from the ventral rami of S1, S2, and S3 nerves. It distributes to the skin of the posterior thigh, buttocks, and the posterior scrotum/labia. Irritation of this nerve would not produce the symptoms seen in this patient.

Refer to the following image for answer 5:

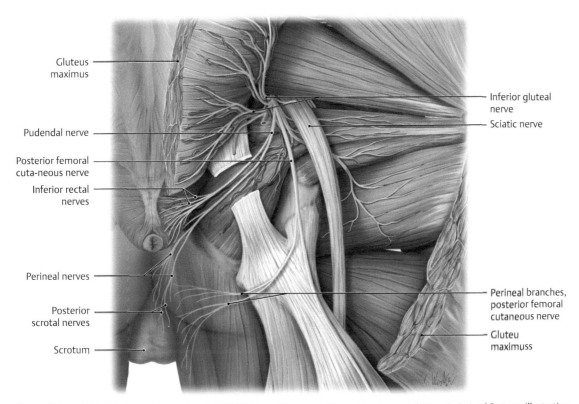

Source: Schuenke M, Schulte E, Schumacher U. THIEME Atlas of Anatomy. General Anatomy and Musculoskeletal System, Illustrations by Voll M and Wesker K. 2nd ed. New York: Thieme Medical Publishers; 2016

6. Correct: Internal pudendal (D)

Refer to the following image for answer 6:

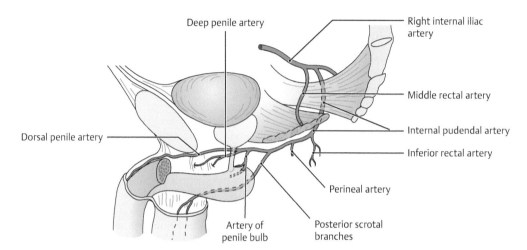

(**D**) The internal pudendal arteries supply the erectile tissue including the bulb of the penis, the corpus spongiosum, and the corpora cavernosa via the artery to the bulb of the penis, the deep artery of the penis, and the dorsal artery of the penis, respectively. Atherosclerosis in these vessels can lead to erectile dysfunction. (**A**) The deferential artery is a branch of the internal iliac artery and supplies blood to the ductus (vas) deferens, not to the erectile tissues. (**B, C, E**) The external iliac, inferior epigastric, and lateral sacral arteries do not supply blood to any reproductive structures in the pelvis or perineum.

7. Correct: Skin, superficial penile fascia, deep penile (Buck's) fascia, tunica albuginea (C)

Refer to the following image for answer 7:

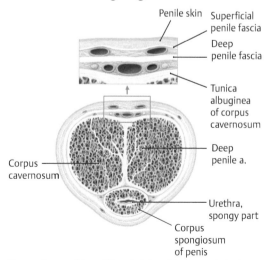

Source: Source: Gilroy AM et al. Atlas of Anatomy. 3rd ed. 2016. Based on: Schuenke M, Schulte E, Schumacher U. THIEME Atlas of Anatomy. Volumes 1-3. Illustrations by Voll M and Wesker K. 2nd ed. New York: Thieme Medical Publishers; 2016

(**C**) The needle would pass, sequentially through the skin, superficial fascia of the penis, deep (Buck's) fascia of the penis, and tunica albuginea. (**A**) The superficial fascia of the penis is superficial to the deep (Buck's) fascia of the penis. Dartos fascia is continuous with the superficial fascia of the penis as well as the superficial fascia of the scrotum and would not be the deepest layer pierced by the needle. (**B, E**) The perineal membrane is not found in the body of the penis and, while it is associated with the root of the penis, it is located deep to the erectile bodies and does not form one of the coverings of the erectile bodies. (**D**) The tunica albuginea is the deepest layer surrounding the corpora cavernosa.

8. Correct: Seminal fluid and prostatic fluid (B)

(**B**) Secretions from the seminal glands (vesicles), the prostate gland and the testes (sperm) are combined in the prostatic part of the urethra to form semen. Typically, the ductus (vas) deferens is ligated in the superior scrotum during a vasectomy. Since the ligation occurs in the scrotum proximal to the seminal glands and prostate, only sperm would be expected to be missing from semen. (**A**) The prostate gland and the seminal glands release their secretions into the prostatic part of the urethra and would not be affected by ligation of the ductus deferens. Thus, secretions from both glands would be present in the post-vasectomy ejaculate. (**C–E**) Sperm would not be found in the ejaculate because the ductus deferens carries sperm from the tail of the epididymis to the ejaculatory duct. When the ductus deferens is ligated, sperm will not reach the ejaculatory duct and will not be included as part of semen.

9. Correct: Subperitoneal (infraperitoneal) (D)

(**D**) Urethral injuries located in the membranous and prostatic urethra are considered posterior urethral injuries. Often they are the result of blunt trauma during a motor vehicle collision or from serious falls. They may be accompanied by pelvic fractures. Since the rupture occurred distal and inferior to the prostatic urethra and at the perineal membrane, blood and urine would collect primarily in the subperitoneal space of the pelvis, superior to the perineal spaces (pouches). (**A**) When there is urethral trauma distal to the perineal membrane and membranous urethra, which does not involve the deep (Buck's) fascia, extravasation is confined by Buck's fascia. In this case, edema and extravasated urine and blood will be restricted to the shaft of the penis. This is called an eggplant deformity or the aubergine sign. (**B, C, E**) When there is injury to the urethra distal to the perineal membrane and Buck's fascia is compromised, patients typically have a "butterfly" hematoma. This results from blood collecting in the superficial perineal space and lower anterior abdominal wall. Scrotal enlargement is also common in this injury, as extravasated fluids follow the reflections of the membranous layer (Colles') of superficial fascia.

Refer to the following image for answer 9:

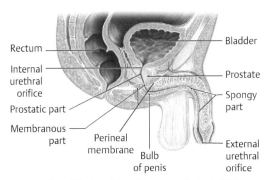

Source: Gilroy AM et al. Atlas of Anatomy. 3rd ed. 2016. Based on: Schuenke M, Schulte E, Schumacher U. THIEME Atlas of Anatomy. Volumes 1-3. Illustrations by Voll M and Wesker K. 2nd ed. New York: Thieme Medical Publishers; 2016

10. Correct: Sacral splanchnic (E)

(**E**) During orgasm, the initial step in emission is contraction of the internal urethral sphincter at the urinary bladder neck due to sympathetic innervation. This action prevents retrograde flow of semen into the urinary bladder. With retrograde ejaculation, the urethral sphincter does not constrict properly and semen can enter the bladder (hence the cloudy urine and low volume of ejaculate expressed from the penis). Preganglionic sympathetic fibers arise from T1–L1/L2 spinal cord levels and synapse in the sympathetic chain. Postganglionic sympathetic fibers leave the sacral sympathetic chain as sacral splanchnic nerves to join the inferior hypogastric plexus that then course to the internal urethral sphincter via the pelvic plexuses. (**A**) The least splanchnic nerves contain preganglionic sympathetic axons that arise from T11–T12 spinal segments and travel to the aorticorenal plexus, where they synapse with postganglionic neurons. These do not supply the internal urethral sphincter. (**B**) The lumbosacral trunk is comprised of part of the L4 ventral ramus and all of the L5 ventral ramus. These nerve fibers join the sacral plexus and are mostly involved in the sensory and motor innervation of the lower extremity. (**C**) The pelvic splanchnic nerves contain parasympathetic preganglionic fibers that arise from S2–S4 spinal segments and do not innervate the internal urethral sphincter. (**D**) The somatic pudendal nerve is also derived from S2–S4 spinal segments and conveys motor and sensory innervation to and from the perineum. It does not innervate the internal urethral sphincter.

11. Correct: Left renal (E)

(**E**) The cancer cells from the left testis would travel first within the testicular vein to the left renal vein and then into the inferior vena cava. On the right side, the testicular vein drains directly into the inferior vena cava. (**A**) The left testicular vein drains into the left renal vein, so cancer cells in the left testicular vein would not directly enter the inferior vena cava. (**B–D**) The inferior epigastric, internal iliac and internal pudendal vessels do not play a role in venous drainage of the testes.

Refer to the following image for answer 11:

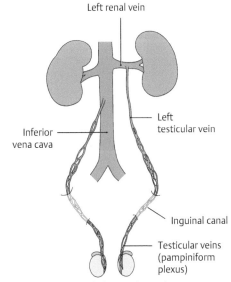

Source: Schuenke M, Schulte E, Schumacher U. THIEME Atlas of Anatomy. Internal Organs. Illustrations by Voll M and Wesker K. 2nd ed. New York: Thieme Medical Publishers; 2016

12. Correct: Epididymis (D)

Refer to the following images for answer 12:

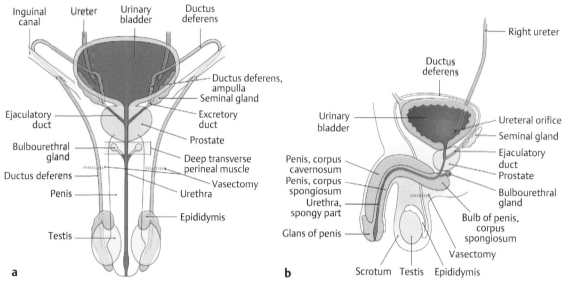

Source: Gilroy AM et al. Atlas of Anatomy. 3rd ed. 2016. Based on: Schuenke M, Schulte E, Schumacher U. THIEME Atlas of Anatomy. Volumes 1-3. Illustrations by Voll M and Wesker K. 2nd ed. New York: Thieme Medical Publishers; 2016

(**D**) The epididymis is the only location listed where mature sperm are likely to be found following a vasectomy. Normally, the ductus deferens is ligated in the superior aspect of the scrotum. Therefore, mature sperm can only travel from the testis through the epididymis and into the most proximal ductus deferens. (**A, C, E**) The ampulla of the ductus deferens, ejaculatory duct, and prostatic urethra are all distal to the site of ligation and would not contain viable sperm. (**B**) The duct of the seminal gland conveys only seminal fluid and would not be expected to ever contain sperm.

13. Correct: Smaller subpubic angle (D)

(**D**) The subpubic angle of the male pelvis is smaller than that of the female. Generally, one can use the angle formed between the spread index (second) and middle (third) fingers to approximate the subpubic angle in a male and the angle formed between the thumb (first) and index (second) fingers to approximate the subpubic angle in a female. (**A–C, E**) These are all features of a female pelvis. Generally, the subpubic angle and pubic arch are greater in the female pelvis than in the male pelvis. The pelvic inlet for females is rounded, while for males it is heart shaped. The pelvic outlet for females is larger than in males.

Refer to the following image for answer 13:

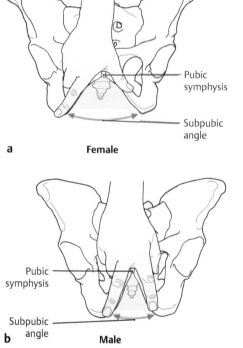

Source: Gilroy AM et al. Atlas of Anatomy. 3rd ed. 2016. Based on: Schuenke M, Schulte E, Schumacher U. THIEME Atlas of Anatomy. Volumes 1-3. Illustrations by Voll M and Wesker K. 2nd ed. New York: Thieme Medical Publishers; 2016

Refer to the following image for answers 14 and 15:

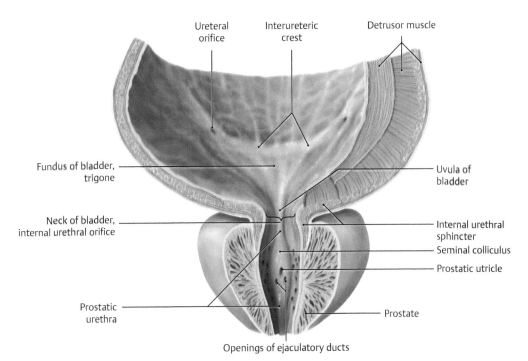

Ureteral orifice

Intereureteric crest

Detrusor muscle

Fundus of bladder, trigone

Neck of bladder, internal urethral orifice

Prostatic urethra

Uvula of bladder

Internal urethral sphincter

Seminal colliculus

Prostatic utricle

Prostate

Openings of ejaculatory ducts

Source: Gilroy AM et al. Atlas of Anatomy. 3rd ed. 2016. Based on: Schuenke M, Schulte E, Schumacher U. THIEME Atlas of Anatomy. Volumes 1-3. Illustrations by Voll M and Wesker K. 2nd ed. New York: Thieme Medical Publishers; 2016

14. Correct: Uvula of the bladder (E)

(**E**) The uvula is a median projection of the mucosa on the posterior wall of the urinary bladder near the internal urethral orifice. Because the uvula overlies the middle lobe of the prostate, enlargement of the prostate, as in benign prostatic hyperplasia (BPH), can result in constriction of the urethra by an impinging uvula, resulting in difficulties with urination. (**A**) The external urethral sphincter (sphincter urethrae) is a skeletal muscle in the perineum that encircles the membranous and portions of the prostatic urethra and functions in the voluntary control of urination. It would not be enlarged in BPH. (**B**) The intereureteric crest is an elevation on the posterior wall of the bladder that courses transversely between the two ureteric orifices. It is unrelated to the prostate gland and would not be enlarged in BPH. (**C**) The prostatic utricle is a small, blind, epithelium-lined diverticulum in the posterior wall of the prostatic urethra at the cranial end of the seminal colliculus. It is located between the openings of the ejaculatory ducts and is believed to be a remnant of the fused caudal ends of the Müllerian ducts, and thus the male homolog of the upper vagina and uterine cervix. It would not be enlarged in BPH. (**D**) The seminal colliculus is an elevation on the urethral crest of the posterior wall of the prostatic urethra where the two ejaculatory ducts and the prostatic utricle open.

15. Correct: Ejaculatory duct (C)

(**C**) The ejaculatory duct on each side opens onto the posterior wall of the prostatic urethra. Each duct forms from the union of the duct of the respective seminal gland and ductus deferens, and courses through the prostate gland to open on either side of seminal colliculus (also referred to as the veromontanum). Removal of the posterior wall of the prostatic urethra likely also removes a portion of the ejaculatory ducts. (**A**) The ampulla of the ductus deferens is a distal enlargement of the ductus deferens just proximal to where it joins the duct of the seminal gland to form the ejaculatory duct. It does not traverse the prostate gland and would not be affected by the surgery. (**B**) The bulbourethral glands are located in the perineum distal to the prostatic urethra. The ducts of the bulbourethral glands on each side open into the bulbar portion of the spongy urethra. They are not associated with the prostatic urethra and are unlikely to be affected by the surgery. (**D**) The navicular fossa is a dilation in the portion of the spongy urethra as it passes through the glans penis. It would not be affected by surgery in the prostatic urethra. (**E**) The seminiferous tubules are the system of tubules within each testis where spermatogenesis takes place. They are not associated with the prostatic urethra and would not be affected by the surgery.

16. Correct: Subcutaneous (dartos) fascia, external spermatic fascia, cremaster muscle and fascia, internal spermatic fascia (D)

(**D**) The correct order of layers after the skin would be the subcutaneous (dartos) fascia, external spermatic fascia, cremaster muscle and fascia, internal spermatic fascia. (**A, B**) The subcutaneous (dartos) fascia is a superficial layer of fascia continuous with the superficial fascia of the abdominal wall and the perineum. It is external to the spermatic cord and its layers. (**C, E**) The tunica vaginalis testis is a double layer of serous membrane that encloses the anterior and lateral aspects of the testis. It is the distal remnant of the processus vaginalis, and would not normally be found in the upper scrotum.

Refer to the following image for answer 16:

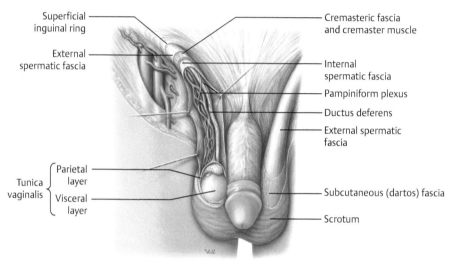

Source: Gilroy AM et al. Atlas of Anatomy. 3rd ed. 2016. Based on: Schuenke M, Schulte E, Schumacher U. THIEME Atlas of Anatomy. Volumes 1-3. Illustrations by Voll M and Wesker K. 2nd ed. New York: Thieme Medical Publishers; 2016

17. Correct: Deep to the deep penile (Buck's) fascia (D)

Refer to the following image for answer 17:

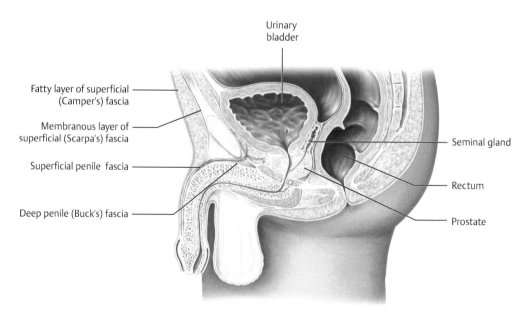

Source: Gilroy AM et al. Atlas of Anatomy. 3rd ed. 2016. Based on: Schuenke M, Schulte E, Schumacher U. THIEME Atlas of Anatomy. Volumes 1-3. Illustrations by Voll M and Wesker K. 2nd ed. New York: Thieme Medical Publishers; 2016

(**D**) Because the injury is confined to the urethra, it will be retained beneath (deep to) the deep (Buck's) fascia. (**A**) In order for the urine to extravasate between the deep (Buck's) and the superficial fascia, there would have to be injury to Buck's fascia in addition to injury to the urethra. (**B**) For there to be extravasation of urine into the anterior abdominal wall, there would have to be damage to Buck's fascia as well as the urethra and the extravasated urine would be deep to the superficial fascia (both fatty [Camper's] and membranous [Scarpa's] layers). (**C**) For there to be extravasation of urine into the superficial perineal space, between the deep and superficial fascia, there would have to be damage to Buck's fascia as well as the urethra.

18. Correct: Between the parietal and visceral layers of the tunica vaginalis (C)

(**C**) A hydrocele develops when there is fluid accumulation in the potential space between the visceral and parietal layers of the tunica vaginalis of the testes. During development, this space results from the processus vaginalis, a diverticulum of peritoneum on each side that precedes the descent of the testes into the scrotum. During the perinatal period (a few weeks before or after birth), the connection between the peritoneal cavity and the processus is lost and a distal remnant of the processus vaginalis persists as the tunica vaginalis, which envelops the testicle. The tunica has parietal and visceral layers separated by a potential space containing a thin layer of serous fluid. (**A, B, D, E**) Because this represents a hydrocele, it would not be located outside the potential space of the tunica vaginalis or between the other individual layers of the spermatic cord.

Refer to the following image for answer 18:

19. Correct: Subperitoneal (infra- or retroperitoneal) (E)

(**E**) Rupture at the bladder neck would be inside the pelvic cavity, but not the peritoneal cavity, and therefore urine from the ruptured urinary bladder would leak into the extraperitoneal tissues around the subperitoneal bladder, as seen in the accompanying cystogram (*arrows*). (**A, C, D**) Extravasation into the lower abdominal wall deep to the superficial (Colles' and Scarpa's) fascia or deep to the superficial (dartos) fascia of the scrotum and penis, is more likely to occur if there is injury to the urethra distal to the perineal membrane and involving the deep (Buck's) fascia. (**B**) Extravasation deep to the deep (Buck's) fascia is more likely to occur if there is injury to the urethra distal to the perineal membrane and *not* involving Buck's fascia.

20. Correct: Pelvic splanchnic (C)

(**C**) The pelvic splanchnic nerves arise from S2–S4 spinal segments and convey preganglionic parasympathetic fibers. The parasympathetic preganglionic fibers involved with the bladder join the vesical plexus on the bladder wall to synapse with postganglionic neurons. These nerves mediate the "detrusor reflex" involving both visceral afferent impulses resulting from distension of the wall of the urinary bladder and parasympathetic motor fibers to the detrusor muscle. (**A**) The ilioinguinal nerve arises from the L1 spinal cord. It passes along the inguinal canal and exits through the superficial inguinal ring to supply the skin of the upper medial thigh and anterior scrotum. It has no role in bladder function. (**B, E**) The lumbar splanchnic nerves arise from the abdominal part of the sympathetic trunk. They travel to the intermesenteric, inferior mesenteric, and superior hypogastric

Covering layer		Derived from
①	Scrotal skin	Abdominal skin
②	Tunica dartos	Dartos fascia and muscle
③	External spermatic fascia	External oblique
④	Cremaster muscle and cremasteric fascia*	Internal oblique
⑤	Internal spermatic fascia	Transversalis fascia
⑥a	Tunica vaginalis, parietal layer	Peritoneum
⑥b	Tunica vaginalis, visceral layer	

* The transversus abdominis has no contribution to the spermatic cord or covering of the testis.

Source: Source: Gilroy AM et al. Atlas of Anatomy. 3rd ed. 2016. Based on: Schuenke M, Schulte E, Schumacher U. THIEME Atlas of Anatomy. Volumes 1-3. Illustrations by Voll M and Wesker K. 2nd ed. New York: Thieme Medical Publishers; 2016

plexuses and convey preganglionic sympathetic fibers to associated prevertebral ganglia. Postganglionic sympathetic fibers travel to targets in the abdomen and pelvis. Sympathetic innervation of the bladder is from T10–L2 spinal cord segments and causes the internal urethral sphincter to contract and the bladder wall to relax. (**D**) The pudendal nerve also arises from S2–S4 spinal nerves; however, it conducts somatic efferent and afferent fibers to and from the perineal region and does not play a role in bladder function. Somatic control of urination is through the external urethral sphincter that is innervated by a branch of the pudendal nerve.

Refer to the following image for answer 20:

21. Correct: Pubis (E)

(**E**) The vertically oriented fracture crosses the body of the pubic bone. (**A–D**) The fracture is not present in these other parts of the bony pelvis (acetabulum, body of ilium, iliac fossa, ischium).

22. Correct: Ala of sacrum and auricular surface of ilium (A)

(**A**) The diastasis is at the sacro-iliac joint, which separates the ala of the sacrum and the auricular surface of the ilium. (**B–E**) The diastasis is not located between any of these other pelvic bones (apex of sacrum and coccyx, inferior pubic ramus and ramus of ischium, right and left pubic bodies, superior pubic ramus and ilium).

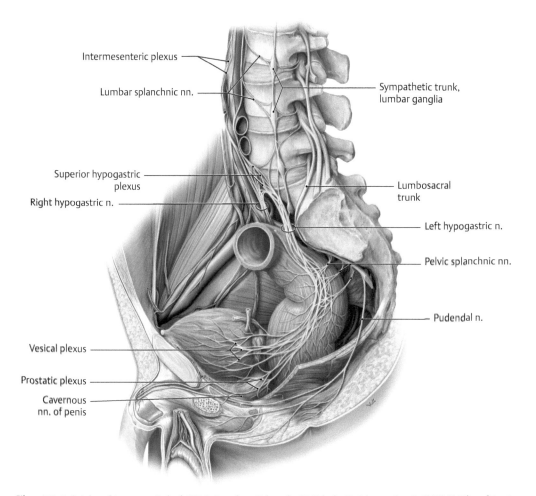

Intermesenteric plexus

Lumbar splanchnic nn.

Sympathetic trunk, lumbar ganglia

Superior hypogastric plexus

Right hypogastric n.

Lumbosacral trunk

Left hypogastric n.

Pelvic splanchnic nn.

Pudendal n.

Vesical plexus

Prostatic plexus

Cavernous nn. of penis

Source: Gilroy AM et al. Atlas of Anatomy. 3rd ed. 2016. Based on: Schuenke M, Schulte E, Schumacher U. THIEME Atlas of Anatomy. Volumes 1-3. Illustrations by Voll M and Wesker K. 2nd ed. New York: Thieme Medical Publishers; 2016

23. Correct: Intraperitoneal (B)

(**B**) This is an example of an intraperitoneal urinary bladder rupture. There is contrast within the peritoneal cavity as evidenced by its outlining the loops of bowel. Intraperitoneal bladder rupture is often caused by a direct blow on a full bladder. Other causes are cystoscopy, surgery, and penetrating trauma. An intraperitoneal bladder rupture implies rupture of the dome, which is the only part of the bladder covered by peritoneum. Intraperitoneal bladder ruptures, as opposed to extraperitoneal bladder ruptures, almost always require surgical repair. (**A**) The retropubic space (cave of Retzius or Retzius' space), is the extraperitoneal space between the pubic symphysis and urinary bladder. (**C, E**) The perineal and subpubic spaces are located in the perineum. The contrast medium and, thus, the extravasated urine in this individual are within the peritoneal cavity and unrelated to the perineal or subpubic space. (**D**) The majority of bladder ruptures are into the extraperitoneal tissues and the contrast medium and urine would tend to outline the urinary bladder. An extraperitoneal rupture is usually located at the base of the urinary bladder.

24. Correct: It may pass through the superficial inguinal ring (C)

(**C**) An indirect inguinal hernia will enter the inguinal canal via the deep inguinal ring and the hernia's neck will be located at this point (i.e., lateral to the inferior epigastric vessels). The hernial sac may extend the entire length of the inguinal canal and may protrude through the superficial inguinal ring and course along the spermatic cord into the scrotum. This usually develops over a period of time. Indirect inguinal hernias are almost always associated with a patent processes vaginalis and manifest within the first few decades of life. (**A**) An indirect hernia does pass through the deep inguinal ring. (**B**) The median umbilical fold is a peritoneal fold created by the underlying median umbilical ligament, a remnant of the urachus. Indirect and direct inguinal hernias will lie lateral to this midline structure. (**D**) The deep inguinal ring is located lateral to the inferior epigastric vessels. An indirect inguinal hernia enters the inguinal canal via the deep inguinal ring, thus the neck of the hernia will lie lateral to the inferior epigastric vessels. (**E**) Indirect inguinal hernias will always involve the deep inguinal ring. Over time they may progress for variable lengths along the inguinal canal to reach and protrude through the superficial inguinal ring and even enter the scrotum. Indirect inguinal hernias do not always reach the superficial inguinal ring. This is somewhat dependent on how much of the processus vaginalis remains patent as this type of hernia follows the course of a patent processus vaginalis.

25. Correct: Gubernaculum testis (B)

(**B**) The gubernaculum testis is a fibromuscular cord that is attached to the lower pole of the testicle and to the floor of the scrotum. It is responsible for "guiding" the testicle along its descent along the posterior abdominal wall, through the inguinal region, and into the scrotum. This is accomplished through a combination of shortening of the gubernaculum and lengthening of the trunk of the fetus. If the testicle is located in the inguinal canal, a portion of the gubernaculum will persist between the testicle and the scrotal wall. Thus, the gubernaculum will pass through the superficial inguinal ring in this patient. If the testicle completes its migration into the scrotum, only a small tuft of gubernaculum persists between the lower pole of the testicle and the scrotal wall. (**A, C, D, E**) The testicle carries all of these structures with it as it migrates to the scrotum. If the testicle is located in the inguinal canal, the vas deferens, epididymis, and testicular vessels will not pass through the superficial inguinal ring.

26. Correct: Genital branch of genitofemoral (B)

(**B**) The cremasteric reflex is elicited by stroking the superior medial aspect of the thigh. The normal response is contraction of the cremaster muscle and elevation of the testis on that side. The genital branch of the genitofemoral nerve (L1–L2) is the efferent limb of the cremasteric reflex as it is motor to the cremaster muscle. Since this branch passes along the inguinal canal, it is susceptible to injury during a herniorrhaphy. (**A**) The cremasteric reflex involves both sensory and motor fibers of the genitofemoral nerve. Sensory information from the superior aspect of the thigh is conveyed via the femoral branch of the genitofemoral nerve (L1–L2) and the ilioinguinal nerve (L1). (**C**) The iliohypogastric nerve (L1) conveys sensory information from the skin superior to and parallel with the inguinal ligament and is not involved in the cremasteric reflex. (**D**) Sensory information for the cremasteric reflex from the anterior scrotum and medial aspect of the thigh is conveyed via the femoral branch of the genitofemoral nerve (L1–L2) and the ilioinguinal nerve (L1). The ilioinguinal nerve enters the inguinal canal, and is susceptible to injury during a herniorrhaphy (**E**) The posterior scrotal nerves convey sensory information from the posterior aspect of the scrotum and do not supply motor fibers to the cremaster muscle.

27. Correct: Abdominal aorta (A)

(**A**) The major arteries that would be clamped are the testicular arteries that are direct branches from the abdominal aorta. (**B–E**) Because the testicular vessels arise from the level of embryological origin of the testes, none of these other vessels (external iliac, inferior epigastric, internal iliac, internal pudendal) provide arterial supply to the testes. While the internal pudendal and femoral arteries do provide blood supply to scrotum, these vessels do not supply the testis.

28. Correct: T10–T11 (E)

(E) Developmentally, the testes originate from the same level to which the kidneys ascend and share a common level of innervation. Visceral afferent fibers from the testes enter the T10–T11 spinal cord levels and pain is referred to those dermatomes on the anterior abdominal wall. (A) The L1 spinal cord level receives primarily somatic sensory innervation from the anterior scrotal skin via the ilioinguinal and genitofemoral nerves. (B) The L4–L5 spinal cord levels receive primarily somatic sensory innervation from the lower extremity and pain would be referred to those dermatomes. (C) Somatic sensory information from the skin of the posterior portion of the scrotum is via the posterior scrotal branches of the pudendal nerves (S2–S4). (D) The T5–T9 dermatomes receive pain sensations from the organs supplied by the celiac plexus.

29. Correct: Cremasteric reflex (A)

(A) The genital branch of the genitofemoral nerve (L1–L2) provides motor innervation to the cremaster muscle and sensory innervation from the anterior scrotum. The femoral branch of the genitofemoral provides sensory innervation from the anterior thigh over the femoral triangle. (B) Hip flexion would not be affected following injury to the genitofemoral nerve, as the hip flexors are innervated by branches of the ventral rami of L2–L4 spinal nerves (femoral nerve). (C) The pyramidalis muscle is supplied by the subcostal nerve (T12) and would not be affected by injury to the genitofemoral nerve. (D) Sensation from the lateral aspect of the thigh is conveyed via the lateral femoral cutaneous nerve (L2–L3) and would not be affected by injury to the genitofemoral nerve. (E) Sensory innervation from the dorsum of the penis is conveyed by the dorsal nerve of the penis, a branch of the pudendal nerve (S2–S4).

30. Correct: Inferior rectal nerve (C)

(C) The inferior rectal nerve, a branch of the pudendal nerve, supplies the external anal sphincter muscle. It courses through the ischioanal fossa and is susceptible to injury when draining a perianal abscess. Injury could result in fecal incontinence. (A) The bulbourethral glands are located deep to the perineal membrane in the male urogenital triangle of the perineum and are not likely to be in jeopardy when a perianal abscess is drained. (B) The inferior gluteal nerve innervates gluteus maximus muscle and does not enter the perineum. (D) The membranous portion of the male urethra exits the pelvis by passing through the pelvic floor in the urogenital (anterior) division of the perineum. It is not associated with the ischioanal fossa. (E) The obturator nerve courses on the lateral wall of the pelvis to exit through the obturator canal and innervate muscles in the medial compartment of the thigh. It is unlikely to be in jeopardy when a perianal abscess is drained.

31. Correct: Skin of the medial thigh (D)

(D) The skin of the medial thigh conveys sensory impulses via the ilioinguinal (L1), and femoral branch of the genitofemoral (L1–L2) nerves that would not be affected by injury to the pudendal nerve. The erectile dysfunction and hypoesthesia of the penis imply that the pudendal nerve was traumatized. Pudendal nerve injury would also result in sensory deficit from the posterior aspect of the scrotum, along with motor deficits for muscles of the perineum. The pudendal nerve lies medial to, and in close proximity with, the sciatic nerve in the gluteal region. Therefore, it is possible that delivery of a sciatic nerve block may injure the pudendal nerve. (A) The external anal sphincter is supplied by the inferior rectal branch of the pudendal nerve and, therefore, would be affected by pudendal nerve injury. (B) The external urethral sphincter (formed by the deep transverse perineal and sphincter urethrae muscles) is supplied by the deep branch of the perineal nerve, a branch of the pudendal nerve. It would be affected by pudendal nerve injury. (C) The ischiocavernosus muscle is supplied by the perineal branch of the pudendal nerve and, therefore, would be affected by pudendal nerve injury. (E) The skin of the scrotum is supplied by the posterior scrotal branch of the pudendal nerve and, therefore, would be affected by pudendal nerve injury.

32. Correct: Prostate (D)

(D) The prostate develops from the prostatic urethra, which is a derivative of the endodermal-lined urogenital sinus. Endodermal outgrowths from the prostatic urethra grow into the surrounding mesoderm to form the glandular epithelium of the prostate. The surrounding mesoderm will form the stroma and the smooth muscle of the prostate. The paramesonephric (Müllerian) ducts of female and the mesonephric (Wolffian) ducts of male are homologous. (A–C, E) The mesonephric (Wolffian) ducts will form the epididymis, ductus deferens, ampulla of the ductus deferens, and the seminal gland. The ejaculatory duct, which passes through the prostate, forms from the ductus deferens and the duct of the seminal gland and is, thus, also derived from the mesonephric ducts.

33. Correct: Anal triangle (A)

(**A**) The extravasation of fluid will not extend into the anal triangle as the extravasation will be deep to Colles' fascia. Since Colles' fascia fuses with the posterior edge of the perineal membrane, the ischiopubic rami on each side, and is continuous with Scarpa's fascia of the anterior abdominal wall, the extravasation will be restricted to the superficial space (pouch) of the urogenital triangle in the perineum. (**B**) Because Colles' is continuous with Scarpa's fascia, the extravasation of blood and urine can spread upward into the anterior abdominal wall deep to Scarpa's fascia. (**C**) Since the rupture pierced the deep penile fascia, extravasation can extend beyond the penis. If Buck's fascia had not been breached, the blood and urine would have been confined to the penis. (**D**) Colles' fascia is continuous with dartos fascia in the scrotum, so extravasation beneath Colles' fascia could result in blood and urine in the scrotum. (**E**) Since Colles' fascia fuses with the posterior edge of the perineal membrane and the ischiopubic rami on each side, and is continuous with Scarpa's fascia of the anterior abdominal wall, the extravasation will be restricted in the perineum to the superficial space of the urogenital triangle.

34. Correct: Hydrocele (A)

Refer to the following image for answer 34:

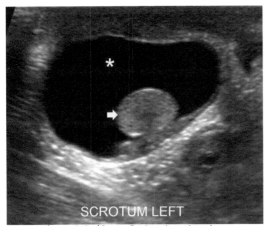

Source: Chopra S. RadCases. Genitourinary Imaging. 1st Edition. Thieme; 2011.

(**A**) A hydrocele is formed when there is patency of the processus vaginalis, allowing accumulation of fluid between layers of the tunica vaginalis (*asterisk* in the accompanying image). The processus vaginalis normally closes spontaneously at the deep inguinal ring, sealing the internal entrance to the inguinal canal. There are different types of hydrocele: if fluid is restricted to the tunica vaginalis it is a noncommunicating or scrotal hydrocele; if the processus vaginalis fuses proximally and distally but remains open in between, the isolated fluid collection is referred to as a hydrocele of the spermatic cord. Because the hydrocele is fluid-filled, it transilluminates. (**B**) Testicular cancer is rare in a newborn and is unlikely to transilluminate. (**C**) Testicular torsion is an acute event, and a urological emergency. The infant would be in considerable pain and would likely have presented sooner. (**D**) An undescended testis would not create a bulge in the scrotal sac that could be transilluminated. (**E**) A varicocele is a swelling in the scrotum due to varicosities in the pampiniform plexus of veins that drain the testis. Varicoceles are most common among teenagers and adult men and have the appearance of "a bag of worms."

35. Correct: Parasympathetic efferent (A)

(**A**) The pelvic splanchnic nerves, also known as nervi erigentes, are preganglionic parasympathetic nerve fibers that arise from the S2–S4 spinal cord. Fibers from the pelvic splanchnics pass through the inferior hypogastric (pelvic) plexus to the cavernous nerves that distribute to the erectile tissue. The cavernous nerves stimulate smooth muscle in the helicine arteries to relax and allow blood to fill the corpora cavernosa and the corpus spongiosum, causing tumescence. (**B**) Somatic afferents, conveyed via the pudendal nerve, transmit sensory innervation from the penis and do not cause vasodilation. (**C**) Somatic efferents are conveyed to the muscles of the external genitalia via the pudendal nerve (S2–S4). These innervate perineal muscles (e.g., bulbospongiosus and ischiocavernosus) and their contraction assists in maintaining an erection. (**D**) Sympathetic efferents cause peristalsis in the ductus deferens and closure of the internal urethral sphincter to prevent reflux of semen into the bladder. (**E**) Visceral afferent fibers are not involved in the vascular engorgement.

36. Correct: Median lobe of the prostate (D)

Refer to the following image for answer 36:

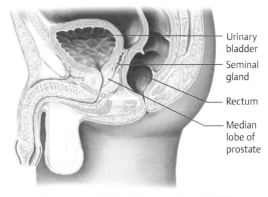

Source: Gilroy AM et al. Atlas of Anatomy. 3rd ed. 2016. Based on: Schuenke M, Schulte E, Schumacher U. THIEME Atlas of Anatomy. Volumes 1-3. Illustrations by Voll M and Wesker K. 2nd ed. New York: Thieme Medical Publishers; 2016

(**D**) The median lobe (sometimes called the middle lobe) of the prostate surrounds the urethra and does not extend to the posterior surface of the prostate. Therefore, it cannot be readily palpated in a digital examination. (**A–C, E**) A full bladder, inflamed seminal glands, and the lateral and posterior lobes of the prostate can all be palpated in a digital examination per anum.

37.   Correct: Lumbar (lateral aortic) (D)

(**D**) The testes begin development high on the posterior abdominal wall. Their blood and lymphatic supply form at this level and, when the testicle migrates to its adult position these vessels elongate to accompany it. The lymphatic vessels of the testes generally follow the testicular veins, eventually emptying into the lumbar (lateral aortic) lymph nodes. Testicular tumors tend to first metastasize to these lymph nodes. The right testis drains into the interaortocaval node, which is located at the level of the L2 vertebral body. In contrast, the left testis drains into lymph nodes in the para-aortic region in an area bounded by the renal vein superiorly, the aorta medially, the ureter laterally, and the origin of the inferior mesenteric artery inferiorly. (**A**) Lymphatic vessels of the scrotum drain to the inguinal lymph nodes. The glans penis, glans clitoris, labia minora, and terminal inferior end of the vagina drain into deep inguinal nodes and external iliac nodes. The deep inguinal lymph nodes drain superiorly to the external iliac lymph nodes then to the pelvic lymph nodes and on to the para-aortic lymph nodes. (**B**) The external iliac nodes receive lymph directly from pelvic structures, especially the superior parts of the middle to anterior pelvic organs and lymph from the inguinal lymph nodes. The external iliac lymph nodes are located above the pelvic brim, along the external iliac vessels. (**C**) The internal iliac nodes cluster around the internal iliac artery and receive lymph from the inferior pelvic viscera, deep perineum and deep gluteal region. Lymphatic vessels from deep parts of the perineum accompany the internal pudendal blood vessels and drain mainly into internal iliac nodes in the pelvis. (**E**) Lymphatic channels from superficial tissues of the penis or clitoris accompany the superficial external pudendal blood vessels and drain mainly into superficial inguinal nodes, as do lymphatic channels from the scrotum or labia majora.

Refer to the following image for answer 37:

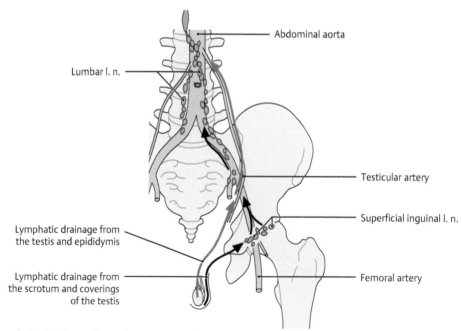

Abdominal aorta

Lumbar l. n.

Testicular artery

Superficial inguinal l. n.

Lymphatic drainage from the testis and epididymis

Lymphatic drainage from the scrotum and coverings of the testis

Femoral artery

Source: Schuenke M, Schulte E, Schumacher U. THIEME Atlas of Anatomy. General Anatomy and Musculoskeletal System. Illustrations by Voll M and Wesker K. 2nd ed. New York: Thieme Medical Publishers; 2016

38. Correct: Ilioinguinal (D)

(**D**) The ilioinguinal and iliohypogastric nerves arise from the L1 ventral ramus. The ilioinguinal nerve is predominantly a sensory nerve and passes through the superficial inguinal ring to provide cutaneous sensation to the upper medial thigh, mons pubis, and labium majus in women, and to the root of the penis and anterior surface of the scrotum in men. (**A**) The femoral nerve (L2–L4) provides sensory innervation over the anterior aspect of the thigh, with its terminal saphenous branch providing sensory innervation along the medial side of the leg and foot. (**B**) The genitofemoral nerve (L1–L2) is motor to the cremaster muscle in the spermatic cord and sensory to the medial thigh. (**C**) The iliohypogastric nerve (L1) is sensory to the hypogastric region, above the inguinal canal. (**E**) The posterior scrotal nerve (primarily S3), a sensory branch of the pudendal nerve (S2–S4), supplies the posterior scrotum.

39. Correct: Abnormal attachment of tunica vaginalis (A)

(**A**) Of the two types of testicular torsion (intravaginal and extravaginal), intravaginal torsion is usually related to abnormal suspension of the testis. Normally, the tunica vaginalis attaches to the posterior wall of the scrotum and allows for very little mobility of the testis. An abnormally high attachment of the tunica vaginalis allows the testis to rotate freely on the spermatic cord within the tunica vaginalis (intravaginal testicular torsion). Failure of normal posterior anchoring of the gubernaculum, epididymis, and testis allows the testes to swing and rotate within the tunica vaginalis, like the clapper of a bell (hence the designation of a "bell clapper deformity"). This deformity is usually present bilaterally. (**B**) If the processes vaginalis does not close completely, a "communication" persists which allows abdominal fluid to pass freely between the peritoneal cavity and the scrotum (and vice versa depending on body position). This congenital condition is termed a communicating hydrocele. This does not predispose to torsion. (**C**) A direct (acquired) inguinal hernia occurs when a weakness develops in the lower anterior abdominal musculature (i.e., the posterior floor of the inguinal canal). It may result from stress

resulting from lifting heavy objects, frequent coughing or straining, pregnancy, or constipation. The neck of a direct hernia lies medial to the inferior epigastric vessels and is not associated with a patent processus vaginalis. (**D**) An indirect (congenital) inguinal hernia is associated with a patent processes vaginalis. The herniated tissues follow the "indirect" course through the inguinal region taken by the patent processus vaginalis. Indirect hernias extend through the internal or deep inguinal ring and their neck lies lateral to the inferior epigastric vessels. (**E**) A patent processus vaginalis predisposes to an indirect inguinal hernia, not testicular torsion.

40. Correct: Mesonephric duct (A)

(**A**) The genital ducts in male arise from the mesonephric (Wolffian) ducts. The mesonephric ducts are paired structures that develop into the epididymis, ductus deferens, and seminal glands (vesicles). (**B**) The mesonephric tubules are the excretory tubules of the intermediate embryonic kidney, the mesonephros. While most of the mesonephric tubules degenerate during development, some persist and form the efferent ductules that connect the rete testis to the epididymis. (**C**) The paramesonephric (Müllerian) ducts form the female genital ducts: the uterine tubes, uterus, and upper vagina. These degenerate in males in response to anti-Müllerian hormone produced by the sustentacular (Sertoli) cells of the developing testis. (**D**) The seminiferous cords are the precursors of the seminiferous tubules. These cords are formed from sustentacular (Sertoli) cells that surround the developing male germ cells. (**E**) The urogenital sinus, the anterior derivative of the cloaca, is lined with endoderm and will develop into the urinary bladder and urethra in the male.

41. Correct: Pelvic splanchnic (A)

(**A**) Referred pain from the pelvic viscera is conveyed via visceral afferent fibers accompanying either the sympathetic or parasympathetic fibers. Afferent fibers from pelvic viscera that are not in contact with the peritoneum (i.e., inferior to the pelvic pain line) accompany parasympathetic fibers via pelvic splanchnic nerves to reach the S2–S4 spinal cord. Pain sensation from the prostate would follow this course. Afferent fibers from pelvic viscera that are in contact with the peritoneum (i.e., superior to the pelvic pain line) course retrogradely with sympathetic efferents to those organs. The superior surface of the bladder and uterine fundus and body are considered to be above the pelvic pain line. (**B, D**) The perineal nerve, a branch of the pudendal nerve, conveys motor and somatic sensory innervation for structures within the urogenital triangle, but not pelvic viscera. (**C**) The posterior scrotal nerve is a branch of the perineal nerve and is a cutaneous nerve of the scrotum. (**E**) Sacral splanchnic nerves arise from the sacral part of the sympathetic trunk and contain a mix of preganglionic and postganglionic sympathetic fibers. They also contain visceral afferent fibers that convey visceral sensory information from pelvic viscera above the pelvic pain line. Afferent impulses from structures below the pelvic pain line follow the course of parasympathetic nerves.

Refer to the following image for answer 41:

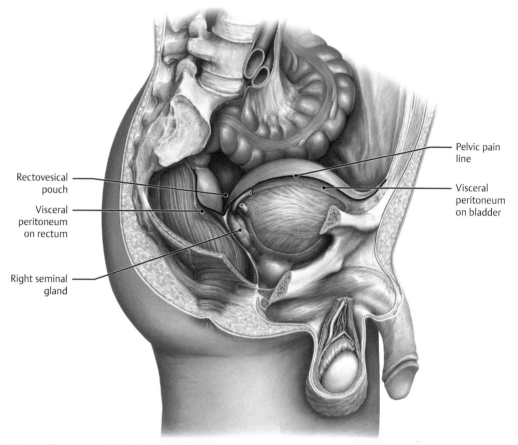

Source: Gilroy AM et al. Atlas of Anatomy. 3rd ed. 2016. Based on: Schuenke M, Schulte E, Schumacher U. THIEME Atlas of Anatomy. Volumes 1-3. Illustrations by Voll M and Wesker K. 2nd ed. New York: Thieme Medical Publishers; 2016

42. Correct: Hypospadias (C)

(**C**) Hypospadias is a congenital defect in the development of the penis where the urethral folds fail to fully fuse during development. This penile anomaly can present with the urethral meatus located anywhere along the ventral penile shaft from the glans to the perineum. (**A**) Epispadias refers to the condition in which the urethral meatus is located on the dorsal surface of the penis. Epispadias is a rare congenital anomaly that may be mild or severe. It often accompanies bladder exstrophy. (**B**) In exstrophy of the bladder, the bladder mucosa is exposed through the anterior abdominal wall. The exstrophy-epispadias complex comprises a spectrum of congenital abnormalities affecting the bladder, penis and pelvic bones. (**D**) Paraphimosis is a condition in which the foreskin is retracted proximal to the corona of the glans penis and cannot be returned to its normal position as a hood over the glans penis when the penis is flaccid. (**E**) Priapism is the state of a continuous erection of at least 4-hour duration. Neonatal priapism is rare.

43. Correct: Varicocele (E)

Refer to the following image for answer 43:

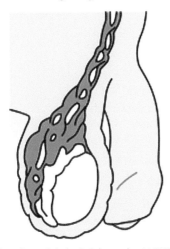

Source: Schuenke M, Schulte E, Schumacher U. THIEME Atlas of Anatomy. General Anatomy and Musculoskeletal System. Illustrations by Voll M and Wesker K. 2nd ed. New York: Thieme Medical Publishers; 2016

(**E**) A varicocele is an enlargement of the veins within the scrotum (pampiniform venous plexus) and often presents as cord-like structures visible in the scrotum that resembles "bag of worms." Varicoceles are a common cause of low sperm production and decreased sperm quality, which can cause infertility. (**A**) A hematocele is a collection of blood within the tunica vaginalis and is usually the result of trauma to the scrotum. (**B**) A hydrocele is formed when there is patency of the processus vaginalis, allowing accumulation of fluid between layers of the tunica vaginalis. The processus vaginalis normally closes spontaneously at the deep inguinal ring sealing the entrance to the inguinal canal. There are different types of hydroceles: if fluid is restricted to the tunica vaginalis it is a noncommunicating or scrotal hydrocele; if the processus vaginalis fuses proximally and distally but remains open in between, the isolated fluid collection is referred to as a hydrocele of the cord. Because the hydrocele is fluid-filled, it can be transilluminated. (**C**) A spermatocele is a painless, fluid-filled cyst of the epididymis that feels like a smooth, firm lump in the scrotum at the superior pole of the testis. The fluid in the cyst may contain sperm that are no longer alive. (**D**) Testicular torsion occurs when the spermatic cord twists, causing ischemia of the testis. Torsion typically presents as rapid onset and acute testicular pain. The most common underlying cause is "bell-clapper deformity," a congenital anomaly where the testis is inappropriately attached to the scrotum, allowing the testis to move freely, thus making it more susceptible to twisting of the spermatic cord.

44. Correct: Phimosis (D)

(**D**) Phimosis, the inability to retract the prepuce (foreskin) that covers the glans of the penis, may occur as the result of infection, inflammation, or scarring. It is more common in uncircumcised adult men. (**A**) Epispadias, the condition where the urethral meatus is located on the dorsal surface of the penis, is a rare congenital anomaly that may be mild or severe, and often accompanies bladder exstrophy. It would present at birth. (**B**) In exstrophy of the bladder the bladder mucosa is exposed through the anterior abdominal wall. The exstrophy-epispadias complex comprises a spectrum of congenital abnormalities affecting the bladder, penis, and pelvic bones. It would present at birth. (**C**) Hypospadias is a congenital defect in the development of the penis where the urethral folds fail to fully fuse during development. This penile anomaly can present with the urethral meatus located anywhere along the ventral penile shaft from the glans to the perineum. (**D**) Priapism is the state of a continuous erection.

45.   Correct: Sacral splanchnic and perineal (E)

(**E**) The event that is absent in this patient is ejaculation and this is influenced by both the autonomic and somatic portions of the nervous system. The sympathetic part of the autonomic nervous system is responsible for peristaltic contractions of the smooth muscle in the walls of the organs and ducts of the male reproductive tract (epididymis, vas deferens, prostate, seminal gland, urethra). The presynaptic nerve cell bodies are located in the T10–L2 segments of the spinal cord. The delivery of sperm from the epididymis, prostatic secretions, and seminal gland secretions into the prostatic urethra forms semen and this event is termed emission. Emission will cause the sensation of orgasm. Ejaculation is the delivery of semen from the prostatic urethra to the external urethral orifice. Ejaculation will be facilitated by continued peristaltic contractions along the urethra, as well as contractions of perineal skeletal muscles, especially the bulbospongiosus. These perineal muscles are innervated by the perineal branch of the pudendal nerve (S2–S4).

(**A**) The genitofemoral nerve originates from the lumbar plexus (L1–L2) and has two branches. The genital branch passes through the deep inguinal ring to enter the inguinal canal and the spermatic cord where it supplies the cremaster muscle and scrotal skin. The femoral branch passes deep to the inguinal ligament and supplies the skin of the proximal anterior thigh. (**B**) The ilioinguinal nerve (L1) accompanies the spermatic cord through the superficial inguinal ring and is distributed to the skin of the proximal anterior and medial thigh. It also forms the anterior scrotal nerve to the anterior scrotum and skin over the root of the penis. (**C**) The lesser splanchnic nerve contains preganglionic sympathetic fibers that arise in the thorax and are distributed primarily to the superior mesenteric ganglion to travel with the tributaries of the superior mesenteric arteries to the midgut. (**D**) Pelvic splanchnics convey the parasympathetic fibers that are responsible for erection. Note the classic mnemonic: "point" (parasympathetic) and "shoot" (sympathetic).

Refer to the following image for answer 45:

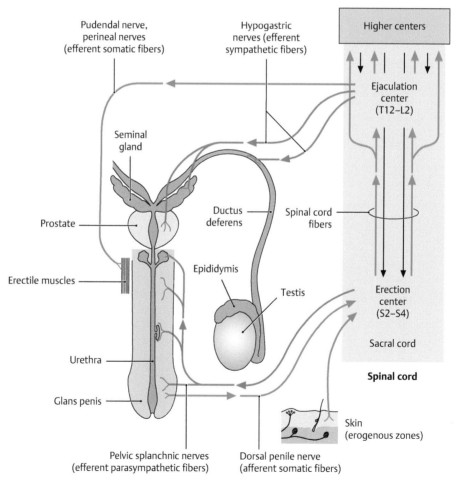

Source: Schuenke M, Schulte E, Schumacher U. THIEME Atlas of Anatomy. Internal Organs. Illustrations by Voll M and Wesker K. 2nd ed. New York: Thieme Medical Publishers; 2016

46. Correct: Seminal gland (vesicle) (C)

Refer to the following image for answer 46:

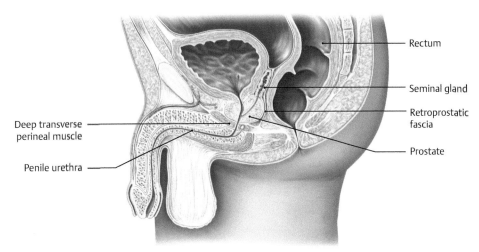

Source: Gilroy AM et al. Atlas of Anatomy. 3rd ed. 2016. Based on: Schuenke M, Schulte E, Schumacher U. THIEME Atlas of Anatomy. Volumes 1-3. Illustrations by Voll M and Wesker K. 2nd ed. New York: Thieme Medical Publishers; 2016

(**C**) The seminal gland (vesicle) is located immediately superior to the posterior aspect of the prostate. Therefore, anesthesia injected into the periprostatic region would affect this structure sooner than others. (**A**) The deep transverse perineal muscle is located in the perineum and is unlikely to be affected by the anesthesia. (**B**) The hemorrhoidal plexus lies deep to the rectal mucosa, being separated from the prostate by the walls of the rectum and retroprostatic (Denonvillier's) fascia. (**D**) The spongy (penile) urethra is found in the perineum and is too far removed to be immediately affected by the anesthesia. (**E**) The ureters enter the urinary bladder superior to the prostate and seminal glands.

47. Correct: Retropubic (B)

(**B**) In an open prostatectomy, the most direct surgical approach to the prostate is via the retropubic space (prevesical space or the cave of Retzius). This extraperitoneal space is located posterior to the pubic symphysis and anterior to the urinary bladder and allows access to the prostate without entering the peritoneal cavity. (**A, C**) The intraperitoneal and supravesical approaches would not be good choices as they would require entry into the peritoneal cavity to access the prostate gland. (**D**) While a transurethral approach is a direct route to the prostate, it is not used generally for total prostatectomy. It is commonly used for resection of portions of the prostate as in benign prostatic hyperplasia.

Refer to the following image for answer 47:

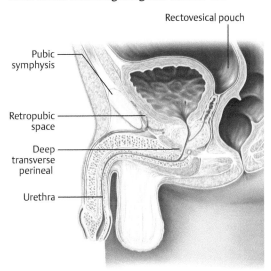

Source: Gilroy AM et al. Atlas of Anatomy. 3rd ed. 2016. Based on: Schuenke M, Schulte E, Schumacher U. THIEME Atlas of Anatomy. Volumes 1-3. Illustrations by Voll M and Wesker K. 2nd ed. New York: Thieme Medical Publishers; 2016

48. Correct: Vestibule and penile urethra (E)

(**E**) The penile urethra develops in the male from the fusion of the urethral folds to enclose the urethral plate. In the female, the vaginal vestibule is formed because the urethral folds do not fuse in the midline. In an individual with congenital adrenal hyperplasia (CAH), excess androgens cause virilization of the urethral folds. Where the labia minora fuse in the midline and the clitoris is enlarged. (**A**) The bulbs of the vestibule are the female erectile tissues that underlie the labia minora; they are the homolog of the corpus spongiosum of male. The bulbourethral (Cowper's) glands are the male homologs of the greater vestibular glands in females. (**B**) The greater vestibular glands and bulb of the penis are not homologous structures. (**C**) The labia majora and bulb of the penis are not homologous structures. (**D**) The labia majora are the homologs of the scrotum in male. The penile urethra develops from the fusion of the urethral folds in the midline to encircle the urethral plate.

49. Correct: Corpus spongiosum (A)

Refer to the following image for answer 49:

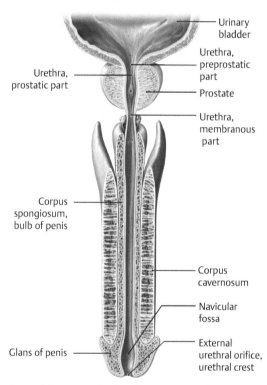

Source: Gilroy AM et al. Atlas of Anatomy. 3rd ed. 2016. Based on: Schuenke M, Schulte E, Schumacher U. THIEME Atlas of Anatomy. Volumes 1-3. Illustrations by Voll M and Wesker K. 2nd ed. New York: Thieme Medical Publishers; 2016

(**A**) The external urethral orifice is located at the tip of the glans penis, which is the distal expansion of the corpus spongiosum. Within the glans penis, the external urethral orifice leads to the expanded navicular fossa. (**B**) The external urethral sphincter muscle is located in the perineum superior to and adjacent to the perineal membrane. It surrounds the membranous urethra. (**C**) The pelvic diaphragm forms the muscular floor of the pelvis and roof of the perineum. The urogenital hiatus is the anterior opening between the two sides of the pelvic diaphragm. The membranous portion of the urethra will pass through the urogenital hiatus as it leaves the pelvis and enters the perineum. (**D**) The prostate is located in the pelvis and surrounds the more proximal and pelvic portion of the urethra, the prostatic urethra. (**E**) The seminal colliculus (referred to clinically as the veromontanum) is an elevation in the prostatic urethra and is not related to the distal penile urethra.

50. Correct: Communicating hydrocele (A)

(**A**) A congenital hydrocele (communicating hydrocele) is an accumulation of fluid within a patent processus vaginalis. In this condition, there is a persistent communication between the peritoneal cavity and the lumen of the processus vaginalis that extends into the scrotum. This communication will cause the scrotum to enlarge when pressure is applied to the anterior abdominal wall. Normally, the processus vaginalis degenerates along most of its length prior to birth. The only remaining part will form the tunica vaginalis, which envelops the testicle. (**B**) In femoral hernias, a small part of the intestine protrudes through the femoral ring into the femoral canal. The hernial sac can protrude through the saphenous hiatus and become subcutaneous. It would not be found in the scrotum. (**C**) A maldescended testis travels along an abnormal route and fails to reach the scrotum. Aberrant locations include: superior to the superficial inguinal ring; at the root of penis; or in the thigh. (**D**) An umbilical hernia in a newborn is caused by a failure of part of the midgut to return to the abdominal cavity during fetal life. It does not extend into the scrotum. (**E**) In a varicocele, the pampiniform venous plexus becomes dilated. On palpation, a varicocele is often described as having the consistency of a "bag of worms."

51. Correct: Visceral and parietal layers of tunica vaginalis (E)

(**E**) At the level of the testicle, the distal end of the patent processus vaginalis will envelop the testicle to form a tunica vaginalis with visceral and parietal layers. The fluid of the communicating hydrocele will be located between these layers. (**A–D**) Fluid of a hydrocele does not accumulate between any of these other layers (cremasteric and internal spermatic fascia, dartos and external spermatic fascia, ductus deferens and internal spermatic fascia, internal and external spermatic fascia).

Chapter 9

Endocrine System

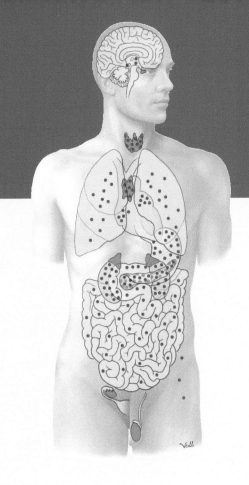

ANATOMICAL LEARNING OBJECTIVES

▶ Describe the anatomy of the pineal gland, including its anatomical relationships.

▶ Describe the anatomy of the pituitary gland, including its anatomical relationships and development.

▶ Describe the anatomy of the thyroid gland, including its neurovasculature, anatomical relationships, and development.

▶ Describe the anatomy of the parathyroid glands, including their neurovasculature, anatomical relationships, and development.

▶ Describe the anatomy of the thymus, including its anatomical relationships and development.

▶ Describe the anatomy of the pancreas, including its neurovasculature, anatomical relationships, and development.

▶ Describe the anatomy of the suprarenal (adrenal) glands, including their neurovasculature, anatomical relationships, and development.

▶ Describe the anatomy of the male reproductive organs, including their neurovasculature, anatomical relationships, and development.

▶ Describe the anatomy of the female reproductive organs, including their neurovasculature, anatomical relationships, and development.

▶ Describe the developmental anatomy of the pharyngeal arches and list structures derived from each pharyngeal arch, pouch, and cleft.

9.1 Questions

Easy   Medium   Hard

Consider the following case for questions 1 and 2:

A 2-month-old boy with a known ventricular septal defect is admitted to the emergency department with symptoms of a seizure. Chest radiographs are ordered (refer to the accompanying images). Laboratory tests reveal a serum calcium level of 6.0 mg/dL (normal: 8.0–10.0 mg/dL). These and further studies and clinical features confirm a diagnosis of DiGeorge syndrome.

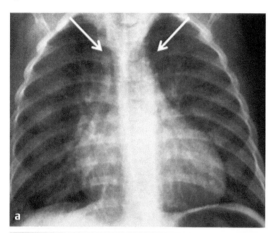

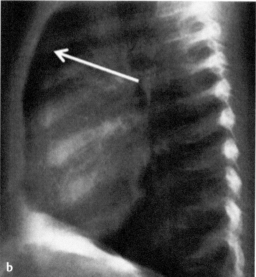

Source: Burgener F, Kormano M, Pudas T. The Chest X-Ray. Differential Diagnosis in Conventional Radiology. 2nd revised Edition. Thieme; 2005.

1. Which of the following structures typically seen on radiographs is missing (translucent areas indicated by the *arrows*) in this infant?

A. Inferior parathyroid gland
B. Superior parathyroid gland
C. Thoracic esophagus
D. Thymus
E. Thyroid gland

2. What is the most likely explanation for the radiographic findings and reduced calcium levels?

A. The parathyroid and thyroid glands failed to descend into the neck via the thyroglossal duct
B. The thymus and parathyroid glands failed to descend into the neck via the thyroglossal duct
C. The thymus and parathyroid glands failed to develop from the pharyngeal pouch 3
D. The thymus and thyroid glands failed to descend into the neck via the thyroglossal duct
E. The thymus and thyroid glands failed to develop from the same pharyngeal pouch

3. A 43-year-old woman with a 3-month history of intermittent headaches, palpitations, sweating, and severe hypertension presents to her primary care physician. Ultrasound reveals an 8 cm mass consistent with a pheochromocytoma on her left adrenal gland. An adrenalectomy is performed via a dorsal laparoscopic approach, during which the arteries that supply the superior part of the gland are ligated. From which of the following arteries do the ligated arteries arise?

A. Aorta
B. Greater pancreatic
C. Inferior phrenic
D. Renal
E. Superior mesenteric

4. A 61-year-old man presents with epigastric pain and nausea for the last 36 hours. Laboratory results show elevated serum lipase and amylase. An abdominal CT reveals inflammatory changes to the tail of the pancreas consistent with acute pancreatitis. Which of the following arteries supplies the inflamed portion of the pancreas?

A. Gastroduodenal

B. Inferior pancreaticoduodenal

C. Left gastro-omental

D. Splenic

E. Superior mesenteric

F. Superior pancreaticoduodenal

5. A 12-year-old boy with acute onset of left scrotal pain is brought to the emergency department. The scrotal pain is only relieved with testicular elevation. The testicle itself is not tender; however, the epididymis is palpable and tender. A cremasteric reflex is present and a characteristic "blue dot" sign in the skin of the scrotum is noted. This "blue dot" is due to venous congestion of which of the following?

A. Appendix testis

B. Epididymis

C. Hydrocele

D. Testis

E. Tunica vaginalis

6. A 37-year-old man who underwent a thyroidectomy for Graves' disease presents postoperatively with hoarseness. The nerve that was most likely iatrogenically damaged supplies which of the following pharyngeal arches?

A. First pharyngeal arch

B. Second pharyngeal arch

C. Third pharyngeal arch

D. Fourth pharyngeal arch

E. Sixth pharyngeal arch

Consider the following case for questions 7 and 8:

A 24-year-old woman who was recently involved in an automobile accident is referred to the neurosurgeon because of an incidentally discovered pituitary adenoma. Physical examination reveals a right medial gaze palsy. An MRI performed to evaluate her head trauma reveals a 7 mm mass on the right side of her pituitary.

7. Which of the following nerves is most likely to be compressed initially when the adenoma expands laterally?

A. Abducens (CN VI)

B. Maxillary (CN V2)

C. Oculomotor (CN III)

D. Ophthalmic (CN V1)

E. Trochlear (CN IV)

8. With anterosuperior expansion of the ademoma, which of the following signs or symptoms would be most likely?

A. Lateral gaze palsy

B. Loss of sensation from the forehead

C. Loss of sensation from the upper lip

D. Loss of vision

E. Medial gaze palsy

9. A 37-year-old woman undergoes thyroidectomy on the right side. Postoperatively, she complains of hoarseness. Which of the following statements is correct regarding the nerve that is most likely damaged during surgery?

A. It courses inferior and posterior to the subclavian artery

B. It is accompanied by the superior laryngeal artery

C. It pierces the thyrohyoid membrane

D. It provides sensory innervation to the larynx

E. It travels inferior and then posterior to the arch of the aorta

10. A 52-year-old woman is admitted to the hospital with hypertension, tachycardia, headache, and anxiety. An abdominal CT reveals a 2.5 × 2.0 cm mass on the left suprarenal (adrenal) gland and a diagnosis of a left pheochromocytoma is made. During a laparoscopic procedure to remove the tumor, which of the following is within the surgical field and should be mobilized to prevent injury?

A. Gallbladder

B. Head of the pancreas

C. Liver

D. Proximal duodenum

E. Tail of the pancreas

11. A 16-year-old girl with primary amenorrhea is brought to the gynecologist. Physical examination reveals underdeveloped breasts and immature external genitalia. A rudimentary vagina is evident, and a mass is palpable in each labium majus. Ultrasound reveals the absence of a uterus. Karyotyping reveals a 46 XY genotype. Which of the following structures is most likely to be present in this individual?

A. Cervix

B. Uterine tubes

C. Ovaries

D. Testes

E. Upper vagina

12. A 27-year-old woman with a history of amenorrhea presents with hirsutism (excessive male pattern facial and body hair in a woman), hoarseness, rudimentary breasts, and clitoromegaly. Although testosterone levels are elevated, genetic analysis reveals a female karyotype (46 XX), and MRI indicates that testes are not present. Which of the following structures is likely to be missing in this individual?

A. Ovaries

B. Uterine tubes

C. Uterus and uterine tubes

D. Vagina and cervix

E. Vas deferens

13. A 6-year-old girl with a sore throat is brought to the clinic. Physical examination reveals that her stature is short for her age and that she exhibits edema of the hands and feet, redundant nuchal skin, and a low hairline. An endocrinology consult confirms a diagnosis of Turner syndrome. Which of the following structures would be most likely affected in this individual?

A. Clitoris

B. Fallopian tubes

C. Ovaries

D. Uterus

E. Vagina

14. A 40-year-old woman reports for a postsurgical visit with tingling and numbness throughout her body. The surgeon is concerned that this is a consequence of postsurgical hypocalcemia resulting from iatrogenic injury during surgery. Which of the following was the target most likely structure for the surgery?

A. Carotid artery

B. Larynx

C. Superior cervical ganglion

D. Thyroid gland

E. Trachea

15. A 38-year-old man is taken to the emergency department after losing consciousness. An MRI of his head reveals a walnut-sized solid mass on his pituitary gland. Profuse bleeding occurs during transphenoidal resection of the mass. Which of the following arteries is most vulnerable to injury during this procedure?

A. Basilar

B. Internal carotid

C. Middle meningeal

D. Ophthalmic

E. Posterior cerebral

16. A 40-year-old woman with a history of severe pain in her left forearm presents to her primary care physician. Radiologic imaging reveals fractures of both the radius and ulna, and MRI of her neck reveals a soft tissue hypoechoic lesion with calcification (refer to the *arrow* in the accompanying image). Laboratory results indicate hypercalcemia. Adenoma of which of the following structures is most likely?

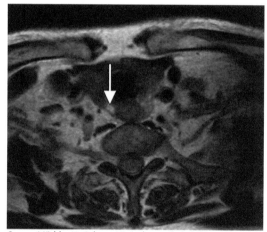

Source: Mödder U, Cohnen M, Andersen K et al. Direct Diagnosis in Radiology. Head and Neck Imaging. 1st Edition. Thieme; 2007.

A. Parathyroid gland

B. Pituitary gland

C. Submandibular gland

D. Suprarenal (adrenal) gland

E. Thymus

17. A 45-year-old woman with headache and blurred vision presents to her physician. A suprasellar mass (refer to the *arrow* in the accompanying image) with a mixed solid and cystic appearance is identified by MRI as a craniopharyngeoma. The tissue encroaching on her optic chiasm is derived from the embryonic precursor of which structure?

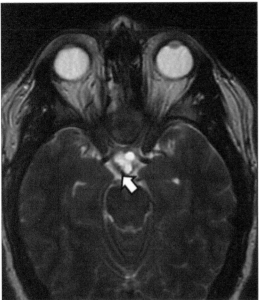

Source: Riascos R, Bonfante E. RadCases: Neuro Imaging. 1st Edition. Thieme; 2010.

A. Anterior pituitary gland

B. Epithalamus

C. Hypothalamus

D. Pineal body (gland)

E. Posterior pituitary gland

18. A 12-year-old boy presents with acute scrotal pain and vomiting. Ultrasound images demonstrate an enlarged left testicle with engorgement. On Doppler ultrasound, minimal flow can be seen in the left testicle (refer to the accompanying images). Which of the following is the most likely cause of the testicular pain?

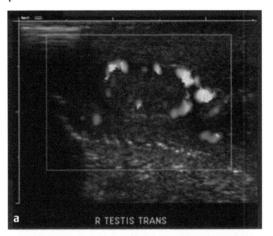

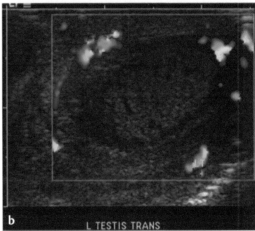

Source: Gunderman R, Delaney L. RadCases. Pediatric Imaging. 1st Edition. Thieme; 2010.

A. Epididymitis

B. Hydrocele

C. Indirect hernia

D. Testicular neoplasm

E. Testicular torsion

19. A 35-year-old man presents with increasing headaches and paralysis of upward gaze. Imaging shows a heterogeneous mass in the region of the pineal gland, with obstructive hydrocephalus and dilatation of the third and lateral ventricles. Which of the following is likely to be the site of the obstruction?

A. Cerebral aqueduct

B. Interventricular foramina (of Munro)

C. Median aperture (foramen of Magendie)

D. Spinal (central) canal

Consider the following case for questions 20 to 22:

A 50-year-old man presents with a 3-day history of worsening abdominal pain, nausea, and vomiting. He has had four similar episodes over the previous five years, each of which lasted 3 to 5 days. A diagnosis of recurrent, acute pancreatitis with pancreatic necrosis is made after an exploratory laparotomy. Debridement of the pancreatic head is undertaken.

20. During debridement, branches of which of the following arteries are most likely cauterized?

A. Dorsal pancreatic

B. Gastroduodenal

C. Great pancreatic

D. Inferior mesenteric

E. Splenic

21. Which of the following describes the relationship of the necrotic portion of the pancreas to neighboring vascular structures?

A. Inferior to the portal vein

B. Lateral and anterior to the gastroduodenal artery

C. Posterior to the inferior vena cava

D. To the left of the superior mesenteric vein

22. Which of the following structures located posterior to the pancreas should be protected during the surgery?

A. First part of duodenum

B. Inferior vena cava

C. Lesser sac

D. Stomach

E. Transverse mesocolon

Consider the following case for questions 23 and 24:

A 45-year-old woman with abdominal pain for the past 2 to 3 weeks presents to her primary care provider. She describes the pain as a dull, continuous ache, and localized to her right side (flank). Ultrasonography of her abdomen reveals bilateral adrenal masses. She is diagnosed with multiple endocrine neoplasia and is scheduled for bilateral adrenalectomy. The pathology report shows a pheochromocytoma.

23. Which of the following is the embryonic origin of cells that formed the masses?

A. Hematopoetic stem cells

B. Metanephric blastema

C. Nephrogenic cord

D. Neural crest

E. Primordial germ cells

24. Which of the following contribute to the innervation of the neoplastic cells?

A. Lumbar splanchnic nerves

B. Pelvic splanchnic nerves

C. Sacral splanchnic nerves

D. Thoracic splanchnic nerves

Consider the following case for questions 25 and 26:

A 38-year-old woman with a family history of ovarian cancer undergoes elective prophylactic bilateral oophorectomy.

25. During the procedure, the surgeon must bilaterally transect which of the following structures?

A. Ligament of the ovary

B. Round ligament of the uterus

C. Transverse cervical (cardinal) ligament

D. Uterine tube

E. Uterosacral ligament

26. During the procedure, the ovarian arteries must be ligated/cauterized. The vessels that must be ligated/cauterized during the procedure are associated with which of the following structures?

A. Ligament of the ovary

B. Mesosalpinx

C. Round ligament of the uterus

D. Suspensory ligament of the ovary

E. Transverse cervical ligament

27. A 52-year-old man is hospitalized with recurrent upper abdominal pain during the past 1.5 years. The pain is severe and usually lasts for 1 to 2 hours, but can be relieved by flexing his trunk. His urine and serum amylase are significantly elevated. Both CT and MRI demonstrate pancreatitis and show that the descending duodenum is being compressed. Which of the following conditions is suggested by these findings?

A. Annular pancreas

B. Duodenal atresia

C. Intestinal malrotation

D. Meckel's diverticulum

E. Volvulus

28. A 25-year-old woman with hirsutism (excessive male pattern facial and body hair in a woman), obesity, severe acne, and oligomenorrhea (infrequent menses) reports to her gynecologist because she is unable to conceive after several years of trying. Transvaginal sonographic imaging of her pelvis shows enlarged ovaries (refer to the accompanying image). Which of the following is the most likely cause of her infertility?

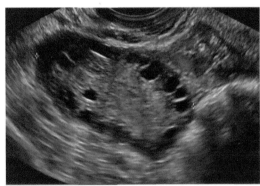

Source: Merz E. Ultrasound in Obstetrics and Gynecology. 2nd Edition. Thieme; 2004.

A. Androgen insensitivity syndrome

B. Congenital adrenal hyperplasia

C. Hypothyroidism

D. Ovarian tumor

E. Polycystic ovarian syndrome

29. A 19-year-old woman with vaginal bleeding, severe nausea and vomiting presents to the emergency department. Physical examination and ultrasonography reveal an enlarged uterus with numerous small vesicles (refer to the accompanying image). Her serum human chorionic gonadotropin (hCG) level is elevated. Which of the following is the most likely diagnosis?

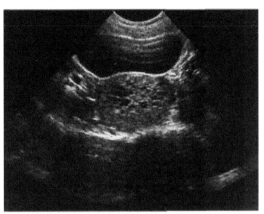

Source: Merz E. Ultrasound in Obstetrics and Gynecology. 2nd Edition. Thieme; 2004.

A. Ectopic pregnancy

B. Molar pregnancy

C. Normal pregnancy

D. Uterine fibroid

E. Uterine polyp

Consider the following case for questions 30 and 31:

A 19-year-old woman presents for treatment of chronic pelvic pain. At age 15, she was diagnosed with dysmenorrhea (difficult or painful menstruation), which has now worsened and lasts throughout the month. She became sexually active six months ago and reports experiencing severe pain with intercourse (dyspareunia). Laparoscopy of her right ovary detects a "chocolate cyst" characteristic of an endometrioma.

30. With which of the following anatomical spaces is the endometrioma most closely associated?

A. Anterior vaginal fornix

B. Posterior vaginal fornix

C. Rectouterine pouch

D. Retropubic space

E. Vesicouterine pouch

31. Laparoscopy also reveals endometriosis in the rectouterine pouch near the rectovaginal septum (rectovaginal endometriosus). With which of the following is the endometriosis in this patient most closely associated?

A. Anterior vaginal fornix

B. Posterior vaginal fornix

C. Retropubic space

D. Vesicouterine pouch

32. A 24-year-old woman with complaints of feeling "something" in her throat, difficulty swallowing, snoring, and sleep apnea presents to her primary care physician. Her history reveals that these symptoms have become more severe over the last year. Physical examination shows vascularized, pink-purple, globular mass on the root of the tongue, and soft tissues normally palpable on either side of the inferior larynx superior trachea are not detected. CT reveals a mass with smooth contours and dense contrast localized to the root of tongue. Which of the following is the most likely cause of this patient's symptoms?

A. Branchial cyst

B. Ectopic thymus

C. Enlarged palatine tonsil

D. Lingual thyroid

E. Lingual tonsil

F. Thyroglossal duct cyst

33. A 5-year-old boy presents to his pediatrician with a nontender, mobile, submental swelling (refer to the accompanying images). Physical examination reveals that the swelling moves upward when the patient protrudes his tongue. Ultrasound shows an anechoic structure in the submental triangle. Which of the following is the most likely cause of the swelling?

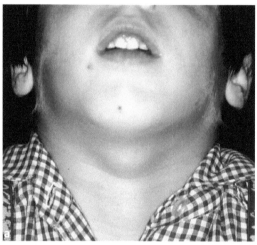

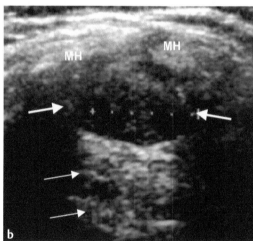

Source: Valvassori G, Mafee M, Becker M. Imaging of the Head and Neck. 2nd Edition. Stuttgart: Thieme; 2004.

A. Branchial cyst

B. Ectopic thymus

C. Enlarged palatine tonsil

D. Lingual thyroid

E. Thyroglossal duct cyst

9.2 Answers and Explanations

Easy	Medium	Hard

1. Correct: Thymus (D)

(**D**) The thymus is a lymphoid organ located in the inferior neck and anterior portion of the superior mediastinum. In radiographs of infants, the thymus is typically seen as a shadow in the superior mediastinum. The thymus continues to grow until puberty, and then involutes. In the adult, it lies posterior to the manubrium and may extend inferiorly in front of the pericardium. DiGeorge syndrome is classified as an immune deficiency because of thymic aplasia or agenesis. Since this patient has DiGeorge syndrome, the radiograph does not show a thymic shadow at the sites indicated by the arrows. DiGeorge syndrome usually presents initially with congenital heart disease, hypocalcemic seizures or tetany, and aortic defects, hypoplastic mandible, as well as defective ears and other abnormal facial features. (**A, B**) The parathyroid glands, not usually visualized in radiographs, are located on the dorsal aspect of the thyroid gland in the anterior neck. (**C**) The thoracic esophagus, although found in the superior mediastinum, is not implicated in DiGeorge syndrome. (**E**) The thyroid gland is not implicated in DiGeorge syndrome. It is located in the anterior neck, with right and left lobes at the C5–T1 vertebral levels, and an isthmus anterior to the second and/or third tracheal cartilage.

Refer to the following images for answer 1:

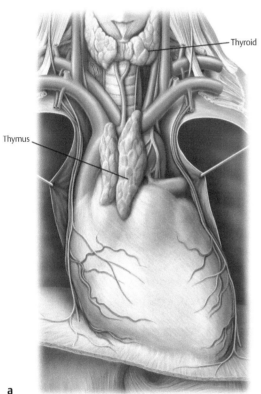

a

Source: Gilroy AM et al. Atlas of Anatomy. 3rd ed. 2016. Based on: Schuenke M, Schulte E, Schumacher U. THIEME Atlas of Anatomy. Volumes 1-3. Illustrations by Voll M and Wesker K. 2nd ed. New York: Thieme Medical Publishers; 2016

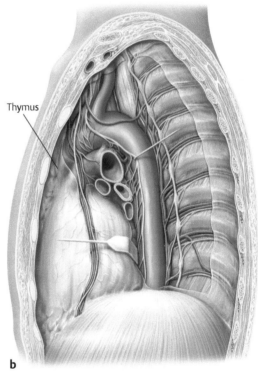

b

Source: Gilroy AM et al. Atlas of Anatomy. 3rd ed. 2016. Based on: Schuenke M, Schulte E, Schumacher U. THIEME Atlas of Anatomy. Volumes 1-3. Illustrations by Voll M and Wesker K. 2nd ed. New York: Thieme Medical Publishers; 2016

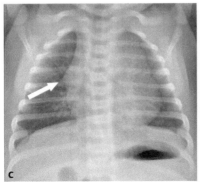

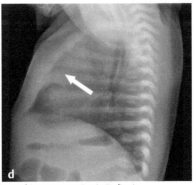

Source: Yoo S, MacDonald C, Babyn P, Chest Radiographic Interpretation in Pediatric Cardiac Patients. 1st Edition. Thieme; 2010.

2. Correct: The thymus and parathyroid glands failed to develop from the pharyngeal pouch 3 (C)

Refer to the following images for answer 2:

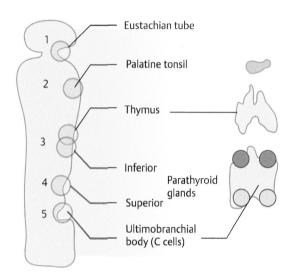

Features of DiGeorge Syndrome

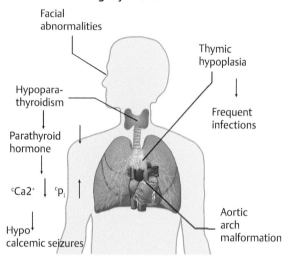

(C) The thymus and inferior parathyroid glands originate from the third pharyngeal pouch. Thymic aplasia with hypocalcemia due to parathyroid hypoplasia is highly indicative of DiGeorge syndrome. (A, B, D, E) The thyroid gland develops as a diverticulum of endoderm (thyroglossal duct) in the floor of the pharynx at the foramen cecum, whereas the parathyroid glands are derivatives of the endoderm of the third and fourth pharyngeal pouches. Neither the thymus nor the parathyroid glands descend through the tongue during development.

3. Correct: Inferior phrenic (C)

(C) The left and right superior suprarenal arteries branch from the respective inferior phrenic artery. The left and right inferior phrenic arteries supply the diaphragm and are the first branches of the abdominal aorta. (A) The middle suprarenal arteries (middle capsular arteries) arise from either side of the abdominal aorta, opposite the superior mesenteric artery. (B, E) The greater pancreatic and superior mesenteric arteries do not supply the suprarenal gland. (D) The renal arteries give rise to the inferior suprarenal arteries.

Refer to the following image for answer 3:

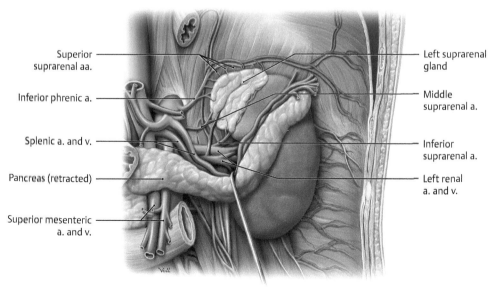

Source: Gilroy AM et al. Atlas of Anatomy. 3rd ed. 2016. Based on: Schuenke M, Schulte E, Schumacher U. THIEME Atlas of Anatomy. Volumes 1-3. Illustrations by Voll M and Wesker K. 2nd ed. New York: Thieme Medical Publishers; 2016

4. Correct: Splenic (D)

Refer to the following image for answer 4:

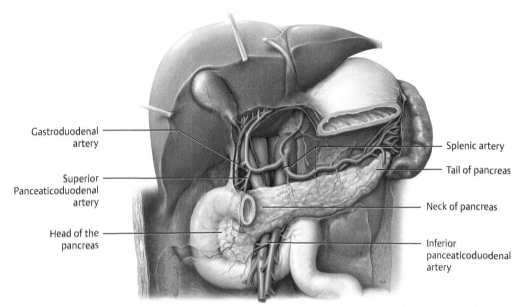

Source: Gilroy AM et al. Atlas of Anatomy. 3rd ed. 2016. Based on: Schuenke M, Schulte E, Schumacher U. THIEME Atlas of Anatomy. Volumes 1-3. Illustrations by Voll M and Wesker K. 2nd ed. New York: Thieme Medical Publishers; 2016

(**D**) The tail of the pancreas is supplied by the pancreatic branches of the splenic artery. The splenic artery courses along the upper surface of the pancreas and supplies the neck, body, and tail. (**A**) The gastroduodenal artery provides the superior pancreaticoduodenal (anterior and posterior) branches that supply the head of the pancreas. (**B**) The inferior pancreaticoduodenal artery, a branch of the superior mesenteric, distributes to the anterior and posterior surfaces of the head of the pancreas. (**C**) The left gastro-omental (gastroepiploic) artery does not supply the pancreas. (**E**) The superior mesenteric artery supplies inferior pancreaticoduodenal branches to the pancreas. (**F**) The superior pancreaticoduodenal artery, a branch of the gastroduodenal, also distributes to the anterior and posterior surfaces of the head of the pancreas.

5. Correct: Appendix testis (A)

(**A**) The appendix testis is a remnant of the cranial end of the paramesonephric duct. Torsion of this structure presents as tenderness near upper pole of the testes. A characteristic "blue dot," due to venous congestion of the twisted appendix testis, can be observed through the skin of the scrotum. (**B**) Torsion of the epididymis is not common. (**C**) A hydrocele is usually associated with a patent processus vaginalis

and presents as a painless swelling. (**D**) Testicular torsion usually presents with sudden severe scrotal pain, a testicle positioned higher than normal, and an absent cremasteric reflex with no change in pain in response to testicular elevation. (**E**) The tunica vaginalis is the remnant of the processus vaginalis, an outpocketing of the peritoneum that precedes testicular descent into the scrotum. The processus vaginalis is normally apposed to the testis and independent torsion of the processus is unlikely.

Refer to the following image for answer 5:

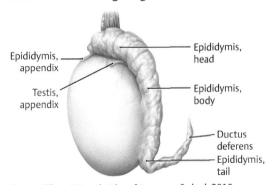

Source: Gilroy AM et al. Atlas of Anatomy. 3rd ed. 2016. Based on: Schuenke M, Schulte E, Schumacher U. THIEME Atlas of Anatomy. Volumes 1-3. Illustrations by Voll M and Wesker K. 2nd ed. New York: Thieme Medical Publishers; 2016

6. Correct: Sixth pharyngeal arch (E)

(**E**) The recurrent laryngeal branches of the vagus nerve (CN X) distribute to derivatives of the sixth pharyngeal arch. The recurrent laryngeal branches are close to the bifurcation of the inferior thyroid artery and are at risk during thyroid and parathyroid surgery. Because the recurrent laryngeal nerve supplies most intrinsic laryngeal muscles, injury to the nerve will cause hoarseness and dyspnea (difficulty in breathing). (**A–C**) Derivative of pharyngeal arches 1 to 3 are not supplied by the recurrent laryngeal nerve. (**D**) Derivatives of pharyngeal arch 4 are supplied by the superior laryngeal branch of the vagus.

Refer to the following image for answer 6:

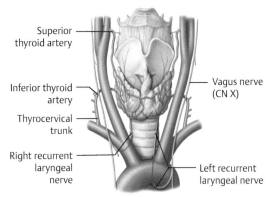

Source: Gilroy AM et al. Atlas of Anatomy. 3rd ed. 2016. Based on: Schuenke M, Schulte E, Schumacher U. THIEME Atlas of Anatomy. Volumes 1-3. Illustrations by Voll M and Wesker K. 2nd ed. New York: Thieme Medical Publishers; 2016

7. Correct: Oculomotor (CN III) (C)

(**C**) The oculomotor nerve is the most medial (and superior) of the cranial nerves that traverse the cavernous sinus (see the presented image) and is subject to a mass effect from a laterally expanding pituitary adenoma. (**A, B, D, E**) The abducens, ophthalmic, trochlear, and maxillary nerves are all located more lateral or inferior within the cavernous sinus than the oculomotor nerve and are, therefore, less likely to be affected by a laterally expanding pituitary adenoma.

8. Correct: Loss of vision (D)

(**D**) Expansion of a pituitary adenoma in a anterosuperior direction would likely create a mass effect on the optic chiasm leading to bitemporal hemianopia, a partial blindness in which vision is diminished or lost in the temporal (outer) halves of both the right and left visual fields. (**A**) A lateral gaze palsy would indicate involvement of the abducens nerve, which courses inferior and slightly lateral to the internal carotid artery. Both of these structures are located lateral to the sella turcica and pituitary gland. (**B, C**) Loss of sensation from the forehead and/or upper lip would indicate involvement of the ophthalmic (CN V1) or maxillary (CN V2) nerves, respectively. In such a case, the tumor would have expanded laterally to impact these nerves as they course along the lateral wall of the cavernous sinus. (**E**) A medial gaze palsy would indicate involvement of the oculomotor nerve. Among the cranial nerves that are associated with the cavernous sinus, this nerve is located most medially (and superiorly) and may be affected by a laterally expanding pituitary adenoma.

Refer to the following image for answers 7 and 8:

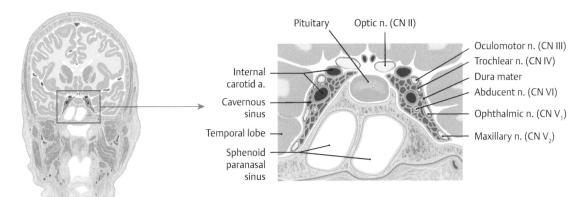

Source: Gilroy AM et al. Atlas of Anatomy. 3rd ed. 2016. Based on: Schuenke M, Schulte E, Schumacher U. THIEME Atlas of Anatomy. Volumes 1-3. Illustrations by Voll M and Wesker K. 2nd ed. New York: Thieme Medical Publishers; 2016

9. Correct: It courses inferior and posterior to the subclavian artery (A)

(**A**) Hoarseness after a thyroidectomy is consistent with an iatrogenic injury to the recurrent laryngeal nerve. The recurrent laryngeal nerves are branches of the vagus (CN X) and supply all intrinsic laryngeal muscles except the cricothyroid. The right and left recurrent laryngeal nerves are not symmetrical in their course: the left loops under the arch of the aorta and the right loops under the right subclavian artery before they ascend in the neck along their respective tracheoesophageal grooves. The course of the recurrent laryngeal nerves is of particular clinical significance as they may be injured by a number of conditions or during a variety of procedures: an aortic aneurysm may compress the left recurrent laryngeal nerve as it passes inferior to the arch of the aorta; lymph node metastases of bronchial carcinoma may compress the left recurrent laryngeal nerve as it passes close to the left main bronchus; and, as in this case, the right or left recurrent laryngeal nerve may be injured during thyroid operations as they pass close to the dorsolateral aspects of the thyroid gland. (**B–D**) The superior laryngeal nerve, also a branch of the vagus, divides into external and internal branches. The internal branch, accompanied by the superior laryngeal artery, is sensory and pierces the thyrohyoid membrane to provide innervation to the supraglottic laryngeal mucosa (i.e., superior to the vocal folds). Injury to the external branch of the superior laryngeal nerve near the superior pole of the thyroid, or during isolation of the superior parathyroid glands is also possible during such procedures; however, injury to this nerve is more likely to cause a problem in producing high-pitched sounds. (**E**) The left recurrent laryngeal nerve travels inferior and posterior to arch of the aorta to take a recurrent course to the larynx.

Refer to the following image for answer 9:

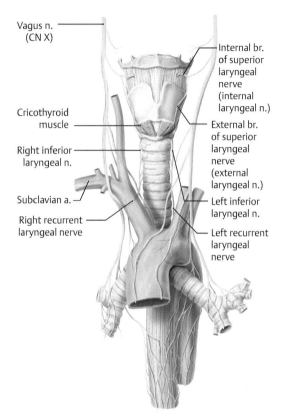

Source: Gilroy AM et al. Atlas of Anatomy. 3rd ed. 2016. Based on: Schuenke M, Schulte E, Schumacher U. THIEME Atlas of Anatomy. Volumes 1-3. Illustrations by Voll M and Wesker K. 2nd ed. New York: Thieme Medical Publishers; 2016

10. Correct: Tail of the pancreas (E)

(**E**) The tail of the pancreas, the spleen, and the blood vessels that supply the kidney are at risk of damage during a left laparoscopic adrenalectomy. (**A–D**) The gallbladder, head of the pancreas, liver, and the superior part of the duodenum are located on the right side and would not be involved in a left adrenalectomy.

Refer to the following image for answer 10:

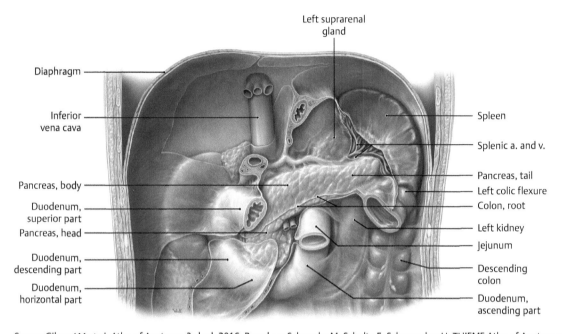

Source: Gilroy AM et al. Atlas of Anatomy. 3rd ed. 2016. Based on: Schuenke M, Schulte E, Schumacher U. THIEME Atlas of Anatomy. Volumes 1-3. Illustrations by Voll M and Wesker K. 2nd ed. New York: Thieme Medical Publishers; 2016

11. Correct: Testes (D)

Refer to the following image for answer 11:

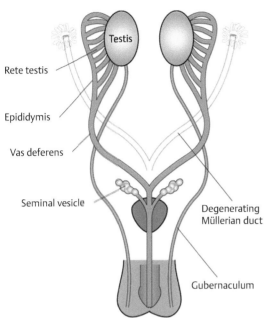

Source: Michael J, Sircar S. Fundamentals of Medical Physiology. 1st Edition. Thieme; 2010.

(**D**) The findings are consistent with complete androgen insensitivity syndrome (CAIS, or testicular feminization syndrome). Male hormones are produced by the testes, but are not recognized by the individual's genital tissues because these lack androgen receptors. Because the testes produce normal amounts of Müllerian-inhibiting factor, also known as Müllerian-inhibiting substance or anti-Müllerian hormone, affected individuals do not have female genital ducts. (**A–C, E**) The paramesonephric (Müllerian) ducts, which form the female genital ducts (uterine/fallopian tubes, uterus, and proximal/upper vagina), are inhibited from further development in these individuals because the testes produce Müllerian-inhibiting factor.

12. Correct: Vas deferens (E)

(**E**) The vas deferens would be missing in this individual because, in the absence of testicular development and production of testosterone from the testes, the male reproductive ducts fail to differentiate. (**A–C**) Because there are no testes, the female internal genitalia will develop. In the absence of Müllerian-inhibiting factor, normally produced by the testes, female genital ducts will be retained. (**D**) In this XX individual, primordial germ cells would develop into oogonia and influence the indifferent gonad to differentiate into an ovary.

Refer to the following image for answer 12:

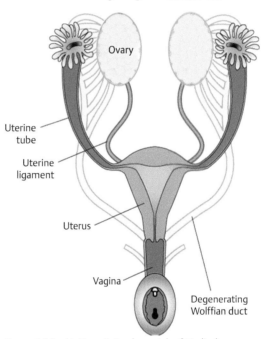

Source: Michael J, Sircar S. Fundamentals of Medical Physiology. 1st Edition. Thieme; 2010.

13. Ovaries (C)

(**C**) Turner (Ullrich–Turner) syndrome (also known as gonadal dysgenesis or 45 X0) is a condition in which a female is missing part or all of an X chromosome. In these individuals, the ovaries are often represented by fibrous streaks (streak gonads). (**A, B, D, E**) Because this individual lacks a Y chromosome, female genital ducts form because Müllerian-inhibiting hormone is not produced (testes are absent).

14. Correct: Thyroid gland (D)

Refer to the following images for answer 14:

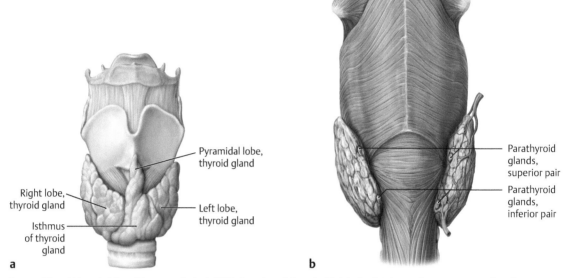

Source: Gilroy AM et al. Atlas of Anatomy. 3rd ed. 2016. Based on: Schuenke M, Schulte E, Schumacher U. THIEME Atlas of Anatomy. Volumes 1-3. Illustrations by Voll M and Wesker K. 2nd ed. New York: Thieme Medical Publishers; 2016

(**D**) This individual is most likely suffering from hypoparathyroidism due to iatrogenic injury to, or removal of, the parathyroid glands during thyroid surgery. Because the parathyroid glands are located on the posterior aspect of the thyroid gland (image b), any surgery of the thyroid gland can result may impact function of the parathyroid glands. (**A–C, E**) Surgeries involving the carotid artery (e.g., carotid endarterectomy), larynx, superior cervical ganglion, and trachea are unlikely to injure the parathyroid glands because they are not as intimately related to the thyroid gland, as are the parathyroids.

15. Correct: Internal carotid (B)

(**B**) The cavernous part of the internal carotid artery lies between the layers of the dura mater that form the cavernous sinus. Within this sinus, this artery is located lateral to the body of the sphenoid bone and pituitary gland. (**A**) The basilar artery is not located within the cavernous sinus. It is part of the posterior cerebral circulation and arises from the union of the left and right vertebral arteries at the base of the pons. (**C**) The middle meningeal artery does traverse the cavernous sinus. This epidural artery courses in a groove on the inside of the cranium. (**D**) The ophthalmic artery, which is the first branch of the internal carotid artery, arises from the internal carotid after this vessel leaves the cavernous sinus. It supplies the structures in the orbit, nose, face, and meninges. (**E**) The posterior cerebral arteries are not associated with the cavernous sinus. They supply the posterior aspect of the occipital lobe of the brain.

Refer to the following image for answer 15:

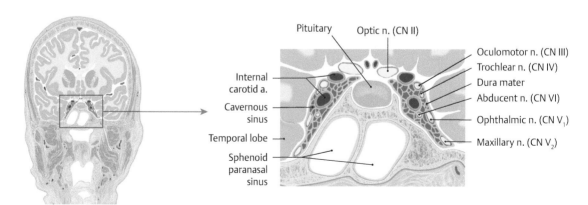

Source: Gilroy AM et al. Atlas of Anatomy. 3rd ed. 2016. Based on: Schuenke M, Schulte E, Schumacher U. THIEME Atlas of Anatomy. Volumes 1-3. Illustrations by Voll M and Wesker K. 2nd ed. New York: Thieme Medical Publishers; 2016

16. Correct: Parathyroid gland (A)

(**A**) The location of the tumor and laboratory results indicate a parathyroid adenoma. A parathyroid adenoma is a benign tumor of the parathyroid that leads to calcium and phosphorus imbalances due to increased levels of parathyroid hormone. Hyperparathyroidism can result in fragile and brittle bones that may lead to fractures. (**B–E**) An adenoma in the pituitary, submandibular, suprarenal (adrenal), and thymus glands would not be found in this location and would not account for the physical and laboratory findings.

17. Correct: Anterior pituitary gland (A)

(**A**) Craniopharyngiomas are epithelial neoplasms arising from remnants of Rathke's pouch, the embryonic precursors to the anterior pituitary gland derived from the oral ectoderm. The clinical presentation includes visual disturbance (blurred vision), endocrine dysfunction, and raised intracranial pressure. (**B–E**) The epithalamus, hypothalamus, pineal glands, and posterior pituitary are all derived from neuroectoderm and are not related to Rathke's pouch.

18. Correct: Testicular torsion (E)

(**E**) The combination of an enlarged testis and no demonstrable internal color Doppler signal is essentially diagnostic of testicular torsion. Color Doppler ultrasound is used to assess the vascular supply to the testis and is the key in the evaluation of suspected testicular torsion. (**A**) No abnormality was observed within the epididymis. (**B–D**) No hydrocele, indirect hernia, or testicular mass was evident in this individual.

19. Correct: Cerebral aqueduct (A)

(**A**) This individual has a tumor of the pineal gland (pinealoma) blocking the cerebral aqueduct. CSF normally flows through the cerebral ventricular system in order from: lateral ventricles → interventricular foramina (Munro) → third ventricle → cerebral aqueduct (Sylvius) → fourth ventricle → median (Magendie) and/or lateral apertures (Lushka). Since the lateral and third ventricles are dilated, the obstruction is in the cerebral aqueduct, between the third and fourth ventricles. (**B**) The interventricular foramina (foramina of Monro) connect the lateral ventricles with the third ventricle at the midline of the brain. Since the third ventricle is dilated, the obstruction must be distal to this location. (**C**) The median aperture (foramen of Magendie) allows CSF to leave the fourth ventricle and enter the subarachnoid space. (**D**) Blockage of the spinal canal (central canal of the spinal cord) is likely to have minimal impact on flow within the ventricular system because CSF would still be able to enter the subarachnoid space via the medial and lateral apertures from the fourth ventricle.

Refer to the following image for answer 19:

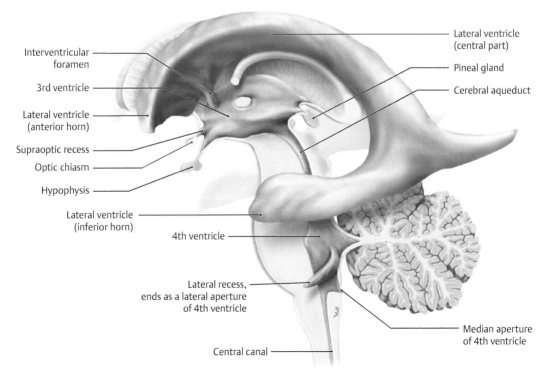

Source: Gilroy AM et al. Atlas of Anatomy. 3rd ed. 2016. Based on: Schuenke M, Schulte E, Schumacher U. THIEME Atlas of Anatomy. Volumes 1-3. Illustrations by Voll M and Wesker K. 2nd ed. New York: Thieme Medical Publishers; 2016

20. Correct: Gastroduodenal (B)

Refer to the following image for answer 20:

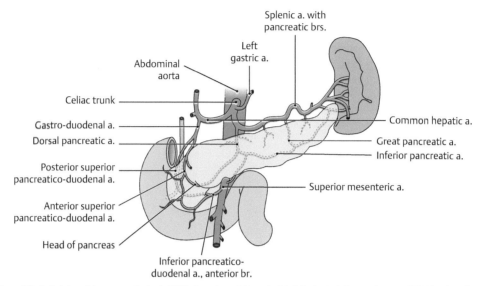

Source: Gilroy AM et al. Atlas of Anatomy. 3rd ed. 2016. Based on: Schuenke M, Schulte E, Schumacher U. THIEME Atlas of Anatomy. Volumes 1-3. Illustrations by Voll M and Wesker K. 2nd ed. New York: Thieme Medical Publishers; 2016

(**B**) To prevent excessive bleeding during the surgery, the surgeon would cauterize the pancreaticoduodenal branches of the gastroduodenal artery, which supply the head of the pancreas. These arteries anastomose with the anterior and posterior inferior pancreatico-duodenal arteries, which are branches of the superior mesenteric. (**A, C, E**) The dorsal and great pancreatic arteries are branches of the splenic artery. The splenic artery courses along the superior margin of the pancreas to supply the neck, body, and tail of the pancreas. (**D**) The inferior mesenteric artery does not supply the pancreas.

21. Correct: Inferior to the portal vein (A)

(**A**) The head of the pancreas is located inferior to the portal vein. (**B**) The head of the pancreas is located medial and inferior to the gastroduodenal artery. The gastroduodenal artery, a branch of the common hepatic, descends anterior to the neck of the pancreas. (**C**) The head of the pancreas is anterior to the inferior vena cava. (**D**) The head of the pancreas is located to the right of the superior mesenteric vein. The pancreas lies to the right side of the superior mesenteric vessels so that its neck is anterior, its head is to the right, and its uncinate process is posterior to the vessels.

Refer to the following image for answer 21:

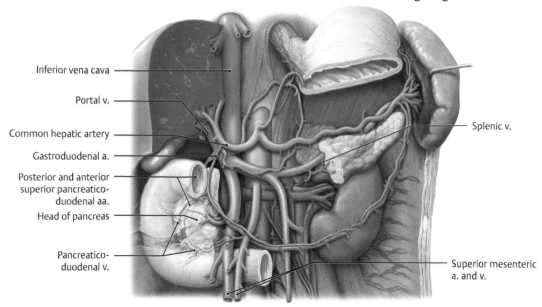

Source: Gilroy AM et al. Atlas of Anatomy. 3rd ed. 2016. Based on: Schuenke M, Schulte E, Schumacher U. THIEME Atlas of Anatomy. Volumes 1-3. Illustrations by Voll M and Wesker K. 2nd ed. New York: Thieme Medical Publishers; 2016

22. Correct: Inferior vena cava (B)

(**B**) The inferior vena cava lies posterior to the pancreas. (**A**) The first part of the duodenum lies anterior to the head of the pancreas. (**C**) The lesser sac lies anterior to the pancreas. (**D**) The stomach is located anterior and to the left of the pancreatic head. (**E**) The transverse mesocolon is inferior and to the left of the head of the pancreas.

23. Correct: Neural crest (D)

(**D**) Pheochromocytomas are tumors originating from chromaffin cells of the suprarenal gland. Chromaffin cells (also called pheochromocytes) in the medulla of the suprarenal glands are derived from neural crest cells. In contrast, the cortical cells of the suprarenal gland are derived from the intermediate mesoderm. (**A**) Hematopoietic stem cells are the precursors to all blood cell types. They originate initially in blood islands of the yolk sac and are later thought to develop from the aorta-gonad-mesonephros, a region that develops from the lateral plate mesoderm. (**B**) The metanephric blastema, another derivative of the intermediate mesoderm, will form the excretory units of the definitive kidney. (**C**) The nephrogenic cord, which also forms from intermediate mesoderm, will ultimately give rise to parts of the urogenital system. (**E**) Primordial germ cells are the precursors of gonocytes (gametes). They migrate from the yolk sac (where they can initially be identified) into the developing ovary and testes to form oogonia and spermatogonia, respectively.

Refer to the following images for answer 23:

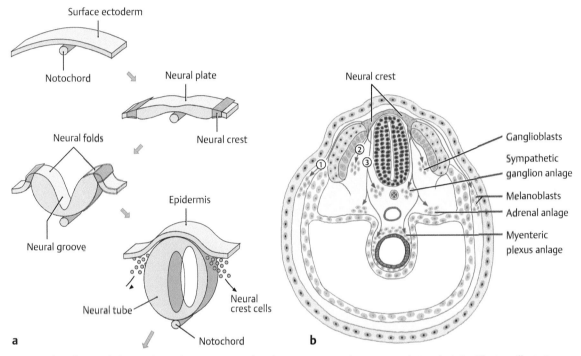

Source: Schuenke M, Schulte E, Schumacher U. THIEME Atlas of Anatomy. General Anatomy and Musculoskeletal System. Illustrations by Voll M and Wesker K. 2nd ed. New York: Thieme Medical Publishers; 2016

24. Correct: Thoracic splanchnic nerves (D)

Refer to the following image for answer 24:

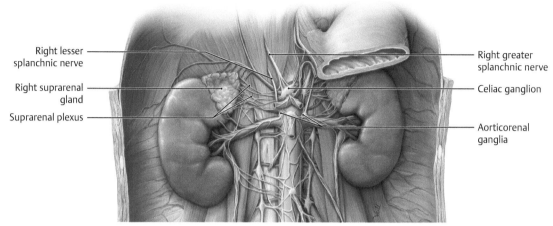

Right lesser splanchnic nerve — Right suprarenal gland — Suprarenal plexus — Right greater splanchnic nerve — Celiac ganglion — Aorticorenal ganglia

Source: Schuenke M, Schulte E, Schumacher U. THIEME Atlas of Anatomy. Internal Organs. Illustrations by Voll M and Wesker K. 2nd ed. New York: Thieme Medical Publishers; 2016

(**D**) The thoracic (also referred to as thoracoabdominal) splanchnic nerves, which include the greater (T5–T9), lesser (T10–T11), and least (T12) splanchnic nerves, innervate abdominal organs of the foregut and midgut, and the chromaffin cells of the suprarenal gland. The chromaffin cells of the suprarenal glands resemble postganglionic sympathetic neurons. They are derived from neural crest cells and are innervated by preganglionic sympathetic neurons whose axons reach the suprarenal glands via the greater splanchnic nerve. (**A**) The lumbar splanchnic nerves arise from the lumbar part of the sympathetic trunk. They contain preganglionic sympathetic fibers that synapse in the inferior mesenteric ganglion or in ganglia in the inferior hypogastric (pelvic) plexus. The latter innervate smooth muscles and glands in the distal portion of the gastrointestinal tract and pelvic viscera. (**B**) The pelvic splanchnic nerves arise from the S2-S4 spinal cord and transmit preganglionic parasympathetic fibers to target organs. (**C**) The sacral splanchnic nerves arise from the sacral sympathetic trunk and provide postganglionic sympathetic innervation to pelvic viscera and the lower limb.

25. Correct: Ligament of the ovary (A)

(**A**) The ligament of the ovary (proper ovarian ligament) is a fibromuscular band that extends from the medial aspect of the ovary to the lateral aspect of the uterine body, just inferior to the junction of the uterine tube and uterus. It is the proximal remnant of the gubernaculum ovary. (**B**) On each side, the round ligament of the uterus (the distal remnant of the gubernaculum ovary) courses anterolaterally in the broad ligament and passes along the inguinal canal to the labium majus and mons pubis. It does not connect to the ovary. (**C**) The transverse cervical (cardinal) ligament is a condensation of endopelvic fascia in the base of the broad ligament on each side that extends from the supravaginal cervix to the lateral pelvic walls. It contains the uterine vessels, but does not connect to the ovary. (**D**) The uterine tubes lie in the superior edge of the broad ligament. Except for the fimbria ovarica (a single fimbria that is attached to tubal pole of the ovary), this tube does not connect directly to the ovary. (**E**) The uterosacral ligaments, also condensations of endopelvic fascia, extend from the uterus to the sacrum and do not connect to the ovary.

26. Correct: Suspensory ligament of the ovary (D)

(**D**) The suspensory ligament of the ovary, also called the infundibulopelvic (IP) ligament, is a fold in the pelvic peritoneum that conveys the ovarian vessels and nerves to the ovary. (**A**) The ligament of the ovary (proper ovarian ligament) is a fibromuscular band that extends from the medial aspect of the ovary to the lateral aspect of the uterine body, just inferior to the junction of the uterine tube and uterus. It is the proximal remnant of the gubernaculum ovary. (**B**) The mesosalpinx is the portion of the broad ligament that encloses the uterine tubes. The mesosalpinx is a mesentery and conveys branches of uterine and ovarian vessels. However, it is not the position at which the ovarian vessels would be ligated in an oophorectomy. (**C**) The round ligament of the uterus, the distal remnant of the gubernaculum ovary, courses anterolaterally in the broad ligament and passes along the inguinal canal to the labia majus and mons pubis. It does not convey the ovarian vessels to the ovary. (**E**) The transverse cervical (cardinal) ligament is a condensation of endopelvic fascia in the base of the broad ligament on each side that extends from the supravaginal cervix to the lateral pelvic walls. It conveys the uterine, not ovarian, vessels.

Refer to the following image for answers 25 and 26:

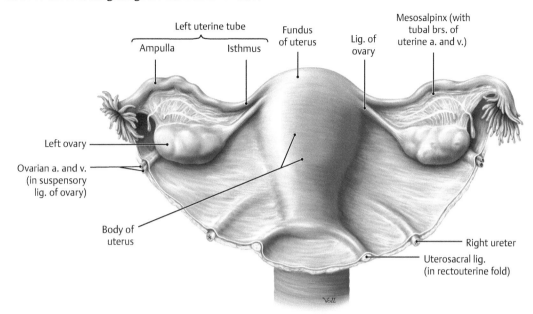

Source: Gilroy AM et al. Atlas of Anatomy. 3rd ed. 2016. Based on: Schuenke M, Schulte E, Schumacher U. THIEME Atlas of Anatomy. Volumes 1-3. Illustrations by Voll M and Wesker K. 2nd ed. New York: Thieme Medical Publishers; 2016

27. Correct: Annular pancreas (A)

(**A**) Pancreatic tissue is most likely encircling the duodenum in this individual, resulting from a congenital annular pancreas. The pancreas develops from ventral and dorsal buds of the foregut: the dorsal bud forms most of the head, neck, and body of the pancreas, whereas the ventral bud rotates around the bile duct to form part of the pancreatic head and the uncinate process. If the ventral bud splits (becomes bifid), the two segments may encircle the duodenum forming an annular pancreas. Usually, an annular pancreas is an isolated developmental anomaly and does not occur with other types of intestinal malrotation. (**B**) While duodenal atresia may result from an annular pancreas, the finding of pancreatic tissue encircling the duodenum and the resultant inflammation of the pancreatic tissue is indicative of an annular pancreas. (**C**) Intestinal malrotation is a developmental anomaly that results from abnormal rotation of the midgut as it returns to the abdominal cavity during embryogenesis. The finding of pancreatic tissue encircling the duodenum, and the resultant inflammation of the pancreatic tissue, is indicative of an annular pancreas. (**D**) A Meckel's diverticulum results from a failure of the vitelline duct to degenerate. It does not affect the pancreas but may contain ectopic pancreatic tissue. The finding of pancreatic tissue encircling the duodenum, and the resultant inflammation of the pancreatic tissue, is indicative of an annular pancreas. (**E**) Volvulus usually results from intestinal malrotation during development that leads to twisting of the intestines and can result in intestinal obstruction and/or ischemia. Symptoms include abdominal pain and bloating, nausea, bloody stools, and constipation.

Refer to the following images for answer 27:

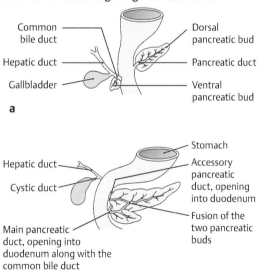

Source: Gilroy AM et al. Atlas of Anatomy. 3rd ed. 2016. Based on: Schuenke M, Schulte E, Schumacher U. THIEME Atlas of Anatomy. Volumes 1-3. Illustrations by Voll M and Wesker K. 2nd ed. New York: Thieme Medical Publishers; 2016

28. Correct: Polycystic ovarian syndrome (E)

(**E**) This individual has polycystic ovarian syndrome (PCOS), a condition that results from elevated androgen levels. Ultrasonography shows multiple, small follicles peripherally placed in her enlarged right ovary. PCOS is indicated when combined with her other symptoms (hirsutism, obesity, acne, and oligomenorrhea). (**A**) In androgen insensitivity syndrome, the body cannot use androgens. Individuals with this syndrome have the external sex characteristics of females but do not have a uterus or ovaries and, therefore, do not menstruate and are unable to conceive. Since this individual does have ovaries, this is not a likely diagnosis. (**B**) Although individuals with congenital adrenal hypoplasia may develop hirsutism and oligomenorrhea, they generally have ambiguous external genitalia with normal internal reproductive organs. The polycystic nature of this patient's ovaries and her other symptoms are more indicative of PCOS. (**C**) Although hypothyroidism can present with menstrual disturbances and impaired fertility, the polycystic nature of this patient's ovaries and her other symptoms are more indicative of PCOS. (**D**) Symptoms of an ovarian tumor include: abdominal bloating, pressure and pain; abnormal fullness after eating and difficulty eating; and increased urination or urge. The polycystic nature of this patient's ovaries and her other symptoms are more indicative of PCOS.

29. Correct: Molar pregnancy (B)

(**B**) The enlarged uterus with numerous, small vesicles is indicative of a molar pregnancy. A molar pregnancy, also known as hydatidiform mole, is a benign uterine tumor that occurs when the placenta becomes a mass of cysts. In a complete molar pregnancy, neither an embryo nor normal placental tissue is present. In a partial molar pregnancy, an abnormal embryo is present and, possibly, some normal placental tissue. However, growth of the embryo is usually retarded and it fails to develop fully. (**A, C–E**) An ectopic and normal pregnancy would unlikely present with cystic structures in the uterus, and neither uterine polyps nor fibroids would cause the elevated hCG. Because the uterus is filled with small cysts, and there is no evidence of embryonic development, the individual is most likely to have a complete molar pregnancy.

30. Correct: Rectouterine pouch (C)

(**C**) The rectouterine pouch (cul-de-sac; pouch of Douglas) is a recess in the peritoneal cavity located between the uterus and the rectum (see the presented image). The ovaries are attached to the ligament of the ovary (proper ovarian ligament) on the posterior aspect of the broad ligament and are, therefore, most closely associated with the rectouterine pouch. Chocolate cysts are endometrial cysts that occur when endometrial tissue abnormally attaches to the ovary. The endometrial cells multiply and form cysts when stimulated by menstrual hormones. Because the endometrial tissue inside the cyst responds to monthly elevated hormone levels, it bleeds and fills the interior of the cysts with unclotted blood. The presence of cysts on the ovaries can cause dyspareunia (pain during sexual intercourse). (**A, B**) The vaginal fornices are formed by the projection of the uterine cervix into the vaginal lumen. They are not associated with the ovaries. (**D**) The retropubic space is located between the pubis and urinary bladder and is not related to the ovaries. (**E**) The vesicouterine pouch is a peritoneal recess that lies between the urinary bladder and the uterus. Since the ovaries are suspended from the posterior aspect of the broad ligament, this space is not related to the ovaries.

Refer to the following image for answer 30:

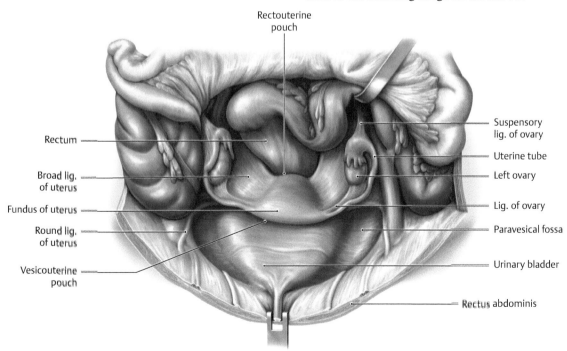

Rectouterine pouch

Rectum

Broad lig. of uterus

Fundus of uterus

Round lig. of uterus

Vesicouterine pouch

Suspensory lig. of ovary

Uterine tube

Left ovary

Lig. of ovary

Paravesical fossa

Urinary bladder

Rectus abdominis

Source: Gilroy AM et al. Atlas of Anatomy. 3rd ed. 2016. Based on: Schuenke M, Schulte E, Schumacher U. THIEME Atlas of Anatomy. Volumes 1-3. Illustrations by Voll M and Wesker K. 2nd ed. New York: Thieme Medical Publishers; 2016

31. Correct: Posterior vaginal fornix (B)

(**B**) Endometriosis involving the rectovaginal septum would be most closely associated with the posterior vaginal fornix. This region lies within the superior portion of the vagina, posterior to the cervix and lies adjacent to the rectouterine pouch. (**A**) The anterior vaginal fornix lies anterior to the uterine cervix and is, therefore, associated with the anterior most aspect of the superior vagina. (**C**) The retropubic space is located between the pubis and urinary bladder and, therefore, unrelated to the posterior vaginal wall. (**D**) The vesicouterine pouch lies between the urinary bladder and the uterus and is a peritoneal recess.

Refer to the following image for answer 31:

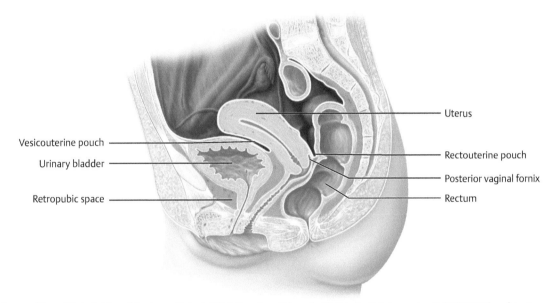

Source: Gilroy AM et al. Atlas of Anatomy. 3rd ed. 2016. Based on: Schuenke M, Schulte E, Schumacher U. THIEME Atlas of Anatomy. Volumes 1-3. Illustrations by Voll M and Wesker K. 2nd ed. New York: Thieme Medical Publishers; 2016

32. Correct: Lingual thyroid (D)

Refer to the following images for answers 32 and 33:

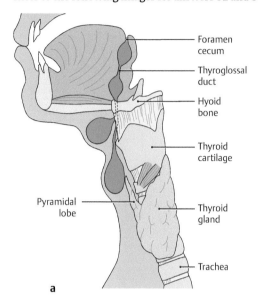

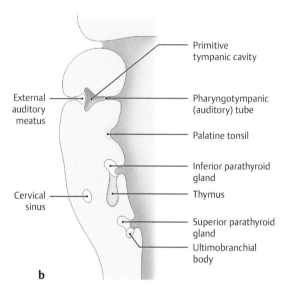

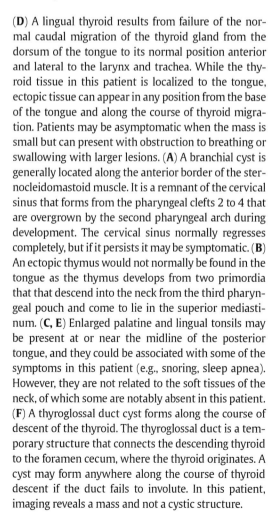

a

Source: Schuenke M, Schulte E, Schumacher U. THIEME Atlas of Anatomy. Head, Neck, and Neuroanatomy. Illustrations by Voll M and Wesker K. 2nd ed. New York: Thieme Medical Publishers; 2016

b

Source: Gilroy AM et al. Atlas of Anatomy. 3rd ed. 2016. Based on: Schuenke M, Schulte E, Schumacher U. THIEME Atlas of Anatomy. Volumes 1-3. Illustrations by Voll M and Wesker K. 2nd ed. New York: Thieme Medical Publishers; 2016

(**D**) A lingual thyroid results from failure of the normal caudal migration of the thyroid gland from the dorsum of the tongue to its normal position anterior and lateral to the larynx and trachea. While the thyroid tissue in this patient is localized to the tongue, ectopic tissue can appear in any position from the base of the tongue and along the course of thyroid migration. Patients may be asymptomatic when the mass is small but can present with obstruction to breathing or swallowing with larger lesions. (**A**) A branchial cyst is generally located along the anterior border of the sternocleidomastoid muscle. It is a remnant of the cervical sinus that forms from the pharyngeal clefts 2 to 4 that are overgrown by the second pharyngeal arch during development. The cervical sinus normally regresses completely, but if it persists it may be symptomatic. (**B**) An ectopic thymus would not normally be found in the tongue as the thymus develops from two primordia that that descend into the neck from the third pharyngeal pouch and come to lie in the superior mediastinum. (**C, E**) Enlarged palatine and lingual tonsils may be present at or near the midline of the posterior tongue, and they could be associated with some of the symptoms in this patient (e.g., snoring, sleep apnea). However, they are not related to the soft tissues of the neck, of which some are notably absent in this patient. (**F**) A thyroglossal duct cyst forms along the course of descent of the thyroid. The thyroglossal duct is a temporary structure that connects the descending thyroid to the foramen cecum, where the thyroid originates. A cyst may form anywhere along the course of thyroid descent if the duct fails to involute. In this patient, imaging reveals a mass and not a cystic structure.

33. Correct: Thyroglossal duct cyst (E)

(**E**) A thyroglossal duct cyst forms along the course of descent of the thyroid gland primordium. The thyroglossal duct is a temporary structure that connects the dorsum of the tongue, where the thyroid originates, with the gland as it descends into the neck. A cyst may form anywhere along the course of thyroid descent if the duct fails to involute. The swelling moves upwards when the patient protrudes the tongue because of its association between the cystic remnant of the thyroglossal duct and the tongue. (**A**) A branchial cyst, which is located along the anterior border of the sternocleidomastoid muscle, is a remnant of the cervical sinus that forms from the pharyngeal clefts 2 to 4 that are overgrown by the second pharyngeal arch during development. The cervical sinus normally regresses completely, but if it persists it may be symptomatic. (**B**) An ectopic thymus would not normally be found in the tongue as the thymus develops from two primordia that that descend into the neck from the third pharyngeal pouch and come to lie in the superior mediastinum. (**C**) An enlarged palatine tonsil may extend from the tonsillar fossa toward the midline of the pharynx (near the posterior tongue). An enlarged palatine tonsil would not move upwards when the patient protrudes the tongue because this tonsil is not attached to the tongue. (**D**) A lingual thyroid results from failure of the normal caudal migration of the thyroid gland from the dorsum of the tongue to its normal position anterior and lateral to the larynx and trachea.

Chapter 10

Lymphatic System

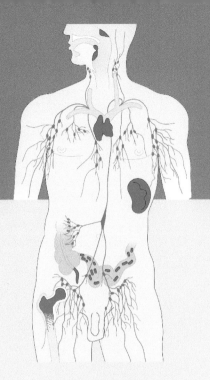

ANATOMICAL LEARNING OBJECTIVES

▶ Describe the anatomy of the lymphoid system, including specific lymphoid tissues and organs, the distribution of major groups of lymph nodes.

▶ Describe the lymphatic drainage from the head and neck as it relates to metastatic disease and the spread of infection.

▶ Describe the lymphatic drainage from the upper and lower limbs as it relates to metastatic disease and the spread of infection.

▶ Describe the lymphatic drainage from the thorax, including the breasts, thoracic walls, and internal organs, as it relates to metastatic disease and the spread of infection.

▶ Describe the lymphatic drainage from the abdomen, including its walls and organs, as it relates to metastatic disease and the spread of infection.

▶ Describe the lymphatic drainage from the urinary organs as it relates to metastatic disease and the spread of infection.

▶ Describe the lymphatic drainage from the pelvis, including its walls and organs, as it relates to metastatic disease and the spread of infection.

10.1 Questions

Easy	Medium	Hard

1. A 37-year-old woman with a history of constipation describes the recent onset of painful bowel movements and bright red blood on toilet tissue. Physical examination reveals a longitudinal fissure in her lower anal canal. Which of the following major groups of lymph nodes first receives lymph from the area of the fissure?

A. Deep inguinal

B. Internal iliac

C. Paracolic

D. Pararectal

E. Superficial inguinal

2. A 28-year-old woman presents with a small ulcer on her left nipple to her gynecologist. She noticed the ulcer 2 weeks ago and it has become painful. Physical examination indicates that the lesion is restricted to the nipple and lymph nodes in the area are not palpable. Further testing leads to a diagnosis of Paget's disease of the nipple. Lymph from the affected area initially drains to which of the following?

A. Interpectoral lymphatic plexus

B. Parasternal lymph nodes

C. Pectoral lymph nodes

D. Subareolar lymphatic plexus

E. Subclavian lymphatic trunk

3. A 44-year-old woman comes to her primary care physician because she has noticed changes in her right breast over the past several weeks. The patient indicates that the nipple has become progressively inverted and painful and now produces a blood-tinged discharge. She believes she can feel a lump in the breast. A mammogram indicates a mass in the upper medial quadrant of the right breast and biopsy results show malignancy. If metastasis occurs from this tumor, which of the following groups of lymph nodes will the malignant cells most likely reach first?

A. Apical axillary

B. Central axillary

C. Parasternal

D. Pectoral

E. Subscapular

4. A 63-year-old man arrives on referral at an oncology clinic with a chronic cough and recent hemoptysis (coughing up blood). A patient history shows that he has been a smoker for 20 years, and currently smokes a pack each day. Bronchoscopy shows a widening of the trachea at its bifurcation with posterior displacement of the main bronchi. A PET CT scan confirms bronchogenic carcinoma. Which of the following lymph nodes are responsible for the airway alteration revealed during bronchoscopy?

A. Anterior mediastinal

B. Hilar

C. Lobar

D. Paratracheal

E. Tracheobronchial

5. An 89-year-old man with dysphagia (difficulty swallowing), progressive weight loss, and chest pain presents to a gastroenterologist. The patient's history reveals that he is a chronic smoker and suffers from obesity. An endoscopic esophageal ultrasound reveals enlarged paratracheal lymph nodes. Additional tests lead to a diagnosis of cancer in the upper digestive tract. Which of the following is the most likely site of the cancer?

A. Abdominal esophagus

B. Cardia of stomach

C. Cervical esophagus

D. Fundus of stomach

E. Thoracic esophagus

6. A 48-year-old man with progressive dysphagia (difficulty swallowing), odynophagia (painful swallowing), and rapid weight loss is referred to a gastroenterologist. A double-contrast barium swallow shows a mass in the proximal esophagus. Further tests confirm malignancy of the mass. The cancer may spread to which of the following groups of lymph nodes?

A. Celiac

B. Deep cervical

C. Parahiatal

D. Paratracheal

E. Pulmonary hilar

7. A 56-year-old man presents to his primary care physician with concerns of progressive upper abdominal discomfort, anorexia (loss of appetite), and weight loss. An abdominal examination is normal, but laboratory results indicate iron deficiency anemia. He is referred to a gastroenterologist and an esophagogastroscopy reveals a lesion along the gastric canal. Biopsy of the lesion shows it to be an adenocarcinoma. To which of the following lymph nodes would the cancer initially spread?

A. Celiac and splenic

B. Pancreaticoduodenal

C. Right and left gastric

D. Right and left gastro-omental

E. Supra- and subpyloric

8. An 87-year-old man presents with the chief concern of jaundice (yellowish discoloration of the skin). The initial assessment is inconclusive and he is referred to a gastroenterologist. Endoscopy shows an ulcerative tumor mass at the major duodenal papilla and biopsy leads to a diagnosis of adenocarcinoma affecting the hepatopancreatic ampulla (of Vater). Which of the following lymph nodes should be considered for metastatic spread?

A. Celiac

B. Inferior mesenteric

C. Gastro-omental

D. Paracolic

E. Splenic

9. A 47-year-old man with melena (black stool) presents to the primary care physician. The physical examination is not remarkable and an MRI of the abdomen is ordered. The imaging reveals a mass in the proximal jejunum with enlarged preaortic lymph nodes. A biopsy of the mass is taken and the pathology report shows adenocarcinoma of the jejunum. Through which of the following structures did this cancer spread to preaortic lymph nodes?

A. Gastrocolic ligament

B. Gastrosplenic ligament

C. Hepatoduodenal ligament

D. Mesentery (of small intestine) proper

E. Transverse mesocolon

10. A 28-year-old man is brought to the emergency department after a car accident. He is in severe pain and his vital signs suggest that he has intra-abdominal bleeding. Physical examination confirms pain and tenderness in the epigastric and left flank regions. He also exhibits a left-sided Kehr's sign (acute shoulder pain). CT imaging shows a fracture of the left 10th rib near its angle, fluid in the abdominal cavity, and a ruptured abdominal organ. Which of the following organs is most likely ruptured?

A. Kidney

B. Liver

C. Pancreas

D. Spleen

E. Stomach

11. A 28-year-old woman presents to her primary care physician with fever, night sweats, and weight loss. The physical examination shows generalized lymphadenopathy (lymph node swelling) and jaundice (yellowish discoloration of the skin). Biopsy of enlarged cervical lymph nodes results in a diagnosis of Hodgkin's lymphoma. Enlargement of lymph nodes in which of the following structures is most likely responsible for the jaundice?

A. Greater omentum

B. Hepatoduodenal ligament

C. Hepatogastric ligament

D. Mesentery proper

E. Transverse mesocolon

12. A 58-year-old man with changes in bowel habits and abdominal pain of several weeks' duration presents to a gastroenterologist. A fecal occult blood test is positive. A follow-up CT scan shows a mass in the distal portion of the sigmoid colon which is subsequently determined to be malignant. Which of the following lymph nodes would appear enlarged in the CT scan if there was metastasis?

A. Celiac

B. Ileocolic

C. Inferior mesenteric

D. Splenic

E. Superior mesenteric

13. An 88-year-old woman presents to the emergency department with fever, vomiting, and pain at McBurney's point. Ultrasound reveals a swollen appendix. A laparoscopic appendectomy is performed and, per standard procedure, the resected tissue is sent to pathology for evaluation. The pathology report indicates the presence of a mucinous cystadenocarcinoma. To which of the following lymph nodes will this cancer spread initially?

A. Celiac

B. Ileocolic

C. Inferior mesenteric

D. Splenic

E. Superior mesenteric

14. A 68-year-old man with hematuria (blood in urine) and left flank pain presents to a primary care physician. Physical examination reveals an abdominal mass in the left lumbar region. CT imaging shows a mass in the left kidney and a laparoscopic nephrectomy is performed. Cytological studies of the resected specimen indicate a renal cell carcinoma with infiltration to the surrounding tissue. Malignant cells from the affected organ would initially spread to which of the following lymph nodes?

A. Celiac

B. Inferior mesenteric

C. Lumbar

D. Splenic

E. Superior mesenteric

15. A 22-year-old man with scrotal pain and swelling presents to his primary care physician. The patient claims he cut himself while shaving his pubic hair. Physical examination reveals a superficial, red, tender swelling confined to the dartos layer of the scrotum. Which of the following lymph nodes will initially enlarge due to the infection?

A. Common iliac

B. Deep inguinal

C. External iliac

D. Internal iliac

E. Superficial inguinal

16. A 48-year-old man with a severe cough and hemoptysis (coughing up blood-stained mucus) presents to his primary care physician. The patient history indicates that he is a chronic smoker. Bronchoscopy shows a growth on the left main bronchus and biopsy confirms malignancy. Cancer cells from the affected structure will metastasize through which of the following?

A. Left bronchomediastinal trunk

B. Left pulmonary (intrapulmonary) lymph nodes

C. Right pulmonary lymph nodes

D. Superficial lymphatic plexus

E. Thoracic duct

17. A 12-year-old boy with a high fever of the past 2 days is brought to his pediatrician. A history shows that he injured his left leg when he tried to cross a barbed wire fence 5 days ago. He kept the injury secret from his parents as he feared they would ground him. Physical examination shows a laceration limited to the skin, which is oozing pus on the lateral aspect of the leg. Which of the following lymph nodes should the physician initially assess to rule out lymphadenitis?

A. Deep inguinal

B. External iliac

C. Horizontal group of superficial inguinal

D. Popliteal

E. Vertical group of superficial inguinal

18. A 38-year-old man with the chief concern of discharge from his nipple presents to his primary care physician. The patient tells the physician that he noticed this several months ago, but did not think it was serious. Physical examination reveals a subareolar mass and enlarged axillary lymph nodes. A biopsy of the mass confirms cancer. Which of the following fasciae did the cancer most likely infiltrate?

A. Axillary

B. Brachial

C. Clavipectoral

D. Deltoid

E. Pectoral

19. A 64-year-old man presents with pain when opening his mouth and a severe burning sensation in his mouth when eating spicy food. The patient history shows he is a chronic alcoholic and physical examination reveals an ulcerated mass in the central portion of the body of the tongue. The mass is biopsied and malignant cells are found. In which of the following neck triangles might enlarged lymph nodes be palpable because of a primary/initial metastasis?

A. Carotid

B. Digastric

C. Occipital

D. Omoclavicular

E. Submental

20. An 88-year-old woman is referred to a colorectal surgeon because of anal bleeding and an anal mass. The surgeon identifies thrombosed internal hemorrhoids and performs a hemorrhoidectomy. Cytological analysis of the resected anal mass indicates malignant cells. Which of the following lymph nodes will first receive lymphatic drainage from the malignant tissue?

A. Common iliac

B. Deep inguinal

C. External iliac

D. Internal iliac

E. Superficial inguinal

21. A 36-year-old woman presents to her primary care physician with a puncture wound on her right hypothenar eminence. The patient history indicates that she received the injury 5 days ago from a thorn in her rose garden. Physical examination reveals subcutaneous red streaks emanating from the wound, a sign that is characteristic of lymphangitis. Which of the following lymph nodes will first receive lymph from the area of the wound?

A. Cubital

B. Humeral

C. Parasternal

D. Pectoral

E. Subscapular

22. A 76-year-old woman with itching, burning, and raised skin lesions in her vulva presents to her primary care physician. Physical examination reveals a pink skin lesion on the right labium majus. A biopsy leads to a diagnosis of vulvar intraepithelial neoplasia. Which of the following lymph nodes should be assessed to rule out initial metastasis from the affected area?

A. Common iliac

B. Deep inguinal

C. External iliac

D. Internal iliac

E. Superficial inguinal

23. A 56-year-old woman with a distended and painful abdomen presents to her primary care physician. Physical examination reveals right lower abdominal tenderness. A CT scan shows a mass on the right ovary and her serum CA-125 (a biomarker for tumor cells) is elevated. Which of the following lymph nodes might appear enlarged on the CT, suggesting an initial metastasis from the affected organ?

A. Common iliac

B. External iliac

C. Inferior mesenteric

D. Internal iliac

E. Lumbar

24. A 56-year-old woman presents to her gynecologist with vaginal bleeding and urinary difficulty. A Papanicolaou test (Pap test/smear, cervical smear) and ultrasonography are performed. Malignant cells are present in the Pap smear and the ultrasound shows ureteral compression by a mass in the supravaginal part of the cervix that has extended into the base of the broad ligament of the uterus. Cancer cells from the affected organ will initially metastasize to which of the following lymph nodes?

A. Common iliac

B. Inferior mesenteric

C. Internal iliac

D. Lumbar (para-aortic and paracaval)

E. Obturator

25. A 26-year-old woman with vulvar pain during walking, sitting, and sexual intercourse (dyspareunia) presents to her primary care physician. Physical examination reveals a 4 cm diameter abscess associated with the posterior aspect of the right labium minus. A greater vestibular (Bartholin) gland abscess is diagnosed. Which of the following lymph nodes should be examined to determine any initial spread of the infection from the affected area?

A. Common iliac

B. External iliac

C. Internal iliac

D. Sacral

E. Superficial inguinal

26. A 71-year-old man with a chief concern of difficulty in urination is referred to the urologist. The urologist performs a digital rectal examination and detects an irregularly enlarged, hard prostate. Laboratory tests reveal an elevated serum prostate-specific antigen. A transurethral biopsy shows adenocarcinoma of the prostate. Cancer cells from the affected organ initially metastasizes to which of the following lymph nodes?

A. Common iliac

B. Deep inguinal

C. Lumbar

D. Obturator

E. Superficial inguinal

27. A 32-year-old woman with throbbing clitoral pain for the last 2 weeks presents to her gynecologist. The patient used an over-the-counter ointment on the affected area, which decreased the pain, but the clitoris is still swollen and she feels like it is constantly aroused. Physical examination reveals white patches on the glans of the clitoris consistent with a yeast infection. Which of the following lymph nodes should be evaluated to determine any initial spread of infection from the affected area?

A. Common iliac

B. Deep inguinal

C. External iliac

D. Sacral

E. Superficial inguinal

28. A 28-year-old woman in the postpartum period presents to her gynecologist with a fever and a swelling in her perineum. Physical examination reveals that her mediolateral episiotomy is infected and purulent (producing pus). Which of the following lymph nodes should be examined to assess any initial spread of the infection from the affected area?

A. Common iliac

B. Deep inguinal

C. External iliac

D. Internal iliac

E. Superficial inguinal

29. A 35-year-old woman with a swollen, painful, and tender tip of her tongue presents to her primary care physician. Patient history shows she had a tongue piercing 1 week prior. Physical examination confirms a red, swollen tongue. She is diagnosed with glossitis. Which of the following lymph nodes should be evaluated to assess any initial spread of infection?

A. Deep cervical

B. Jugulodigastric

C. Jugulo-omohyoid

D. Submandibular

E. Submental

30. A 9-year-old girl with fever, sore throat, and difficulty swallowing is brought by her parents to the pediatrician. Examination of her oral cavity reveals bilateral swellings between the palatoglossal and palatopharyngeal folds. The area is swabbed for culture and the results indicate infection of the lymphoid tissue between the folds. Which of the following lymph nodes should be evaluated to assess for initial spread of the infection from the affected lymphoid tissue?

A. Deep parotid

B. Jugulodigastric

C. Submandibular

D. Submental

E. Superficial parotid

31. A 29-year-old man with a swollen upper eyelid presents to a primary care physician. The patient reveals that he was mugged 6 days ago, during which he sustained this injury. Physical examination shows a left swollen, red, upper eyelid that has tenderness. Which of the following lymph nodes should be evaluated to determine any initial spread of the infection from the affected region?

A. Mastoid

B. Occipital

C. Parotid

D. Submandibular

E. Submental

32. A 9-year-old boy with severe itching on the back of the head and restless sleep for the past several weeks is brought to a pediatrician. Physical examination of the scalp shows red spots superior to the inion that resembles insect bites. Examination of this region with a hand lens reveals live lice. A diagnosis of pediculosis capitis (head lice infestation) is made. Which of the following lymph nodes may be enlarged from the initial spread of infection from the affected site?

A. Mastoid

B. Occipital

C. Parotid

D. Submandibular

E. Submental

33. A 32-year-old man presents to the emergency department with a fever and an infected wound on his forehead. The patient history reveals that a deep laceration on the forehead, superior to the glabella, occurred as a result of a motor vehicle accident, and that the wound was sutured. Which of the following lymph nodes should be evaluated to determine any initial spread of the infection from the affected region?

A. Mastoid

B. Occipital

C. Parotid

D. Submandibular

E. Submental

34. A 50-year-old man with a lesion on the tip of his nose presents to a primary care physician. Physical examination reveals scaly skin on the nose and a 1 cm diameter, deep, "punched-out" ulcer at the tip. The ulcer is biopsied and the pathology report indicates squamous cell carcinoma. Which of the following lymph nodes should be evaluated to determine any initial metastasis from the affected region?

A. Mastoid

B. Occipital

C. Parotid

D. Submandibular

E. Submental

35. A 63-year-old man with a blister on his lip of several weeks duration presents to a primary care physician. The patient admits that he is a chronic smoker. The blister is on the upper lip close to right nasolabial sulcus. A biopsy of the lesion reveals a basal cell carcinoma. The cancer is most likely to first metastasize to which of the following lymph nodes?

A. Mastoid

B. Occipital

C. Parotid

D. Submandibular

E. Submental

36. A 58-year-old man with an infection on his lower lip presents to a primary care physician. A history indicates that he had a piercing done 2 weeks ago. Physical examination shows a purulent (pus producing) wound on the lower lip at right labial commissure. Which of the following lymph nodes should be evaluated to rule out initial lymphadenitis?

A. Left submandibular

B. Parotid

C. Right and left submandibular

D. Right submandibular

E. Submental

37. A 57-year-old man describes to a primary care physician a tender area on the "back of my tongue" that has been present for approximately 3 weeks. The patient history indicates an earlier diagnosis of type 16 human papillomavirus (HPV) infection. Physical examination reveals an ulcerated area surrounded by leukoplakia (white patches) on the posterior tongue. This area also has paresthesia (tingling or numbness). A biopsy of the area leads to a diagnosis of carcinoma of the root of the tongue. Which of the following lymph nodes should be evaluated to determine any initial metastasis from the affected region?

A. Inferior deep cervical

B. Parotid

C. Submandibular

D. Submental

E. Superior deep cervical

38. A 74-year-old man with a history of hypertension visits a primary care physician for severe, "tearing," abdominal pain that radiates to his back. Physical examination detects a large, mobile pulsatile mass in his left lower abdominal quadrant, near the midline. Imaging reveals the superior limit of the mass is in the aortic hiatus of the diaphragm (T12 vertebral level). Which of the following structures is most likely compressed at the superior limit of the mass?

A. Cisterna chyli

B. Hemi-azygos vein

C. Phrenic nerve

D. Thoracic duct

E. Vagal trunks

39. A 48-year-old woman presents to the emergency department with fever and acute, severe pain in the right lower abdominal quadrant. A CT of the abdomen shows an enlarged appendix and she is diagnosed with acute appendicitis. After a laparoscopic appendectomy, pathological examination of the resected appendix shows adenocarcinoma. If metastasis has occurred, which of the following lymph nodes will be initially involved in this patient?

A. Ileocolic and inferior mesenteric

B. Ileocolic and superior mesenteric

C. Left colic and inferior mesenteric

D. Left colic and superior mesenteric

E. Right colic and inferior mesenteric

F. Right colic and superior mesenteric

40. A 68-year-old man with a skin lesion on the anterior abdominal wall, inferior to the umbilicus, presents to a primary care physician. Physical examination confirms an asymmetrical nodule with variegated color (refer to the accompanying image). Further evaluation determines that the lesion is a malignant melanoma confined to the layers of the skin. Which of the following lymph nodes should be evaluated first to establish if there is metastasis?

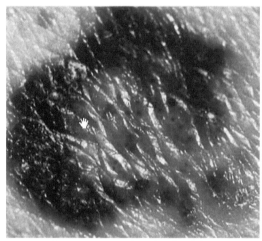

Source: Riede U, Werner M. Color Atlas of Pathology. 1st Edition. Thieme; 2004.

A. Axillary

B. Deep cervical

C. External iliac

D. Lumbar

E. Superficial inguinal

41. A 28-year-old man presents to his primary care physician because he recently discovered an "extra" lump in his scrotum. Physical examination reveals a mass on the right testicle and ultrasound shows the mass to be solid and within the testicular tissue. The patient is referred to the urology clinic for further evaluation. A biopsy shows the mass to be malignant and a diagnosis of seminoma (germ cell carcinoma) is made. A CT scan is performed to assess for metastasis. Which of the following groups of lymph nodes may be enlarged as a sign of initial metastasis?

A. Deep inguinal

B. External iliac

C. Lumbar

D. Sacral

E. Superficial inguinal

42. A 38-year-old man with fever, pain during urination and ejaculation, and urgency presents to his urologist. His history reveals that eight months ago he was referred with similar symptoms by his primary care physician. At the time, he was diagnosed with chronic bacterial prostatitis, and despite treatment with antibiotics, has had two recurrences since the original diagnosis. Which of the following groups of lymph nodes would be the first to show signs of lymphatic spread of the infection?

A. Aortic and caval

B. Ileocolic and lumbar

C. Internal iliac and sacral

D. Pararectal and inferior mesenteric

E. Superficial inguinal and deep inguinal

Consider the following case for questions 43 and 44:

A 29-year-old man presents with nausea, postprandial (after a meal) epigastric pain, and significant weight loss over the past 3 months. On physical examination, a 3 × 4 cm, firm, nontender lump is noted in the left supraclavicular fossa (refer to the *arrow* in the accompanying image), which the patient indicates has been enlarging for a couple of months. This is recognized as a positive Troisier's sign (Virchow's node) and fine-needle aspiration biopsy reveals adenocarcinoma.

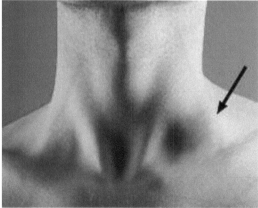

Source: Schmidt G, Greiner L, Nürnberg D. Differential Diagnosis in Ultrasound Imaging. 2nd Edition. Thieme; 2014.

43. Which of the following structures is the most likely source of the malignancy?

A. Left lung

B. Left main bronchus

C. Left ventricle

D. Mediastinal portion of esophagus

E. Stomach

44. CT imaging reveals the tumor as a focal circular thickening in the wall of an upper digestive organ located just inferior to the diaphragm. Which of the following groups of lymph nodes would most likely be the first to receive carcinoma cells from the region of the stomach involved (refer to the *arrows* in the accompanying image)?

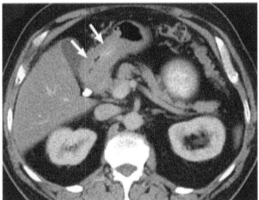

Source: Burgener F, Zaunbauer W, Meyers S et al. Differential Diagnosis in Computed Tomography. 2nd Edition. Stuttgart: Thieme; 2011.

A. Celiac

B. Left gastric

C. Left gastro-omental

D. Mesenteric

E. Right gastro-omental

45. A 58-year-old man presents to the emergency department with abdominal pain and distension as well as nausea and vomiting. History reveals he had an abdominal aortic aneurysm reconstruction one month ago. During the physical examination a fluid wave test is positive for abdominal ascites and subsequent paracentesis returns milky fluid that contains elevated triglycerides (> 180 mg/dL). Injury to which of the following structures during the reconstruction is most likely responsible for the ascites?

A. Bronchomediastinal trunk

B. Cisterna chyli

C. Jugular trunk

D. Right lymphatic duct

E. Subclavian trunk

46. Three days after surgery to correct a congenital heart defect, a 14-month-old boy presents with tachypnea (rapid breathing), dyspnea (difficulty breathing), and cough. Physical examination shows decreased breath sounds and a chest radiograph reveals an opaque shadow on the left. Thoracentesis (pleural tap) returns a milky white fluid, which confirms a chylothorax. The damaged structure responsible for this condition typically enters the posterior mediastinum at which vertebral level?

A. T8

B. T9

C. T10

D. T11

E. T12

47. A 68-year-old man undergoes esophageal resection for carcinoma. On the second postoperative day, the patient develops dyspnea and chest pain, especially on deep inhalation. A pleural effusion that contains high triglyceride levels (> 110 mg/mL) is collected by thoracentesis. Which of the following conditions is most likely in this patient?

A. Chylothorax

B. Hemothorax

C. Pneumonia

D. Pneumothorax

10.2 Answers and Explanations

Easy	Medium	Hard

1. Correct: Superficial inguinal (E)

Refer to the following image for answer 1:

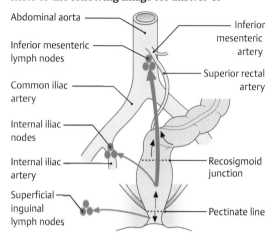

Source: Gilroy AM et al. Atlas of Anatomy. 3rd ed. 2016. Based on: Schuenke M, Schulte E, Schumacher U. THIEME Atlas of Anatomy. Volumes 1-3. Illustrations by Voll M and Wesker K. 2nd ed. New York: Thieme Medical Publishers; 2016

(**E**) Lymph from the lower portion of the anal canal (inferior to the pectinate line) first enters superficial inguinal nodes. Superficial structures in the lower limb and lower anterior abdominal wall, as well as the urogenital region of the perineum (scrotum and skin of the penis; skin of the clitoris and labia), also drain to superficial inguinal lymph nodes. (**A**) Deep inguinal lymph nodes drain portions of the external genitalia (glans penis and clitoris, corpora cavernosa, corpus spongiosum and bulb of the penis in the male, and the vestibular bulb in the female) and deeper structures of the lower limb. They receive lymph from the superficial inguinal lymph nodes secondarily. (**B**) Some lymph from the lower rectum (as well as most pelvic organs) drains through lymphatics that follows the middle and inferior rectal arteries to internal iliac nodes. (**C**) Paracolic lymph nodes form a large group of lymph nodes that lie adjacent to the colon. They are found along the medial aspect of the ascending, descending, and sigmoid colon and along the inferior border of the transverse colon. (**D**) Pararectal lymph nodes drain lymph from the rectum and anal canal above the pectinate (dentate) line. Lymph from these nodes drains through lymphatics along the superior rectal artery to inferior mesenteric nodes.

2. Correct: Subareolar lymphatic plexus (D)

(**D**) Lymph from the nipple, areola, and lobules of the breast drains initially to the subareolar lymphatic plexus. From there, lymph will drain into axillary lymph nodes. Paget's disease of the nipple, also known as Paget's disease of the breast, is a form of breast malignancy characterized by infiltration of the nipple epidermis by malignant cells. (**A**) Some lymph from lateral breast quadrants may drain directly to interpectoral, deltopectoral, supraclavicular, or inferior deep cervical lymph nodes. (**B**) Lymph, particularly from medial breast quadrants, drains to parasternal lymph nodes or to the opposite breast. (**C**) Most lymph from lateral breast quadrants drains initially to the pectoral group of axillary lymph nodes. (**E**) Lymph from the axillary nodes lymph drains into supraclavicular and infraclavicular nodes, and then into the subclavian lymphatic trunk.

Refer to the following image for answer 2:

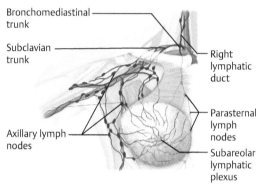

Source: Gilroy AM et al. Atlas of Anatomy. 3rd ed. 2016. Based on: Schuenke M, Schulte E, Schumacher U. THIEME Atlas of Anatomy. Volumes 1-3. Illustrations by Voll M and Wesker K. 2nd ed. New York: Thieme Medical Publishers; 2016

3. Correct: Parasternal (C)

Refer to the following image for answer 3:

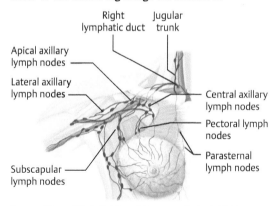

Source: Gilroy AM et al. Atlas of Anatomy. 3rd ed. 2016. Based on: Schuenke M, Schulte E, Schumacher U. THIEME Atlas of Anatomy. Volumes 1-3. Illustrations by Voll M and Wesker K. 2nd ed. New York: Thieme Medical Publishers; 2016

(**C**) Most lymph from the medial quadrants of the breast will enter the parasternal group of nodes first. These nodes are within the thoracic cavity and lie along the internal thoracic artery, being most numerous in the upper three intercostal spaces. Some lymph from medial breast quadrants will pass across the midline to the opposite breast and/or parasternal lymph nodes. (**A**) The apical lymph nodes are found at the apex of the axilla along the first part of the axillary artery and they receive lymph from the central group of nodes. (**B**) The central axillary nodes are associated with the second part of the axillary artery (deep to pectoralis minor muscle) and receive efferent lymphatic vessels from the pectoral, subscapular, and humeral groups of nodes. (**D**) Pectoral nodes lie along the medial wall of the axilla and primarily receive lymph from the lateral quadrants (especially the upper lateral) and the subareolar plexus of the breast. (**E**) Subscapular nodes are located along the posterior axillary fold and are not involved in drainage of the breast.

---

4. Correct: Tracheobronchial (E)

(**E**) The inferior tracheobronchial (carinal, subcarinal) lymph nodes are located inferior to the carina in the angle between the trachea and main bronchi. Metastasis to these lymph nodes from a bronchogenic carcinoma causes them to enlarge and results in structural changes near the carina including distortion, widening, and/or immobility of the airways. These alterations can be identified on bronchoscopy. (**A**) Anterior mediastinal lymph nodes are located on the anterior surface of the pericardium. Enlargement of these lymph nodes will not cause widening of the carina. (**B**) Hilar lymph nodes are located along the main bronchi in the hila of the lungs. Enlargement of these lymph nodes is not likely to cause structural changes in the carina. (**C**) Lobar lymph nodes are located along the lobar bronchi. Enlargement of these lymph nodes will not cause a distortion of the carina. (**D**) Paratracheal lymph nodes are located in the superior mediastinum on either side of the trachea. Enlargement of these lymph nodes will not cause a structural change in the carina.

Refer to the following image for answer 4:

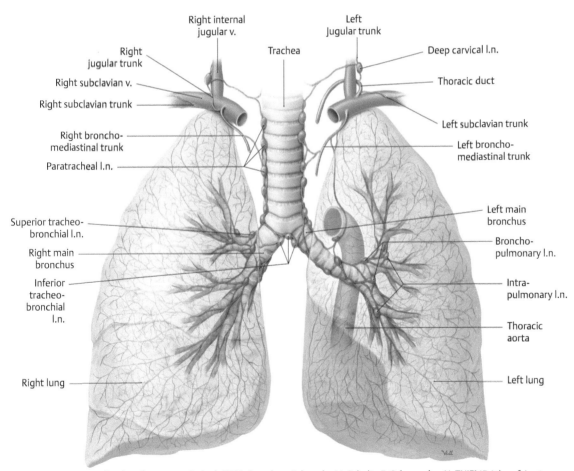

Source: Gilroy AM et al. Atlas of Anatomy. 3rd ed. 2016. Based on: Schuenke M, Schulte E, Schumacher U. THIEME Atlas of Anatomy. Volumes 1-3. Illustrations by Voll M and Wesker K. 2nd ed. New York: Thieme Medical Publishers; 2016

5. Correct: Thoracic esophagus (E)

Refer to the following image for answer 5:

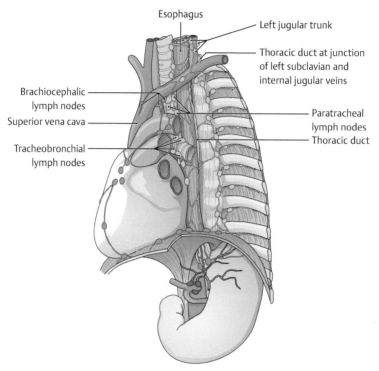

Source: Schuenke M, Schulte E, Schumacher U. THIEME Atlas of Anatomy. Internal Organs.
Illustrations by Voll M and Wesker K. 2nd ed. New York: Thieme Medical Publishers; 2016

(**E**) The thoracic part of the esophagus may drain lymph cranially or caudally, but primarily it drains to lymph nodes in the posterior mediastinum. (**A, B, D**) The abdominal esophagus, such as the stomach (fundus and cardia), first drains lymph into the left gastric, and then into the celiac lymph nodes. (**C**) The cervical part of the esophagus drains lymph cranially, mainly to deep cervical lymph nodes and then to the jugular trunks.

6. Correct: Deep cervical (B)

(**B**) Cancers in the cervical (proximal) part of the esophagus spread cranially, mainly to deep cervical lymph nodes and then to the jugular lymph trunks. In contrast, cancer in the middle part of the esophagus will metastasize to lymph nodes in the thorax, and cancer in the inferior (distal) part will metastasize to lymph nodes in the abdomen. (**A, C**) Left gastric, celiac, and parahiatal lymph nodes collect lymph from the abdominal esophagus (as well as from the fundus and cardia of the stomach). (**D, E**) Paratracheal and pulmonary hilar lymph nodes in the posterior mediastinum collect lymph from the thoracic part of the esophagus.

Refer to the following image for answer 6:

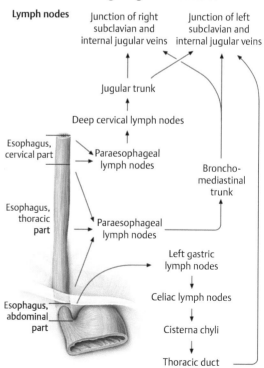

Source: Schuenke M, Schulte E, Schumacher U. THIEME Atlas of Anatomy. Internal Organs. Illustrations by Voll M and Wesker K. 2nd ed. New York: Thieme Medical Publishers; 2016

7. Correct: Right and left gastric (C)

Refer to the following image for answer 7:

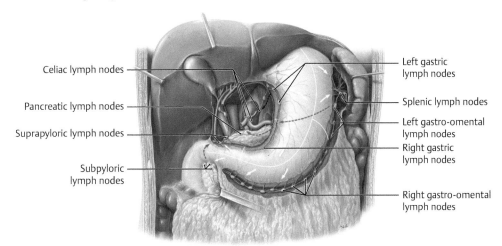

Source: Gilroy AM et al. Atlas of Anatomy. 3rd ed. 2016. Based on: Schuenke M, Schulte E, Schumacher U. THIEME Atlas of Anatomy. Volumes 1-3. Illustrations by Voll M and Wesker K. 2nd ed. New York: Thieme Medical Publishers; 2016

(**C**) Cancer along the lesser curvature of the stomach, including the gastric canal, will first metastasize to the right and left gastric lymph nodes. The gastric canal is a furrow that is formed during swallowing. It follows the lesser curvature between the longitudinal gastric rugae. (**A**) Efferent lymph vessels from lymph nodes of the stomach will drain into celiac lymph nodes. (**B**) Lymph from the duodenum initially drains into pancreaticoduodenal nodes. (**D**) Lymph from the greater curvature of the stomach initially drains into right and left gastro-omental nodes. (**E**) Lymph from the pylorus of the stomach initially drains into supra- and subpyloric lymph nodes.

8. Correct: Celiac (A)

(**A**) Efferent lymphatic vessels from lymph nodes draining most of the duodenum (pancreaticoduodenal lymph nodes and pyloric lymph nodes) enter the celiac lymph nodes. Some lymph from the posterior aspect of the duodenum drains into superior mesenteric lymph nodes. Duodenal adenocarcinomas that involve the hepatopancreatic ampulla (of Vater) may cause obstruction of the biliary system leading to obstructive jaundice and/or pancreatitis. (**B**) Lymph from hindgut-derived structures drains into inferior mesenteric lymph nodes. Since the duodenum is a foregut/midgut-derived structure, it would not drain to inferior mesenteric lymph nodes. (**C**) Gastro-omental lymph nodes receive lymph from the greater curvature of the stomach. (**D**) Paracolic lymph nodes drain most of the colon. (**E**) Splenic lymph nodes receive lymph from the spleen.

Refer to the following image for answer 8:

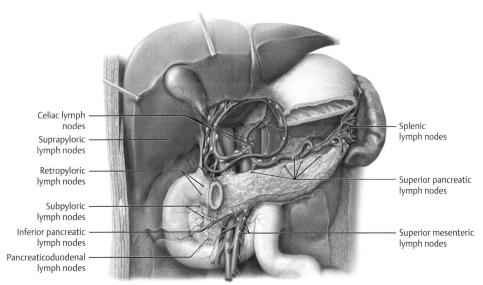

Source: Gilroy AM et al. Atlas of Anatomy. 3rd ed. 2016. Based on: Schuenke M, Schulte E, Schumacher U. THIEME Atlas of Anatomy. Volumes 1-3. Illustrations by Voll M and Wesker K. 2nd ed. New York: Thieme Medical Publishers; 2016

9. Correct: Mesentery (of small intestine) proper (D)

(**D**) Cancer cells from the jejunum can pass through lymph vessels and nodes within the mesentery proper (mesentery of the small intestine) and spread to Preaortic lymph nodes in the retroperitoneal area. (**A**) The gastrocolic ligament is the apron-like part of the greater omentum that extends between the greater curvature of the stomach and the transverse colon. It does not contain lymphatic vessels that drain the jejunum. (**B**) The gastrosplenic ligament extends between the greater curvature of the stomach and the hilum of the spleen. It is a subdivision of the greater omentum and would not contain lymphatic vessels that drain the jejunum. (**C**) The hepatoduodenal ligament, a subdivision of the lesser omentum, extends between the lesser curvature of the stomach and the hilum of the liver. It does not contain lymphatic vessels that drain the jejunum. (**E**) The transverse mesocolon suspends the transverse colon from the posterior abdominal wall. It would not contain lymphatic vessels draining the jejunum.

Refer to the following image for answer 9:

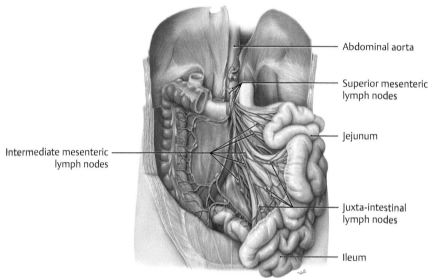

Source: Schuenke M, Schulte E, Schumacher U. THIEME Atlas of Anatomy. Internal Organs. Illustrations by Voll M and Wesker K. 2nd ed. New York: Thieme Medical Publishers; 2016

10. Correct: Spleen (D)

(**D**) The spleen is the largest lymphatic organ and the most commonly ruptured abdominal organ. A fractured left 9th, 10th, or 11th rib may lacerate the spleen, causing intra-abdominal bleeding and pain. Epigastric and left flank pain is due to trauma to the spleen stimulating pain receptors in its capsule. Referred pain to the left shoulder region (Kehr's sign) is due to irritation of the diaphragmatic parietal peritoneum by extravasated blood. A Kehr's sign on the left shoulder when the patient is supine and the legs elevated is a classical symptom of spleen rupture. (**A–C, E**) None of these organs (kidney, pancreas, liver, stomach) are related directly to left 10th rib.

Refer to the following image for answer 10:

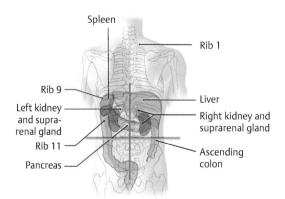

Source: Gilroy AM et al. Atlas of Anatomy. 3rd ed. 2016. Based on: Schuenke M, Schulte E, Schumacher U. THIEME Atlas of Anatomy. Volumes 1-3. Illustrations by Voll M and Wesker K. 2nd ed. New York: Thieme Medical Publishers; 2016

11. Correct: Hepatoduodenal ligament (B)

(**B**) Enlarged lymph nodes within the hepatoduodenal ligament, due to their relationship to the porta hepatis, can compress or obstruct the bile duct, resulting in jaundice. Fever, night sweats, and weight loss are characteristic of Hodgkin's lymphoma.

(**A, C–E**) None of these peritoneal folds (greater omentum, hepatogastric ligament, transverse mesocolon, mesentery of the small intestine proper) contain ducts of the biliary system.

Refer to the following image for answer 11:

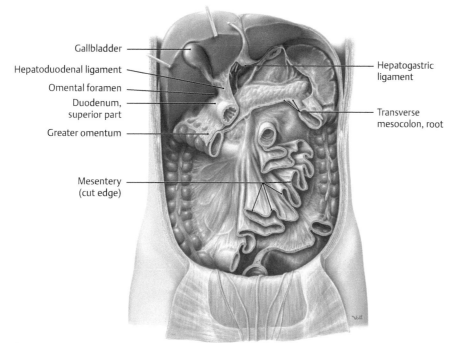

Source: Gilroy AM et al. Atlas of Anatomy. 3rd ed. 2016. Based on: Schuenke M, Schulte E, Schumacher U. THIEME Atlas of Anatomy. Volumes 1-3. Illustrations by Voll M and Wesker K. 2nd ed. New York: Thieme Medical Publishers; 2016

12. Correct: Inferior mesenteric (C)

(**C**) Lymphatic drainage from the distal part of the descending and sigmoid colon (both hindgut-derived structures) is initially to sigmoid, paracolic and intermediate colic lymph nodes (located along branches of the left colic artery). Efferent vessels from these lymph nodes enter the inferior mesenteric lymph nodes. (**A**) Celiac lymph nodes receive lymphatic drainage from foregut-derived structures. (**B**) Ileocolic nodes receive lymphatic drainage from the cecum and appendix. (**D**) Splenic lymph nodes receive lymph from the spleen, stomach, and pancreas. (**E**) Superior mesenteric lymph nodes receive lymph from midgut derivatives.

Refer to the following image for answer 12:

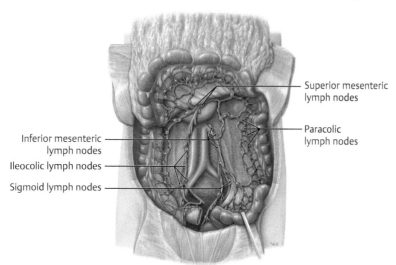

Source: Schuenke M, Schulte E, Schumacher U. THIEME Atlas of Anatomy. Internal Organs. Illustrations by Voll M and Wesker K. 2nd ed. New York: Thieme Medical Publishers; 2016

13. Correct: Ileocolic (B)

(**B**) Ileocolic lymph nodes receive lymph from the cecum and appendix. Efferent lymphatics follow the course of the ileocolic vessels and drain to the superior mesenteric lymph nodes. Therefore, the malignant cells from the appendix will initially spread to ileocolic and then superior mesenteric lymph nodes. (**A**) Celiac lymph nodes receive lymph from foregut-derived structures. (**C**) The lymphatic drainage from the distal one-third of the transverse colon, and the descending and sigmoid colon, all hindgut derivatives, is to the inferior mesenteric lymph nodes. (**D**) The lymphatic drainage from the spleen is to the splenic lymph nodes. (**E**) The appendix and cecum are derived from the midgut and, hence, lymphatic drainage from these organs eventually (after ileocolic lymph nodes) passes to superior mesenteric nodes.

Refer to the following image for answer 13:

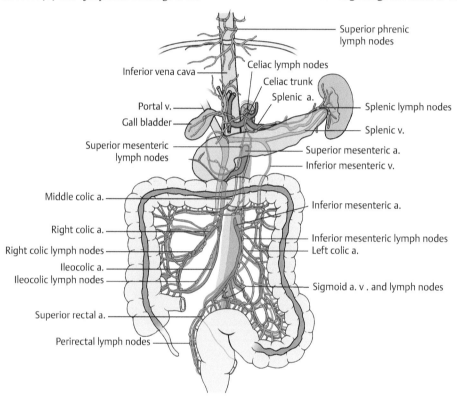

14. Correct: Lumbar (C)

(**C**) Lymphatic drainage from the left kidney follows the left renal vein to the left lumbar lymph nodes. (**A**) Celiac lymph nodes drain foregut derivatives, which does not include the kidneys. (**B**) Lymphatic drainage from the descending and sigmoid colon, both hindgut derivatives, is to the inferior mesenteric lymph nodes. (**C**) Splenic lymph nodes drain the spleen. (**D**) Superior mesenteric lymph nodes receive lymphatic drainage from midgut derivatives which does not include the kidneys.

Refer to the following image for answer 14:

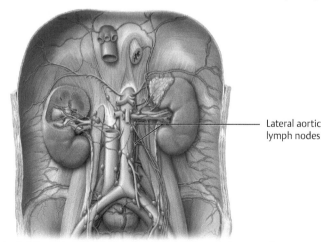

Source: Schuenke M, Schulte E, Schumacher U. THIEME Atlas of Anatomy. Internal Organs. Illustrations by Voll M and Wesker K. 2nd ed. New York: Thieme Medical Publishers; 2016

15.   Correct: Superficial inguinal (E)

Refer to the following image for answer 15:

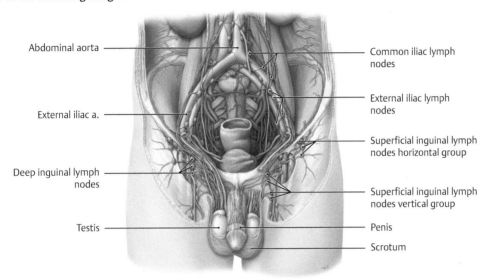

Source: Gilroy AM et al. Atlas of Anatomy. 3rd ed. 2016. Based on: Schuenke M, Schulte E, Schumacher U. THIEME Atlas of Anatomy. Volumes 1-3. Illustrations by Voll M and Wesker K. 2nd ed. New York: Thieme Medical Publishers; 2016

(**E**) The scrotum is an outpocketing of the skin of the anterior abdominal wall and, as such, drains lymph into the superficial inguinal lymph node. (**A–D**) These lymph nodes (common iliac, deep inguinal, external iliac, internal iliac) would not initially be enlarged as they do not receive the lymph directly from the scrotum.

16.   Correct: Left bronchomediastinal trunk (A)

(**A**) Lymph from the left main (primary) bronchus would first drain into the inferior tracheobronchial (carinal) lymph nodes and, eventually, into the left bronchomediastinal trunk which usually terminates in the left subclavian vein. (**B**) The left pulmonary (intrapulmonary) lymph nodes, located along the left lobar bronchi, drain the lymph from the submucosa of the bronchi and the peribronchial connective tissue on that side. (**C**) Right pulmonary lymph nodes, located along the right lobar bronchi, drain lymph from the submucosa of the bronchi and peribronchial connective tissue on that side. (**D**) The superficial (subpleural) lymphatic plexus receives lymph from the visceral pleura and the lung parenchyma. Malignant cells from a tumor on the main bronchus will not enter this plexus. (**E**) Most of the lymph from the left side of the thorax and left side of the head and neck and the remainder of the body below the diaphragm eventually drains into the thoracic duct to reach the venous circulation. The left bronchomediastinal trunk usually joins the left subclavian vein independently, bypassing the thoracic duct.

Refer to the following image for answer 16:

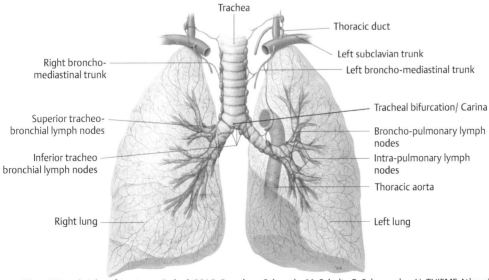

Source: Gilroy AM et al. Atlas of Anatomy. 3rd ed. 2016. Based on: Schuenke M, Schulte E, Schumacher U. THIEME Atlas of Anatomy. Volumes 1-3. Illustrations by Voll M and Wesker K. 2nd ed. New York: Thieme Medical Publishers; 2016

17.   Correct: Popliteal (D)

Refer to the following image for answer 17:

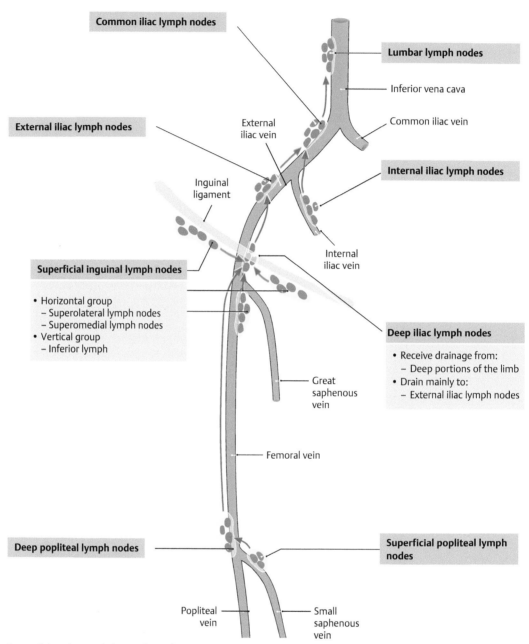

Common iliac lymph nodes

Lumbar lymph nodes

Inferior vena cava

Common iliac vein

External iliac lymph nodes

External iliac vein

Internal iliac lymph nodes

Inguinal ligament

Internal iliac vein

Superficial inguinal lymph nodes

• Horizontal group
  – Superolateral lymph nodes
  – Superomedial lymph nodes
• Vertical group
  – Inferior lymph

Deep iliac lymph nodes

• Receive drainage from:
  – Deep portions of the limb
• Drain mainly to:
  – External iliac lymph nodes

Great saphenous vein

Femoral vein

Deep popliteal lymph nodes

Superficial popliteal lymph nodes

Popliteal vein

Small saphenous vein

Source: Schuenke M, Schulte E, Schumacher U. THIEME Atlas of Anatomy. General Anatomy and Musculoskeletal System. Illustrations by Voll M and Wesker K. 2nd ed. New York: Thieme Medical Publishers; 2016

(D) Popliteal nodes receive lymph from the lateral leg and foot. The superficial lymphatic vessels accompany the small saphenous vein, while deep lymphatics vessels accompany the anterior and posterior tibial vessels. (A) Deep inguinal nodes receive lymph from deep lymphatic vessels in the lower limb, the superficial inguinal and popliteal nodes, and the glans and body of the clitoris/penis. Efferent lymphatic vessels from the deep inguinal nodes will drain to external iliac nodes. (B) External iliac lymph nodes receive lymph from the superficial and deep inguinal lymph nodes and some pelvic viscera. (C) The horizontal group of superficial inguinal lymph nodes (superolateral and superomedial) receives lymph from the gluteal region, lower anterior abdominal wall, and the perineum. (E) The vertical group of superficial inguinal nodes (inferior) receives lymph from the medial aspects of the superficial thigh, leg, and foot.

18. Correct: Pectoral (E)

Refer to the following image for answer 18:

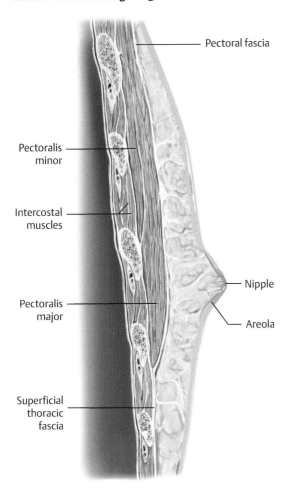

(**E**) The posterior aspect of the breast lies on the pectoral (deep) fascia that covers the pectoralis major and serratus anterior muscles. Carcinoma of the breast in either sex may infiltrate the underlying pectoral fascia, the pectoralis major, and spread to axillary lymph nodes. (**A**) Axillary fascia forms the floor of the axilla. While it is continuous with the pectoral fascia, most of the axillary fascia is located posterior to the pectoralis major and minor muscles. (**B**) Brachial fascia is located in the arm. (**C**) Clavipectoral fascia is attached to the clavicle and descends to become continuous with the axillary fascia. It encloses the subclavius and pectoralis minor muscles. (**D**) Deltoid fascia is located superficial to the deltoid muscle in the shoulder region.

19. Correct: Carotid (A)

(**A**) Lymph from the central portion of the body of the tongue drains into the inferior deep cervical lymph nodes bilaterally. These lymph nodes form a chain along the course of the internal jugular vein and, if enlarged, are palpable in the carotid triangle. (**B**) Lymph from the lateral parts of body of the tongue drains into ipsilateral submandibular lymph nodes. These lymph nodes, when enlarged can be palpated along the inferior border of the mandible in the submandibular (digastric) triangle. (**C**) The occipital triangle is located posterior to the sternocleidomastoid. The deep cervical lymph nodes are not found in this triangle. (**D**) The omoclavicular (subclavian) triangle is located posterior to the sternocleidomastoid. The deep cervical lymph nodes are not found in this triangle. (**E**) Lymph from the apex of the tongue and the frenulum drain to the submental lymph nodes. These lymph nodes, when enlarged, are palpable in the submental triangle.

Refer to the following image for answer 19:

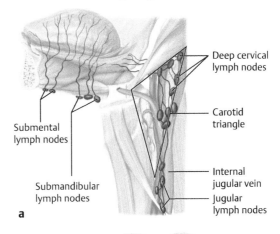

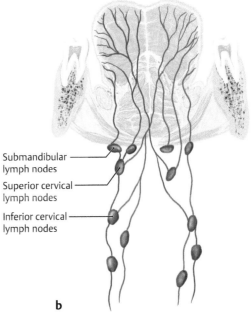

Source: Gilroy AM et al. Atlas of Anatomy. 3rd ed. 2016. Based on: Schuenke M, Schulte E, Schumacher U. THIEME Atlas of Anatomy. Volumes 1-3. Illustrations by Voll M and Wesker K. 2nd ed. New York: Thieme Medical Publishers; 2016

20. Correct: Internal iliac (D)

Refer to the following image for answer 20:

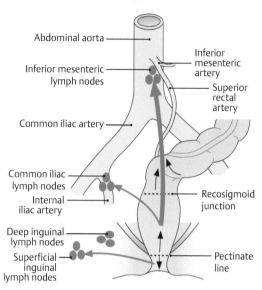

Source: Schuenke M, Schulte E, Schumacher U. THIEME Atlas of Anatomy. Internal Organs. Illustrations by Voll M and Wesker K. 2nd ed. New York: Thieme Medical Publishers; 2016

(**D**) Internal hemorrhoids involve submucosal veins (tributaries of superior rectal veins) located superior to the pectinate line of the anal canal. Lymphatic drainage from the anal canal superior to the pectinate line (as well as the inferior rectum) follows efferent lymphatic vessels along middle rectal blood vessels to internal iliac lymph nodes. In contrast, drainage inferior to the pectinate line follows external pudendal vessels to superficial inguinal nodes. (**A**) Common iliac nodes receive efferent vessels from the internal and external iliac nodes. Thus, the common iliac nodes would not be the first to receive malignant cells from the upper anal canal. (**B**) The deep inguinal nodes do not receive lymph from the anal canal superior to the pectinate line. These nodes may receive some lymph from the anal canal inferior to the pectinate line due to their communication with superficial inguinal nodes. (**C**) The external iliac nodes do not receive lymph from the anal canal superior to the pectinate line. These nodes will receive lymph from the anal canal inferior to the pectinate line, via the inguinal lymph nodes. (**E**) Superficial inguinal nodes receive lymph from most of the skin of the perineum and the anal canal inferior to the pectinate line, gluteal region, lower anterior abdominal wall, and superficial tissues of the medial lower limb.

21. Correct: Cubital (A)

(**A**) Lymphatic vessels from the hypothenar eminence and medial aspect of the forearm follow the basilic vein and drain into cubital nodes, located proximal to the medial epicondyle of the humerus. From

there, lymph will eventually reach the axillary lymph nodes. Lymphangitis is an inflammation of the walls of lymphatic vessels and appears as subcutaneous red streaks. (**B**) Lymphatic vessels from the thenar eminence and lateral aspect of the forearm follow the cephalic vein and drain into humeral (lateral axillary) lymph nodes. From there, lymph will eventually reach the central group of axillary lymph nodes. (**C**) Lymphatic vessels from the medial quadrants of the breast drain into parasternal lymph nodes. (**D**) Lymphatic vessels from the anterior aspect of the chest wall and lateral quadrants of the breast drain into the pectoral (anterior) group of axillary lymph nodes. (**E**) Lymphatic vessels from the posterior aspect of the thoracic wall and scapular region drain into the subscapular (posterior) group of axillary nodes.

Refer to the following image for answer 21:

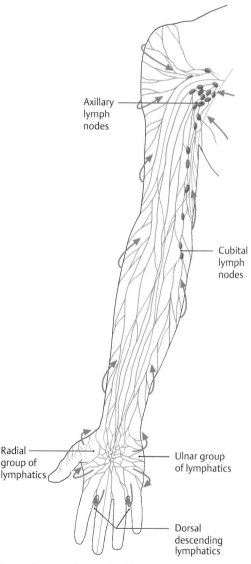

Source: Schuenke M, Schulte E, Schumacher U. THIEME Atlas of Anatomy. General Anatomy and Musculoskeletal System. Illustrations by Voll M and Wesker K. 2nd ed. New York: Thieme Medical Publishers; 2016

22. Correct: Superficial inguinal (E)

Refer to the following image for answer 22:

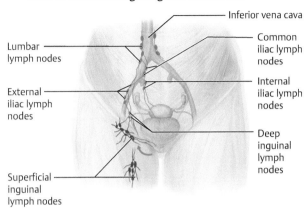

Source: Schuenke M, Schulte E, Schumacher U. THIEME Atlas of Anatomy. General Anatomy and Musculoskeletal System. Illustrations by Voll M and Wesker K. 2nd ed. New York: Thieme Medical Publishers; 2016

(**E**) Lymph from skin of the perineum (including the vulva) drains first into the superficial inguinal group of lymph nodes. (**A**) Lymph from internal and external iliac lymph nodes drains into the common iliac lymph nodes. While external iliac and common iliac lymph nodes will contain lymph from the vulva (via inguinal lymph nodes), these lymph nodes are not the first to receive vulvar lymph. (**B**) Deep inguinal lymph nodes receive lymph from deep lymphatic vessels in the lower limb, the superficial inguinal and popliteal nodes, and the glans and body of the clitoris/penis. Efferent lymphatic vessels from the deep inguinal lymph nodes will join external iliac lymph nodes. (**C**) Lymph from anterosuperior pelvic structures (superior bladder, superior pelvic ureter, upper vagina, lower body of uterus and supravaginal cervix) and the deep inguinal lymph nodes drains into external iliac lymph nodes. (**D**) Lymph from inferior pelvic structures (base of bladder, inferior pelvic ureter, anal canal above pectinate line, inferior rectum, all of vagina except portion in vulva, most of the body of the uterus, vaginal part of cervix), and sacral lymph nodes drains into internal iliac lymph nodes. Some female pelvic organs drain lymph into more than one group of lymph nodes, for example, the uterus and vagina.

23. Correct: Lumbar (E)

(**E**) The ovaries, uterine tube (except the isthmus and intrauterine parts), and the fundus of the uterus drain into lumbar (caval on left; aortic on right) lymph nodes because they follow the course of the ovarian vessels as they course along the posterior abdominal and lateral pelvic walls. (**A–D**) Lymph from the ovary does not enter any of these groups of lymph nodes (common iliac, external iliac, inferior mesenteric, internal iliac).

Refer to the following image for answer 23:

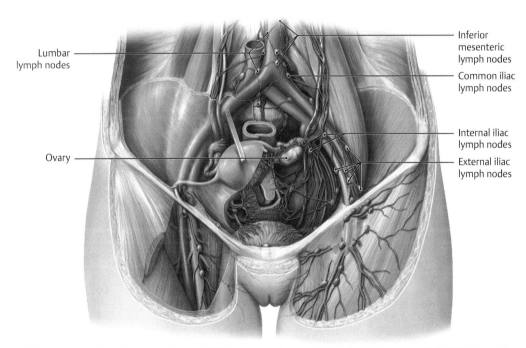

Source: Gilroy AM et al. Atlas of Anatomy. 3rd ed. 2016. Based on: Schuenke M, Schulte E, Schumacher U. THIEME Atlas of Anatomy. Volumes 1-3. Illustrations by Voll M and Wesker K. 2nd ed. New York: Thieme Medical Publishers; 2016

24. Correct: Internal iliac (C)

Refer to the following image for answer 24:

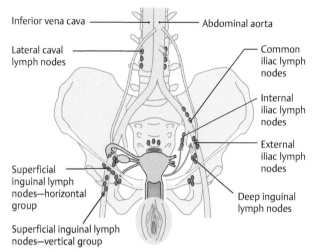

Source: Schuenke M, Schulte E, Schumacher U. THIEME Atlas of Anatomy. Internal Organs. Illustrations by Voll M and Wesker K. 2nd ed. New York: Thieme Medical Publishers; 2016

(**C**) Lymph from the supravaginal cervix drains into internal and external iliac nodes, as well as sacral lymph nodes. (**A, B, D, E**) None of these nodal groups (common iliac, inferior mesenteric, lumbar, obturator) initially receive lymph from the supravaginal cervix.

25. Correct: Superficial inguinal (E)

Refer to the following image for answer 25:

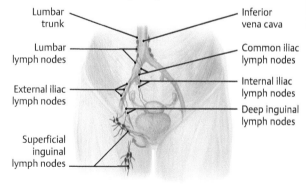

Source: Schuenke M, Schulte E, Schumacher U. THIEME Atlas of Anatomy. General Anatomy and Musculoskeletal System. Illustrations by Voll M and Wesker K. 2nd ed. New York: Thieme Medical Publishers; 2016

(**E**) Superficial inguinal lymph nodes drain most structures of the female perineum, including the greater vestibular (Bartholin's) glands (secondarily, these structures drain to deep inguinal lymph nodes, which may be difficult to distinguish on palpation from superficial inguinal lymph nodes). Other perineal structures, including the body and glans of the clitoris, corpora cavernosa, the vestibular bulbs, and the anterior labia minora drain directly to deep inguinal lymph nodes. Structures of the deep perineum (including membranous urethra, inferior-most vagina, and the upper part of anal canal) drain to internal iliac lymph nodes (these lymphatics likely follow internal pudendal vessels). (**A–D**) None of these lymph node groups (common iliac, external iliac, internal iliac, sacral) receives lymph directly from the greater vestibular gland.

26. Correct: Obturator (D)

Refer to the following image for answer 26:

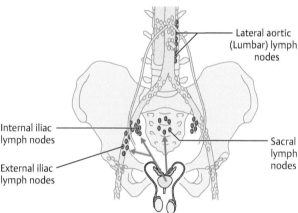

Source: Schuenke M, Schulte E, Schumacher U. THIEME Atlas of Anatomy. Internal Organs. Illustrations by Voll M and Wesker K. 2nd ed. New York: Thieme Medical Publishers; 2016

(**D**) Lymphogenous metastasis (lymphatic dissemination) of adenocarcinoma cells from the prostate spreads primarily to internal iliac or obturator lymph nodes, although drainage of lateral prostate to external iliac nodes and from posterior prostate to sacral lymph nodes may occur. Malignant prostate cells may also enter a series of valveless veins (Batson's plexus) to enter the internal vertebral venous plexus of the vertebral column. (**A**) Lymph from internal and external iliac nodes enters the common iliac nodes. While common iliac nodes may contain lymph from the prostate, via the internal iliac nodes, common iliac nodes do not initially receive lymph from the prostate. (**B, C, E**) None of these groups of lymph nodes (deep inguinal, lumbar, superficial inguinal) initially receive lymph from the prostate.

27. Correct: Deep inguinal (B)

Refer to the following image for answer 27:

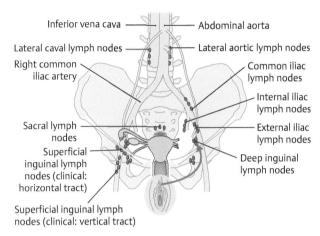

Source: Schuenke M, Schulte E, Schumacher U. THIEME Atlas of Anatomy. Internal Organs. Illustrations by Voll M and Wesker K. 2nd ed. New York: Thieme Medical Publishers; 2016

(**B**) The glans and corpora cavernosa of the clitoris drain directly to deep inguinal lymph nodes. In contrast, the skin of the clitoris, as well as the labia and remainder of the perineum drain into superficial inguinal lymph nodes (and from there to deep inguinal lymph nodes). (**A, C, D**) None of these lymph node groups (common iliac, external iliac, sacral) receives initial infection spread from the glans of the clitoris. (**E**) The vulva, except for the glans and corpora cavernosa of the clitoris, drain to superficial inguinal lymph nodes (and from there, to deep inguinal lymph nodes).

28. Correct: Superficial inguinal (E)

Refer to the following image for answer 28:

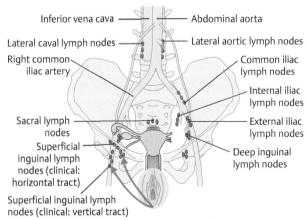

Source: Schuenke M, Schulte E, Schumacher U. THIEME Atlas of Anatomy. Internal Organs. Illustrations by Voll M and Wesker K. 2nd ed. New York: Thieme Medical Publishers; 2016

(**E**) Superficial inguinal lymph nodes drain the skin of the perineum, including that over the perineal body

and the anal canal inferior to the pectinate line. During vaginal delivery, a skin incision from the posterior aspect of the vaginal opening (episiotomy) may be made to minimize tearing of perineal skin and muscles. A mediolateral episiotomy is preferred over a median episiotomy as the former has decreased incidence of damage to the anal sphincters. (**A–D**) None of these groups of lymph nodes (common iliac, deep inguinal, external iliac, internal iliac) receives initial lymph from the skin of the perineum.

29. Correct: Submental (E)

Refer to the following images for answer 29:

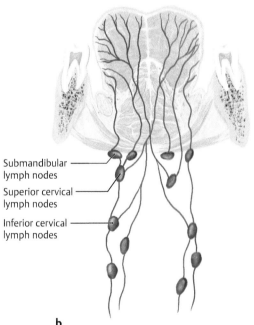

Source: Gilroy AM et al. Atlas of Anatomy. 3rd ed. 2016. Based on: Schuenke M, Schulte E, Schumacher U. THIEME Atlas of Anatomy. Volumes 1-3. Illustrations by Voll M and Wesker K. 2nd ed. New York: Thieme Medical Publishers; 2016

(**E**) The apex (tip) of the tongue and its frenulum together with the central portion of the lower lip drain initially to submental lymph nodes (see the presented image a). All lymph from the tongue eventually reaches the deep cervical nodes. (**A**) The root of the tongue drains bilaterally into superior deep cervical lymph nodes. The medial part of the body of the tongue drains bilaterally and directly to inferior deep cervical lymph nodes. (**B**) The jugulodigastric node is part of the deep cervical nodes located close to the angle of the mandible. It receives lymph from the tongue and pharynx. (**C**) The jugulo-omohyoid lymph node, part of the deep cervical nodes, is located close to the intermediate tendon of the omohyoid muscle. All lymph from the tongue eventually drains to the deep cervical nodes. (**D**) The lateral part of the body of the tongue drains to the ipsilateral submandibular lymph nodes (see the presented image b).

30. Correct: Jugulodigastric (B)

(**B**) The jugulodigastric lymph node (tonsillar lymph node) is located near the angle of the mandible where the posterior belly of digastric muscle crosses the internal jugular vein. It receives lymph from the tongue and pharynx and is commonly enlarged with tonsillitis. (**A**) Deep parotid lymph nodes (preauricular lymph nodes) are located on the deep side of the parotid gland. They are part of the deep cervical chain of lymph nodes. (**C**) Most of the skin of the face, lateral part of the body of the tongue, and the floor of the mouth drain into the submandibular lymph nodes. These lymph nodes lie superficial to the submandibular gland and, when enlarged, can be palpated along the inferior border of the body of the mandible. (**D**) The apex of the tongue, frenulum, and central part of the lower lip drain into submental lymph nodes that can be palpated, when enlarged, in the submental triangle. (**E**) Superficial parotid lymph nodes are located on the capsule of the parotid gland and drain the lateral aspect of the face, scalp, and eyelids.

Refer to the following image for answer 30:

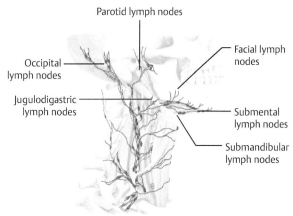

Source: Gilroy AM et al. Atlas of Anatomy. 3rd ed. 2016. Based on: Schuenke M, Schulte E, Schumacher U. THIEME Atlas of Anatomy. Volumes 1-3. Illustrations by Voll M and Wesker K. 2nd ed. New York: Thieme Medical Publishers; 2016

31. Correct: Parotid (C)

(**C**) The temporal and frontal regions, some of the face (including the eyelids), and anterior auricle drain initially into superficial parotid lymph nodes. Most of the scalp and face eventually drain into lymph nodes located at the junction of the head with the neck, referred to as the "pericervical collar" of lymph nodes. This includes submental, submandibular, parotid, mastoid, and occipital lymph nodes. (**A, B, D, E**) None of these groups of lymph nodes (mastoid, occipital, submandibular, submental) will receive lymph from the upper eyelid directly.

Refer to the following image for answer 31:

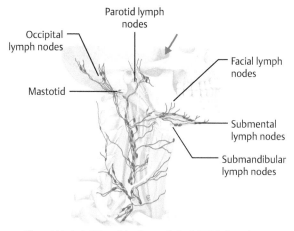

Source: Gilroy AM et al. Atlas of Anatomy. 3rd ed. 2016. Based on: Schuenke M, Schulte E, Schumacher U. THIEME Atlas of Anatomy. Volumes 1-3. Illustrations by Voll M and Wesker K. 2nd ed. New York: Thieme Medical Publishers; 2016

32. Correct: Occipital (B)

Refer to the following image for answer 32:

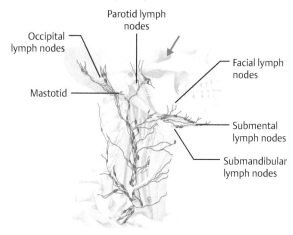

Source: Gilroy AM et al. Atlas of Anatomy. 3rd ed. 2016. Based on: Schuenke M, Schulte E, Schumacher U. THIEME Atlas of Anatomy. Volumes 1-3. Illustrations by Voll M and Wesker K. 2nd ed. New York: Thieme Medical Publishers; 2016

(**B**) The posterior part of the scalp (occipital region), including the skin close to the inion (external occipital protuberance), drains initially into occipital lymph nodes. Infection of the head hair and scalp by the head louse Pediculus humanus capitis is called pediculosis capitis. Most of the scalp and face drain into lymph nodes located at the junction of the head with the neck, referred as the "pericervical collar" of lymph nodes that includes submental, submandibular, parotid, mastoid, and occipital lymph nodes. (**A**) Skin of the scalp close to the mastoid process, and the cranial surface of the posterior half of the auricle, drains to mastoid and deep cervical lymph nodes. (**C**) The temporal and frontal regions, lateral face (including the eyelids), and auricle (anterior part) drain directly lymph into superficial parotid lymph nodes. (**D**) Most of the skin of the face, lateral part of the body of the tongue, and the floor of the mouth drain into the submandibular nodes. These lymph nodes lie superficial to the submandibular gland and when enlarged can be palpated along the inferior border of the body of the mandible. (**E**) The apex of the tongue, frenulum, and central part of the lower lip drain into submental lymph nodes that can be palpated, when enlarged, in the submental triangle.

33. Correct: Parotid (C)

Refer to the following image for answer 33:

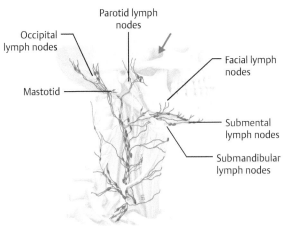

Source: Gilroy AM et al. Atlas of Anatomy. 3rd ed. 2016. Based on: Schuenke M, Schulte E, Schumacher U. THIEME Atlas of Anatomy. Volumes 1-3. Illustrations by Voll M and Wesker K. 2nd ed. New York: Thieme Medical Publishers; 2016

(**C**) The temporal and frontal regions, lateral face (including the eyelids), and anterior auricle, drain lymph into superficial parotid lymph nodes. Most of the scalp and face eventually drains into lymph nodes located between the junction of the head and the neck, referred to as the "pericervical collar" of lymph nodes that includes submental, submandibular, parotid, mastoid, and occipital lymph nodes. (**A**) Skin of the scalp, close to the mastoid process and the cranial surface of the posterior half of the auricle, drains to mastoid and deep cervical lymph nodes (**B**) The posterior part of the scalp (occipital region), including the skin close to the inion (external occipital

protuberance), drains into occipital lymph nodes. (**D**) Most of the skin of the lower face, lateral part of the body of the tongue, and the floor of the mouth drain into the submandibular lymph nodes. These lymph nodes lie superficial to the submandibular gland and when enlarged can be palpated along the inferior border of the body of the mandible. (**E**) The apex of the tongue, frenulum, and central part of the lower lip drain into submental lymph nodes that can be palpated, when enlarged, in the submental triangle.

Refer to the following image for answers 34 to 36:

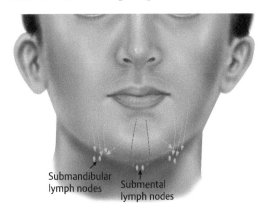

34. Correct: Submandibular (D)

(**D**) Most of the skin of the face (including the nose), lateral part of the body of the tongue, and the floor of the mouth drain into the submandibular nodes. These nodes lie superficial to the submandibular gland and when enlarged can be palpated along the inferior border of the body of the mandible. (**A**) Skin of the scalp close to the mastoid process and the cranial surface of the posterior half of the auricle drains to the mastoid and deep cervical lymph nodes. (**B**) The posterior part of the scalp (occipital region), including the skin close to the inion (external occipital protuberance), drains into occipital lymph nodes. (**C**) The temporal and frontal regions, lateral face (including the eyelids), and anterior auricle drain lymph into superficial parotid nodes. Most of the scalp and face eventually drain into lymph nodes located between the junction of the head and the neck, referred to as the "pericervical collar" (or superficial ring) of lymph nodes. This includes submental, submandibular, parotid, mastoid, and occipital lymph nodes. (**E**) The apex of the tongue, frenulum, and central part of the lower lip drain into submental nodes that can be palpated, when enlarged, in the submental triangle.

35. Correct: Submandibular (D)

(**D**) Most of the skin of the face (including the upper lip), lateral part of the body of the tongue, and the floor of the mouth drain into the submandibular nodes. These nodes lie superficial to the submandibular gland and, when enlarged, can be palpated along the inferior border of the body of the mandible. (**A**) Skin of the scalp close to the mastoid process and the cranial surface of the posterior half of the auricle drains to the mastoid lymph nodes and deep cervical lymph nodes. (**B**) The posterior part of the scalp (occipital region), including the skin close to the inion (external occipital protuberance), drains into occipital lymph nodes. (**C**) The temporal and frontal regions, lateral face (including the eyelids), and auricle (anterior part) drain lymph into superficial parotid nodes. Most of the scalp and face drain eventually into lymph nodes located between the junction of the head and the neck, referred as the "pericervical collar" of lymph nodes that includes submental, submandibular, parotid, mastoid, and occipital lymph nodes. (**E**) The apex of the tongue, frenulum, and central part of the lower lip drain into submental nodes that, when enlarged, can be palpated in the submental triangle.

36. Correct: Right and left submandibular (C)

(**C**) Lateral parts of the lower lip drain bilaterally into submandibular lymph nodes, whereas the middle part of the lower lip drains into submental nodes. Therefore, it is essential that both the left and right submandibular nodes be examined. Submandibular lymph nodes lie superficial to the submandibular gland and when enlarged can be palpated along the inferior border of the body of the mandible. (**A, D**) The lateral portions of the lower lip drain bilaterally into the submandibular lymph nodes, so it is necessary to palpate the nodes on both sides to assess for infection spread. (**B**) The temporal and frontal regions, lateral face (including the eyelids, and anterior auricle drain lymph into superficial parotid nodes. Most of the scalp and face eventually drain into lymph nodes located between the junction of the head and the neck, referred to as the "pericervical collar" or superficial ring) of lymph nodes. This includes submental, submandibular, parotid, mastoid, and occipital lymph nodes. (**E**) The apex of the tongue, frenulum, and central part of the lower lip drain into submental nodes that can be palpated, when enlarged, in the submental triangle.

37. Correct: Superior deep cervical (E)

(**E**) Lymph from the root of the tongue drains bilaterally into the superior deep cervical nodes. HPV 16 is a risk factor for carcinoma of the tongue. Leukoplakia (white patches on mucous membranes of the oral cavity) and paresthesia on the tongue may be associated with malignancy. (**A**) Lymph from the medial portion of the body of the tongue drains bilaterally into the inferior deep cervical nodes. (**B**) The temporal and frontal regions, lateral face (including the eyelids and parietal scalp), and anterior auricle drain lymph into superficial parotid nodes. Most of the scalp and face

eventually drains into lymph nodes located between the junction of the head and the neck, referred to as the "pericervical collar" that includes submental, submandibular, parotid, mastoid, and occipital lymph nodes. (**C**) Most of the skin of the face (including the upper lip), lateral part of the body of the tongue, and the floor of the mouth drain into the submandibular nodes. These lymph nodes lie superficial to the submandibular gland and when enlarged can be palpated along the inferior border of the body of the mandible. (**D**) Lymph from the apex of the tongue and the frenulum drains to the submental lymph nodes.

38. Correct: Thoracic duct (D)

(**D**) Together with the aorta, the thoracic duct and azygos vein pass through the aortic hiatus (T12). An aortic aneurysm at this level might compress these two structures. (**A–C, E**) The cisterna chyli, hemiazygos vein, phrenic nerve, and vagal trunks are not located in the aortic hiatus and, hence, are not compressed by an aortic aneurysm at this level.

39. Correct: Ileocolic and superior mesenteric (B)

(**B**) Lymph from the appendix tends to follow the arteries and drain primarily into ileocolic and superior mesenteric lymph nodes. Cancer at the base of the appendix can cause obstruction, leading to appendicitis. Appendiceal cancer can sometimes be misdiagnosed as acute appendicitis, so it is essential to have a pathology report for the resected specimen. (**A, C–F**) Lymph from the appendix does not drain into the inferior mesenteric, left colic, or right colic lymph nodes.

40. Correct: Superficial inguinal (E)

Refer to the following image for answer 40:

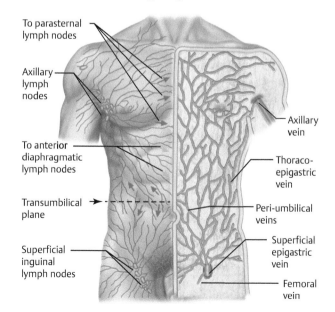

(**E**) A malignant melanoma confined to the skin of the anterior abdominal wall inferior to the umbilicus (inferior to the transumbilical plane) spreads initially via lymphatic vessels to the superficial inguinal lymph nodes. Lesions involving deeper layers of the anterior abdominal wall drain via deep lymphatic channels to external and common iliac, and lumbar lymph nodes. (**A–D**) Lymph from the skin of the anterior abdominal wall inferior to the umbilicus will not first drain into axillary, deep cervical, external iliac, or lumbar lymph nodes.

41. Correct: Lumbar (C)

Refer to the following image for answer 41:

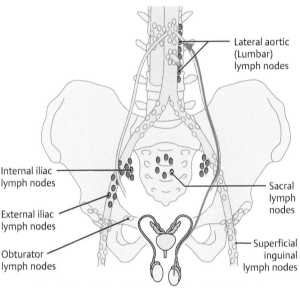

Internal iliac lymph nodes

External iliac lymph nodes

Obturator lymph nodes

Lateral aortic (Lumbar) lymph nodes

Sacral lymph nodes

Superficial inguinal lymph nodes

Source: Gilroy AM et al. Atlas of Anatomy. 3rd ed. 2016. Based on: Schuenke M, Schulte E, Schumacher U. THIEME Atlas of Anatomy. Volumes 1-3. Illustrations by Voll M and Wesker K. 2nd ed. New York: Thieme Medical Publishers; 2016

(**C**) Lymph from the testes will first enter the lumbar group of lymph nodes located just inferior to the renal veins. The testes develop initially in the upper abdomen and their blood and lymphatic vessels, as well as their nerve supply, are established before they descend along the posterior abdominal wall, through the inguinal region, and into the scrotum. Thus, lymph from the testes drains to lumbar nodes that lie near the origin of the testicular vessels (arteries from the abdominal aorta or veins that drain to the inferior vena cava or left renal vein). Consequently, a stage II seminoma (metastasis beyond the testicle) may show enlargement of lumbar nodes on

a CT. (**A, B, D, E**) None of these groups of nodes (deep inguinal, external iliac, sacral, superficial inguinal) receive lymph from the testes. The superficial inguinal nodes receive lymph from the scrotum (a diverticulum of skin from the anterior abdominal wall), but not the testes.

42. Correct: Internal iliac and sacral (C)

(**C**) Lymph from the prostate gland first enters the internal iliac and sacral lymph nodes and these nodes could be enlarged with chronic infection of the gland. (**A, B, D, E**) None of these groups of lymph node (aortic, caval, ileocolic, lumbar, pararectal, inferior mesenteric, superficial inguinal, deep inguinal) receives initial lymph from the prostate gland.

Refer to the following image for answer 42:

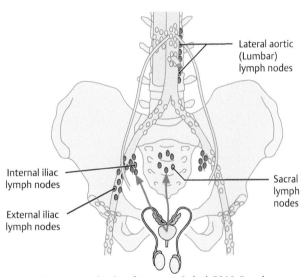

Lateral aortic (Lumbar) lymph nodes

Internal iliac lymph nodes

External iliac lymph nodes

Sacral lymph nodes

Source: Gilroy AM et al. Atlas of Anatomy. 3rd ed. 2016. Based on: Schuenke M, Schulte E, Schumacher U. THIEME Atlas of Anatomy. Volumes 1-3. Illustrations by Voll M and Wesker K. 2nd ed. New York: Thieme Medical Publishers; 2016

43. Correct: Stomach (E)

(**E**) An enlarged left supraclavicular lymph node (known commonly as Virchow's node, but also as Trosier's node), combined with gastric symptoms, is considered a positive Trosier sign and indicates metastasis from the stomach. The lymphatic pathway from the stomach passes through the thoracic duct to the left supraclavicular nodes in the root of the neck, near the termination of the thoracic duct at the left venous angle. Clinical evidence indicates that abdominal and pelvic tumors have a propensity to metastasize to the left supraclavicular lymph node, whereas metastases from the thorax, breast, head, neck, skin, or lymphomas do not show a laterality preference. (**A–D**) All of these organs (left lung, left main bronchus, left ventricle, mediastinal portion of esophagus) are located in the thorax and lymph from these organs do not show a laterality preference in metastasis to supraclavicular lymph nodes.

Refer to the following image for answer 43:

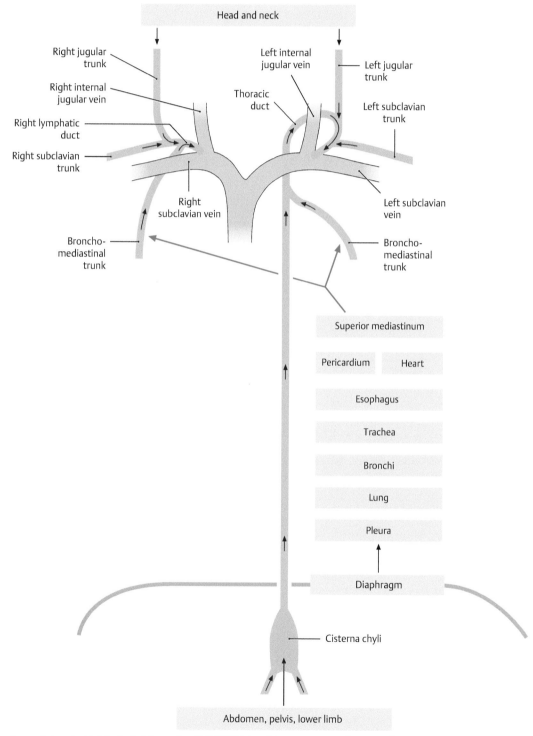

Source: Schuenke M, Schulte E, Schumacher U. THIEME Atlas of Anatomy. Internal Organs. Illustrations by Voll M and Wesker K. 2nd ed. New York: Thieme Medical Publishers; 2016

44.   Correct: Right gastro-omental (E)

Refer to the following image for answer 44:

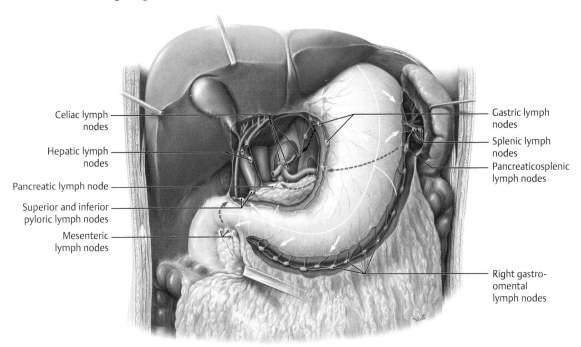

Celiac lymph nodes

Hepatic lymph nodes

Pancreatic lymph node

Superior and inferior pyloric lymph nodes

Mesenteric lymph nodes

Gastric lymph nodes

Splenic lymph nodes

Pancreaticosplenic lymph nodes

Right gastro-omental lymph nodes

Source: Schuenke M, Schulte E, Schumacher U. THIEME Atlas of Anatomy. Internal Organs. Illustrations by Voll M and Wesker K. 2nd ed. New York: Thieme Medical Publishers; 2016

(**E**) Lymphatic dissemination of cancer cells from the pyloric antrum and canal, which have the highest incidence of carcinoma of the stomach, is to right gastro-omental and pyloric lymph nodes. (**A**) Celiac lymph nodes receive lymph secondarily from lymph nodes of the stomach (gastric and gastro-omental). Lymph from these nodes is carried by abdominal lymph trunks in to the cisterna chyli, and then into the thoracic duct. (**B**) The cardia, fundus, and abdominal part of the esophagus drain to left gastric lymph nodes. (**C**) The left part of the greater curvature drains to left gastro-omental, and pancreaticosplenic lymph nodes. (**D**) Mesenteric lymph nodes, both those within the mesentery itself as well as those clustered around the roots of the superior and inferior mesenteric arteries, receive lymph from respective regions of the small and large intestine.

45. Correct: Cisterna chyli (B)

(**B**) The cisterna chyli is the expanded, inferior part of the thoracic duct that receives lymph from intestinal and lumbar lymph trunks in the abdomen. Because of its close proximity to the abdominal aorta, abdominal aortic reconstruction surgery can result in iatrogenic injury to the cisterna chyli. Rupture of this structure will result in extravasation of milky chyle into the peritoneal cavity, termed chylous ascites. (**A, C–E**) None of these structures (bronchomediastinal trunk, jugular trunk, right lymphatic duct, subclavian trunk) are located in the abdominal cavity and will not be injured during abdominal aortic reconstruction.

Refer to the following image for answer 45:

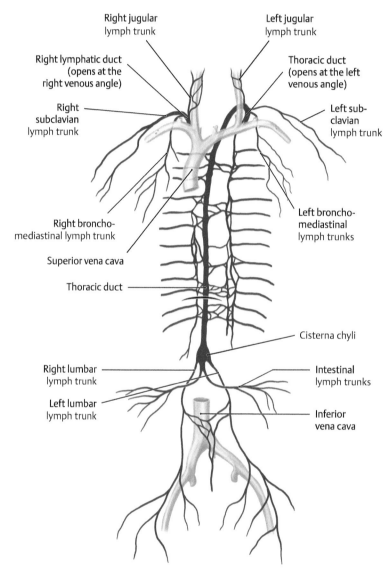

Source: Schuenke M, Schulte E, Schumacher U. THIEME Atlas of Anatomy. General Anatomy and Musculoskeletal System. Illustrations by Voll M and Wesker K. 2nd ed. New York: Thieme Medical Publishers; 2016

46. Correct: T12 (E)

Refer to the following image for answer 46:

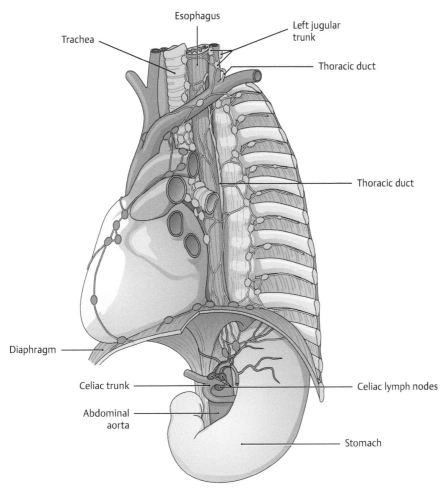

Source: Schuenke M, Schulte E, Schumacher U. THIEME Atlas of Anatomy. Internal Organs. Illustrations by Voll M and Wesker K. 2nd ed. New York: Thieme Medical Publishers; 2016

(**E**) The thoracic duct originates from the cisterna chyli, which typically lies at the L1–L2 vertebral level. The duct passes through the aortic hiatus at the T12 vertebral level to enter the posterior mediastinum. Because the thoracic duct is thin-walled and may be difficult to identify, it is thus susceptible to iatrogenic injury in the posterior mediastinum. (**A–D**) The aortic hiatus (T12 vertebral level), through which the thoracic duct passes, is not located at any of these vertebral levels (T8-T11).

47. Correct: Chylothorax (A)

(**A**) Chylothorax is a type of pleural effusion that can result from iatrogenic injury to the thoracic duct during thoracic surgery (e.g., in procedures such as thoracic aorta repair and esophagectomy) or from lymphoma or lung carcinoma. A milky pleural effusate with high levels of triglyceride and a protein concentration great than that of plasma (> 3 gm/dL) helps confirm a diagnosis of chylothorax. (**B**) A hemothorax is defined as the presence of blood in the pleural cavity. (**C**) Pneumonia is a lung infection caused by bacteria, viruses, or fungi that results in inflammation of the lower respiratory tract (lower trachea, bronchi, alveoli, and lung interstitium). (**D**) A pneumothorax is defined as the presence of air in the pleural cavity. (**E**) A fibrothorax typically is a result of a severe pleural inflammation from asbestosis, empyema, hemothorax, TB, allergic reaction to drug, or pleurodesis performed for malignant pleural effusion.

Index

A

abdominal aorta 180, 227, 261, 324
abdominal esophagus 368
abdominal oblique 256
abducens nerve 17
   CN VI 20
abducent nerve
   palsy 124
abduction 23
   finger 27
   of index finger 93
   shoulder 29
   thumb 32
abductor hallucis 109
abductor pollicis brevis 32
   muscles 89
abductor pollicis longus 32, 89, 91
abnormal smooth muscle development
   273
accessory nerve (CN XI) 21, 121, 128
accessory oculomotor nucleus 20
acinus 211
acoustic neuroma 26
ACPO see acute colonic pseudo-obstruction (ACPO)
acromioclavicular injury 81
acromion 79
acute appendicitis 34
acute colonic pseudo-obstruction
   (ACPO) 257
adduction 23
   finger 27
   thumb 93
adductor longus muscle 104
adductor pollicis 93
AIN see anterior interosseous nerve
   (AIN)
aldosterone 180
allantois 272
Allen's test 89
alveolar epithelial cells type II 212
alveolar period 212
alveoli 210
ampulla, blockage of 269
anal canal 294
anal cushions 267
anal fissures 271
anal reflex 30
anal wink 16, 30
androgen insensitivity syndrome 353
angiotensinogen 180
annular pancreas 263
anocutaneous reflex 30
anoderm 271
ansa cervicalis 121
anteflexion 284

anterior cerebral arteries 159
anterior displacement of hindfoot 108
anterior drawer (Lachman) test 106
anterior ethmoidal nerve 17, 23
anterior fontanelle 126
anterior intercostal artery 169
anterior interosseous nerve (AIN) 73,
   74, 90
   lesion 74, 90, 93
anterior interventricular artery 172,
   177
anterior longitudinal ligament 94
anterior longitudinal ligament courses
   122
anterior mediastinal lymph nodes 367
anterior scalene 83
anterior scrotal nerve 314
anterior shoulder dislocation 76, 80
anterior superior iliac spine (ASIS) 109
anterior talofibular ligament 108
anterior tibial artery 184, 185
anterior tibial vein 107, 186
anterior vaginal fornix 355
anterosuperior pelvic structures 377
anteversion 284
anti-Müllerian hormone 300, 347
antirefl ux mechanism of urinary system 228
aortic hiatus 387
aortopulmonary window 210
apex of tongue 379, 381
apical lymph nodes 366
aponeurosis of transversus abdominis
   muscle 131
appendectomy 35
appendicular artery 178
appendix 372
   testis 343
arcuate ligament 75
arcuate line 136
arterial cannula 107
articular tubercle 121
arytenoid cartilage 126
ASIS see anterior superior iliac spine
   (ASIS)
asterisk 79
auditory ossicles 26
Auerbach's plexuses of bowel wall 35
auricular nerve 25
auriculotemporal nerve 24
auscultation
   of aortic valve 172
   left atrioventricular valve 172
   of pulmonary valve 172
autonomic nervous system 330
axillary artery 82, 176

axillary fascia 375
axillary lymph nodes, dissection of 76
axillary nerve 84
   injury 76
axillary veins 86
axons of accessory nerve (CN XI) 21
azygos vein 201

B

backfire fracture 90
bag of worms 329
baroreceptors 37
Barton's fracture 90
basilic veins 86
bell-clapper deformity 327, 329
Bell's palsy 19, 22–23
biceps brachii 84, 93
   muscle flexes 85
biceps brachii reflex 89
biceps femoris 110, 184
biceps femoris border 113
biceps femoris muscle 28
bicipital aponeurosis 87
biconvex shape 160
bilateral blindness 23
bilateral contraction of splenius capitis
   muscles 129
bilateral hypesthesia 27
bilateral involvement 17
bilateral maxillary sinuses 37
bilateral paralysis 27
bimanual examination 223
bipolar olfactory neurons 17
bladder exstrophy 272
blink reflex 19
blockage of spinal canal 349
blowout fractures 21
   medial orbital wall 23
blunt force trauma 160
Bow hunter's syndrome 96
bow-legged 109
brachial fascia 375
brachialis 84
brachial plexus 28
   block 89
brachial veins 86
brachiocephalic artery 176
brachiocephalic trunk 169–170, 170
brachiocephalic vein 82
brachioradialis reflex 89
branchial cyst 355, 356
branchial motor 26
   axons 22
   fibers 26
broad ligament 225, 287, 300
bronchial carcinoma 122

bronchial vein 201
bronchopulmonary (hilar) nodes 209
bronchopulmonary segments 206
buccal nerve 24
buccopharyngeal membrane 213
bucket handle movements 211
Buck's fascia 317, 320
bulbospongiosus muscles 138
bulbourethral gland 302
bulbourethral glands 319, 324

C

CAIS see complete androgen insensitivity syndrome (CAIS)
calcaneal (Achilles) tendon 103
calcaneal (Achilles') tendon reflex 22, 28
calcaneofibular ligaments 108
calcaneus 106
calculi 269
calculus (sialolith) 269
Camper's fasciae 133
Cannon–Böhm point 257
cardiac conduction system 177
cardinal ligament 228, 298
carina 201
carotid bifurcation 37
carotid sinus 37
carotid sinus syncope 37
Carpal tunnel syndrome 94
carpal tunnel syndrome 74, 84, 93
caudal epidural anesthesia 32
cavernous dural venous sinus 163
cavernous nerves 30, 313
cavernous sinus 19
cecum 257, 372
celiac ganglion 28
celiac lymph nodes 371, 372, 385
celiac trunk 227, 253
central axillary nodes 367
central retinal artery 18
cephalic veins 86
cerebrospinal fluid (CSF) 35
cervical canal 294
cervical dystonia 121
cervical myelopathy 27
cervix 292
chauffeur's fracture 90
cherry-red spot 18
chickenpox 17
choana 208
chocolate cysts 355
cholecystectomy 253
chorda tympani 19, 23, 25, 26
chorda tympani nerve 258
chronic constipation 257
chronic exertional compartment syndrome 107, 186
chronic inflammatory bowel disease 272
chylothorax 387
chylous ascites 386
ciliary body 20
ciliary ganglion 17, 19
ciliary nerves 19

circular folds 266
cirrhosis 252
cisterna chyli 386
clavicle fractures 80, 81
clitoris 299
cloacal extrophy 35
coarctation of aorta 169
coccygeus 292
cochlea 24
cochlear nerve 26
Colles' fascia 325
Colles' fracture 80, 81, 89, 94
color doppler ultrasound 349
communicating hydrocele 327
complete androgen insensitivity syndrome (CAIS) 347
conducting bronchioles 211
cone photoreceptor cells 18, 20
congenital adrenal hyperplasia 299
congenital adrenal hypoplasia 354
congenital defect 272
congenital diaphragmatic hernia 211
congenital hydrocele 332
congenital malformation 35
congenital megacolo 35
conjoint tendon 131
constricted pupil 21
contralateral receptors 17
conus medullaris 36
coracobrachialis 85
corneal reflex 19, 21
coronary arteries 173
coronary sinus 172
costodiaphragmatic recess 203
costodiaphragmatic recesses 261
coxa valga 109
craniopharyngiomas 349
cremasteric reflex 28, 323
cricoid cartilage 164
cricothyroid 121
cricothyrotomy 208
Crohn's disease 272
CSF see cerebrospinal fluid (CSF)
cubital fossa 87
cubital tunnel syndrome 75, 93
culdocentesis 263, 295
cutaneous areas 234
cystic artery 258
cystocele 288
cystourethrogram 229

D

dartos 132
deep brachial artery 176
deep branch of perineal nerve 314
deep circumfl ex iliac artery 185, 186
deep dorsal vein of penis 181
deep femoral artery 180, 184
deep fibular nerve 99
deep gluteal muscles 101
deep inguinal lymph nodes 366, 377
deep inguinal nodes 374, 376
deep inguinal ring 323
deep lymphatic plexus of lungs 209

deep parotid lymph nodes 380
deep penile fascia 30
deep perineal nerves 228
deep petrosal nerve 20
deep temporal artery 165
deep transverse perineal muscle 331
deep vein thromboembolus 201
deferential artery 316
deltoid fascia 375
deltoid muscle 80, 91
denticulate ligament 96
De Quervain tenosynovitis 94
dermatome 16
  C5 27
  C6 85
  C7 27
  C8 27, 204
  L4 22, 27
  S2–S4 27
  T1 27
detrusor reflex 314, 321
detumescence 30
diastasis 322
digastric muscle 127
DiGeorge syndrome 341
dinner fork deformity 89, 94
diplopia 20
direct (acquired) inguinal hernia 327
distal ileum 258
distal median nerve lesion 74
distal urethra 228
divergent rami 141
dominant artery 167
donor hepatectomy 252
dorsal artery of foot 185
dorsal artery of penis 182
dorsal horn of spinal cord 17
dorsal lingual artery 165
dorsal nerve of penis 30
dorsal (posterior) root ganglia 17
dorsal scapular 21
dorsal scapular nerve 21, 76, 78
dorsiflexion 34
dorsiflexors 27
double bubble sign 35, 273
double vision 20
dual blood supply 18
ductus arteriosus 174, 235
ductus venosus 235
duodenal atresia 35, 273, 353
duodenal papilla 266
duodenum 232
  C-shaped 257
  descending 235
  horizontal pat of 261
duplicated renal pelvis 227
Dupuytren's contracture 74, 81, 93, 94
dysphagia 126

E

eccentric action 104
ectopia cordis 272
ectopic implantation 291
ectopic kidney 223
  ureter of 223

ectopic pregnancy 354
ectopic thymus 355, 356
ectopic ureter 227
efferent ductules 302
efferent lymphatic vessels 369
ejaculation 330
ejaculatory duct 319
embolus
    in arterial arcade 253
    in mesenteric artery 253
emergency decompression 202
emphysema 202
endometriosis 355
endometrium 295
endothoracic fascia 206–207
enlarged palatine 355
enlarged palatine tonsil 356
epicardium 169
epicranial hematoma 160
epididymis 318
epidural hematoma 160
episiotomy 294
epispadias 329
Erb's palsy 36, 204
erectile dysfunction 324
erectile tissues of penis 181
erection 30
erector spinae muscles 97
esophageal tributaries 252
esophagus 132
excessive bleeding 350
excessive ureteric distension 234
exstrophy of bladder 329
external abdominal oblique 132
external acoustic meatus 26
external anal sphincter 324
external carotid artery 162, 164,
        166, 168
external iliac artery 180, 186
external iliac lymph nodes 374
external iliac nodes 117, 326, 376
external laryngeal nerve 31
external nasal nerve 23
external pudendal artery 182, 185
external pudendal vein 181
external urethral orifice 332
external urethral sphincter 228, 291,
        318, 324
    muscle 229
extraperitoneal fat 133
extravasated contrast 231
extravasation of urine 320
eyelid closure 19

F

facial artery 162, 166
facial canal 24
facial nerve 19
    CN VII 26, 27
facial (CN VII) nerves 128
facial pain syndrome 23
falciform ligament 259
fall on an outstretched hand
        (FOOSH) 80, 89, 94
falx inguinalis 131
fascia lata 107

female genitourinary organs 292
female homologue of hydrocele 300
female internal genital structures
        300
female pelvic organs 225
female ureters 228
femoral artery 101, 113, 187
femoral branch 136
femoral canal 106
femoral hernia 114, 332
femoral nerve 327
femoral neuropathy 34
femoral ring 106
fertilization of ovum 288
fetal ventral mesentery 259
fibromuscular band 353
fibrothorax 387
fibrous pericardium 169
fibular nerve 34
Finkelstein test 94
flaccid penis 30
flank pain 224
flexion 284
flexor carpi radialis tendon 33
flexor pollicis brevis 84
    muscles 89
flexor pollicis longus 73
foramen rotundum 126
forearm compartment syndrome 81
forearm pronators 85
fracture
    of cribriform plate 17
    of right jugular foramen 27
Froment's sign tests 89
frontal nerves 19
frontonasal duct 208
fundus of stomach 258

G

gag reflex 26
gallbladder 232
    removal 253
ganglion cyst 33, 81
gastric adenocarcinoma 264
gastric ischemia 132
gastric ulcer 262
gastrocnemius muscle 103
gastrocolic ligament 370
gastroduodenal artery 252, 265, 343
gastroesophageal junction 132
gastroesophageal reflux disease
        (GERD) 255
gastro-omental lymph nodes 369
gastrophrenic ligament 262
gastroschisis 229, 273
gastrosplenic ligament 262, 370
generalized periumbilical pain 256
genioglossus 22, 124
geniohyoid 124
genitofemoral nerve 16, 28, 136,
        233, 234, 327, 330
    distribution of 28
genu vara 109
GERD see gastroesophageal reflux
        disease (GERD)
glenoid cavity superiorly 91

glossopharyngeal nerve 128, 258
    (CN IX) 26, 207
gluteus maximus 101, 109
gluteus medius gait 101
gluteus medius muscle 101, 109
gluteus minimus 112
golfer's elbow 91
gonadal dysgenesis 347
great cardiac vein 172
greater palatine nerve 258
great saphenous vein 181
gubernaculum testis 323

H

halitosis 126
hangman's fracture 96
hard stools 271
head of pancreas 257–258
hematocele 329
hematopoietic stem cells 351
hemifacial paralysis 19
hemorrhage 160
hemorrhoidal plexus 331
hemothorax 204
hepatic artery 252, 253
hepatoduodenal ligament 252, 262,
        370
hepatorenal (Morrison's)
        pouch 35
hepatorenal recess (Morison's
        pouch) 252, 262
hernia sac 106
herniated disc projects 27
herniation
    of intervertebral disc 22
    of urinary bladder 229
herpes zoster 17
Hesselbach's triangle 134, 260
high steppage gait 95
hilar lymph nodes 367
hip flexion 324
    weakness in 29
Hirschsprung's disease 35
hissing of air 202
Horner's syndrome 204
horseshoe kidney 224, 227
Hutchinson's fracture 90
hydatidiform mole 354
hydrocele 321, 329
17-hydroxyprogesterone 299
hymen 291
hyoglossus muscle 124, 270
hyperacusis 19, 26
hyperkyphosis 96
hyperparathyroidism 349
hypertension 291–292
hypertrophied piriformis 115
hypesthesia 32
hypoesthesia of penis 324
hypogastric nerve 28, 30, 35, 36
hypoglossal nerve
    CN XII 22, 27, 128
hypoparathyroidism 348
hypopharynx 126
hypospadias 329
hypothyroidism 354

I

ICA *see* internal carotid artery (ICA)
ileocolic artery 179
ileocolic lymph nodes 372
ileocolic nodes 371
iliac fossa 134
iliococcygeus muscle 295
iliohypogastric nerve 16, 35, 327
   distribution of 28
   L1 28
iliohypogastric nerves 296, 327
ilioinguinal nerve 16, 134
ilioinguinal nerves 296, 327
iliopsoas 104
impaired adduction 20
incomplete canalization 212
indirect inguinal hernia 323
indirect (congenital) inguinal hernia 327
indirect inguinal hernias 323
inferior alveolar artery 167
inferior alveolar nerve 22, 24, 124
inferior epigastric artery 178
inferior gluteal artery 181, 183, 186
inferior gluteal nerve 315, 324
inferior gluteal vein 183
inferior hypogastric plexus 29, 36
inferior mesenteric arteries 257
inferior mesenteric artery 179, 180
inferior nasal concha 208
inferior oblique 20
inferior pancreaticoduodenal artery 343
inferior parathyroid glands 342
inferior pelvic structures 377
inferior perineal nerves 137
inferior pole 223
inferior pubic rami 141
inferior rectal nerve 137, 228, 313, 315, 324
inferior rectus 20
inferior thyroid artery 166
inferior thyroid veins 208
inferior tracheobronchial lymph nodes 367
inferior vena cava 132, 226, 227, 252, 351
inferior vesical vein 267
inflatable prosthesis 138
infraglenoid tubercle 80
infraorbital foramen 126
infraorbital nerve 17, 19, 21, 23
infraspinatus 78
infratemporal fossa 24, 161
infundibulopelvic ligament 298, 353
inguinal hernia 135
inguinal region 31
intercostal nerve 16, 31, 201
intercostal neurovascular bundle 129
intermuscular septae 107
internal abdominal oblique fibers 132
internal acoustic meatus 19, 26
internal anal sphincter 140

internal carotid artery (ICA) 18, 163, 164, 168, 348
internal hemorrhoids 376
internal iliac artery 180, 181, 186
internal iliac nodes 117, 326
internal laryngeal nerve 31, 32, 258
internal pudendal artery 105–106, 182, 185, 316
internal thoracic artery 169
interureteric crest 318
interventricular foramina 349
intervertebral disc 27
intestinal malrotation 353
intra-articular fracture 90
intracranial hemorrhages 160
intracranial pressure 20
intraperitoneal urinary bladder rupture 323
intravaginal testicular torsion 327
intravaginal torsion 327
intrinsic hand muscles 74
intrinsic laryngeal muscles 27
involuntary urinary bladder empty-ing 228
ipsilateral recurrent laryngeal nerve 126
ischial tuberosity 110
ischioanal fossa 134
ischiocavernosus muscle 291, 324
ischiococcygeus 139, 140
ischiococcygeus muscle 292
ischium 141
isthmus of fauces 26

J

jejunum 258
jugular foramen 24, 26
jugulodigastric lymph node 380
jugulodigastric node 380

K

Kehr's sign 370
Kiesslebach's area 208
Klumpke's palsy 36
knee flexion 103
knee jerk 22
knock-knee 109
kyphosis 95, 96

L

labia majora 332
lacrimal bone 23
lacrimal nerves 19
lamina papyracea 23
laryngeal branches 27
laryngeal muscles, actions of 126
laryngeal musculature 122
laryngeal ventricle 208
laryngeal vestibule 208
laryngopharynx 126
lateral circumflex femoral artery 108, 185, 186
lateral collateral ligament 109
lateral cricoarytenoid muscle 126

lateral cutaneous nerve 136
lateral epicondylitis 91
lateral gaze 21
lateral gaze palsy 344
lateral horn of spinal cord 17
lateral inguinal fossa 134
lateral pectoral nerves 28
lateral pterygoid 127
lateral pterygoid muscle 121
lateral rectus 20
   muscle 123
lateral winging 78
latissimus dorsi 97
least splanchnic nerve 29
left atrioventricular valve sound 171
left colic artery 179
left colic vein 267
left coronary artery 176, 177
left gastric artery (LGA) 252, 265, 270
left gastro-omental (gastroepiploic) artery 265, 343
left hypoglossal palsy 22
left marginal artery 172, 176
left subphrenic recess 252
left suprarenal gland 226
left testicular vein 317
left vagus nerve 26
lesser occipital nerve 25, 121
lesser omentum 268
lesser petrosal nerve 26
lesser sac (omental bursa) 252
lesser splanchnic nerve 256, 330
lesser tubercle of humerus 80
levator ani 139
   pubococcygeus and puborectalis portions of 292
levator palpebrae superioris 20, 21
LGA *see* left gastric artery (LGA)
ligamentum flavum 96
ligation of splenic artery 261
linea alba 136
linea nigra 136
linea semilunaris 136
lingual artery 165, 166
lingual branch of glossopharyngeal nerve 258
lingual nerve 22
lingual thyroid 355, 356
lingual tonsils 355
lingula 24
lobar lymph nodes 367
locomotion 101, 116
long ciliary nerves 20
longitudinal arches of foot 118
longitudinal ridges 212
long thoracic nerve 28, 76
longus capitis 129
lordosis 95
loss of finger extension 93
loss of flexion
   of distal interphalangeal joint of index finger 93
   interphalangeal joint of thumb 93
loss of thumb opposition 93
lower respiratory tract 212

lower subscapular nerve 21, 76, 78
lower ureteric obstruction 224
lumbar lymph nodes 372
lumbar nerve plexus 111
lumbar paraspinal abscesses 111
lumbar plexus 136
lumbar puncture needle 36, 96
lumbar splanchnic nerves 29, 321, 352
lumbar vertebrae 96, 111
lumbosacral trunk 28, 117, 317
lung hypoplasia 274
lung parenchyma 210
lymphatic channels 326
lymphatic drainage 372
lymphatic vessels 326, 376
lymphogenous metastasis 378

M

Mackenrodt's ligament 228, 298
macular region 18
maldescended testis 332
male hormones 347
malignant melanoma 382
mallet finger 81
mandibular nerve
    CN V2 24
    CN V3 24, 26
marginal artery 178
masticator 22
maxillary artery 161, 165
maxillary nerve 24
    CN V2 26
maxillary sinuses 37
McBurney's point 261
Meckel's diverticulum 35, 229, 267,
    272, 353
medial circumfl ex femoral arteries
    108
medial deviation of femur 109
medial epicondyle 75
medial gaze 21
medial gaze palsy 345
medial inguinal fossa 134
medial meniscus tears 106
medial plantar nerve, cutaneous
    branches of 98
medial rectus 20
medial thigh conveys sensory 324
medial umbilical fossa 134
medial winging 78
median aperture 349
median cubital vein 86
median nerve 73, 74, 84
    recurrent branch of 84
median neuropathy 85
median umbilical fold 323
mediastinal shift 202
mediolateral episiotomy 379
Meissner's plexuses of bowel wall 35
membranous interventricular septal
    defect 173
meningomyelocele 35
menisci 103
mental artery 167
meralgia paresthetica 114
mesenteric lymph nodes 385

mesodermal migration 35
mesonephric ducts 327
mesonephric (Wolffian) ducts 227,
    299
mesonephric tubules 299
mesosalpinx 353
metanephric blastema 227, 351
middle cardiac vein 172
middle cerebral arteries 159
middle colic artery 179
middle cranial fossa 161
middle meningeal artery 160, 161,
    168
middle nasal concha 208
middle rectal artery 181
middle suprarenal arteries 342
midgut rotation (malrotation) 273
midline abdominal wall defect 272
midline episiotomy 291
midshaft humeral fracture 93
minimal lung sounds 202
miosis 21
molar pregnancy 354
Morison's pouch 252, 262
motor axons 21
motor vehicle collisions 96
mucosa
    of oropharynx and oropharyngeal
        isthmus 26
Müllerian-inhibiting substance 347
multiple bronchial profiles 210
multiple rib fractures 210
Murphy's sign 262
musculocutaneous nerve 84, 85, 204
musculophrenic artery 187
musculotendinous junction 104
musculus uvulae 270
mydriasis 17, 20, 21
myelomeningocele 35, 36
mylohyoid muscle 270
myocardium 169
myometrium 295

N

nasociliary nerve 19, 20
nasopalatine nerve 24
navicular fossa 319
needle insertion 202
nephrogenic cord 351
nephroptosis 223
nerve fibers 21
nerve trauma 105
nervi erigentes 325
nervus intermedius 26
neural tissue 36
neural tube defect 35
neuronal cell bodies 17
normal pregnancy 354
nucleus solitarius 22
nursemaid's elbow 81
nutcracker syndrome 231

O

obesity 291–292
obliquus capitis 97

obturator artery 101, 180, 183, 185,
    186
obturator artery branches 181
obturator externus 104
obturator hernia 114
obturator internus 119, 140
obturator nerve 28, 34, 136, 315,
    324
    L2–L4 28
occipital artery 166, 167
occipital triangle 375
occipitofrontalis 129
occlusive pressure 89
occulta 36
oculomotor nerve 17, 344
    CN III 17, 20
oculomotor nerve (CN III) 23
oculomotor palsies 124
odontoid process 128
Ogilvie's syndrome 257
olfaction 17
olfactory mucosa 209
olfactory nerve 37
omental appendices 266
omental bursa 29
omoclavicular (subclavian) triangle
    375
omohyoid muscles 122
omphalocele 229, 272, 274
open pneumothorax 202
open prostatectomy 331
ophthalmic artery 163, 168, 348
ophthalmic nerve (CN V1) 16–17,
    26, 37
ophthalmic veins 17
opponens pollicis 73
optic canal 22
optic nerve (CN II) 17
orbital blowout fracture 23, 209
orbital edema 21
orbital floor fracture 21
orbital surface of maxilla 23
oropharyngeal membrane 213
otic ganglia 23
otic ganglion 37
ovarian tumor 354
overuse syndrome 91

P

Paget's disease of nipple 366
paired bulbospongiosus muscles 296
paired cricothyroid muscles 122
paired greater vestibular (Bartholin's)
    glands 288
paired levator veli palatini muscles
    128
paired posterior cerebral arteries
    159
paired pubovesical ligaments 225
palatine nerve 24
palatoglossus muscle 270
palmar fascia 74, 93
palmaris longus 73
palpebral fissure 20
pancreas 232
pancreatic tissue 353

paracentesis 256
paracolic gutters 261
paracolic lymph nodes 366
paraesophageal hernia 255
paralysis
    left vocal fold 26–27
    long digital extensor muscles 91
    of posterior cricoarytenoid muscle
        206, 207
    of serratus anterior palsy 78
    of stapedius 26
    of thumb adduction 91
    of vocal cord 89
paramedian approach 96
paramesonephric (Müllerian) ducts
    227–228
paraphimosis 329
pararectal lymph nodes 366
parasympathetic fibers 313
parasympathetic involvement 20
parasympathetic preganglionic
    fibers 321
parasympathetic pterygopalatine
    ganglion 24
parathyroid adenoma 349
parathyroid glands 208
paratracheal hilar lymph nodes 368
paratracheal lymph nodes 367
paratracheal nodes 209
paresis 27
parietal peritoneum 34, 131, 133
parietal pleura 31
parietal serous pericardium 169
parotid (Stensen's) duct 258
patellofemoral syndrome 118
patent ductus arteriosus 169
patent processus vaginalis 135, 332
patent urachus 235
PCOS see polycystic ovarian syn-
    drome (PCOS)
pectinate (dentate) line 266
pectineus 28, 104, 117
pectoral nodes 367
pelvic diaphragm 332
pelvic splanchnic nerves 35, 37, 228,
    317, 321, 325, 352
pelvic splanchnics 330
penile urethra 331
perforating arteries 185
perianal venous nodules 35
pericardiacophrenic artery 169, 187
pericervical collar 381, 382
    of lymph nodes 380
perineal body 295
perineal nerve 328
perineal nerve of penis 30
perineal structures 378
perirenal fat 226, 229
peritoneal cavity 35
peritoneal recesses 290
periumbilical pain 34
petrosal nerve 26
Peyer's patches 257
pharyngeal constrictor muscles
    force 127
pharyngeal muscles 26
pharyngeal plexus 31

pharyngeal recesses 201
pharynx 126
pheochromocytomas 351
phimosis 329
phrenic nerve 89, 206
phrenic nerves 28
physiological herniation 272, 273
piriform fossae 208
piriformis 101, 140
piriformis muscles 109
piriformis syndrome 115
piriform recesses 268
plantar aponeurosis 102
plantar deep fascia 102
plantar fasciitis 102
plantarflexion 34
pleuritic chest pain 31
pleuritic (sharp) chest pain 201
pleuropericardial membranes
    211–212
pneumocytes type II 212
pneumonia 202, 204, 387
pneumothorax 387
polycystic ovarian syndrome (PCOS)
    353
popliteal artery 101, 180, 187
popliteal nodes 374
popliteal vein 107, 186
popliteus 184
popliteus muscle 113
portal hypertension 252
portal vein 253
portosystemic anastomosis 252
posterior auricular artery 167
posterior cerebral arteries 348
posterior communicating artery 159
posterior cricoarytenoid muscle 126
posterior cruciate ligament 106
posterior drawer test 106
posterior ethmoidal nerve 23
posterior femoral cutaneous nerve
    315
posterior intercostal artery 169
posterior interosseous nerve 73,
    74, 90
posterior interventricular arteries
    177
posterior labial branches of puden-
    dal nerve 296
posterior longitudinal ligament 95,
    96, 122
posterior nasal aperture 208
posterior scrotal nerve 314, 327, 328
posterior scrotal nerves 324
posterior superior alveolar nerve 24
posterior talofibular ligaments 108
posterior tibial arteries 184
posterior tibial artery 184
posterior tibial vein 107, 186
posterior urethral valves 227
posterolateral herniation 27
posterolateral herniation of inter-
    vertebral disc 95
postganglionic axons 17
postganglionic sympathetic fibers
    21, 36, 314, 322
postoperative dyspnea 89

post-polio syndrome 101
posttraumatic swelling 34
preganglionic parasympathetic
    fibers 17, 20, 23, 25, 314
preganglionic sympathetic fibers
    28–29, 317
pregnancy line 136
priapism 329–330
primary forearm pronators 93
primary sensory neuronal cell
    bodies 17
primary sensory neurons 17
primordial germ cells 299, 351
pringle maneuver 252
processus vaginalis 135
pronator syndrome 84
proper ovarian ligament 298
prostate 332
prostatic urethra 228
prostatic utricle 318
prostatitis 31
proximal internal carotid artery 37
proximal median nerve lesions 92
proximal portion of brachial plexus
    89
proximal ureter 233
psoas major 111
pterygoid canal traverses 126
pterygopalatine fossa 24
pterygopalatine ganglia 23, 24
ptosis 20
pubis 141
pubocervical ligaments 285
pubococcygeus 292
pubococcygeus form 140
puborectalis 292
puborectalis muscle 291
pubovesical ligaments 285
pudenal nerve 35
pudendal nerve 16, 119
pudendal nerve block 295
pudendal nerve injury 324
pudendal nerve of penis 30
pulled elbow 81
pulmonary hilar lymph nodes 368
pulmonary hypertension 174
pulmonary hypoplasia 211
pulmonary (intrapulmonary) lymph
    nodes 373
pulmonary sequestration 211
pulmonary vein 201
pump handle movements 211
pupillary dilation 17
pyloric stenosis 273
pylorus of stomach 258

Q

Q-angle 109
quadrangular space 77
quadratus femoris 101
quadriceps femoris complex 118

R

radial artery 89
radial nerve 32, 83
    superficial branch of 83, 85

radial neuropathy 85
radicular pain 96
rectouterine pouch 252, 262, 263, 290, 354
rectum 292
rectus abdominis 132
recurrent laryngeal branches of vagus nerve 344
recurrent laryngeal nerve 31, 122
recurrent laryngeal nerves 345
referred pain 201, 327
Remnants of Gartner's duct 288
renal arteries 342
renal cysts 224
renal fascia 226
renal hilum 223
renal papilla 227
renal pelvis 223, 227
repetitive movements 94
respiratory bronchioles 211
retinal ganglion cells 18
retroesophageal (aberrant) right subclavian artery 170
retroflexion 284, 294
retromandibular vein 165
retroperitoneal gas 263
retroperitoneal organ 252
retropharyngeal abscess 204
retropubic space 262, 323, 355
retroversion 284, 294
Retzius space 323
reverse Colles' fracture 80, 90
rhinoscleroma 211
rhomboid 91
rhomboid paralysis 21
rhomboids act 78
right brachiocephalic vein 208
right colic artery 178
right inferior lobe 201
right marginal artery 177
right marginal vessel 172
right renal artery 178, 226
right subclavian artery 169, 176
rod photoreceptors 20
rotator cuff weakness 204
round ligaments 287
    of uterus 298, 353
ruptured appendix 35
ruptured urinary bladder 321

S

saccular (berry) aneurysm 159
sacral promontory 140
sacral splanchnic nerves 30, 35, 37, 228, 328, 352
sacrotuberous ligaments 285
sagging kidney 223
salivation, decreased 25
saphenous nerve 33, 34, 98, 99
scaphoid fracture 74, 90, 94
scapular winging 21
Scarpa's fasciae 133
sciatic nerve 34, 119
sciatic notch borders 105
scoliosis 95, 96
scrotal ligament 300

scrotum 373
segmental bronchi 210
semilunar line 136
seminal colliculus 318, 332
seminal gland (vesicle) 331
seminiferous tubules 319
semispinalis capitis 97
sensory deficits 92
sensory fibers 23
    C6 85
sensory ganglia 17
sensory innervation
    medial forearm 77
    proximal medial forearm 77
sensory innervation of laryngeal mucosa superior 207
sensory nucleus 22
septum secundum 212
serratus anterior 78
serratus anterior muscle protracts 91
serratus anterior paralysis 21
serratus anterior protracts 75
serratus posterior superior 97
shingles 17
short gastric arteries 180, 265
shoulder abduction, weakness in 29
shoulder dislocation 81
shoulder dystocia 36
shoulder separation 80
sigmoid arteries 179
sigmoid colon 257
sigmoid dural venous sinus 162
single basilar artery 159
situs inversus 272
six pack 136
skeletal tuberculosis 95
skin dimpling of breast 287
skull base fracture 26
sliding hiatal hernia 255
SMA see superior mesenteric (SMA)
small cardiac vein 172
Smith's fracture 80, 81, 90
snuff box muscle 91
soleus 103, 116, 184
solitary tract nucleus 22
somatic afferent fibers 28
somatic afferents 325
somatic efferents 325
somatic pudendal nerve 317
somatosensation 17
somatosensory cortex 17
special sensory fibers 26
spermatocele 329
sphenoidal sinuses 208
sphenoid bone 23
sphenopalatine artery 167
sphincter pupillae muscle 17
sphincter urethrae 318
spina bifida 35, 96, 97
spina bifida occulta 36, 95
spinal cord
    C7 22
    injury of 97
    L4 28
    S1 28
spinal nerve 32

C7 89
    unilateral compression of 27
splanchnic nerve 29
splanchnic nerve (T5–T9) 28
spleen 232
splenectomy 261
splenic artery 265
splenic lymph nodes 371, 372
splenic veins 254
splenius muscles 97
spondylolisthesis 95, 96
spondylolysis 96
spongy urethra 228
spongy (penile) urethra 331
stapedius muscle 26
    paralysis of 26
stellate ganglion 37
stenosis 168
    of renal artery 180
step deformity 81
sternal angle 210
sternocleidomastoid 21, 129
sternocostal portion of pectoralis major 92
sternohyoid 121
sternothyroid muscle 121
styloglossus muscle 270
styloglossus retrudes 270
stylohyoid 26, 124
stylohyoid chain 127
styloid process 127
stylopharyngeus muscle 270
subarachnoid hemorrhages 160
subclavian artery 130
subclavian venous catheterization 204
subclavius muscle 83
subcostal nerve 16, 136
subcutaneous fascia 320
subcutaneous hematoma 160
subcutaneous tissue layer 207
subdural hematoma 160
subhepatic space 261
sublingual gland 269
submandibular lymph nodes 382
submucosal internal rectal venous plexus 267
subperitoneal 231
subphrenic recess 262
subscapularis adducts 76
subscapular nodes 367
subtendinous bursae 113
superficial abdominal reflex 16
superficial anal reflex 22
superficial branches of perineal nerve 228
superficial branch of radial nerve 73, 74
superficial cutaneous reflex 16
superficial dorsal vein of penis 181
superficial epigastric artery 178
superficial fascia 107
    of penis 316, 317
superficial fibular nerve 34, 98, 99
superficial inguinal lymph nodes 374, 378
superficial inguinal nodes 376

superficial inguinal ring 135
superficial (subpleural) lymphatic
    plexus 373
superficial parotid lymph nodes 380
superficial perineal nerve 314
superficial structures 366
superficial temporal artery 168
superficial transverse perineal
    muscle 291
superficial vein of clitoris 183
superior cervical ganglion 23, 37
superior epigastric artery 178
superior gluteal artery 186
superior gluteal nerve 115, 119
superior laryngeal nerve 32
superior mesenteric (SMA) 264
superior mesenteric artery 178, 227,
    257
superior mesenteric lymph nodes
    371, 372
superior mesenteric plexus 34
superior mesenteric veins 254
superior nasal concha 208
superior oblique 20
superior oblique muscle 123
superior orbital fissure 17
superior pancreaticoduodenal artery
    264, 343
superior phrenic 187
superior phrenic artery 169
superior pole of kidney 223
superior rectal artery 179
superior rectal veins 183
superior rectus 20
superior suprarenal arteries 342
superior tarsal muscle 20
superior thyroid artery 163, 164,
    166, 208
    branches 166
superior vena cava 170, 205
superior vesical artery 186, 228
supracristal plane 36
supraglenoid tubercle 80
supraorbital nerve 17, 23
suprapubic cystostomy 229
suprapubic pain 29
suprarenal gland 234
suprascapular nerve 21, 75, 76
suprascapular nerves 291
supraspinatus 91
supraspinatus abducts 21, 75, 92
supraspinatus muscle 78
supratrochlear nerve 17, 23
supravesical fossa 134
surfactant 212
suspensory ligament 287, 300
    of ovary 353
sympathetic chain 204
sympathetic efferents 325
sympathetic fibers 28, 31
synovial membrane 103

T

taeniae coli 266
tendinous intersections 136
tendonitis 94

tendon of extensor
    hallucis longus 109
tendon of flexor
    carpi radialis 73, 88
    pollicis longus 73
tendons of extensor
    digitorum brevis 109
    digitorum longus 109
tensor fasciae latae 101
tensor tympani 26
teres minor 75, 78
terminal bronchioles 210, 211
tertiary (segmental) bronchi 211
testicular artery branches 179
testicular cancer 325
testicular feminization syndrome
    347
testicular torsion 325, 327, 329, 343
thoracic duct 387
thoracic nerve 21, 76
thoracic splanchnic nerves 352
thoracoabdominal nerve 16
    T10 16
thoracodorsal nerve 76, 78
thromboembolus 201
thrombus formation 177
thumb abduction, unilateral paresis
    of 27
thymic tumor 201
thymus 341
thyrocervical trunk 166
thyroglossal duct 213, 269
    cyst 355, 356
thyrohyoid muscle 122
thyroidectomy 207, 345
tibialis anterior 109
tibialis anterior muscle 28, 100
tibialis posterior reflex 22
tibial nerve 34, 99, 105
tibial tuberosities 106
tibiofibular ligaments 108
tic douloureux 23
tight bicipital aponeurosis 92
Tinel's sign 75, 93
Tinel's test 89
tonsillar artery 165
torticollis 121
torus tubarius 208
tracheobronchial nodes 209
tracheoesophageal ridges 212
tracheoesophageal septum 212
traction 36
transition zone 35
transurethral approach 331
transversalis fascia 107, 131
transverse cervical ligament 225,
    298, 300, 353
transverse cervical (cardinal) liga-
    ment 353
transverse cervical nerves 121
transverse dural venous sinus 162
transverse fibers 126
transverse mesocolon 268, 351, 370
transversus abdominis 132
transversus abdominis muscle fibers
    132
trapezius 21, 91, 97, 129

trapezius acts 92
trapezius muscle 91
Trendelenburg 101
triangular ligament 262
triceps reflex 89
trigeminal (Meckel's) cave 24
trigeminal ganglion 23
trigeminal motor nucleus 22
trigeminal nerve 24
trigeminal neuralgia 23
trochlear nerve 17
    CN IV 20
trochlear nerve (CN IV) 23
trochlearnerve palsy 124
tunica albuginea 316
tunica vaginalis 327, 343
tunica vaginalis testis 320
Turner syndrome 300
Turner (Ullrich–Turner) syndrome
    347
typhoid fever 257

U

ulcerative colitis 266
ulnar artery 89
ulnar (Guyon's) canal syndrome 74
ulnar nerve 32, 73, 74
    deep branch of 84
    entrapment 81
    palmar cutaneous branch of 33
ulnar neuropathy 85
umbilical hernia 332
umbilicus 132
undescended testis 325
unhappy triad 106
unilateral action of sternocleido-
    mastoid muscle 121
unilateral compression of spinal
    nerve 27
unilateral contraction 129
unilateral deficit 17
unilateral facial paralysis 19
unilateral hypesthesia 27
unilateral injury of vagus nerve 128
unilateral oculomotor palsy 123
unilateral paresis of thumb abduc-
    tion 27
unmyelinated axons 17
upper brachial plexus injury 92
upper brachial plexus palsy 91
upper subscapular nerve 76, 78
upward gaze 20
urachus 229
ureteric buds 228
ureteric pain 234
urethral injuries 317
urinary bladder neck 228
urinary stress incontinence 139
urogenital folds 301
urogenital sinus 227, 235, 299, 301
urogenital triangle of perineum 182
urorectal septum 235
uterine artery 286
    ligation of 289
uterine tubes 353
uterosacral ligament 298

uterosacral ligaments 285, 353
uterus masculinus 302
uvula 318

V

vaginal delivery 36
vaginismus 295
vagus nerve 25, 29, 207
  CN X 26
valga 109
varicella zoster virus 17
varicocele 325, 329, 332
varicosities of vein 300
vasa rectae 253
vascular entrapment 184
vas deferens 347
vastus medialis muscle 118
venipuncture 86
ventral horn 17
  of spinal cord 17
ventrogluteal placement site 112

veromontanum 332
vertebral artery 96, 164
vertebral bodies collapse 95
vertebral defect 35
vertebral flexor muscles 97
vesicoureteric junction (VUJ) 228
vesicouterine pouch 262, 355
vestibular nerve 26
vestibulocochlear (CN VIII) nerves
  27
Virchow's node 383
visceral afferent axons 22
visceral afferent fibers 28, 34, 35
visceral afferents 325
visceral peritoneum of uterus 131
visceral sensory fibers 256
visceral serous pericardium 169
vitelline duct 272
Volkmann's ischemic contracture 81
volvulus 353
VUJ *see* vesicoureteric junction (VUJ)
vulva 379

W

waddle gait 28
weakened elbow flexion 92
weakened glenohumeral abduction
  92
weak forearm flexion 85
whiplash injury 122
winged scapula 76
wrist drop 32, 83
wry neck 121

X

xiphoid process 16
xiphoid process of sternum 130

Z

zygomatic bone 23
zygomatic nerve 17